PERSONAL INFORMATION

Name _GAYLE CROCKART_

Address _3 GRAY ROW_
RUTHVENFIELD
PERTH PH13JR

Tel No _PERTH 20537_

Training School/College of Nursing _PERTH_
GLASGOW ROAD

Date of entry _10/8/87_

Date of Completion _30/9/90_

Personal Identification No _____

State Examination pass date _____

Additional qualifications and dates

1985/6 HANDBOOK OF COMMUNITY NURSING

Sixth edition, fully revised and expanded, published July 1985

The sole national source of information on Community Nursing Services in the UK, the Handbook is published annually in a convenient A5 format (softback). The 1985/6 edition, comprising c. 240 pages, will provide names of Senior Nurse Managers and addresses and telephone numbers, including emergency out-of-hours and night contact details, for the following services throughout the UK:

- *DISTRICT NURSING   *HEALTH VISITING
- *SCHOOL NURSING   *COMMUNITY MIDWIFERY
- *COMMUNITY PSYCHIATRIC NURSING
- *COMMUNITY MENTAL HANDICAP NURSING
- *SOCIAL SERVICES & SOCIAL WORK DEPARTMENTS

Also covered will be names, addresses and contact telephone numbers for *Specialist Liaison Staff and Geriatric, Stoma-Care and other Nurse Visitors/ Advisors*. The 1985/6 Handbook will also contain useful and comprehensive guides to:

- *Towns/Areas covered by each Health Authority in the UK.
- *Nursing Qualifications.
- *Statutory, professional, voluntary bodies of interest to Nurses.
- *Future Nursing Events.

Plus authoritative review articles on *Aids and Nursing Care; and the Role of the Voluntary Sector in Primary Health Care*.

Copies available from the publishers at £6.00 each, including postage.

ASGARD PUBLISHING COMPANY LTD
FOXCOMBE HOUSE, SOUTH HARTING
PETERSFIELD, HANTS GU31 5PL
TEL: HARTING (073085) 662

Baillière's
Nurses'
Dictionary

NURSING CAREERS IN THE RAF

The Princess Mary's Royal Air Force Nursing Service is looking for qualified men and women to join them as Enrolled Nurses (General) to fill vacancies in our hospitals. Hospitals that are among the most modern and best equipped anywhere; and are small enough for you to spend all the time you need with all your patients.

There are also opportunities for you to apply to join the PMRAFNS on a commission if you are an RGN with at least one year's post registration experience and preferably with a second certificate.

Later on you could also be offered training in specialist areas, such as intensive care or aeromedical nursing.

For further information call in at your nearest RAF Careers Information Centre; the address is in the Phone Book.

Formal applications must be made in the U.K.

THE PRINCESS MARY'S ROYAL AIR FORCE NURSING SERVICE

Baillière's Nurses' Dictionary

REVISED BY

KAY KASNER
SRN, RCNT, DipN (London)

AND

DENNIS H. TINDALL
BA (Oxon)

TWENTIETH EDITION

Baillière Tindall
LONDON   PHILADELPHIA   TORONTO

Baillière Tindall   1 St Anne's Road
                     Eastbourne, East Sussex BN21 3UN, England

                     West Washington Square
                     Philadelphia, PA 19105, USA

                     1 Goldthorne Avenue
                     Toronto, Ontario M8Z 5T9, Canada

First published 1912
Ninteenth edition 1979
   Reprinted 1981, 1982
Twentieth edition 1984
   Reprinted 1985, 1986

English Language Book Society edition of 20th edition 1984
Spanish edition of 18th edition (Elicien, Barcelona) 1977
Italian edition of 18th edition (Editorial Ermes, Milan) 1977
French edition of 18th edition (Libraire Maloine, Paris) 1978

Printed and bound in Great Britain by
William Collins, Glasgow

British Library Cataloguing in Publication Data

Baillière's nurses dictionary.—20th ed.
   1 Nursing—Dictionaries
   I. Kasner, Kay   II. Tindall, Dennis
   610 73 03 21   RT21

ISBN (paperback) 0–7020–1035–9
ISBN (cased) 0–7020–1046–4
ISBN (ELBS) 0–7020–1045–6

CONTENTS

Contents

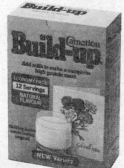

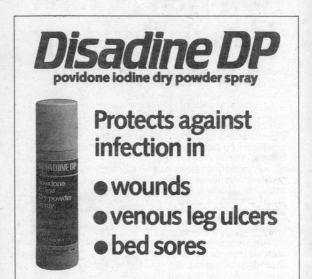

PREFACE

For its twentieth edition this well-known dictionary has been radically revised and enlarged. Although the book has been kept up to date by regular revision every three or four years, we both felt that something more fundamental was required to give homogeneity to the work of a succession of revisers covering several decades. Most of the entries therefore have been amended or totally rewritten, and there are numerous entirely new entries. While many of these new definitions cover recent developments in medicine and the nursing care associated with them, we are glad to have been able to include for the first time a number of terms used by the paramedical professions of physiotherapy, radiography and speech therapy. We know that students of these disciplines make considerable use of this dictionary and we hope that these additions will be welcomed by them. We have also included a number of specialized ophthalmic terms.

The appendixes, edited and revised by Richard Wells, provide a wealth of information to which nurses need to have access. Those dealing with nursing research and the nursing process are new, whilst that covering Dietetics has been rewritten and entitled 'Nutrition'.

The many new illustrations add to the usefulness of this comprehensive dictionary and work of reference for practising nurses and for those employed in related disciplines. We hope that in its revised form the book will continue to be as valuable and as widely used as it has been for so many years.

Kay Kasner
Dennis H. Tindall

January 1984

ACKNOWLEDGEMENTS

During preliminary discussions on the proposed content of the 20th edition of *Baillière's Nurses' Dictionary* it was decided to increase the amount of specialist words included. For this reason we sought the help of various experts in their specialized fields.

We would like to acknowledge the contributions to this edition made by the following people: Miss Vera Goodson, formerly Ophthalmic Department Sister, W Norfolk and King's Lynn General Hospital, for supplying ophthalmic words and their definitions; Mrs Vivien Golding, Superintendent Physiotherapist, Royal Marsden Hospital, for supplying physiotherapy words and definitions; Miss Susan Ashworth, Clinical Teacher, Royal Marsden Hospital, for revising the radiography and radiotherapy words and definitions; Mrs Anne Christopherson, Speech Therapist, Royal Marsden Hospital, and Mrs Rita Twiston-Davies, Research and Speech Therapist, Charing Cross Hospital, for supplying speech pathology words and definitions. We would also like to thank the many professional colleagues who gave freely of their time and expertise in the definition of individual words.

Miss Elizabeth Jones, Nurse Nutritionist, Royal Marsden Hospital, revised the appendix on nutrition.

Mr Graham Smith, Medical Editor, Baillière Tindall, provided the appendix on prefixes and suffixes.

Mr Richard Wells, Assistant Director of Nursing Services, Royal Marsden Hospital, extensively revised all the other appendixes.

The illustrations have been produced by Mr Kevin Marks and Mr Philip Wilson, Medical Artists, and Miss Caroline Tomb, Medical Artist, Royal Marsden Hospital. The illustrations on pp. 35, 99, 385 and 393 are taken from *Orthopaedic Nursing* (6th edition) by Edward Pinney (Baillière Tindall, 1983).

We would also like to acknowledge the support and invaluable assistance offered throughout by Miss Rosemary Long, Nursing Editor, Baillière Tindall, and to thank Mr Clifford Morgan, Production Editorial Manager, for his meticulous house-editing. We extend our grateful thanks to them both, and our thanks also go to Mrs Theresa Shorter and Mrs Edith Vardy for painstakingly typing the manuscript.

Last, but by no means least, the never failing support of our spouses deserves recognition and thanks. Without them this edition would not have been possible.

Kay Kasner
Dennis H. Tindall

PRONUNCIATION

Stress

Each headword is broken up into syllables by hyphens (e.g. *nu-ro'-sis* for 'neurosis'). The stress mark (') follows the stressed syllable.

Consonants

Most consonants are straightforward and do not need to be described further. Note the following:

c—a hard 'c' is represented by 'k', and a soft 'c' by 's'
g—always used to represent the hard 'g'; soft 'g' is represented by 'j'
q—represented by 'k'; 'qu' by 'kw'
r—often swallowed when following a vowel, although there are regional exceptions to this
x—represented by 'ks'

Some consonant sounds are not represented in the English alphabet by single letters, and require two letters to represent a single sound, e.g.:

ch—as in *ch*eese
ng—as in ri*ng*
sh—as in *sh*ip
th—as in too*th* or *th*is
zh—as in vi*sion* (vizh'-un)

Vowels

The following vowels can be pronounced either long or short: a (fat, fate), e (bet, beet), i (din, dine), o (got, goat) and u (cut, cute). If the long form is to be used, then the hyphen in the pronunciation guide comes directly after the vowel (e.g. *a'-jent* for 'agent'); if the short form is to be used, the hyphen will follow the consonant (e.g. *ak-ute'* for 'acute'). If the final syllable contains a long vowel, then this is represented by the addition of a final 'e' (e.g. *band'-aje* for 'bandage'). If the final syllable ends with a vowel sound, then the long form will be represented by the vowel itself (e.g. *ba'-be* for 'baby') and the short form by the addition of an 'h' (e.g. *ma'-ne-ah* for 'mania').

Note also the following vowel sounds:

aw—as in s*aw*
oi—as in p*oi*nt

oo—as in t*oo*th or b*oo*k
ow—as in c*ow*

Some vowel sounds are associated with the letter 'r'. If preceding a vowel, the 'r' may be pronounced.

ar—as in f*ar*
er—as in p*er*
or—as in f*or*
air—as in f*air*

ABBREVIATIONS

abbrev. = abbreviation
adj. = adjective
b. = born
cap. = capital letter
Gk = Greek

n. = noun
pl. = plural
sing. = singular
v. = verb

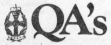

A

A. Abbreviation for the SI unit, the *ampere*.

abacterial (*a-bak-te'-re-al*). Indicating a condition not caused by bacteria.

abarticulation (*ab-ar-tik-u-la'-shun*). Dislocation of a joint.

abatement (*ab-ate'-ment*). A decrease in the severity of a pain or a symptom.

abdomen (*ab-do'-men* or *ab'-do-men*). The belly. The cavity between the diaphragm and the pelvis, lined by a serous membrane, the peritoneum, and containing the stomach, intestines, liver, gall-bladder, spleen, pancreas, kidneys, suprarenal glands, ureters and bladder.

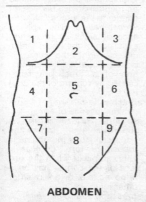

ABDOMEN

For descriptive purposes, its area can be divided into nine regions:
1. *Right hypochondriac.*
2. *Epigastric.*
3. *Left hypochondriac.*
4. *Right lumbar.*
5. *Umbilical.*
6. *Left lumbar.*
7. *Right iliac.*
8. *Hypogastric.*
9. *Left iliac.*

Acute a. Any abdominal condition urgently requiring treatment, usually surgical. *Pendulous a.* A condition in which the anterior part of the abdominal wall hangs down over the pubis. *Scaphoid (navicular) a.* A hollowing of the anterior wall commonly seen in grossly emaciated people.

abdominal (*ab-dom'-in-al*). Pertaining to the abdomen. *A. aneurysm.* A dilatation of the abdominal aorta. *A. aorta.* That part of the aorta below the diaphragm. *A. breathing.* Deep breathing—hyperpnoea. *A. reflex.* Reflex contraction of abdominal wall muscles observed when skin is lightly stroked. *A. section.* Incision through the abdominal wall.

abdominopelvic (*ab-dom'-in-o-pel'-vik*). Concerning the abdomen and the pelvic cavity.

abdominoperineal (*ab-dom'-in-o-per-in-e'-al*). Pertaining to the abdomen and the perineum. *A. excision.* An operation performed through the abdomen and the perineum for the excision of the rectum or bladder. Often done as a synchronized operation by two surgeons, one working at each approach.

abdominoposterior (*ab-dom'-in-o-pos-te'-re-or*). Indicating a position of the fetus with its abdomen turned towards the maternal back.

abducent (*ab-du'-sent*). Leading away from the midline. *A. muscle.* The external rectus muscle of the eye, which rotates it outward. *A. nerve.* The cranial nerve, which supplies this muscle.

abductor (*ab-duk'-tor*). A muscle which draws a limb away from the midline of the body. The opposite of adductor.

aberrant (*ab-er'-ant*). Taking an unusual course. Used of blood vessels and nerves.

aberration (*ab-er-a'-shun*). Deviation from the normal. In optics, failure to focus rays of light. *Mental a.* Mental disorder of an unspecified kind.

ability (*ab-il'-it-e*). The power to perform an act, either mental or physical, with or without training. *Innate a.* The ability with which a person is born.

ablation (*ab-la'-shun*). Removal or destruction by surgical or radiological means of neoplasms or other body tissue.

ablepharia (*a-blef-ar'-e-ah*). Congenital reduction or absence of eyelids.

ablutomania (*ab-lu-to-ma'-ne-ah*). Compulsion to wash oneself frequently.

abnormal (*ab-nor'-mal*). Varying from what is regular or usual.

abort (*ab-ort'*). (1) To terminate a process or disease before it has run its normal course. (2) To give birth to a fetus earlier than the 28th week of pregnancy.

abortifacient (*ab-or-te-fa'-shent*). An agent or drug which may induce abortion.

abortion (*ab-or'-shun*). (1) Premature cessation of a normal process. (2) Emptying of the pregnant uterus before the end of the 28th week. (3) The product of such an abortion. *Complete a.* One in which the contents of the uterus are expelled intact. *Criminal a.* The termination of pregnancy for reasons other than those permitted by law (i.e. danger to mental or physical health of mother or child or family), and without medical approval. *Incomplete a.* That in which some part of the fetus or placenta is retained in the uterus. *Induced a.* The intentional emptying of the uterus. *Inevitable a.* Abortion where bleeding is profuse and accompanied by pains, the cervix is dilated and the contents of the uterus can be felt. *Missed a.* One where all signs of pregnancy disappear and later the uterus discharges a blood clot surrounding a shrivelled fetus, i.e. a carneous mole. *Septic a.* Abortion associated with infection. *Therapeutic a.* One induced on medical advice because of danger to the mother's health. *Threatened a.* The appearance of signs of premature expulsion of the fetus; bleeding is slight, the cervix is closed. *Tubal a.* The termination of a tubal pregnancy caused by rupture of the uterine tube.

abrachia (*a-bra'-ke-ah*). Congenital absence of arms.

abrasion (*ab-ra'-zhun*). A superficial injury, where the skin or mucous membrane is rubbed or torn. *Corneal a.* This can occur when the surface of the cornea has been removed, e.g. by a scratch or other injury.

abreaction (*ab-re-ak'-shun*). A form of psychotherapy in which a patient relives a past painful experience, with the release of repressed emotion.

abruptio placentae (*a-brup'-te-o plas-ent'-e*). Premature detachment of the placenta, causing maternal shock.

abscess (*ab'-ses*). A collection of pus in a cavity. Caused by the disintegration and replacement of tissue damaged by mechanical, chemical or bacterial injury. *Alveolar a.* An abscess in a tooth socket. *Brodie's a.* A bone abscess, usually on the head of the tibia. *Cold a.* The result of chronic tubercular infection, and so called because there are few, if any, signs of inflammation. *Psoas a.* A cold abscess that has tracked down the psoas muscle from caries of the lumbar vertebrae. *Subphrenic a.* One situated under the diaphragm.

absorbent (*ab-sor'-bent*). (1) *adj.* Having tendency to suck in. (2) *n.* Any agent that takes up liquids or gases by suction.

absorption (*ab-sorp'-shun*). (1) In physiology, the taking up by suction of fluids or other substances by the tissues of the body. (2) In psychology, great mental concentration on a single object or activity. (3) In radiology, uptake of radiation by body tissues.

abulia (*a-bu'-le-ah*). Loss of will-power.

acanthoma (*ak-an-tho'-mah*). A tumour originating in the prickle-cell layer of the epidermis. Usually applied to benign epithelial tumours.

acanthosis (*ak-an-tho'-sis*). Hyperplasia of the prickle-cell layer of the epidermis, as seen in psoriasis.

acapnia (*a-kap'-ne-ah*). A deficiency of carbon dioxide in the blood.

acaricide (*ak'-ar-is-ide*). An agent which destroys mites.

Acarus (*ak'-ar-us*). A genus of small mites. *A. scabiei* (*Sarcoptes scabiei*). The cause of scabies.

acatalasia (*a-kat-al-a'-ze-ah*). A condition in which there is absence of the enzyme catalase in the patient's cells. Many of these patients may suffer from oral sepsis.

acatalepsy (*a-kat-al-ep'-se*). Lack of understanding.

acataphasia (*a-kat-ah-fa'-ze-ah*). Loss of the ability to express connected thought, resulting from a cerebral lesion.

accessory (*ak-ses'-or-e*). Supplementary. *A. nerve.* The 11th cranial nerve. It is made up of two portions, the cranial and the spinal.

accommodation (*ak-om'-o-da'-shun*). Adjustment. In ophthalmology, the term refers specifically to adjustment of the ciliary muscle, which controls the shape of the lens. In *negative a.* the ciliary muscle relaxes and the lens becomes less convex, giving long-distance vision; in *positive a.* the ciliary muscle contracts and the lens becomes more convex, giving near vision.

accouchement (*ak-oosh-mon'*). Childbirth.

accountable (*ak-ownt'-abl*). Liable to be held responsible for a course of action. In nursing this refers to the responsibility the trained nurse takes for prescribing and initiating nursing care. The nurse is accountable to his/her patient, his/her peers, his/her employing authority.

accretion (*ak-re'-shun*). Growth. The accumulation of deposits, e.g. of salts to form a calculus in the bladder. In dentistry, the growth of tartar on the teeth.

accumulator (*ak-u'-mu-la-tor*). An apparatus for the collection and storage of electricity.

A battery that can be recharged.

acephalic (*a-kef'-al-ik*). Without a head.

acetabuloplasty (*as-et-ab-u-lo-plas'-te*). An operation performed to improve the depth and shape of the hip socket in correcting congenital dislocation of the hip or in treating osteoarthritis of the hip.

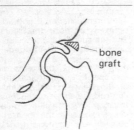

bone graft

ACETABULOPLASTY

acetabulum (*as-et-ab'-u-lum*). The cup-like socket in the innominate bone, in which the head of the femur moves.

acetate (*as'-et-ate*). A· salt of acetic acid.

acetazolamide (*as-et-ah-zol'-am-ide*). A sulphonamide compound which is an oral diuretic and is used in the treatment of congestive heart failure and of glaucoma.

acetic acid (*as-e'-tik as'-id*). The acid of vinegar. It may be used as an antidote to alkaline poisons or as a reagent in urine testing.

acetoacetic acid (*as-et-o-as-e'-tik as'-id*). Diacetic acid. A product of fat metabolism. It occurs in excessive amounts in diabetes and starvation, giving rise to acetone bodies in the urine.

acetonaemia (*as-e-to-ne'-me-ah*). The presence of acetone bodies in the blood.

acetone (*as'-e-tone*). A colourless inflammable liquid with a characteristic odour. Traces are found in the blood and in normal urine. *A. bodies*. Ketones found in the blood and urine of diabetic patients as a result of the incomplete breakdown of fatty and amino acids. Also found in the urine of people who are fasting.

acetonuria (*as-e-to-nu'-re-ah*). The presence of an excess quantity of acetone bodies in the urine which gives it a peculiar sweet smell.

acetylcholine (*as-et-il-ko'-leen*). A chemical transmitter that is released by some nerve endings at the synapse between one neurone and the next or between a nerve ending and the effector organ it supplies. These nerves are said to be cholinergic, e.g. the parasympathetic nerves and the lower motor neurones to skeletal muscles. It is rapidly destroyed in the body by cholinesterase.

acetylcoenzyme A (*as-et-il-ko-en'-zime a*). Active form of acetic acid, to which carbohydrates, fats and amino acids not needed for protein synthesis are converted.

acetylsalicylic acid (*as-et-il-sal-e-sil'-ik as'-id*). Aspirin. An analgesic and antipyretic, usually given in tablet form.

achalasia (*a-kal-a'-ze-ah*). Failure of relaxation of a muscle sphincter causing dilatation of the part above, e.g. of the oesophagus above the cardiac sphincter.

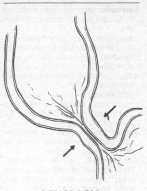

ACHALASIA

ache (*ake*). A dull continuous pain.

Achilles (*ak-il'-eez*). Greek mythological hero who could be wounded only in the heel. *A. tendon*. Tendocalcaneus, connecting the soleus and gastrocnemius muscles of the calf to the heel bone (os calcis).

achillorrhaphy (*ak-il-or'-raf-e*). Repair of the Achilles tendon after it has been torn.

achillotomy (*ak-il-ot'-om-e*). The subcutaneous division of the Achilles tendon, performed in order to lengthen it.

achlorhydria (*a-klor-hi'-dre-ah*). The absence of free hydrochloric acid in the stomach. May be found in pernicious anaemia and gastric cancer.

acholia (*a-ko'-le-ah*). A lack of secretion of bile.

acholuria (*a-ko-lu'-re-ah*). Deficiency or lack of bile from the urine.

acholuric (*a-ko-lu'-rik*). Pertain-

ing to acholuria. *A. jaundice*. Jaundice without bile in the urine.

achondroplasia (*a-kon-dro-pla'-ze-ah*). An inherited condition in which there is early union of the epiphysis and diaphysis of long bones. Growth is arrested and dwarfism is the result.

achromasia (*a-kro-ma'-ze-ah*). (1) Lack of colour in the skin. (2) Absence of normal reaction to staining in a tissue or cell.

achromatopsia (*a-kro-mat-op'-se-ah*). Complete colour blindness caused by disease or trauma. It may be congenital.

achylia (*a-ki'-le-ah*). Absence of chyle. *A. gastrica*. A condition in which gastric secretion is reduced or absent.

acid (*as'-id*). (1) *adj*. Sour or sharp in taste. (2) *n*. A substance which, when combined with an alkali, will form a salt. Any acid substance will turn blue litmus red. Individual acids are given under their specific names. *A.–base balance*. The normal ratio between the acid ions and the basic or alkaline ions required to maintain the pH of the blood and body fluids. *A.-fast*. Descriptive of those microorganisms not easily decolorized when once stained. *A.–alcohol-fast*. Descriptive of stained bacteria that are resistant to decolorization by both acid and alcohol.

acidaemia (*as-id-e'-me-ah*). Abnormal acidity of the blood, which contains an excess of hydrogen ions.

acidity (*as-id'-it-e*). (1) Sourness or sharpness of taste. (2) The state of being acid.

acidosis (*as-id-o'-sis*). A condition in which the relation of alkalinity to acidity of the blood is disturbed, with an increase in the hydrogen ion concentration. It is characterized by vomiting, drowsiness, hyperpnoea, acetone odour of breath (of 'new-mown hay') and acetone bodies in the urine. It may occur in diabetes mellitus owing to incomplete metabolism of fat. *See also* Ketosis.

acidotic (*as-id-ot'-ik*). (1) *adj.* Pertaining to acidosis. (2) *n.* One suffering from acidosis.

aciduria (*as-id-u'-re-ah*). A condition in which acid urine is excreted.

acinus (*as'-in-us*). *pl.* acini. A minute saccule or alveolus lined by secreting cells. The secreting portion of the mammary gland consists of acini.

acme (*ak'-me*). (1) The highest point. (2) The crisis of a fever when the symptoms are fully developed.

acne (*ak'-ne*). An inflammatory condition of the sebaceous glands in which blackheads (comedones) are usually present together with papules and pustules. *A. keratitis.* Inflammation of the cornea associated with acne rosacea. *A. rosacea.* A redness of the forehead, nose and cheeks due to chronic dilatation of the subcutaneous capillaries, which becomes permanent with the formation of pustules in the affected areas. *A. vulgaris.* Form that occurs commonly in adolescents and young adults, affecting the face, chest and back. Its primary cause is thought to be endocrine.

acneiform (*ak-ne'-e-form*). Resembling acne.

acousma (*ak-oos'-mah*). The hearing of imaginary sounds.

acoustic (*ak-oos'-tik*). Relating to sound or the sense of hearing.

acquired (*ak-wi'-rd*). Pertaining to disease, habits or immunity developed after birth; not congenital.

acrid (*ak'-rid*). Bitter; pungent; irritating.

acriflavine (*ak-re-fla'-veen*). A powerful antiseptic derived from coal tar and used in an aqueous solution.

acroarthritis (*ak'-ro-ar-thri'-tis*). Arthritis in the joints of the hands and feet.

acrocentric (*ak-ro-sen'-trik*). Descriptive of chromosomes which have the centromere near to one end.

acrocephalia (*ak-ro-kef-a'-le-ah*). Malformation of the head, in which the top is pointed. Oxycephaly.

acrocyanosis (*ak-ro-si-an-o'-sis*). A blue appearance of the hands and feet often associated with a vasomotor defect.

acrodynia (*ak-ro-din'-e-ah*). An allergic reaction to mercury in children causing pain and erythema in the fingers and toes. Pink disease.

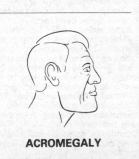

ACROMEGALY

acromegaly (*ak-ro-meg'-al-e*). A chronic condition producing gradual enlargement of the hands, feet and bones of the head and chest. Associated with overactivity of the anterior lobe of the pituitary gland in adults.

acromioclavicular (*ak-ro'-me-o-klav-ik'-u-lah*). Pertaining to the joint between the acromion process of the scapula and the lateral aspect of the clavicle.

acromion (*ak-ro'-me-on*). The outward projection of the spine of the scapula, forming the point of the shoulder.

acronyx (*ak'-ron-iks*). A toe- or finger-nail which becomes ingrown.

acroparaesthesia (*ak-ro-par-es-the'-ze-ah*). Condition in which pressure on the nerves of the brachial plexus causes numbness, pain and tingling of the hand and forearm.

acrophobia (*ak-ro-fo'-be-ah*). Morbid terror of being at a height.

acrosclerosis (*ak'-ro-skler-o'-sis*). A type of scleroderma which affects the hands, feet, face or chest.

acrosome (*ak'-ro-some*). Part of the head of a spermatozoon.

acrylics (*ak-ril'-iks*). Synthetic plastic materials derived from acrylic acid, from which dental and medical prostheses may be made. Used in eye surgery for reconstituting a socket and for making artificial eyes, implants and lenses.

ACTH Adrenocorticotrophic hormone. Corticotrophin.

actin (*ak'-tin*). The protein of myofibril responsible for contraction and relaxation of muscles.

actinism (*ak'-tin-izm*). The ability of rays of light to produce chemical changes.

actinodermatitis (*ak-tin-o-der-mat-i'-tis*). Inflammation of the skin, due to the action of ultraviolet or X-rays.

Actinomyces (*ak-tin-o-mi'-seez*). A genus of branching, spore-forming, vegetable parasites, which may give rise to actinomycosis and from which many antibiotic drugs are produced, e.g. streptomycin.

actinomycin (*ak-tin-o-mi'-sin*). A group of cytotoxic drugs used in the treatment of malignant disease, e.g. Wilms' tumour and lymphadenoma.

actinomycosis (*ak-tin-o-mi-ko'-sis*). A chronic infective disease of cattle which is also found in man. Granulated tumours occur, chiefly on the tongue and jaws.

actinotherapy (*ak-tin-o-ther'-ap-e*). Treatment of disease by rays of light, e.g. artificial sunlight.

action (*ak'-shun*). The operation or function of any part of the body. *A. potential.* The electrical change which takes place when a nerve conducts an impulse or a muscle fibre contracts.

activator (*ak'-ti-va-tor*). A substance, hormone or enzyme, that stimulates a chemical change though it may not take part in the change. In chemistry, a catalyst. (1) Yeast is the activator in the process by which sugar is converted into alcohol. (2) The digestive secretions are activated by hormones to carry out normal digestion.

active (*ak'-tiv*). Causing change; energetic. *A. immunity.* An immunity in which the individual has been stimulated to produce his or her own antibodies. *A. movements*. Movements made by the patient as distinct from passive movements. *A. principle*. The ingredient in a drug which is primarily responsible for its therapeutic action.

actomyosin (*ak-to-mi'-o-sin*). Muscle protein complex; the myosin component acts as an enzyme which causes the release of energy.

acuity (*ak-u'-it-e*). Sharpness. *A. of hearing*. An acute perception of sound. *A. of vision*. Clear focusing ability.

acupuncture (*ak'-u-punkt-chur*). A system, which originated in China, in which the insertion of special needles in particular parts of the body is used for the production of anaesthesia, the relief of pain and the treatment of certain conditions.

acus (*a'-kus*). A needle (*Latin*).

acute (*ak-ute'*). A term applied to a disease in which the attack is sudden, severe and of short duration. *A. yellow atrophy*. Necrosis of the liver cells caused by a toxic agent.

acyclic (*a-si'-klik*). Occurring independently of a natural cycle of events, as of the menstrual cycle.

acystia (*a-sis'-te-ah*). Absence of the bladder.

adactylia (*a-dak-til'-e-ah*). Congenital absence of fingers or toes.

Adam's apple (*ad'-amz ap'-l*). The laryngeal prominence, a protrusion of the front of the neck formed by the thyroid cartilage.

adaptation (*ad-ap-ta'-shun*). (1) The process of modification which a living organism undergoes when adjusting itself to new surroundings or circumstances. (2) The process of overcoming difficulties and adjusting to changing circumstances. Neuroses and psychoses are often associated with failure of adaptation.

addiction (*ad-ik'-shun*). The habitual taking of drugs or alcohol, for which a craving develops that is beyond the will of the person addicted to control. *See* Drug dependence.

Addison's anaemia (*T. Addison, British physician, 1793–1860*). Pernicious anaemia.

Addison's disease. Deficiency disease of the suprarenal cortex; often tuberculous. There is wasting, brown pigmentation of the skin and extreme debility.

adducent (*ad-u'-sent*). Leading toward the midline. *A. muscle*. The medial rectus muscle of the eye which turns it inward.

adductor (*ad-ukt'-or*). A muscle which draws a limb towards the midline of the body. The opposite of abductor.

adenectomy (*ad-en-ek'-tom-e*). Excision of a gland.

adenine (*ad'-en-een*). One of the purine bases found in deoxyribonucleic acid.

adenitis (*ad-en-i'-tis*). Inflammation of a gland.

adenocarcinoma (*ad-en-o-kar-sin-o'-mah*). A malignant new growth of glandular epithelial tissue.

adenofibroma (*ad-en-o-fi-bro'-mah*). A benign tumour of connective tissue which contains glandular structures.

adenoid (*ad'-en-oid*). Resembling a gland. Generally applied to abnormal lymphoid growth in the nasopharynx.

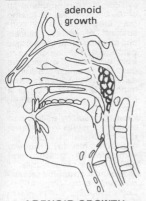

adenoid growth

ADENOID GROWTH

adenoidectomy (*ad-en-oid-ek'-tom-e*). The surgical removal of adenoid tissue from the nasopharynx.

adenoma (*ad-en-o'-mah*). A non-malignant tumour of glandular tissue.

adenomatome (*ad-en-o'-mat-ome*). An instrument for the removal of adenoids.

adenomyoma (*ad-en-o-mi-o'-mah*). An innocent new growth involving both glandular and muscle tissue; usually applied to benign growths of the uterus.

adenopathy (*ad-en-op'-ath-e*). Any disease of a gland, particularly of the lymphatics.

adenosarcoma (*ad'-en-o-sar-co'-mah*). A malignant tumour of connective and glandular tissue. *Embryonal a.* Nephroblastoma.

adenosclerosis (*ad-en-o-skler-o'-sis*). Hardening of a gland. Usually the result of calcification.

adenosine (*ad-en'-o-seen*). A nucleoside consisting of adenine and D-ribose (a pentose sugar). *A. triphosphate.* ATP. A compound containing three phosphoric acids. It is present in all cells and serves as a store for energy.

adenovirus (*ad-en-o-vi'-rus*). A DNA-containing virus. Many types have been isolated, some of which cause respiratory tract infections, while others are associated with conjunctivitis or epidemic keratoconjunctivitis.

adeps (*ad'-eps*). Lard (*Latin.*) A foundation fat for ointments. *A. lanae hydrosus.* Lanolin.

ADH. Antidiuretic hormone. Vasopressin.

adhesion (*ad-he'-zhun*). Union between two surfaces normally separated. Usually the result of inflammation when fibrous tissue forms, e.g. peritonitis may cause adhesions between organs. A possible cause of intestinal obstruction.

adiaphoresis (*a-di-af-or-e'-sis*). Deficiency in the secretion of sweat.

adiaphoretic (*a-di-af-or-et'-ik*). An anhidrotic agent. A drug that prevents the secretion of sweat.

adipocele (*ad'-ip-o-seel*). A hernia, with the sac containing fatty tissue.

adipocere (*ad'-ip-o-seer*). A waxy substance formed in dead bodies when decomposing.

adipose (*ad'-ip-ose*). Of the nature of fat. Fatty.

adiposity (*ad-ip-os'-it-e*). The state of being too fat. Obesity.

adiposuria (*ad-ip-o-su'-re-ah*). The presence of fat in the urine. Lipuria.

aditus (*ad'-it-us*). An opening

or passageway; often applied to that between the middle ear and the mastoid antrum.

adjustment (*ad-just'-ment*). In psychology, the ability of a person to adapt to changing circumstances or environment.

adjuvant (*ad'-ju-vant*). (1) Any treatment used in conjunction with another to enhance its efficacy. (2) A substance administered with a drug to enhance its effect.

ADL. Aids to Daily Living. Supplied by an occupational therapist to assist a patient in living as independently as possible.

Adler's theory (*A. Adler, Austrian psychiatrist, 1870–1937*). The theory that neuroses develop as a compensation for feelings of inferiority, either social or physical.

adnexa (*ad-neks'-ah*). Appendages. *Uterine a.* The ovaries and tubes.

adolescence (*ad-o-les'-ens*). The period between puberty and maturity. In the male—14 to 25 years. In the female—12 to 21 years.

adrenal (*ad-re'-nal*). (1) *adj.* Near the kidneys. (2) *n.* A triangular endocrine gland, one of which is situated above each kidney.

adrenalectomy (*ad-re-nal-ek'-tom-e*). Surgical removal of the adrenal glands. Replacement therapy by giving cortisone is essential. *Medical a.* Treatment with the drug aminoglutethimide.

adrenaline (*ad-ren'-al-in*). Epinephrine. A hormone secreted by the medulla of the adrenal gland. Has an action similar to normal stimulation of the sympathetic nervous system: (1) causing dilatation of the bronchioles; (2) raising the blood pressure by constriction of surface vessels and stimulation of the cardiac output; (3) releasing glycogen from the liver. It is therefore used to treat such conditions as asthma, collapse and hypoglycaemia. It acts as a haemostat in local anaesthetics.

adrenergic (*ad-ren-er'-jik*). Pertaining to nerves that release the chemical transmitter noradrenaline in order to stimulate the muscles and glands they supply.

adrenocorticotrophin (*ad-re'-no-kor-tik-o-tro'-fin*). ACTH. Corticotrophin.

adrenogenital (*ad-re-no-jen'-it-al*). Relating to both the adrenal glands and the gonads. *A. syndrome.* A condition of masculinization in women caused by overactivity of the adrenal cortex.

adrenolytic (*ad-re-no-lit'-ik*). A drug that inhibits the stimulation of the sympathetic nerves and the activity of adrenaline.

adsorbent (*ad-sorb'-ent*). A substance that has the power of attracting gas or fluid to itself.

adsorption (*ad-sorp'-shun*). The power of certain substances to attach other gases or substances in solution to their surface and so concentrate them there. This is made use of in chromatography.

adult (*ad-ult'*). *adj.* Mature. (*ad'-ult*). *n.* A mature person.

adulteration (*ad-ul-ter-a'-shun*). The addition of unnecessary and usually cheaper substances to a product.

advancement (*ad-vans'-ment*). In surgery, an operation to detach a tendon or muscle and reattach it further forward. Used in the treatment of strabismus and uterine retroversion.

adventitia (*ad-ven-tish'-e-ah*). The outer coat of an artery or vein.

Aëdes (*a-e'-deez*). A genus of mosquitoes. It includes *A. aegypti*, the intermediate host in the transmission of dengue and yellow fever.

aegophony (*e-gof'-on-e*). A sound heard in the chest on auscultation, when the patient speaks. Sometimes compared to 'the bleat of a goat'.

aeration (*air-a'-shun*). Supplying with air. Used to describe the oxygenation of blood which takes place in the lungs.

aerobe (*air'-obe*). An organism that can live and thrive only in the presence of oxygen.

aerogenous (*air-oj'-en-us*). Gas-producing. Applied to micro-organisms that give rise to the formation of gas, usually by the fermentation of lactose or other carbohydrate.

aerophagy (*air-off'-aj-e*). The excessive swallowing of air.

aerosol (*air'-o-sol*). Finely divided particles or droplets. *A. sprays*. Used in medicine to humidify air or oxygen, or for the administration of drugs by inhalation and as a local analgesic.

aetas (*e'-tas*). Age (*Latin*). *Abbrev.* aet.

aetiology (*e-te-ol'-oj-e*). The science of the cause of disease.

afebrile (*a-feb'-rile*). Without fever.

afibrinogenaemia (*a-fi-brin'-o-jen-e'-me-ah*). Absence of fibrinogen in the blood. The clotting mechanism of the blood is impaired as a result.

affect (*af-ekt'*). In psychiatry, the feeling experienced in connection with an emotion or mood.

affection (*af-ek'-shun*). (1) A morbid condition or disease state. (2) A warm feeling for someone or something.

affective (*af-ekt'-iv*). Pertaining to the emotions or moods. *A. psychoses*. Major mental disorders in which there is grave disturbance of the emotions.

afferent (*af'-er-ent*). Conveying towards the centre. *A. nerves*. The sensory nerve fibres which convey impulses from the periphery towards the brain. *A. paths* or *tracts*. The course of the sensory nerves up the spinal cord and through the brain. *A. vessels*. Arterioles entering the glomerulus of the kidney, or lymphatics entering a lymph gland. *See* Efferent.

affiliation (*af-il-e-a'-shun*). The judicial decision of paternity of a child with a view to a maintenance order.

affinity (*af-in'-it-e*). In chemistry, the attraction of two substances to each other, e.g. haemoglobin and oxygen.

African tick fever (*af'-rik-an tik fe'-ver*). Disease caused by a spirochaete, *Borrelia duttonii*. Transmitted by ticks. *See* Relapsing fever.

afterbirth (*ahf'-ter-berth*). The placenta, cord and membranes, expelled after childbirth.

after-care (*ahf'-ter-kair*). Social, medical or nursing care following a period of hospital treatment.

after-image (*ahf'-ter-im'-ij*). A visual impression that remains briefly following the cessation of sensory stimulation.

after-pains (ahf'-ter-pa'-nz). Pains due to uterine contraction after childbirth.

afunctional (a-funk'-shun-al). Lacking function.

Ag. Chemical symbol for *silver* (argentum).

agalactia (a-gal-ak'-te-ah). Absence of the milk secretion after childbirth.

agammaglobulinaemia (a-gam-ah-glob-u-lin-e'-me-ah). A condition found in children in which there is no gammaglobulin in the blood. They are therefore susceptible to infections because of an inability to form antibodies.

agar (a'-gar). A gelatinous substance prepared from seaweed. Used as a culture medium for bacteria and as a laxative because it absorbs liquid from the digestive tract and swells, so stimulating peristalsis.

ageing (a'-jing). The structural changes that take place in time that are not caused by accident or disease.

agenesis (a-jen'-es-is). Failure of a structure to develop properly.

agent (a'-jent). Any substance or force capable of producing a physical, chemical or biological effect. *Alkylating a.* A cytotoxic preparation. *Chelating a.* A chemical compound which binds metal ions. *Wetting a.* A substance which lowers the surface tension of water and promotes wetting.

agglutination (ag-lu-tin-a'-shun). The collecting into clumps, particularly of cells suspended in a fluid and of bacteria affected by specific immune serum. *Cross a.* A simple test to decide the group to which a given blood belongs. (*See* Blood group-ing). A drop of serum of known classification is put on a microscope slide, and to this is added a drop of the blood to be tested. An even admixture indicates compatibility. A flaky spotted appearance shows incompatibility as the corpuscles have clumped together. *A. test.* A means of aiding diagnosis and identification of bacteria. If serum containing known agglutinins comes into contact with the specific bacteria, clumping will take place. *See* Widal reaction.

agglutinative (ag-lu'-tin-a-tiv). (1) *adj.* Adherent or gluing together. (2) *n.* Serum which causes clumping of bacteria, e.g. in Widal reaction.

agglutinin (ag-lu'-tin-in). An antibody formed in blood which causes clumping together of bacteria, so that they are more readily destroyed by phagocytes.

agglutinogen (ag-lu-tin'-o-jen). Any substance that, when present in the blood stream, can cause the production of specific antibodies or agglutinins.

aggregation (ag-reg-a'-shun). The massing together of materials, as in clumping. *Familial a.* The increased incidence of cases of a disease in a family compared with that in control families. *Platelet a.* The clumping together of platelets which may be induced by a number of agents such as thrombin and collagen.

aggressin (ag-res'-in). A substance said to be produced by some bacteria which increases their effect upon the host.

aggression (ag-resh'-un).

Animosity or hostility shown towards another person or object, as a response to opposition or frustration.

agitation (*aj-it-a'-shun*). (1) Shaking. (2) Mental distress causing extreme restlessness.

aglossia (*a-glos'-e-ah*). Absence of the tongue.

aglutition (*a-glu-tish'-un*). Difficulty in the act of swallowing. Dysphagia.

agnathia (*ag-na'-the-ah*). Absence or defective development of the jaw.

agnosia (*ag-no'-ze-ah*). An inability to recognize objects as the sensory stimulus cannot be interpreted in spite of a normal sense organ.

agonist (*ag'-on-ist*). The prime mover. A muscle opposed in action by another (the antagonist).

agony (*ag'-on-e*). Extreme suffering, either mental or physical.

agoraphobia (*ag-or-ah-fo'-be-ah*). A fear of open spaces.

agranulocyte (*a-gran'-u-lo-site*). A white blood cell without granules in the cytoplasm. Includes monocytes and lymphocytes.

agranulocytosis (*a-gran'-u-lo-si-to'-sis*). A condition in which there is a marked decrease or complete absence of granular leucocytes in the blood. May result from: (1) the use of drugs, e.g. gold salts, sulphonamides, thiouracil and benzol preparations; (2) excessive irradiation of the bone marrow. Characterized by a sore throat, ulceration of the mouth and pyrexia. It may result in severe prostration and death.

agraphia (*a-graf'-e-ah*). Absence of the power of expressing thought in writing. It arises from a lack of muscular co-ordination or from a cerebral lesion.

ague (*a'-gu*). Malaria. Intermittent fever, accompanied by recurring fits of shivering and sweating.

AHG. Antihaemophilic globulin.

AID. Artificial insemination of a woman with donor semen.

AIDS. Acquired immune deficiency syndrome. A recently documented but still poorly understood disorder. Parts of the immune system are damaged, in varying degrees of severity, and this results in some sufferers being more susceptible than others to certain serious and sometimes fatal diseases, such as Kaposi's sarcoma.

AIH. Artificial insemination of a woman by her husband's semen.

ailment (*ail'-ment*). Any minor disorder of the body.

air (*air*). A mixture of gases surrounding the earth. It consists of: non-active nitrogen 79%; oxygen 21%, which supports life and combustion; traces of neon, argon, hydrogen, etc.; and carbon dioxide 0.03% except in expired air, when 6% is exhaled, due to diffusion which has taken place in the lungs. Air has weight and exerts pressure. The latter aids in syphonage from body cavities. *Complemental a.* Additional air which can be inhaled with inspiratory effort. *Residual a.* Air remaining in the lungs after deep expiration. *Stationary a.* That retained in the lungs after normal expiration. *Supplemental a.* The extra air forced out of the lungs with expiratory effort. *Tidal a.* That which passes in and out of the lungs in normal respiratory action. *A.-bed*. A rubber mattress inflated with air. *A. embolism*. An embolism caused by air entering the circulatory system. *A. encephalography*. Radiological examination of the brain after the injection of air into the subarachnoid space. *A. hunger*. A form of dyspnoea in which there are deep sighing respirations, characteristic of severe haemorrhage or acidosis.

airway (*air'-wa*). (1) The passage whereby the air enters and leaves the lungs. (2) A metal or rubber tube used in anaesthesia, passing through the mouth or nose.

akinesia (*a-kin-e'-ze-ah*). Loss of muscle power. This may be the result of a brain or spinal cord lesion or temporarily due to anaesthesia.

akinetic (*a-kin-et'-ik*). Relating to states or conditions where there is lack of movement.

Al. Chemical symbol for *aluminium*.

alalia (*al-a'-le-ah*). Loss or impairment of the power of speech due to muscle paralysis or cerebral lesion.

alanine (*al'-an-een*). An amino acid formed by the ingestion of dietary protein.

Albers-Schönberg's disease (*H.E. Albers-Schönberg, German radiologist, 1865–1921*). Osteopetrosis

albinism (*al'-bin-izm*). A condition in which there is congenital absence of pigment in the skin, hair and eyes. It may be partial or complete.

albino (*al-be'-no*). A person affected with albinism.

Albright's syndrome (*F. Albright, American physician, 1900–1969*). Condition in which there is abnormal development of bone, excessive pigmentation of the skin and, in females, precocious sexual development.

albumin (*al-bu'-min*). A protein present in most animal tissues. It is soluble in water and coagulates on heating, e.g. white of egg.

albuminuria (*al-bu-min-u'-re-ah*). The presence of albumin in the urine, occurring e.g. in renal disease, in most feverish conditions and sometimes in pregnancy. *Orthostatic* or *postural a*. A non-pathological form which affects some individuals after prolonged standing but disappears after bedrest for a few hours.

albumose (*al'-bu-mose*). A substance formed during gastric digestion, intermediate between albumin and peptone.

alcohol (*al'-ko-hol*). A volatile liquid distilled from fermented saccharine liquids and forming the basis of all wines and spirits. The official (BP) preparation of ethyl alcohol (ethanol) contains 95% alcohol and 5% water. Used: (1) as an antiseptic; (2) in the preparation of tinctures; (3) as a preservative for anatomical specimens. Taken internally, it acts as a temporary heart stimulant, and in large quantities as a depressant poison. It has some value as a food, 30 ml brandy producing about 400 J. *Absolute a*. That which contains not more than 1% by weight of water. *A.-fast*. Pertaining to bacteria that having once been stained are resistant to decolorization by alcohol.

alcoholic (*al-ko-hol'-ik*). (1) *adj*.

Pertaining to alcohol. (2) *n.* A person addicted to excessive, uncontrolled alcohol consumption. This results in loss of appetite and vitamin B deficiency, leading to peripheral neuritis with eye changes and cirrhosis of the liver and to progressive deterioration in the personality.

alcoholism (*al'-ko-hol-izm*). The state of poisoning by excessive consumption of alcohol.

alcoholuria (*al-ko-hol-u'-re-ah*). The presence of alcohol in the urine. This may be estimated when excess blood levels of alcohol are suspected.

aldosterone (*al-do-steer'-one*). A compound isolated from the adrenal cortex, which aids the retention of sodium and the excretion of potassium in the body and by so doing aids in maintaining the electrolyte balance.

aldosteronism (*al-do-steer'-o-nizm*). An excess secretion of aldosterone caused by an adrenal neoplasm. The serum potassium is low and the patient has hypertension and severe muscular weakness.

aleukaemia (*a-lu-ke'-me-ah*). An acute condition in which there is an absence or deficiency of white cells in the blood.

alexia (*a-leks'-e-ah*). A form of aphasia, when there is inability to recognize written or printed words. Word blindness.

algae (*al'-je*). Simple forms of plant life. These form a slimy film on sand filter beds and aid purification of water.

algesia (*al-je'-ze-ah*). Excessive sensitiveness to pain.

algesimeter (*al-jes-im'-e-ter*). An instrument which indicates the degree of sensitiveness to pain.

algid (*al'-jid*). Chilly and cold. *A. state.* One of severe collapse and prostration which may occur in certain types of malaria and in cholera.

alienation (*a-le-en-a'-shun*). A symptom of schizophrenia where the sufferer feels that his thoughts are under the control of someone else. Depersonalization.

alignment (*al-ine'-ment*). The state of being arranged in a line, i.e. in correct anatomical position.

aliment (*al'-im-ent*). Food or nourishment.

alimentary (*al-im-ent'-ar-e*). Relating to the system of nutrition. *A. canal.* or *tract.* The passage through which the food passes, from mouth to anus. *A. system.* The alimentary tract together with the liver and other organs concerned in digestion and absorption.

alimentation (*al-im-en-ta'-shun*). The process of supplying the patient's need for nutrition.

aliquot (*al'-e-kwot*). One of a number of equal parts forming a compound or solution.

alkalaemia (*al-kal-e'-me-ah*). An increase in the alkali content of the blood. The pH is above 7.4. Alkalosis.

alkali (*al'-kal-i*). A substance capable of uniting with acids to form salts, and with fats and fatty acids to form soaps. Alkaline solutions turn red litmus paper blue. Sodium, potassium and ammonia are the alkalis most used in medicine.

alkaloid (*al'-kal-oid*). One of a group of active nitrogenous compounds that are alkaline

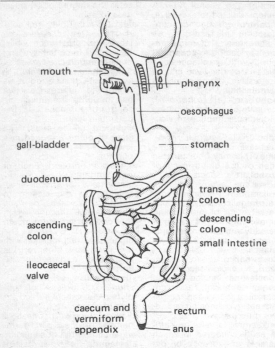

mouth — pharynx

— oesophagus

gall-bladder — stomach

duodenum — transverse colon

ascending colon — descending colon

— small intestine

ileocaecal valve

caecum and vermiform appendix — rectum — anus

ALIMENTARY CANAL

in solution and have a bitter taste. They are of plant origin but many are now made synthetically, e.g. morphine, nicotine, quinine.

alkalosis (al-kal-o'-sis). An increase in the alkali reserve in the blood. It may be confirmed by estimation of the blood carbon dioxide content and treated by giving normal saline or ammonium chloride

intravenously to encourage the excretion of bicarbonate by the kidneys.

alkapton (al-kap'-ton). An abnormal product of protein metabolism, from the amino acid, tyrosine. Homogentisic acid.

alkaptonuria (al-kap-ton-u'-re-ah). The excretion of alkapton in the urine. On standing, oxidation takes place, giving a dark-brown colour to the urine.

alkylating agent (*al'-ki-la-ting a'-jent*). A drug that damages the DNA molecule of the nucleus of malignant tumour cells. Many are nitrogen mustard preparations and may be termed chromosome poisons.

allantois (*al-an'-to-is*). A membranous sac projecting from the ventral surface of the fetus in its early stages. It eventually helps to form the placenta.

allele (*al-eel'*). Allelomorph. One of a pair of genes which occupy the same relative positions on homologous chromosomes and produce different effects on the same process of development.

allelomorph (*al-e'-lo-morf*). Allele.

allergen (*al'-er-jen*). A substance that can produce an allergy.

allergy (*al'-er-je*). A hypersensitivity to some foreign substances which are normally harmless but which produce a violent reaction in the patient. Asthma, hay fever, angioneurotic oedema, migraine, and some types of urticaria and eczema are allergic states. *See* Anaphylaxis.

alloaesthesia (*al-o-es-the'-ze-ah*). Allocheiria. A response or sensation felt on (referred to) the opposite side from that to which a stimulus is applied.

allocheiria (*al-o-ki'-re-ah*). Alloaesthesia.

allograft (*al'-o-graft*). Tissue transplanted from one person to another. *Non-viable a.* Skin taken from a cadaver which cannot regenerate. *Viable a.* Living tissue transplanted.

allokeratoplasty (*al-o-ker'-at-o-plas-te*). Repair of the cornea, using a material foreign to the human body, e.g. a plastic substance.

allopurinol (*al-o-pu'-rin-ol*). A drug which reduces the serum and urinary levels of uric acid. Used in the long-term treatment of gout to lessen the frequency and severity of attacks.

all-or-none law (*orl'-or-nun' lor*). Principle that states that in individual cardiac and skeletal muscle fibres there are only two possible reactions to a stimulus: either there is no reaction at all or there is a full reaction with no gradation of response according to the strength of the stimulus. Whole muscles can grade their response by increasing or decreasing the *number* of fibres involved.

alloy (*al'-oy*). A mixture of two or more metals.

aloes (*al'-oze*). A drug made from the leaves of the aloe. An irritant purgative likely to cause griping. It is contraindicated in pregnancy.

alopecia (*al-o-pe'-she-ah*). Baldness. Loss of hair.

alpha (*al'-fah*). The first letter of the Greek alphabet—α. *A. cells.* Cells found in the islets of Langerhans in the pancreas. They produce the hormone, glucagon. *A. rays.* Particles made up of two protons and two neutrons which are emitted by some radioactive substances. Absorbed by tissue paper. Not used for therapeutic purposes. *A. receptors.* Tissue receptors associated with the stimulation (contraction) of smooth muscle. *A. fetoprotein.* A gammaglobulin originating in the fetal liver and gastrointestinal tract. The level increases in the fetus before birth and falls to very low levels after two years. Serves as a tumour marker for teratomas.

Alport's syndrome (*A.C. Alport, South African physician, 1880–1959*). Congenital glomerulonephritis associated with deafness and sometimes with ocular defects.

alternating current (*awl'-ter-na-ting kur'-ent*). An electrical current that runs alternately from the negative and positive poles.

altitude sickness (*al'-tit-ude sik'-nes*). Condition caused by hypoxia which occurs as a result of lowered oxygen pressure at high altitudes.

alum (*al'-um*). A powerful astringent and styptic, composed of aluminium and potassium or ammonium sulphate. *A. precipitated toxoid.* APT.

aluminium (*al-u-min'-e-um*). *abbrev.* Al. A silver-white metal with a low specific gravity, compounds of which are astringent and antiseptic. *A. hydroxide.* Compound used as an antacid in the treatment of gastric conditions. *A. silicate.* Kaolin; used as a dusting powder or as a poultice. Refined kaolin may be given orally to check diarrhoea.

alveolar (*al-ve-o'-lar*). Concerning an alveolus. *A. air.* Air found in the alveoli or air sacs of the lungs.

alveolitis (*al-ve-o-li'-tis*). Inflammation of the alveoli. *Extrinsic allergic a.* Inflammation of the alveoli of the lung caused by inhalation of an antigen such as pollen.

Alzheimer's disease (*A. Alzheimer, German neurologist, 1864–1915*). Presenile dementia.

amalgam (*am-al'-gam*). A compound of mercury and other metals. *Dental a.* Used for filling teeth.

amastia (*a-mas'-te-ah*). Congenital absence of breast tissue.

amaurosis (*am-aw-ro'-sis*). Loss of vision, sometimes following excessive blood loss; especially after prolonged bleeding, e.g. haematuria. The visual loss may be partial or complete, temporary or permanent.

amaurotic (*am-aw-rot'-ik*). Pertaining to amaurosis. *A. family idiocy.* Tay–Sachs disease. A familial metabolic disorder commencing in infancy or childhood. Characterized by progressive mental deterioration, blindness and spastic paralysis.

ambidextrous (*am-be-deks'-trus*). Equally skilful with either hand.

ambivalence (*am-biv'-al-ens*). The existence of contradictory emotional feelings towards an object, commonly of love and hate for another person. If these feelings occur to a marked degree they lead to psychological disturbance.

amblyopia (*am-ble-o'-pe-ah*). Dimness of vision without any apparent lesion of the eye. Uncorrectable by optical means.

amblyoscope (*am'-ble-o-skope*). An instrument used in orthoptic treatment to aid the correction of strabismus and develop binocular vision.

ambulatory (*am-bu-la'-tor-e*). Having the capacity to walk.

amelia (*a-me'-le-ah*). Congenital absence of a limb or limbs.

amelioration (*am-e-le-or-a'-shun*). Improvement of symptoms; a lessening of the severity of a disease.

amenorrhoea (*a-men-or-e'-ah*). Absence of menstruation. *Primary a.* The non-occurrence of the menses. *Secondary a.* The cessation of the menses after they have been established owing to disease or pregnancy.

amentia (*a-men'-she-ah*). Mental subnormality. May be due to hereditary factors, failure of development of the embryo or birth trauma.

amethocaine (*am-eth'-o-kane*). A local anaesthetic for mucous membranes. *A. pastille.* A lozenge that, when dissolved slowly in the mouth, will aid the passage of a bronchoscope or gastroscope.

ametria (*a-me'-tre-ah*). Congenital absence of the uterus.

ametropia (*a-met-ro'-pe-ah*). Defective vision. A general word applied to incorrect refraction.

amidone (*am'-id-one*). Methadone.

amiloride (*am-il'-or-ide*). A weak diuretic drug which causes retention of potassium.

amino acid (*am'-in-o as'-id*). A chemical compound containing both NH_2 and $COOH$

ESSENTIAL AMINO ACIDS

1	Threonine
2	Lysine
3	Methionine
4	Arginine
5	Valine
6	Phenylalanine
7	Leucine
8	Tryptophan
9	Isoleucine
10	Histidine

groups. The end-product of protein digestion. *Essential a. a.* One required for replacement and growth, which cannot be synthesized in the body in sufficient amounts. *Non-essential a. a.* One necessary for proper growth but which can be synthesized in the body.

aminoglutethimide (*am-in-o-glu-teth'-im-ide*). Formerly used as an anticonvulsant, this drug inhibits adrenal hormone synthesis. Its use is sometimes referred to as 'medical adrenalectomy'. The effects are reversible when the drug is discontinued. Used to treat metastatic breast and prostate cancers.

aminophylline (*am-in-off'-il-in*). An alkaloid from camellia, it relaxes plain muscle spasm of the bronchioles and coronary arteries. It may be given by mouth, intravenously or as a suppository, and is useful in treating asthma and heart failure.

aminosalicylic acid (*am-in-o-sal-is-il'-ik as'-id*). See Para-aminosalicylic acid.

amiphenazole (*am-e-fen'-az-ole*). A drug that stimulates the respiratory system.

amitosis (*a-mi-to'-sis*). Multiplication of cells by simple division or fission.

amitriptyline (*am-e-trip'-til-een*). An antidepressant drug that is chemically related to imipramine. It is useful in relieving tension and anxiety but may cause dizziness and hypotension.

ammonia (*am-o'-ne-ah*). NH_3. A colourless pungent gas. In solution, used as a cardiac stimulant.

ammonium (*am-o'-ne-um*). NH_4^+. A chemical group that combines to form salts similar to those of the alkaline metals. *A. chloride.* Used as a mild diuretic and to render the urine acid. Widely used in mixtures as an expectorant.

amnesia (*am-ne'-ze-ah*). Partial or complete loss of memory. *Anterograde a.* Loss of memory for events that have taken place since an injury or illness. *Retrograde a.* Loss of memory for events prior to an injury. It often applies to the time immediately preceding an accident.

amniocentesis (*am-ne-o-sente'-sis*). The withdrawal of fluid from the uterus through the abdominal wall by means of a syringe and needle. It is used in the diagnosis of chromosome disorders in the fetus and in cases of hydramnios.

amnion (*am'-ne-on*). The innermost membrane enveloping the fetus and enclosing the liquor amnii.

amnioscope (*am'-ne-o-skope*). Instrument for examining the fetus and the amniotic fluid by means of a tube passing through the abdominal wall.

amnioscopy (*am-ne-os'-kop-e*). Inspection of the amniotic sac using an amnioscope.

amniotomy (*am-ne-ot'-om-e*). The surgical rupture of the fetal membranes to induce labour.

amoeba (*am-e'-bah*). A minute unicellular protozoon. It is able to move by pushing out parts of itself (called pseudopodia). Infection of the intestines by *Entamoeba histolytica* causes 'amoebic dysentery'.

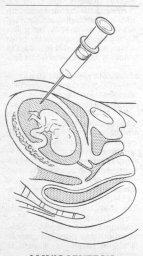

AMNIOCENTESIS

amoebiasis (*am-e-bi'-as-is*). Infection with amoeba, particularly *Entamoeba histolytica.*

amoeboid (*am-e'-boid*). Resembling an amoeba in structure or movement.

amorphous (*a-mor'-fus*). Without definite shape. The term may be applied to fine powdery particles, as opposed to crystals.

ampere (*am'-pair*). *abbrev.* A. The unit of intensity of an electrical current.

amphetamine (*am-fet'-am-een*). A synthetic drug which stimulates the central nervous system. It is addictive and is now seldom used except in the treatment of narcolepsy.

amphiarthrosis (*am-fe-ar-thro'-sis*). A form of joint in which the bones are joined together by fibrocartilage, e.g. the junctions of the vertebrae.

amphibian (*am-fib'-e-an*). Capable of living both on land and in water.

amphoric (*am-for'-ik*). Pertaining to a bottle. Used to describe the sound sometimes heard on auscultation over cavities in the lungs, which resembles that produced by blowing across the mouth of a bottle.

amphotericin (*am-fo-ter'-is-in*). An antifungal drug which is not absorbed by the gut. The only polyene antibiotic which may be given parenterally. Active against most yeasts and other fungi. Side-effects of fever, nausea and vomiting are common when the drug is given parenterally.

ampicillin (*am-pe-sil'-in*). A penicillin with a wide range of action against gram-negative bacteria and some strains of *Escherichia coli*.

ampoule (*am'-pool*). A small glass vessel in which sterile drugs of specified dose for injection are sealed.

ampulla (*am-pul'-ah*). The flask-like dilatation of a canal, e.g. of a uterine tube.

amputation (*am-pu-ta'-shun*). Surgical removal of a limb or other part of the body, e.g. the breast.

amputee (*am-pu-tee'*). A person who has had a limb amputated.

amyl (*am'-il*). The radical C_5H_{11}. *A. nitrite*. Vasodilator and heart stimulant, prescribed for inhalation in cases of angina pectoria. Capsules can be broken into a handkerchief and the fumes inhaled.

amylase (*am'-il-aze*). An enzyme that reduces starch to maltose. Found in saliva (ptyalin) and pancreatic juice (amylopsin).

amylobarbitone (*am-il-o-bar'-bit-one*). A barbiturate hypnotic and sedative.

amyloid (*am'-il-oid*). (1) *adj.* Pertaining to starch. (2) *n.* A waxy starch that forms in certain tissues. *A. degeneration.* Amyloidosis.

amyloidosis (*am-il-oid-o'-sis*). Degenerative changes in the tissues in which amyloid deposits are formed. Notably affects the kidneys, spleen, liver and heart.

amylopsin (*am-il-op'-sin*). An enzyme found in the pancreas. Amylase.

amylum (*am'-il-um*). Starch (*Latin*).

anabolic (*an-ab-ol'-ik*). Relating to anabolism. *A. compound.* A substance that aids in the repair of body tissue, particularly protein. Androgens may be used in this way.

anabolism (*an-ab'-ol-izm*). The building up or synthesis of cell structure from digested food materials. *See* Metabolism.

anacidity (*an-as-id'-it-e*). Decrease in normal acidity.

anacrotic (*an-ak-rot'-ik*). Displaying anacrotism. *A. curve.* An abnormal curve in the ascending line of a pulse tracing by sphygmograph. Typical of aortic stenosis.

anacrotism (*an-ak'-rot-izm*). An abnormal pulse wave embodying a secondary expansion.

anaemia (*an-e'-me-ah*). Deficiency in either quality or quantity of red corpuscles in the blood, giving rise especially to symptoms of anoxaemia. There is pallor, breathlessness on exertion with palpitations, slight oedema of ankles, lassitude, headache, giddiness, albuminuria, indigestion, constipation and amenorrhoea. Anaemia may be due to many different causes. *Aplastic a.* The bone marrow is unable to produce red blood corpuscles. A rare condition of unknown cause in most cases, but it may arise from the administration of certain drugs or from their injudicious use, e.g. benzol preparations or chloramphenicol. *Deficiency a.* Any type which is due to the lack of the necessary factors for cell formation, e.g. hormones or vitamins. *Iron deficiency a.* The commonest anaemia in Great Britain, due to a lack of iron in the diet. It may also be due to excessive blood loss. *Haemolytic a.* A variety in which there is excessive destruction of red blood corpuscles caused by antibody formation in the blood (*see* Rhesus factor) by drugs or by severe toxaemia, as in extensive burns. *Macrocytic a.* A type in which the cells are larger than normal; present in pernicious anaemia. *Microcytic a.* A variety in which the cells are smaller than normal, as in iron deficiency. *Pernicious a.* A variety which is due to the inability of the stomach to secrete the intrinsic factor necessary for the absorption of vitamin B_{12} from the diet. *Sickle-cell a.* A hereditary haemolytic anaemia seen most commonly in Negroes. The red blood cells are sickle shaped. *Splenic a.* A congenital, familial disease in which the red blood cells are fragile and easily broken down.

anaerobe (*an'-air-obe*). A micro-organism which can live and thrive in the absence of free oxygen. These organisms are found in body cavities or wounds where the oxygen tension is very low. Examples are the bacilli of tetanus and gas gangrene.

anaesthesia (*an-es-the'-ze-ah*). Loss of feeling or sensation in a part or in the whole of the body, usually induced by drugs. *Basal a.* Basal narcosis. Loss of consciousness, although supplemental drugs have to be given to ensure complete anaesthesia. *General a.* Unconsciousness produced by inhalation or injection of a drug. *Hysterical a.* A common symptom in hysteria, in which the insensibility to touch or pain has a local distribution unrelated to the nerve supply. *Inhalation a.* The drugs or gas used are administered by a face mask or endotracheal tube to cause general anaesthesia. *Intravenous a.* Unconsciousness is produced by the introduction of a drug, e.g. hexobarbitone, into a vein. *Local a.* Local analgesia. *Rectal a.* A drug is given per rectum. *Spinal a.* Injection into the spinal canal to anaesthetize the lower half of the body.

anaesthetic (*an-es-thet'-ik*). A drug causing anaesthesia.

anaesthetist (*an-ees'-thet-ist*). One who administers an anaesthetic.

anal (*a'-nal*). Pertaining to the anus. *A. eroticism.* Sexual pleasure derived from anal functions. *A. fissure. See* Fissure. *A. fistula. See* Fistula.

analeptic (*an-al-ep'-tik*). A drug that stimulates the central nervous system.

analgesia (*an-al-je'-ze-ah*). Insensibility to pain, especially the relief of pain without causing unconsciousness. *Caudal* *a.* Injection into the sacral epidural space. *Epidural a.* Injection into the space surrounding the spinal cord. *Local or regional a.* The deadening of pain in a small part of the body only, either by infiltration of the operational field with an anaesthetic drug or by injection near the main nerve trunks (nerve block). *Spinal a.* Injection into the intradural or extradural spaces. *Splanchnic a.* Injection into the splanchnic ganglion, which causes complete relaxation of the abdominal viscera.

analgesic (*an-al-je'-zik*). (1) *adj.* Relating to analgesia. (2) *n.* A remedy which relieves pain.

analogous (*an-al'-o-gus*). Having the same function but different in structure and origin.

analogue (*an'-al-og*). (1) An organ with different structure and origin but the same function as another one. (2) A compound with similar structure to another but differing in respect of a particular element.

analysis (*an-al'-is-is*). *pl.* analyses. (1) The act of determining the component parts of a substance. (2) In psychiatry, the method of trying to determine the reasons for an individual's behaviour by understanding his complex mental processes, experiences and relationships with other individuals or groups of individuals.

analyst (*an'-al-ist*). A person who performs analyses.

anaphase (*an'-ah-faze*). Part of the process of mitosis or meiosis.

anaphylaxis (*an-ah-fil-ak'-sis*). Often termed anaphylactic shock. A severe reaction, often fatal, occurring when a second injection of a particular foreign protein is given, e.g. horse serum. The symptoms are severe dyspnoea, rapid pulse, profuse sweating and collapse. The condition may be avoided by giving a test dose before all serum injections. If the patient has any reaction, he may be desensitized by giving repeated small doses.

anaplasia (*an-ah-pla'-ze-ah*). A change in the character of cells, seen in tumour tissue.

anarthrosis (*an-arth'-re-ah*). Inability to articulate speech sounds owing to a brain lesion or damage to peripheral nerves innervating articulatory muscles.

anastomosis (*an-as-to-mo'-sis*). In surgery, any artificial connection of two hollow structures, e.g. gastroenterostomy. In anatomy, the joining of the branches of two blood vessels.

anatomy (*an-at'-om-e*). The science of the structure of the body.

anconeus (*an-ko'-ne-us*). An extensor muscle of the forearm.

Ancylostoma (*an-sil-os'-to-mah*). A genus of nematode roundworms which may inhabit the duodenum and cause extreme anaemia. *A. duodenale.* A hookworm, very widespread in tropical and subtropical areas.

androgen (*an'-dro-jen*). One of a group of hormones secreted by the testes and adrenal cortex. They are steroids which can be synthesized and produce the secondary male characteristics and the building up of protein tissue.

android (*an'-droid*). (1) *adj.* Resembling a man. (2) *n*. A robot in human form. *A. pelvis*. A female pelvis shaped like a male pelvis, with a wedge-shaped entrance and narrow anterior segment.

anencephalous (*an-en-kef'-al-us*). Having no brain. A form of congenital monstrosity.

anergic (*an-er'-jik*). Sluggish, inactive.

aneurine (*an'-u-reen*). Thiamine. An essential vitamin involved in carbohydrate metabolism. The main sources are unrefined cereals and pork. Vitamin B_1.

aneurysm (*an'-u-rizm*). A local dilatation of a blood vessel, usually an artery. It may start as a congenital weakness, be due to chronic inflammation or be caused by trauma. The pressure of blood causes it to increase in size and rupture is likely. Sometimes excision of the aneurysm or ligation of the artery is possible. *Dissecting a.* A condition in which a tear occurs in the aortic lining where the middle coat is necrosed and blood gets between the layers, stripping them apart. *Fusiform a.* A spindle-shaped arterial aneurysm. *Saccular a.* A dilatation of only a part of the circumference of an artery.

angiitis (*an-je-i'-tis*). Inflammation of a blood or lymph vessel.

angina (*an-ji'-nah*). (1) A tight strangling sensation or pain. (2) An inflammation of the throat causing pain on swallowing. *A. cruris.* Intermittent claudication. Severe pain in the leg after walking. *A. of effort* or *a. pectoris.* Cardiac pain which occurs on exertion owing to insufficient blood supply to the heart muscle. It can be relieved by a vasodilator drug. *Ludwig's a.* Acute pharyngitis with swelling and abscess formation. *Vincent's a.* Infection and ulceration of the tonsils by a spirochaete,

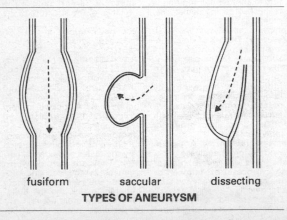

fusiform　　　saccular　　　dissecting

TYPES OF ANEURYSM

Borrelia vincenti, and a bacillus, *Fusiformis fusiformis*.

angiocardiography (*an-je-o-kar-de-og'-raf-e*). Radiological examination of the heart and large blood vessels by means of cardiac catheterization and an opaque contrast medium.

angioectasis (*an-je-o-ek'-tas-is*). Abnormal enlargement of capillaries.

angiography (*an-je-og'-raf-e*). (1) Radiological examination of the blood vessels using an opaque contrast medium. (2) Sphygmography.

angioma (*an-je-o'-mah*). An innocent tumour composed of dilated blood vessels.

angioneurosis (*an-je-o-nu-ro'-sis*). A neurosis affecting the blood vessels, which may produce paralysis.

angioneurotic (*an-je-o-nu-rot'-ik*). Pertaining to angioneurosis. *A. oedema. See* Oedema.

angioplasty (*an'-je-o-plas-te*). Plastic surgery of blood vessels.

angiosarcoma (*an-je-o-sar-ko'-mah*). A malignant vascular growth.

angiospasm (*an'-je-o-spazm*). A spasmodic contration of an artery, causing cramping of the muscles.

angiotensin (*an-je-o-ten'-sin*). A substance that raises the blood pressure. It is a polypeptide produced by the action of renin on plasma globulins. Hypertensin.

Ångström unit (*A.J. Ångström, Swedish physicist, 1814–1874*). One ten-thousand millionth of a metre (10^{-10} m). Wavelengths of light and X-rays are often expressed in Ångström units, but the term is being superseded by the nanometer (1 nm = 10 Å).

anhidrosis (*an-hi-dro'-sis*). Marked deficiency in the secretion of sweat.

anhidrotic (*an-hi-drot'-ik*). An agent that decreases perspiration. An adiaphoretic.

anhydraemia (*an-hi-dre'-me-ah*). Deficiency of water in the blood.

anhydrous (*an-hi'-drus*). Containing no water.

aniline (*an'-il-een*). A chemical compound derived from coal tar, used for making of dyes, e.g. methylene blue. It is a strong antiseptic.

anion (*an'-i-on*). A negatively charged ion which travels against the current towards the anode, e.g. chloride (Cl⁻), carbonate ($CO_3{}^{2-}$). *See* Cation.

aniridia (*an-i-rid'-e-ah*). Lack of part or the whole of the iris.

anisocoria (*an-i-so-ko'-re-ah*). Inequality of diameter of the pupils of the two eyes.

anisocytosis (*an-i-so-si-to'-sis*). Inequality in the size of the red blood cells.

anisomelia (*an-i-so-me'-le-ah*). A congenital condition in which one of a pair of limbs is longer than the other.

anisometropia (*an-i-so-met-ro'-pe-ah*). A marked difference in the refractive power of the two eyes.

ankle (*an'-kl*). The joint between the leg and the foot formed by the tibia and fibula articulating with the talus.

ankyloblepharon (*an-ki-lo-blef'-ar-on*). Adhesions and scar tissue on the ciliary borders of the eyelids, giving the eye a distorted appearance. This may result from burns or from chronic blepharitis.

ankylosis (*an-ki-lo'-sis*). Abnormal consolidation and immobility of the bones of a joint.

Annelida (*an-el'-id-ah*). A phylum of metazoa, segmented worms, which includes the class Hirudinea, the leeches.

annular (*an'-u-lah*). Ring-shaped.

anoci-association (*an-o'-se as-o-se-a'-shun*). The exclusion of pain, fear and shock in surgical operations, brought about by means of local anaesthesia and basal narcosis.

anode (*an'-ode*). The positive pole of an electric battery. *See* Cathode.

anodyne (*an'-o-dine*). A drug which relieves pain.

anomaly (*an-om'-al-e*). Considerable variation from the normal.

anomie (*an'-om-e*). A feeling of hopelessness and lack of purpose.

anonychia (*an-on-ik'-e-ah*). Congenital absence of nails.

Anopheles (*an-off-el-eez*). A genus of mosquito. Many are carriers of the malarial parasite and by their bite infect human beings. Other species transmit filariasis.

anophthalmia (*an-off-thal'-me-ah*). Congenital absence of a seeing eye. Some portion of the eye, e.g. the conjunctiva, is always present.

anorchism (*an-or'-kizm*). A condition in which the testicles have failed to develop or to descend.

anorexia (*an-or-ek'-se-ah*). Loss of appetite for food. *A. nervosa*. A condition in which there is complete lack of appetite, with extreme emaciation. It is generally due to psychological causes and occurs usually in young women.

anosmia (*an-oz'-me-ah*). Loss of the sense of smell.

anovular (*an-ov'-u-lah*). Applied to the absence of ovulation. Usually refers to uterine bleeding when there has been no ovulation.

anoxaemia (*an-oks-e'-me-ah*). Complete lack of oxygen in the blood.

anoxia (*an-oks'-e-ah*). Lack of oxygen to an organ or tissue.

antacid (*ant-as'-id*). A substance neutralizing acidity, particularly of the gastric juices.

antagonist (*an-tag'-on-ist*). (1) A muscle that has an opposite action to another, e.g. the biceps to the triceps. (2) In pharmacology, a drug which inhibits the action of another drug or enzyme, e.g. methotrexate is a folic acid antagonist. (3) In dentistry, a tooth in one jaw opposing one in the other jaw.

anteflexion (*an-te-flek'-shun*). A bending forward, as of the body of the uterus. *See* Retroflexion.

antenatal (*an-te-na'-tal*). Before birth.

antepartum (*an-te-par'-tum*). Shortly before birth, i.e. in the last three months of pregnancy. *A. haemorrhage.* Bleeding occurring before birth. *See* Placenta praevia.

anterior (*an-teer'-e-or*). Situated at or facing towards the front. The opposite of 'posterior'. *A. capsule.* The anterior covering of the lens of the eye. *A. chamber of eye.* The space between the cornea in front and the iris and lens behind.

anteversion (*an-te-ver'-zhun*). The forward tilting of an organ, e.g. the normal position of the uterus. *See* Retroversion.

anthelmintic (*an-thel-min'-tik*). (1) *adj.* Destructive to worms.

(2) *n*. A vermifuge.

anthracosis (*an-thrah-ko'-sis*). A disease of the lungs, caused by inhalation of coal dust. A form of pneumoconiosis. 'Miner's lung'.

anthrax (*an'-thraks*). A contagious disease of cattle, transmitted to man by direct contact or by wool or hide infected with *Bacillus anthracis*, causing malignant pustules of the skin or woolsorters' pneumonia if inhaled.

anthropoid (*an'-thro-poid*). Resembling a man. *A. pelvis*. A female pelvis in which the anteroposterior diameter exceeds the transverse diameter.

anthropology (*an-thro-pol'-o-je*). The study of mankind.

anthropometric (*an'-thro-po-met'-rik*). Pertaining to anthropometry.

anthropometry (*an'-thro-pom'-et-re*). The science which deals with the comparative measurement of parts of the human body, such as height, weight, body fat, etc.

antibacterial (*an-te-bak-te'-re-al*). A substance which destroys or suppresses the growth of bacteria.

antibiotic (*an-te-bi-ot'-ic*). A chemical substance produced by certain bacteria and fungi, which prevents the growth of, or destroys, other bacteria. E.g. penicillin.

antibody (*an'-te-bod-e*). A specific form of blood protein produced in the lymphoid tissue and able to counteract the effects of bacterial antigens or toxins.

anticholinergic (*an-te-ko-lin-er'-jik*). A drug that inhibits the action of acetylcholine.

anticholinesterase (*an-te-ko-lin-est'-er-aze*). A substance that will inhibit the action of cholinesterase.

anticoagulant (*an-te-ko-ag'-u-lant*). A substance which prevents blood from clotting, e.g. heparin.

anticonvulsant (*an-te-kon-vuls'-ant*). A substance which will arrest or prevent convulsions. Anticonvulsant drugs such as phenytoin are used in the treatment of epilepsy and other conditions in which convulsions occur.

antidepressant (*an-te-de-pres'-ant*). One of a group of drugs which elevate mood, often diminish anxiety and increase coping behaviour. Tricyclic and the newer tetracyclic drugs are of value in all types of depression. Monoamine oxidase inhibitors (MAOI) are less commonly used because of the dietary restriction necessary and their incompatibility with other drugs.

antidiuresis (*an-te-di-u-re'-sis*). A reduction in the formation of urine.

antidiuretic (*an-te-di-u-ret'-ik*). A substance that reduces the volume of urine excreted. *A. hormone*. ADH. It is secreted by the posterior pituitary gland. Vasopressin.

antidote (*an'-te-dote*). An agent which counteracts the effect of a poison.

antiemetic (*an-te-em-et'-ik*). A drug that prevents or overcomes nausea and vomiting.

antigen (*an'-te-jen*). Any substance, bacterial or otherwise, which in suitable conditions can stimulate the production of antibodies.

antihistamine (*an-te-hist'-am-een*). Any one of a group of drugs which block the tissue receptors for histamine. They are used to treat allergic conditions, e.g. drug rashes, hay fever and serum sickness. They include promethazine and mepyramine.

anti-lewisite (*an'-te-lu'-is-ite*). Dimercaprol.

antimetabolite (*an-te-met-ab'-ol-ite*). One of a group of chemical compounds which prevent the effective utilization of the corresponding metabolite, and interfere with normal growth or cell mitosis if the process requires that metabolite.

antimony (*an'-tim-on-e*). *abbrev.* Sb. A metallic element especially poisonous to protozoa, the organic compounds of which are now used mainly in the treatment of tropical parasitic infestation, e.g. schistosomiasis and kala-azar.

antimycotic (*an-te-mi-kot'-ik*). A preparation that is effective in treating fungal infections.

antineoplastic (*an-te-neo-plast'-ik*). Effective against the multiplication of malignant cells.

antiperistalsis (*an-te-per-e-stal'-sis*). Contrary contractions which propel the contents of the intestines backwards and upwards.

antipruritic (*an-te-pru-rit'-ik*). An external application or drug that relieves itching.

antipyretic (*an-te-pi-ret'-ik*). An agent which reduces fever.

anti-rhesus serum (*an-te-re'-sus se'-rum*). A substance containing rhesus agglutinins produced in the blood of those who are rhesus-negative if the rhesus-positive antigen obtains access to it, e.g. by blood transfusion. Haemolysis and jaundice are the result. *See* Rhesus factor.

antisepsis (*an-te-sep'-sis*). The

prevention of infection by destroying or arresting the growth of harmful micro-organisms.

antiseptic (*an-te-sep'-tik*). A chemical sterilizing substance for preventing infection. An agent which tends to prevent the growth of organisms causing sepsis in wounds. Antiseptics are commonly applied to the skin before surgery.

antiserum (*an-te-se'-rum*). A serum prepared against a specific disease by immunizing an animal so that antibodies are formed. These can then be used to create a passive immunity or to treat the infection in man.

antisocial (*an-te-so'-shal*). Against society. *A. behaviour.* In psychiatry, the refusal of an individual to accept the normal obligations and restraints imposed by the community upon its members.

antispasmodic (*an-te-spaz-mod'-ik*). A substance used to prevent the occurrence of muscle spasm.

antistatic (*an-te-stat'-ik*). Relating to measures taken to prevent the build-up of static electricity.

antitoxin (*an-te-toks'-in*). A substance produced by the body cells as a reaction to invasion by bacteria, which neutralizes their toxins. Serum from immunized animals contains these antitoxins, and is used in the treatment of specific diseases such as diphtheria, tetanus, etc. *See* Immunity.

antivenin (*an-te-ven'-in*). An antitoxic serum to neutralize the poison injected by the bite of a snake or insect.

antrostomy (*an-tros'-tom-e*).

Surgical opening of an antrum, particularly the maxillary antrum, for drainage purposes.

antrum (*an'-trum*). A cavity in bone. *Mastoid a.* The tympanic antrum, which is an air-containing cavity in the mastoid portion of the temporal bone. *Maxillary a.* Antrum of Highmore. The air sinus in the upper jaw bone.

anuria (*an-u'-re-ah*). Cessation of the secretion of urine.

anus (*a'-nus*). The extremity of the alimentary canal, through which the faeces are discharged. *Imperforate a.* One where there is no opening because of a congenital defect.

anxiety (*ang-zi'-et-e*). A chronic state of tension which affects both mind and body. *A. neurosis. See* Neurosis.

aorta (*a-ort'-ah*). The large artery rising out of the left ventricle of the heart and supplying blood to all the body. *Abdominal a.* That part of the artery lying in the abdomen. *Arch of the a.* The curve of the artery over the heart. *Thoracic a.* That part which passes through the chest.

aortic (*a-or'-tik*). Pertaining to the aorta. *A. incompetence.* Owing to previous inflammation the aortic valve has become fibrosed and is unable to close completely, thus allowing backward flow of blood (*a. regurgitation*) into the left ventricle during diastole. *A. stenosis.* A narrowing of the aortic valve. *A. valve.* The valve between the left ventricle and the ascending aorta, which prevents the backward flow of blood through the artery.

aortitis (*a-or-ti'-tis*). Inflammation of the aorta.

aortography (*a-or-tog'-raf-e*). Radiographic examination of the aorta. A radio-opaque dye is injected into the blood to

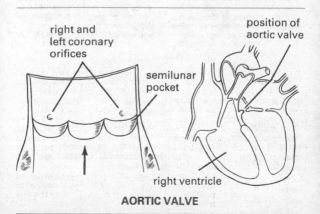

right and left coronary orifices

semilunar pocket

position of aortic valve

right ventricle

AORTIC VALVE

render visible lesions of the aorta or its main branches.

apathy (*ap'-ath-e*). An appearance of indifference, with no response to stimuli or display of emotion.

aperient (*ap-e'-re-ent*). A drug which produces an action of the bowels. A laxative.

aperistalsis (*a-per-e-stal'-sis*). Lack of peristaltic movement of the intestines.

Apert's syndrome (*E. Apert, French paediatrician, 1868–1940*). A congenital abnormality in which there is fusion at birth of all the cranial sutures in addition to syndactyly (webbed fingers).

apex (*a'-peks*). The top or pointed end of a cone-shaped structure. *A. of the heart.* The end enclosing the left ventricle. *A. beat.* The beat of the heart against the chest wall which can be felt during systole. *A. of lung.* The extreme upper part of the organ.

Apgar score (*V. Apgar, American anaesthetist, 1909–1974*). A system used in the assessment of the newborn; reflex irritability and colour.

APH. Antepartum haemorrhage.

aphagia (*a-fa'-je-ah*). Loss of the power to swallow.

aphakia (*a-fa'-ke-ah*). Absence of the lens of the eye. Aphacia.

aphasia (*a-fa'-ze-ah*). A communication disorder due to brain damage; characterized by complete or partial disturbance of language comprehension, formulation or expression. Partial disturbance is also called dysphasia. *Broca's a.* Disorder in which verbal output is impaired, and in which verbal comprehension may be affected as well. Speech is slow and laboured and writing is often impaired. *Developmental a.* A childhood failure to acquire normal language when deafness, mental retardation, motor disability or severe emotional disturbance are not causes.

aphonia (*a-fo'-ne-ah*). Inability to produce sound. The cause may be organic disease of the larynx or may be purely functional.

aphrodisiac (*af-ro-diz'-e-ak*). A

APGAR SCORE

Sign	Score		
	0	1	2
Colour	Blue – pale	Body pink, limbs blue	Completely pink
Respiratory effort	Absent	Slow, irregular, weak cry	Strong cry
Heart rate	Absent	Slow, less than 100 bpm	Over 100 bpm
Muscle tone	Limp	Some flexion of limbs	Active movement
Reflex response to flicking foot	Absent	Facial grimace	Cry

drug which excites sexual desire.

aphthae (*af'-the*). Small greyish-white vesicles, which form ulcers on the tongue and inside the mouth (aphthous stomatitis). They are likely to occur in infants with fever or digestive disorders, but can be prevented by careful regard to mouth hygiene.

apical (*a'-pik-al*). Pertaining to the apex of a structure.

apicectomy (*a-pis-ek'-tom-e*). Excision of the root of a tooth. Root resection.

aplasia (*a-pla'-ze-ah*). Defective development of an organ or tissue.

aplastic (*a-plas'-tik*). Without power of development. *A. anaemia. See* Anaemia.

apnoea (*ap-ne'-ah*). Cessation of respiration. *Cardiac a.* The temporary cessation of breathing caused by a reduction of the carbon dioxide tension in the blood, as seen in Cheyne –Stokes respiration.

apocrine (*ap'-o-krine*). Pertaining to sweat glands that develop in hair follicles, such as are mainly found in the axillary, pubic and perineal areas.

apomorphine (*ap-o-mor'-feen*). A derivative of morphine which produces vomiting.

aponeurosis (*ap-o-nu-ro'-sis*). A sheet of tendon-like tissue which connects some muscles to the parts which they move.

apophysis (*ap-off'-is-is*). A prominence or excrescence, usually of a bone.

apoplexy (*ap'-o-pleks-e*). A sudden fit of insensibility, usually caused by rupture of a cerebral blood vessel or its occlusion by a blood clot. The symptoms are coma, accompanied by stertorous breathing, and a varying degree of paralysis of the opposite side of the body to the lesion.

apparition (*ap-ar-ish'-un*). A hallucinatory vision, usually the phantom appearance of a person. A spectre.

appendectomy (*ap-en-dek'-tom-e*). Appendicectomy.

appendicectomy (*ap-en-dis-ek'-tom-e*). Removal of the vermiform appendix.

appendicitis (*ap-en-dis-i'-tis*). Inflammation of the vermiform appendix.

appendix (*ap-en'-diks*). A supplementary or dependent part. *A. epiploicae.* Small tag-like structures of peritoneum containing fat which are scattered over the surface of the large intestine, especially the transverse colon. *Vermiform a.* A worm-like tube with a blind end, projecting from the caecum in the right iliac region. It may be from 2.5 to 15 cm long.

apperception (*ap-er-sep'-shun*). Conscious reception and recognition of a sensory stimulus.

appliance (*ap-li'-ans*). A device used for performing a particular function.

applicator (*ap'-lik-a-tor*). Any device used to apply medication or treatment to a particular part of the body.

apposition (*ap-o-zish'-un*). The bringing into contact of two structures, e.g. fragments of bone in setting a fracture.

apprehension (*ap-re-hen'-shun*). A feeling of dread or fear.

apraxia (*a-praks'-e-ah*). The inability to perform correct movements because of a brain lesion and not because of sensory impairment or loss

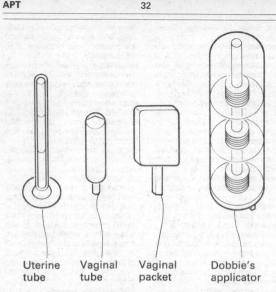

| Uterine | Vaginal | Vaginal | Dobbie's |
| tube | tube | packet | applicator |

RADIOACTIVE SOURCE APPLICATORS

of muscle power in the limbs. *Oral a.* Inability to perform volitional movements of the tongue and lips in the absence of paralysis or paresis. Involuntary movements may be observed however; e.g. the patient may purse lips in order to blow out a match.

APT. Alum precipitated toxoid. A special preparation used for diphtheria immunization.

aptitude (*ap'-tit-ude*). The natural ability or capacity to acquire mental and physical skills.

apyrexia (*a-pi-reks'-e-ah*). The absence of fever.

aqua (*ak'-wah*). Water (*Latin*). *A. destillata.* Distilled water. *A. fortis.* Nitric acid.

aqueduct (*ak'-we-dukt*). A canal for the passage of fluid. *A. of Sylvius.* The canal connecting the third and fourth ventricles of the brain.

aqueous (*a'-kwe-us*). Watery. *A. humour of the eye.* The fluid filling the anterior and posterior chambers of the eye.

Ar. Chemical symbol for *argon*.

Arachis (*ar'-ak-is*). A genus of leguminous plants. *A. oil.* Peanut oil; used as a substitute for olive oil.

arachnodactyly (*ar-ak-no-dak'-til-e*). Abnormally long and thin fingers and toes. A congenital condition.

arachnoid (ar-ak'-noid). (1) adj. Resembling a spider. (2) n. A web-like membrane covering the central nervous system between the dura and pia mater.

arborization (arb-or-i-za'-shun). The branching terminations of many nerve fibres and processes.

arbovirus (ar-bo-vi'-rus). One of a large group of viruses transmitted by insect vectors (arthropod-borne), e.g. mosquitoes, sandflies or ticks. The diseases caused include many types of encephalitis, also yellow, dengue, sandfly and Rift Valley fevers.

arc (ark). A part of the circumference of a circle. In anatomy, a line or structure shaped like a bow. *Electric a.* An electric discharge between two electrodes, producing an intensely bright light. Also used for welding metals.

arch (arch). In anatomy, a structure having a curved shape like a bow.

arcuate (ar'-ku-ate). Arched. Bow-shaped.

arcus (ar'-kus). A bow or arch (Latin). *A. senilis.* An opaque circle appearing round the edge of the cornea in old age.

areola (ar-e-o'-lah). (1) A space in connective tissue. (2) A ring of pigmentation, e.g. that surrounding the nipple.

argentum (ar-jen'-tum). Silver (Latin).

arginine (ar'-jin-een). An essential amino acid produced by the digestion of protein and utilized in the production of creatinine.

argon (ar'-gon). abbrev. Ar. An inert gaseous element in the atmosphere.

Argyll Robertson pupil (D. Argyll Robertson, British ophthalmologist, 1837–1909). See Pupil.

argyria (ar-ji'-re-ah). Poisoning by salts of silver. The skin, the conjunctiva and the internal organs may assume an ashen-grey colour.

Arnold–Chiari deformity (J. Arnold, German pathologist, 1835–1915; H. Chiari, German pathologist, 1851–1916). Herniation of the cerebellum and elongation of the medulla oblongata, associated with spina bifida.

arousal (ar-ow'-zal). A state of alertness and increased response to stimuli.

arrachment (ar-ash'-mon). The extraction of a membranous cataract via a corneal incision.

arrector pili (ar-ek'-tor pi'-li). Pl. Arrectores pilorum. Small muscle attached to the hair follicle of the skin. When contracted causes the hair to become more erect and produces the appearance known as goose-flesh.

arrest (ar-est'). A cessation or stopping. *Cardiac a.* Cessation of ventricular contractions. *Respiratory a.* Cessation of breathing. *Developmental a.* Discontinuation of a child's mental or physical development at a certain stage.

arrhenoblastoma (ar-e-no-blast-o'-mah). A rare ovarian tumour which causes masculinization in the woman, with male distribution of hair and coarsening of the skin.

arrhythmia (a-rith'-me-ah). Lack of rhythm, e.g. in the heart's action. *Sinus a.* An abnormal pulse rhythm due to disturbance of the sino-atrial node, causing quickening of the heart on inspiration and slowing on expiration.

arsenic (*ar'-sen-ik*). *abbrev.* As. A metallic element, organic preparations of which are used in medicine.

artefact (*ar'-te-fakt*). Something that is man-made or introduced artificially.

arteriectomy (*ar-te-re-ek'-tom-e*). The removal of a portion of artery wall usually followed by anastomosis or a replacement graft. *See* Arterioplasty.

arteriography (*ar-te-re-og'-raf-e*). Radiography of arteries after the injection of a radio-opaque contrast medium.

arteriole (*ar-te'-re-ole*). A small artery.

arterioplasty (*ar-te-re-o-plas'-te*). The reconstruction of an artery by means of replacement surgery.

arteriorrhaphy (*ar-te-re-or'-af-e*). Ligature of an artery.

arteriosclerosis (*ar-te-re-o-skler-o'-sis*). A gradual loss of elasticity in the walls of arteries due to thickening and calcification. It is accompanied by high blood pressure, and precedes the degeneration of internal organs associated with old age or chronic disease.

arteriotomy (*ar-te-re-ot'-ome*). An incision into an artery.

arteritis (*ar-ter-i'-tis*). Inflammation of an artery. *Giant-cell a.* A variety of polyarteritis resulting in partial or complete occlusion of a number of arteries. The carotid arteries are often involved. *Temporal a.* Occlusion of the extracranial arteries, particularly the carotid arteries.

artery (*ar'-ter-e*). A tube of muscle and elastic fibres lined with endothelium which distributes blood from the heart to the capillaries, and so throughout the body.

arthralgia (*ar-thral'-je-ah*). Neuralgic pains in a joint.

arthrectomy (*ar-threk'-tom-e*). Excision of a joint.

arthritis (*ar-thri'-tis*). Inflammation of a joint. *Acute rheumatic a.* Rheumatic fever. *Osteo-a.* A degenerative condition attacking the articular cartilage and aggravated by an impaired blood supply, previous injury or overweight, mainly affecting weight-bearing joints and causing much pain. *Rheumatoid a.* A chronic inflammation, usually of unknown origin. The disease is progressive and incapacitating, owing to the resulting ankylosis and deformity of the bones. Usually affects the elderly. A juvenile form is known as Still's disease.

arthroclasia (*ar-thro-kla'-ze-ah*). The breaking down of adhesions in a joint to produce freer movement.

arthrodesis (*ar-thro-de'-sis*). The fixation of a movable joint by surgical operation.

arthrodynia (*ar-thro-din'-e-ah*). Painful joints. Arthralgia.

arthrography (*ar-throg'-raf-e*). The examination of a joint by means of X-rays. An opaque contrast medium may be used.

arthrogryposis (*ar-thro-gri-po'-sis*). (1) A congenital abnormality in which fibrous ankylosis of some or all of the joints in the limbs occurs. (2) A tetanus spasm.

arthroplasty (*ar'-thro-plas-te*). Plastic surgery for the reorganization of a joint, frequently the hip joint. *Cup a.* Reconstruction of the articular surface, which is then covered by a vitallium cup. *Excision a.* Ex-

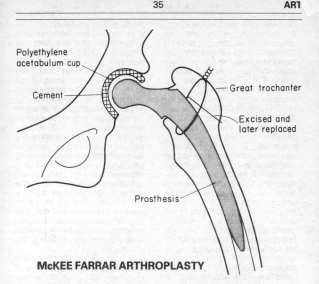

McKEE FARRAR ARTHROPLASTY

Polyethylene acetabulum cup

Cement

Great trochanter

Excised and later replaced

Prosthesis

cision of the joint surfaces affected, so that the gap thus formed then fills with fibrous tissue or muscle. *Girdlestone a.* An excision arthroplasty of the hip. *McKee Farrar a.* Replacement of both the head and the socket of the femur; *Charnley's a.* is similar. *Replacement a.* Partial removal of the head of the femur and its replacement by a metal prosthesis.

arthrotomy (*ar-throt'-om-e*). An incision into a joint.

Arthus phenomenon (*N.M. Arthus, French physiologist, 1862–1945*). Damage to tissue which occurs after repeated exposure to antigens.

articular (*ar-tik'-u-lar*). Pertaining to a joint.

articulation (*ar-tik-u-la'-shun*). (1) A junction point of two or more bones. (2) The enunciation of words.

artificial (*ar-te-fish'-al*). Not natural. *A. feeding.* The giving of food other than by placing it directly in the mouth. It may be provided via the mouth, using an *oesophageal* (Ryle's) *tube*; the food may be introduced into the stomach through a fine tube via the nostril (the *nasal route*) or using a catheter and funnel via the rectum (the *rectal route*, which is only suitable for substances that are ready for absorption, e.g. water, salt, glucose); in cases of oesophageal obstruction, an opening through the abdominal wall into the stomach (i.e. a *gastrostomy*) may allow direct introduction; or food may be injected *intravenously* (*see* Parenteral nutrition). *A. insemination*. The insertion of sperm into the uterus by means of syringe and cannula instead of by coitus. Husband's (AIH) or donor (AID) semen may be used. *A. respiration*. A means of resuscitation from asphyxia.

arytenoid (*ar-e-tee'-noid*). Resembling the mouth of a pitcher. *A. cartilages*. Two cartilages of the larynx, whose function is to regulate the tension of the vocal cords attached to them.

As. Chemical symbol for *arsenic*.

asbestos (*as-bes'-tos*). A fibrous non-combustible silicate of magnesium and calcium, which is a good nonconductor of heat.

asbestosis (*as-bes-to'-sis*). A form of pneumoconiosis caused by the inhalation of asbestos dust.

ascariasis (*as-kar-i'-as-is*). The condition in which roundworms are found in the alimentary tract.

Ascaris (*as'-kar-is*). A genus of roundworm. Some types may infest the human intestine.

Aschoff's nodules or **bodies** (*K.A.L. Aschoff, German pathologist, 1866–1942*). The nodules present in heart muscle in rheumatic myocarditis.

ascites (*as-i'-teez*). Free fluid in the peritoneal cavity. It may be the result of local inflammation, of venous obstruction, or part of a generalized oedema.

ascorbic acid (*as-kor'-bik as'-id*). Vitamin C. This acid is found in many vegetables and

fruits and is an essential dietary constituent for man. It promotes the healing of wounds. Deficiency causes scurvy.

asemia (*a-se'-me-ah*). Inability to understand or to use speech or signs, due to a cerebral lesion. Aphasia.

asepsis (*a-sep'-sis*). Freedom from pathogenic microorganisms.

aseptic (*a-sep'-tik*). Free from sepsis. *A. technique*. A method of carrying out sterile procedures so that there is the minimum risk of introducing infection. Achieved by the sterility of equipment and a non-touch method.

asexual (*a-seks'-u-al*). Without sex. *A. reproduction*. The production of new individuals without sexual union, e.g. by cell division or budding.

aspect (*as'-pekt*). That part of a surface facing in a particular direction. *Dorsal a*. That facing and seen from the back. *Ventral a*. That facing and seen from the front.

aspergillosis (*as-per-jil-o'-sis*). A bronchopulmonary disease in which the mucous membrane is attacked by the fungus, *Aspergillus*.

Aspergillus (*as-per-jil'-us*). A genus of fungi. *A. fumigatus*, found in soil and manure, is a common cause of aspergillosis.

aspermia (*a-sperm'-e-ah*). Absence of sperm.

asphyxia (*as-fiks'-e-ah*). An inability to breathe caused by obstruction of the nose, mouth or throat.

aspiration (*as-pir-a'-shun*). (1) The drawing in of a breath. (2) The drawing off of fluid from a cavity by means of suction.

aspirator (*as'-pir-a-tor*). Any

apparatus for withdrawing fluid or gases from a cavity of the body by means of suction.

aspirin (*as'-pir-in*). Acetyl-salicylic acid. It reduces temperature and relieves pain. *Soluble a.* A combination of aspirin with citric acid and calcium carbonate, which is less irritating to the gastric mucosa.

assay (*as'-a*). A quantitative examination to determine the amount of a particular constituent of a mixture, or of the biological or pharmacological potency of a drug.

assimilation (*as-im-il-a'-shun*). The process of transforming food, so that it can be absorbed into the circulatory system and utilized as nourishment for the tissues of the body.

association (*as-o-se-a'-shun*). Co-ordination of function of similar parts. *A. fibres.* Nerve fibres linking different areas of the brain. *A. of ideas.* A mental impression in which a thought or any sensory impulse will call to mind another object or idea connected in some way with the former. *Free a.* A method employed in psychoanalysis in which the patient is encouraged to express freely whatever comes into his mind. By this method material that is in the unconscious can be recalled.

astasia (*as-ta'-ze-ah*). Inability to stand or walk normally, due to unco-ordination of muscles.

asteatosis (*a-ste-at-o'-sis*). Lack of sebaceous secretion. There is a dry and scaly skin in which fissures may occur.

astereognosis (*a-ster-e-og-no'-sis*). Inability to recognize the shape of objects by feeling or touch.

asthenia (*as-the'-ne-ah*). Want of strength. Debility. Loss of tone.

asthenic (*as-then'-ik*). Descriptive of a type of body build: a pale, lean, narrowly built person with poor muscle development.

asthenopia (*as-then-o'-pe-ah*). Eye strain giving rise to an aching, burning sensation and headache. Likely to arise in long-sighted people when continual effort of accommodation is required for close work in artificial light.

asthma (*asth'-mah*). Paroxysmal dyspnoea. *Bronchial a.* Attacks of dyspnoea in which there is wheezing and difficulty in expiration due to muscular spasm of the bronchi. The attacks may be precipitated by hypersensitivity to foreign substances or associated with emotional upsets. There is often a family history of asthma or other allergic condition. Attacks may accompany chronic bronchitis. *Cardiac a.* Attacks of dyspnoea and palpitation arising most often at night, associated with left-sided heart failure and pulmonary congestion. *Renal a.* Dyspnoea occurring in kidney disease, which may be a sign of developing uraemia. It is unrelated to true asthma.

astigmatism (*as-tig'-mat-izm*). Inequality of the refractive power of an eye, due to defective curvature of its corneal meridians. The curve across the front of the eye from side to side is not quite the same as the curve from above downwards. The focus on the retina is then not a point, but a diffuse and indistinct area.

astringent (*as-trin'-jent*). An

agent causing contraction of organic tissues, thereby checking secretions, e.g. silver nitrate, tannic acid.

astrocytoma (*as-tro-si-to'-mah*). A malignant tumour of the brain or spinal cord. It is usually fast-growing. A glioma.

asymmetry (*a-sim'-et-re*). Inequality in size or shape of two structures normally the same.

asymptomatic (*a-simp-to-mat'-ik*). Without symptoms.

asynergy (*a-sin'-er-je*). Lack of co-ordination of structures which normally act in harmony.

asystole (*a-sis'-to-le*). Absence of heartbeat. Cardiac arrest.

ataraxia (*a-tar-aks'-e-ah*). A state of complete serenity.

atavism (*at'-av-izm*). The reappearance of some hereditary peculiarity which has missed a few generations.

ataxia, ataxy (*a-taks'-e-ah, a-taks'-e*). Failure of muscle co-ordination. *Hereditary a.* Friedreich's ataxia. *Locomotor a.* or *tables dorsalis.* A degenerative disease of the spinal cord; a manifestation of tertiary syphilis allied to general paralysis of the insane. Among signs and symptoms are: unco-ordinated movements of the legs in walking, absence of reflexes, and loss of sphincter control. The disease is chronic and progressive, but can be controlled by antisyphilitic treatment.

atelectasis (*at-el-ek'-tas-is*). Partial collapse of the air vesicles of the lungs (1) from imperfect expansion at birth, (2) as the result of disease or injury.

atheroma (*ath-er-o'-mah*). Patchy degeneration of the walls of large arteries in which fat-like plaques appear.

atherosclerosis (*ath-er-o-skler-o'-sis*). A condition in which the fatty degenerative plaques of atheroma are accompanied by arteriosclerosis, a narrowing and hardening of the vessels.

athetosis (*ath-et-o'-sis*). A recurring series of slow, writhing movements of the hands, usually due to a cerebral lesion, and most often seen in children.

athlete's foot (*ath'-leetz foot*). A fungal infection between the toes which is easily transmitted to others. Tinea pedis.

atlas (*at'-las*). The first cervical vertebra, articulating with the occipital bone of the skull.

atmosphere (*at'-mos-feer*). Air. The gases that surround the earth.

atmospheric pressure (*at-mos-fer'-ik presh'-er*). Pressure exerted by the air in all directions. At sea level it is about 100 kPa (15 lb/in^2).

atom (*at'-om*). The smallest particle of an element that retains all the properties of that element. It is made up of a central positively charged nucleus and, moving around it in orbit, negatively charged electrons.

atomizer (*at'-om-i-zer*). An instrument by which a liquid is very finely divided to form a spray.

atony (*at'-o-ne*). Lack of tone, e.g. in a muscle.

atopen (*at'-o-pen*). An antigen responsible for causing atopy.

atopy (*at'-o-pe*). A state of hypersensitivity to certain antigens. There is an inherited tendency and it includes asthma, eczema, and hayfever.

ATP. Adenosine triphosphate.

atresia (*a-tre'-ze-ah*). Absence of a natural opening, e.g. of the anus or vagina, usually a congenital malformation.

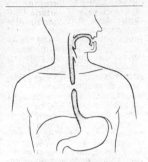

OESOPHAGEAL ATRESIA

atrial (*a'-tre-al*). Relating to the atrium. *A. fibrillation.* Overstimulation of the atrial walls so that many areas of excitation arise and the atrioventricular node is bombarded with impulses, many of which it cannot transmit, resulting in a highly irregular pulse. *A. flutter.* Rapid regular action of the atria. The atrioventricular node transmits alternate impulses or one in three or four. The atrial rate is usually about 300 beats per minute. *A. septal defect.* The non-closure of the foramen ovale at the time of birth giving rise to a congenital heart defect.

atrioventricular (*a'-tre-o-ven-trik'-u-lah*). Pertaining to the atrium and ventricle. *A. bundle. See* Bundle of His. *A. node.* A node of neurogenic tissue situated between the two and transmitting im-

pulses. *A. valves.* The bicuspid and tricuspid valve on the left and right sides of the heart respectively.

atrium (*a'-tre-um*). *pl.* atria. (1) A cavity or passage. (2) One of the two upper chambers of the heart. Formerly called auricle.

atrophy (*at'-ro-fe*). Wasting of any part of the body, due to degeneration of the cells, from disuse, lack of nourishment, or of nerve supply. *Acute yellow a.* Massive necrosis of liver cells. A rare condition that may follow acute hepatitis or eclampsia or be precipitated by certain drugs. *Progressive muscular a.* Degeneration of the motor neurones with wasting of muscle tissue. The condition is usually fatal and its cause is unknown.

atropine (*at'-ro-peen*). The active principle of belladonna. An alkaloid which inhibits respiratory and gastric secretions, relaxes muscle spasm and dilates the pupil. Used preoperatively, and to relieve renal and biliary colic, and as drops to aid examination of the eye.

ATS. Anti-tetanus serum.

attenuation (*at-en-u-a'-shun*). A bacteriological process by which organisms are rendered less virulent by culture in artificial media through many generations, exposure to light, air, etc. Used for vaccine preparations.

attitude (*at'-it-ude*). Position. (1) The posture taken up by the body. (2) A settled disposition of the mind.

atypical (*a-tip'-ik-al*). Not conforming to type.

Au. Chemical symbol for *gold* (aurum).

audiogram (*aw'-de-o-gram*). A graph produced by an audiometer.

audiometer (*aw-de-om'-e-ter*). An instrument for testing hearing, whereby the threshold of the patients' hearing can be measured.

auditory (*aw'-dit-or-e*). Pertaining to the sense of hearing.

Auerbach's plexus (*L. Auerbach, German anatomist, 1828–1897*). The ganglionic neurones of the vagus nerve that supply the muscle fibres of the intestine.

aura (*aw'-rah*). The premonition peculiar to individuals which often precedes an epileptic fit.

aural (*aw'-ral*). Referring to the ear.

auricle (*aw'-rikl*). (1) The external portion of the ear. (2) Obsolete term for the atrium.

auricular (*aw-rik'-u-lar*). Relating to an auricle. *A. fibrillation.* See Atrial fibrillation. *A. flutter.* See Atrial flutter.

auriscope (*aw'-ris-kope*). An instrument for examining the drum of the ear. An otoscope.

aurum (*aw'-rum*). Gold (*Latin*).

auscultation (*aws-kul-ta'-shun*). A method of examining the internal organs by listening to the sounds which they give out. In *direct* or *immediate a.*, the ear is placed directly against the body. In *mediate a.*, a stethoscope is used.

Australia antigen (*aw-stra'-le-ah an'-te-jen*). Antigen found in the blood of patients with serum hepatitis. Originally discovered in Australian aborigines.

autism (*aw'-tizm*). Self-absorption. Abnormal dislike of the society of others. *Infantile a.* Failure of a child to relate to people and situations, leading to complete withdrawal.

autistic (*aw-tis'-tik*). Pertaining to autism.

autoclave (*aw'-to-klave*). A steam-heated sterilizing apparatus in which the temperature is raised by reducing the air pressure inside it and then injecting steam under pressure, so bringing about efficient sterilization.

autoeroticism (*aw-to-e-rot'-is-izm*). Sexual pleasure derived from self-stimulation of erogenous zones (the mouth, the anus, the genitals and the skin).

autogenous (*aw-toj'-en-us*). Generated within the body and not acquired from external sources. *A. vaccine.* Vaccine made from the patient's serum.

autograft (*aw'-to-graft*). The transfer of skin or other tissue from one part of the body to another to repair some deficiency.

autoimmune disease (*aw-to-im-une' diz-eez*). Condition in which the body develops antibodies to its own tissues, as in e.g. autoimmune thyroiditis (Hashimoto's disease).

autoimmunization (*aw'-to-im-mu-ni-za'-shun*). The formation of antibodies against the individual's own tissue.

autoinfection (*aw-to-in-fek'-shun*). Self-infection, transferred from one part of the body to another by fingers, towels, etc.

autoinoculation (*aw-to-in-ok-u-la'-shun*). Inoculation with a micro-organism from the body itself.

autointoxication (*aw-to-in-toks-ik-a'-shun*). Poisoning by toxins generated within the body itself.

autolysis (*aw-tol'-is-is*). A breaking up of living tissues as may occur, e.g., if pancreatic ferments escape into surrounding tissues. It also occurs after death.

automatic (*aw-to-mat'-ik*). Performed without the influence of the will.

automatism (*aw-tom'-at-izm*). Performance of non-reflex acts without apparent volition, and of which the patient may have no memory afterwards, as in somnambulism. *Post-epileptic a.* Automatic acts following an epileptic fit.

autonomic (*aw-to-nom'-ik*). Self-governing. *A. nervous system.* The sympathetic and parasympathetic nerves which control involuntary muscles and glandular secretion over which there is no conscious control.

autoplasty (*aw'-to-plas-te*). Replacement of missing tissue by grafting a healthy section from another part of the body.

autopsy (*aw'-top-se*). Post-mortem examination of a body to determine the cause of death.

autoserum (*aw-to-se'-rum*). A serum derived from the patient's blood.

autosome (*aw'-to-some*). Any chromosome other than the sex chromosomes. In man there are 22 pairs of autosomes and 1 pair of sex chromosomes.

avascular (*a-vas'-ku-lah*). Not vascular. Bloodless. *A. necrosis.* Death of bone owing to deficient blood supply, usually following an injury.

aversion (*av-er'-shun*). Intense dislike. *A. therapy.* A method of treating alcoholism and other addictions by associating the craving for what is addictive with painful or unpleasant stimuli.

avitaminosis (*a-vit-am-in-o'-sis*). A condition resulting from an insufficiency of vitamins in the diet. A deficiency disease.

avulsion (*av-ul'-shun*). The tearing away of one part from another. *Phrenic a.* A tearing away of the phrenic nerve. It paralyses the diaphragm on the affected side.

axilla (*aks-il'-ah*). An armpit.

axis (*aks'-is*). (1) A line through the centre of a structure. (2) The second cervical vertebra.

axon (*aks'-on*). The process of a nerve cell along which electrical impulses travel. The nerve fibre.

axonotmesis (*aks-on-ot-me'-sis*). Partial degeneration of a nerve.

azathioprine (*az-ah-thi'-o-preen*). An immunosuppressive drug, often used in the treatment of renal failure.

azoospermia (*a-zo-o-sperm'-e-ah*). Absence of spermatozoa in the semen.

azygos (*az'-ig-os*). Something that is unpaired. *A. vein.* An unpaired vein that ascends the posterior mediastinum and enters the superior vena cava.

B

Ba. Chemical symbol for *barium.*

Babinski's reflex or **sign** (*J.F.F. Babinski, French neurologist, 1857–1932*). On stroking the sole of the foot, the great toe bends upwards instead of downwards (*dorsal* instead of *plantar* flexion). Present in disease or injury to the upper motor neurone. Babies who have not walked react in the same way, but normal flexion develops later.

baby (*ba'-be*). An infant as yet unable to walk. *Battered b.* One suffering from the result of continued violence; extensive bruising, fractures of limbs, rib and skull, and internal trauma may be found. *Blue b.* One suffering from cyanosis at birth due to atelectasis or congenital heart malformation.

bacillaemia (*bas-il-e'-me-ah*). The presence of bacilli in the blood.

bacilluria (*bas-il-u'-re-ah*). The presence of bacilli in the urine.

bacillus (*bas-il'-us*). pl. bacilli. (1) *cap.* A genus of aerobic, spore-bearing gram-positive bacteria. *B. anthracis.* The cause of anthrax. It is the most serious pathogenic bacillus to man. (2) Loosely, the cause of any bacterial infection by a rod-shaped microorganism, e.g. *B. coli*, the colon bacillus (now known as *Escherichia coli*).

bacitracin (*bas-e-tra'-sin*). An antibiotic drug derived from *Bacillus subtilis.* Bacitracin zinc is now more commonly used, mostly for surface application.

back (*bak*). Dorsum. Posterior trunk from neck to pelvis. *Hunch b.* Kyphosis. *B.bone.* The vertebral column. *B. slab.* Plaster or plastic splint in which a limb is supported.

baclofen (*bak-lo'-fen*). A muscle relaxant, sometimes used in the treatment of multiple sclerosis.

bacteraemia (*bak-ter-e'-me-ah*). The presence of bacteria in the blood stream.

bacterial (*bak-te'-re-al*). Pertaining to bacteria.

bactericidal (*bak-te-ris-i'-dal*). Capable of killing bacteria, e.g. disinfectants, great heat, intense cold or sunlight.

bactericide (*bak-te'-ris-ide*). An agent that kills bacteria.

bacterin (*bak-te'-rin*). (1) Bacterial vaccine. (2) Suspension of bacteria used either prophylactically or therapeutically to stimulate the production of antibodies. (3) Suspension of bacteria used for the production of antisera.

bacteriologist (*bak-te-re-ol'-o-jist*). One who has studied and is skilled in the science of bacteriology.

bacteriology (*bak-te-re-ol'-o-je*). The study of bacteria.

bacteriolysin (*bak-te-re-ol'-is-in*). An antibody produced in the blood to assist in the destruction of bacteria. The action is specific.

bacteriolysis (*bak-te-re-ol'-is-is*). The dissolution of bacteria by a bacteriolytic agent.

bacteriolytic (*bak-te-re-o-lit'-ik*). Capable of destroying or dissolving bacteria.

bacteriophage (*bak-te'-re-o-faje*). A virus which infects only bacteria. Many strains exist, some of which are used for identifying types of staphylococci and salmonellae.

bacteriostat (*bak-te'-re-o-stat*). An agent which inhibits the growth of bacteria.

bacteriostatic (*bak-te-re-o-stat'-ik*). Inhibiting the growth of bacteria.

bacteriotherapy (*bak-te-re-o-ther'-ap-e*). Treatment of disease by the injection of bacteria into the blood, e.g. malaria therapy in the treatment of neurosyphilis.

bacterium (*bak-te'-re-um*). pl.

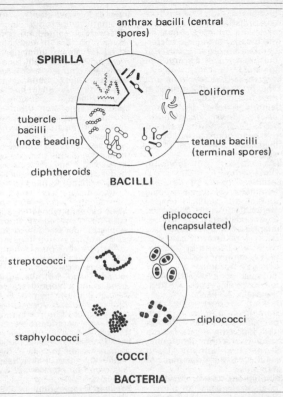

SPIRILLA

anthrax bacilli (central spores)

coliforms

tubercle bacilli (note beading)

tetanus bacilli (terminal spores)

diphtheroids

BACILLI

diplococci (encapsulated)

streptococci

diplococci

staphylococci

COCCI

BACTERIA

bacteria. A general name given to a minute vegetable organism which may live on organic matter. There are many varieties, only some of which are pathogenic to man, animals and plants. Each bacterium consists of a single cell and, given favourable conditions, multiplies by subdivision. Bacteria are classified according to their shape into: (1) *bacilli*, rod-shaped; (2) *cocci*, spherical: (a) streptococci—in chains; (b) staphylococci—in groups; (c) diplococci—in pairs; (3) *spirilla*, *spirochaetes*, spiral-shaped. *Pathogenic b.* One whose growth in the body gives rise to disease, either by destruction of tissue, or by formation of toxins which circulate in the blood. Pathogenic bacteria thrive on organic matter in the presence of warmth and moisture.

bacteriuria (*bak-te-re-u'-re-ah*). The presence of bacteria in the urine.

Bainbridge reflex (*F.A. Bainbridge, British physiologist, 1874–1921*). An increase in the heart rate caused by an increase in right atrial pressure.

BAL. British anti-lewisite. Dimercaprol.

balanitis (*bal-an-i'-tis*). Inflammation of the glans penis and of the prepuce, usually associated with phimosis. Balanoposthitis.

balantidiasis (*bal-an-tid-i'-as-is*). A rare form of colitis or dysentery caused by intestinal infestation by *Balantidium coli*, a protozoon.

baldness (*bawld'-nes*). Absence of hair, especially from the scalp. Alopecia.

Balkan frame (*bawl'-kan frame*). A framework fitted over a bed to carry pulleys and slings or splints for the support of a limb undergoing surgical treatment. Used chiefly in the treatment of fractures.

ballotement (*bal-ot-mon'*). A method of testing for a floating object, e.g. abdominal palpation of the uterus when testing for pregnancy. The uterus is pushed upward by a finger in the vagina, and if a fetus is present it will fall back again like a heavy body in water.

balneotherapy (*bal-ne-o-ther'-ap-e*). The use of baths in the treatment of disease.

balsam (*bawl'-sam*). An aromatic vegetable juice. *Friar's b.* A compound containing tincture of benzoin. Used for steam inhalations. *Peru b.* Used externally as an antiseptic ointment and in *tulle gras. Tolu b.* Used as an expectorant. A constituent of friar's balsam.

bandage (*band'-aje*). A binder to give support or apply pressure to a part or for fixing a dressing in position. There are now available a number of tubular bandages that can be applied to many parts of the body. *Capeline b.* Resembling a cap or hood. Applied to the head, shoulder, or amputation stump. *Many-tailed b.* Wide bandage whose edge is cut into many equal strips. Applied under traction to the abdomen by overlapping strips. *Spica b.* Figure-of-eight bandage. Applied to hips, shoulders, etc.

banding (*band'-ing*). Placing a band round a blood vessel to restrict the flow from it. *Pulmonary arterial b.* A palliative operation used in treating infants with ventricular septal defects.

bank (*bank*). Store of donated human tissues for use in the future by other individuals, e.g. *blood b., human-milk b., sperm b.*

Bankhart's operation (*A.S.B. Bankhart, British orthopaedic surgeon, 1879–1951*). An operation carried out to repair the defect in the glenoid cavity when there is repeated dislocation of the shoulder joint.

Banti's disease (*G. Banti, Italian pathologist, 1852–1925*). A clinical syndrome characterized by splenomegaly, cirrhosis of liver, anaemia,

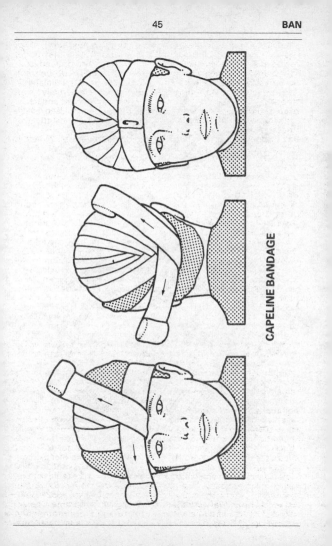

CAPELINE BANDAGE

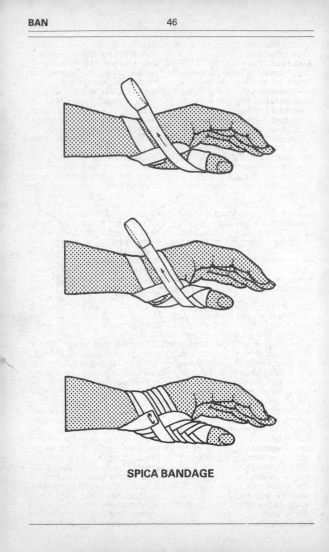

SPICA BANDAGE

leucopenia and gastrointestinal bleeding.

Barbados leg (*bar-ba'-doze leg*). Swelling and enlargement of the leg. A form of elephantiasis.

barbiturate (*bar-bit'-u-rate*). One of a large group of sedative and hypnotic drugs derived from barbituric acid, e.g. phenobarbitone, amylobarbitone. Prolonged use may lead to addiction and they are less used than formerly.

barbotage (*bar'-bo-tahj*). A method of spinal anaesthesia by which some of the anaesthetic is injected followed by partial withdrawal and then reinjection with more of the drug. This process is repeated until the full amount has been given, allowing dilution and mixing with the cerebrospinal fluid.

baritosis (*bar-it-o'-sis*). Inhalation of barite or barium dust resulting in pneumoconiosis.

barium (*bair'-e-um*). *abbrev.* Ba. A soft silvery metallic element. *B. sulphate.* A heavy mineral salt that is comparatively impermeable to X-rays and can therefore be used as contrast medium given as a meal or as an enema. Used to demonstrate abnormality in the stomach or intestines, and to show peristaltic movement. *B. sulphide.* The chief constituent of depilatory preparations, i.e. those which remove hair.

baroreceptors (*bar-o-re-sep'-torz*). The sensory branches of the glossopharyngeal and vagus nerves that influence the blood pressure. The receptors are situated in the walls of the carotid sinus and aortic arch.

Barr body (*M.L. Barr, Canadian anatomist, b. 1908*). Small dark-staining area underneath the nuclear membrane of female cells. Represents an inactive X chromosome.

Barré-Guillain syndrome (*J.A. Barré, French neurologist, b. 1880; G. Guillain, French neurologist, 1876–1961*). Acute febrile polyneuritis.

barrier (*bar'-e-er*). An obstruction. *Blood–brain b.* The selective barrier which separates the circulating blood from the cerebrospinal fluid. *B. contraceptive.* A mechanical barrier preventing the sperm entering the cervical canal, e.g. diaphragm, sheath. *B. nursing.* A method of patient isolation which enables a patient suffering from an infectious disease to be nursed amongst those not so infected. *Placental b.* Semipermeable membrane between maternal and fetal blood. *Protective b.* Radiation-absorbing shield, e.g. lead, concrete, to protect the body against ionizing radiations.

Bartholin's glands (*C.T. Bartholin, Danish anatomist, 1655–1738*). Two glands situated in the labia majora, with ducts opening inside the vulva.

basal (*ba'-sal*). (1) Fundamental. (2) Referring to a base. *B. ganglia.* The collections of nerve cells or grey matter in the base of the cerebrum. They consist of the caudate nucleus and putamen, forming the corpus striatum, and the globus pallidus. Paralysis agitans is associated with degenerative changes in these structures. *B. metabolic rate.* BMR. An indirect method of estimating the rate of metabolism in the body by measuring the O_2 intake and CO_2 output on breathing. The age, weight and size of the patient have to be taken into account. Used as a test of thyroid functioning.

base (*base*). (1) The lowest part or foundation. (2) The main constituent of a mixture. (3) An alkali or other substance which can unite with an acid to form a salt.

basement membrane (*base'-ment mem'-brane*). A thin layer of modified connective tissue supporting layers of cells, found at the base of the epidermis and underlying mucous membranes.

basilar (*bas'-il-ar*). Situated at the base. *B. artery*. Midline artery at the base of the skull, formed by the junction of the vertebral arteries.

basilic (*bas-il'-ik*). Prominent. *B. vein*. A large vein on the inner side of the arm.

basophil(e) (*ba'-zo-fil*). A leucocyte or white blood cell which takes staining by basic dyes.

basophilia (*ba-zo-fil'-e-ah*). Increase of basophils in the blood.

Batchelor plaster (*J.S. Batchelor, British surgeon*). A plas-

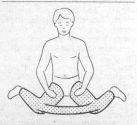

BATCHELOR PLASTER

ter of Paris splint which corrects congenital dislocation of the hip.

bath (*bahth*). Vessel used for cleansing the body and stimulating the circulation. Suggested temperatures for a *cool b.* 18°C (65°F); *tepid b.* 29°C (85°F); *warm b.* 38°C (100°F); *hot b.* 40°C (105°F). Baths containing bran, oatmeal, starch or sodium bicarbonate are soothing for skin diseases. *Air b.* Exposure of the body to a flow of warm air. *Electric b.* One in which a current is passed through the water. *Fucus b.* One containing seaweed. *Sauna b.* Finnish type of steam bath. *Wax b.* The application of warm wax to the small joints of the hands and feet.

battery (*bat-er-e*). A number of connected cells for generating or storing electricity.

BCG. Calmette–Guérin bacillus.

Be. Chemical symbol for *beryllium*.

'bearing down' (*bair'-ing down*). (1) The expulsive pains in the second stage of labour. (2) A feeling of heaviness and downward strain in the pelvis present with some uterine growths or displacements.

beat (*beet*). Pulsation of the heart or an artery. *Apex b.* Pulsation of the heart felt over its apex. The beat of the heart is felt against the chest wall. *Dropped b.* The occasional loss of a ventricular beat. *Ectopic b.* One that originates somewhere other than the sinu-atrial node.

becquerel (*bek'-er-el*). *abbrev.* Bq. The SI unit of radioactivity equal to the quantity of material undergoing one disintegration per second—3.7 × 10^{10} becquerels is equal to 1 curie.

Beer's knife (*G.J. Beer, German ophthalmologist, 1763–1821*). One with a triangular blade used in cataract operations, for incising the cornea preparatory to removal of the lens.

beeswax (*beez'-waks*). Yellow wax secreted by bees, and used in the manufacture of ointments.

behaviour (*be-ha'-vyor*). The way in which an organism reacts to an internal or external stimulus. *Incongruous b.* Behaviour that is out of keeping with the person's normal reaction or has the opposite effect to that consciously desired. *B. disorders* may take many forms, such as truancy, stealing, temper-tantrums, bed wetting, or thumb sucking.

behaviourism (*be-ha'-vyor-izm*). The purely objective study and observation of the behaviour of individuals.

bejel (*ba'-jel*). A non-venereal but infectious form of syphilis caused by a treponema indistinguishable from that causing syphilis.

belching (*belch'-ing*). The noisy expulsion of gas from the stomach through the mouth. Eructation.

belladonna (*bel-ah-don'-ah*). A drug from the deadly nightshade plant. Used as an antispasmodic in colic, to check secretions, and to dilate the pupil of the eye.

belle indifference (*bel in-dif'-er-ons*). An indication of conversion hysteria, in which the patient describes his symptoms appearing not to be distressed by them.

Bell's palsy (*Sir C. Bell, British physiologist, 1774–1842*). Facial paralysis.

bemegride (*bem'-e-gride*). An analeptic, used particularly in cases of barbiturate poisoning.

Bence Jones protein (*H. Bence Jones, British physician, 1813–1873*). *See* Protein.

bendrofluazide (*ben-dro-flu'-az-ide*). An oral diuretic of the thiazide group. Used primarily to treat mild hypertension and cardiac failure.

bends (*bendz*). A colloquial term for caisson disease. Decompression sickness.

benign (*be-nine'*). The opposite to malignant. *B. tumour. See* Tumour. *B. tertian fever.* Fever due to a malarial parasite, more tractable to treatment than that which causes malignant tertian fever.

benzathine penicillin (*benz'-ath-een pen-is-il'-in*). A long-acting antibiotic. Used in treatment of infections and also in rheumatic fever prophylaxis.

benzene (*ben'-zeen*). Benzol. A coal-tar derivative widely used as a solvent of fats and resins.

benzhexol (*benz'-hex-ol*). An antispasmodic drug which helps to overcome the tremors and rigidity of Parkinson's disease.

benzocaine (*ben'-zo-kane*). A surface anaesthetic used for the relief of pain in oral lesions.

benzyl benzoate (*ben'-zil ben'-zo-ate*). An emulsion used in the treatment of scabies.

benzylpenicillin (*benz-il-pen-is-il'-in*). A widely used soluble penicillin that is quickly absorbed. High blood levels can therefore be obtained.

beri beri (*ber'-e ber'-e*). A deficiency disease due to insufficiency of vitamin B_1 in the diet. It is a form of neuritis, with pain, paralysis and oedema of the extremities.

berylliosis (*ber-il-e-o'-sis*). An industrial lung disease due to the inhaling of beryllium. Interstitial fibrosis arises, impairing lung function.

beryllium (*ber-il'-e-um*). *abbrev.* Be. A metallic element, which is used in the manufacture of some aluminium alloys.

Besnier's prurigo (*E. Besnier, French dermatologist, 1831–1909*). Diathetic prurigo, seen in young children.

beta (*be'-tah*). The second letter in the Greek alphabet—β. *B. blockers*. Drugs used to block the action of adrenaline on receptors in cardiac muscle. *B. cells*. Insulin-producing cells found in the islets of Langerhans in the pancreas. *B. rays*. Electrons used therapeutically for treatment of lesions of the cornea and iris. *B. receptors*. Receptors associated with the inhibition (relaxation) of smooth muscle. They also bring an increase in the force of contraction and rate of the heart.

betamethasone (*be-tah-meth'-az-one*). A synthetic glucocorticoid which is the most active of the anti-inflammatory steroids.

betatron (*be'-tah-tron*). An apparatus used to accelerate a stream of electrons into a beam for use in radiotherapy. The electrons move in circular orbits in an evacuated chamber before striking an X-ray target or scattering foil.

bethanidine (*beth-an'-id-een*). An adrenergic blocking agent

used in the treatment of moderate to severe hypertension.

Betz cells (*V.A. Betz, Russian anatomist, 1834–1894*). The pyramidal cells in the precentral area of the cerebrum.

bezoar (*be'-zor*). A mass of hair, fruit or vegetable fibres sometimes found in the stomach or intestines.

Bi. Chemical symbol for *bismuth*.

bicarbonate (*bi-kar'-bon-ate*). Any salt containing the HCO_3^- anion, i.e. a salt of carbonic acid in which only one of the hydrogen atoms has been replaced by another cation, e.g. $NaHCO_3$ (sodium bicarbonate).

bicellular (*bi-sel'-u-lar*). Composed of two cells.

biceps (*bi'-seps*). A muscle with two heads. (1) A flexor of the arm. (2) One of the hamstring muscles of the thigh.

biconcave (*bi-kon'-kave*). Pertaining to a lens or other structure with a hollow or depression on each surface.

biconvex (*bi-kon'-veks*). Pertaining to a lens or other

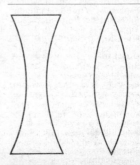

BICONCAVE   BICONVEX

structure that protrudes on both surfaces.

bicornuate (*bi-korn'-u-ate*). Having two horns. *B. uterus.* A congenital malformation in which there is a partial or complete vertical division into two parts of the body of the uterus.

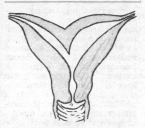

BICORNUATE UTERUS

bicuspid (*bi-kus'-pid*). Having two cusps or projections. *B. teeth.* The premolars. *B. valve.* The mitral valve of the heart between the left atrium and ventricle.

bidet (*be-'da*). A low narrow basin on a stand for washing the perineum and genitalia.

bifid (*bi'-fid*). Divided or cleft into two parts.

bifocal (*bi-fo'-kal*). Having two foci, as with spectacles in which the lenses have two different foci, the lower for close work and the upper for distant vision.

bifurcate (*bi'-fer-kate*). To divide into two branches; arteries bifurcate frequently, thereby getting smaller.

bifurcation (*bi-fer-ka'-shun*). The junction where a vessel divides into two branches, e.g. where the aorta divides

into the right and left iliac vessels.

bigeminal (*bi-jem'-in-al*). Double. *B. pulse.* Two pulse beats which occur together, regular in time and force. A regular irregularity.

biguanide (*bi-gwan'-ide*). An oral hypoglycaemic drug for treating diabetes, most commonly used in overweight diabetics.

bilateral (*bi-lat'-er-al*). Pertaining to both sides.

bile (*bile*). A secretion of the liver, greenish-yellow to brown in colour and with a bitter taste. It is concentrated in the gall-bladder and passes into the small intestine, where it assists digestion by emulsifying fats and stimulates peristalsis. *B. pigments.* Bilirubin and biliverdin, produced by haemolysis in the spleen. Normally these colour the faeces only, but in jaundice the skin and urine may also become coloured. *B. salts.* Sodium taurocholate and sodium glycocholate, which cause the emulsification of fats.

Bilharzia (*T.M. Bilharz, German physician, 1825–62*). A genus of blood fluke now known as *Schistosoma.*

bilharziasis (*bil-harts-i'-as-is*). Schistosomiasis.

biliary (*bil'-e-ar-e*). Pertaining to bile. *B. colic.* Spasm of muscle walls of the bile duct causing excruciating pain when gall stones are blocking the tube. Pain is in the right upper quadrant of the abdomen and referred to the shoulder. *B. ducts.* The tubes through which the bile passes from the liver and gall-bladder to the intestine. *B. fistula.* An abnormal opening between the gall-bladder and the surface of the body.

bilious (*bil'-e-us*). Characterized by biliousness.

biliousness (*bil'-e-us-nes*). A colloquial term for a condition comprising nausea, headache and abdominal discomfort.

bilirubin (*bil-e-ru'-bin*). An orange or yellow bile pigment.

biliuria (*bil-e-u'-re-ah*). Bile or bile salts in the urine.

biliverdin (*bil-e-ver'-din*). A green bile pigment, the oxidized form of bilirubin.

Billroth's operation (*C.A.T. Billroth, Austrian surgeon, 1829–1894*). *See* Gastrectomy.

bimanual (*bi-man'-u-al*). Using both hands. *B. examination*. Examination with both hands. Used chiefly in gynaecology, when the internal genital organs are examined between one hand on the abdomen, and the other hand or a finger within the vagina.

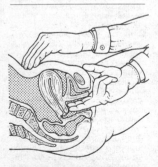

BIMANUAL EXAMINATION OF UTERUS

binary (*bi'-nar-e*). Made up of two parts. *B. fission*. The multiplication of cells by division into two equal parts. *B. scale*. One used in calculating, in which only two symbols, 0 and 1, are used. Digital computers use this scale.

binaural (*bin-aw'-ral*). Pertaining to both ears. *B. stethoscope*. *See* Stethoscope.

binder (*bine'-der*). An abdominal bandage which can be used for support after childbirth or abdominal operation.

Binet's test (*A. Binet, French physiologist, 1857–1911*). A method of ascertaining the mental age of children or young persons by using a series of questions standardized on the capacity of normal children at various ages.

binocular (*bin-ok'-u-lar*). Relating to both eyes.

binovular (*bin-ov'-u-lar*). Derived from two ova. *B. twins*. Twins, which may or may not be of different sexes.

bioassay (*bi-o-as'-a*). Biological assay. The use of animals or an isolated organ preparation to determine the effect of the active power of a sample of a drug. Comparison is made with the effect of a standard preparation.

biochemistry (*bi-o-kem'-is-tre*). The chemistry of living matter.

biofeedback (*bi-o-feed'-bak*). Visual or auditory evidence provided to an individual of the satisfactory performance of an autonomic body function, e.g. sounding a tone when blood pressure is at a satisfactory level, so that, through conditioning, he may assert control over that function.

biogenesis (*bi-o-jen'-es-is*).

The theory that living organisms can originate only from those already living and cannot be artificially produced.

biology (*bi-ol'-o-je*). The science of living organisms, dealing with their structure, function and their relations with one another.

biometrics, biometry (*bi-o-met'-riks, bi-om'-et-re*). (1) Anthropometry. (2) The use of statistics in biological science.

biomicroscopy (*bi-o-mi-kros'-ko-pe*). A microscopic examination of living tissues, e.g. of the structures of the anterior of the eye during life. *See* Slit lamp.

bioplasm (*bi'-o-plazm*). Protoplasm. The active principle in matter which produces living organisms.

biopsy (*bi-op'-se*). Observation of the living body. Used to describe the removal of some tissue or organ, e.g. a lymph gland, for examination to establish a diagnosis. *Aspiration b.* Biopsy in which the tissue is obtained by suction through a needle and syringe. *Excisional b.* Removal of an entire lesion and significant portion of normal-looking tissue for examination. *Needle b.* Tissue obtained by the puncture of a lesion with a needle. Rotation of the needle removes tissue within the lumen of the needle. *Punch b.* Tissue obtained by a punch, e.g. cervical tissue.

biorhythm (*bi'-o-rithm*). A similar concept to the circadian rhythm, but one where biological functions are said to occur according to the individual's pattern, which may be totally independent of the 24-hour cycle. The behaviour of the individual patient will depend on his biorhythms.

biosynthesis (*bi-o-sin'-thes-is*). The creation of a compound within a living organism.

biotin (*bi'-o-tin*). Formerly termed vitamin H, now part of vitamin B complex and present in all normal diets.

biparietal (*bi-par-i'-et-al*). Pertaining to both parietal eminences or bones.

biparous (*bip'-ar-us*). Giving birth to two infants at a time.

bipolar (*bi-po'-lar*). With two poles. *B. nerve cells.* Cells having two nerve fibres, e.g. ganglionic cells.

BIPP. An antiseptic paste composed of bismuth, iodoform and paraffin.

birth (*berth*). The act of being born. *B. control.* Limiting the size of the family by abstention or the use of contraceptives. *B. mark.* A naevus present from birth. *Premature b.* One taking place after 28 weeks of pregnancy but before term. Now all infants under 2500 g weight are considered premature.

bisacodyl (*bis-ak-o'-dil*). A laxative that acts directly on the rectum. Given as tablets or in the form of suppositories.

bisexual (*bi-seks'-u-al*). Possessing characteristics of both sexes; hermaphroditic.

bismuth (*biz'-muth*). *abbrev.* Bi. A greyish metallic element. Certain of its salts are used as gastric sedatives and in the treatment of syphilis.

bistoury (*bis'-too-re*). A slender surgical knife, sometimes curved.

bite (*bite*). (1) *v.* To seize with the teeth. (2) *n.* A wound made by biting. (3) *n.* An impression made by the teeth on a thin sheet of malleable material such as wax.

Bitot's spots (*P.A. Bitot, French physician, 1822–1888*). Collections of dried epithelium, micro-organisms, etc., forming shiny, greyish spots on the cornea. A sign of vitamin A deficiency.

bitters (*bit-ers*). Drugs characterized by bitter taste; used to stimulate the appetite.

bivalve (*bi'-valv*). (1) *adj.* Having two valves, as the shells of molluscs such a oysters. (2) *v.* To cut a plaster cast into an anterior and a posterior section. *B. speculum.* A vaginal one having two blades that can be adjusted for easy insertion.

blackhead (*blak'-hed*). A comedo.

blackout (*blak'-owt*). Momentary failure of vision and unconsciousness due to cerebral circulatory insufficiency.

blackwater fever (*blak'-wawter fe'-ver*). A form of malignant malaria in which severe haemolysis causes a dark discoloration of the urine.

bladder (*blad'-er*). A membranous sac. *B. worm.* A cysticercus. *Atonic b.* A condition in which there is lack of tone in the bladder wall, which may be the result of incomplete emptying over a long period. *Gall-b.* The reservoir for bile. *Irritable b.* A condition in which there is frequent desire to micturate. *Urinary b.* The reservoir for urine.

Blalock–Taussig operation (*A. Blalock, American surgeon, 1899–1964; H.B. Taussig, American paediatrician, b. 1898*). Operation in which the subclavian artery is anastomosed to the pulmonary artery. Performed in cases of Fallot's tetralogy.

bland (*bland*). Non-stimulating. *B. fluids.* Mild and non-irritating fluids such as barley water and milk.

blast (*blast*). (1) An immature cell. (2) A wave of high air pressure caused by an explosion of some kind.

blastocyst (*blas'-to-sist*). Blastula.

blastocyte (*blas'-to-site*). An embryonic cell that has not yet become differentiated into its specific type.

blastoderm (*blas'-to-derm*). The germinal cells of the embryo consisting of three layers, the ectoderm, mesoderm and entoderm.

blastolysis (*blas-tol'-is-is*). The destruction of germ substance.

blastomycosis (*blas-to-mi-ko'-sis*). A fungal infection which after invasion of the skin may cause granulomatous lesions in the mouth, pharynx and lungs.

blastula (*blas'-tu-lah*). Blastocyst. An early stage in the development of the fertilized ovum. This stage precedes the gastrula.

bleb (*bleb*). A blister.

bleeder (*ble'-der*). (1) A popular name for one who suffers from haemophilia. (2) A vessel which is difficult to seal at operation.

bleeding (*ble'-ding*). (1) Escape of blood from an injured vessel. (2) Venesection. *B. time.* The time taken for oozing to cease from a sharp prick of the finger or ear lobe. The normal is 1 to 3 min. *Functional b.* Bleeding from the uterus when no organic lesion is present.

blennorrhagia (*blen-or-aj'-e-ah*). (1) An excessive discharge of mucus, e.g. leucorrhoea. (2) Gonorrhoea.

blennorrhoea (*blen-or-e'-ah*). Blennorrhagia.

bleomycin (*ble-o-mi'-sin*). An anti-tumour antibiotic drug especially effective against squamous cell carcinomas.

blepharitis (*blef-ar-i'-tis*). Inflammation of the eyelids. *Allergic b.* That associated with response to drugs or cosmetics applied to the eye or eyelids. *Squamous b.* That associated with dandruff of the scalp.

blepharon (*blef'-ar-on*). The eyelid.

blepharophimosis (*blef'-ar-o-fi-mo'-sis*). Abnormal narrowing of the aperture between the eyelids. Usually congenital but may arise from chronic inflammation.

blepharoptosis (*blef-ar-op-to'-sis*). Drooping of the upper eyelid.

blepharospasm (*blef'-ar-o-spazm*). Prolonged spasm of the orbicular muscles of the eyelids.

blind (*blind*). Without sight. *B. spot.* The point where the optic nerve leaves the retina, which is insensitive to light. Punctum caecum.

blind loop syndrome (*blind loop sin'-drome*). A condition of stasis in the small intestine which aids bacterial multiplication leading to diarrhoea and salt deficiencies. The cause may be intestinal obstruction or surgical anastomosis.

blindness (*blind'-nes*). Loss of ability to see. May be congenital or acquired. *Colour b.* Colloquial term for misperception of hues.

blister (*blis'-ter*). A bleb or vesicle. A collection of serum

between the epidermis and the true skin. *Blood b.* A blister containing blood, usually caused by a pinch or bruise.

block (*blok*). A stoppage or obstruction. The term is used to describe (1) various forms of regional anaesthesia, e.g. epidural block; (2) obstruction to the passage of a nervous impulse due to disease, e.g. heart block (*see* Heart); (3) an interruption of mental function.

blood (*blud*). The fluid that circulates through the heart and blood vessels, supplying nutritive material to all parts of the body, and carrying off waste products. It is a colourless fluid (*plasma*) in which float myriads of minute bodies (*corpuscles*). These are of three kinds: *red* and *white* (in the proportion of about 500:1), and *platelets*. (1) The red corpuscles or *erythrocytes* contain haemoglobin which combines with oxygen in passing through the lungs. This oxygen is released into the tissues from the capillaries and oxidation takes place. (2) The white corpuscles or *leucocytes* defend against invading micro-organisms, which they have power to destroy. (3) Blood platelets or *thrombocytes* are concerned with the clotting of blood. *See* Normal values. *B. bank.* A collection of various types of blood and blood products obtained from blood donors and stored for use in transfusions. *B. casts.* Minute filaments of coagulated blood found in the urine in some cases of kidney disease. *B. count.* Calculation of the number of red and white corpuscles in one cubic millimetre of

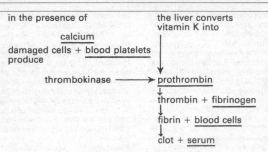

| in the presence of

calcium
damaged cells + _blood platelets_
produce | the liver converts
vitamin K into |

thrombokinase ⟶ prothrombin
                              ↓
                    thrombin + _fibrinogen_
                              ↓
                    fibrin + _blood cells_
                              ↓
                    clot + _serum_

CLOTTING OF BLOOD
Underlined substances are normally present in blood

blood, as seen through the microscope. _Differential b.c._ One which gives the relative number of the different types of normal and abnormal white cells. _B. culture._ The cultivation of bacteria present in a patient's blood in order that a disease may be diagnosed or sensitivity tests carried out. _B. donor._ An individual who gives blood that can be used for transfusion into another person. _B. group._ A type of blood based on compatibility. For transfusion purposes, the ABO system is followed, in which four groups are recognized: A, B, AB and O. If two which are incompatible are mixed, agglutination of cor-puscles results. Therefore in blood transfusion the donor's and recipient's blood must be of the same or a compatible group. Introduction of incompatible blood produces a severe reaction which may be fatal. Theoretically, group O (universal donors) can give to anyone but it is imperative that direct cross-matching should precede blood transfusion. _See_ Rhesus factor. _B. plasma._ The fluid portion of blood that contains proteins, salts, hormones, and the end products of digestion, together with waste and toxic substances for excretion. _B. pressure._ The pressure exerted on the arteries by the

Group	Antigen present in red cell	Antibody present in plasma
AB	A and B	—
A	A	Anti. B (β)
B	B	Anti. A (α)
O	—	Anti. A and Anti. B (α and β)

ABO SYSTEM

blood as it flows through them. It can be measured in millimetres of mercury (mmHg) using a sphygmomanometer. Two readings are made. One records the pressure whilst the heart is in systole and is the higher or *systolic pressure*. The other records the pressure whilst the heart is in diastole and is the lower or *diastolic pressure*. The range of normal readings varies according to age but in a young adult is approximately 100–120/70–80 mmHg. (In S.I. units pressure is measured in pascals (Pa) and blood pressure in kilopascals (kPa). Thus the range would be 15–16/9–11 kPa.) *B. serum*. Plasma without the clotting agents. The fluid that remains after blood or plasma has clotted. *B. sugar*. The amount of glucose present in the blood. The normal range is 2.5–4.7 mmol/litre. When the amount exceeds 10 mmol/litre glucose is excreted in the urine, as in diabetes mellitus. *B. transfusion.* Introduction of blood from the vein of one person (*donor*) or from a blood bank into the vein of another (*recipient*), in cases of severe loss of blood, trauma, septicaemia, etc. It is used to supplement the volume of blood and also to introduce constituents, such as clotting factors or antibodies, which are deficient in the patient. Clotting must be prevented in the transition stage. This is usually done by admixture with sodium citrate (1 g to 450 ml of blood). Too much sodium citrate tends to produce a reaction, and rigor and shock may occur. *B. urea*. Excretory product of protein present in the blood. The normal range is 3–7 mmol/litre. This increases in renal failure when the kidneys cease to function normally.

'blue baby' (*bloo ba'-be*). A child born with a very blue colour. The colour may be due to atelectasis or to a defect in the heart, in consequence of which arterial and venous blood become mixed. *See* Fallot's tetralogy.

blue paint (*bloo paint*). An antiseptic made from aniline dyes. It consists of 1% *brilliant green* and 1% *gentian violet* in 25% *spirit*. Both skin and linen are badly stained by it. Bonney's blue.

blush (*blush*). Growing redness of the face, usually a reaction to emotion or heat.

BMR. Basal metabolic rate.

Boeck's disease (*C.P.M. Boeck, Norwegian dermatologist, 1845–1917*). A form of sarcoidosis.

boil (*boil*). An acute staphylococcal inflammation of the skin and subcutaneous tissues round a hair follicle. It causes a painful swelling with a central core of dead tissue (*slough*), which is eventually discharged. A furuncle.

bolus (*bo'-lus*). (1) A large pill. (2) A rounded mass of masticated food immediately before being swallowed or one passing through the intestines. (3) A small quantity of a drug injected directly and rapidly into a vital organ where maximal concentrations are required.

bone (*bone*). The dense connective tissue forming the skeleton. It is composed of cartilage or membrane impregnated with mineral salts, chiefly calcium phosphate and calcium carbonate. This is arranged as an outer hard *compact* tissue and an inner network of cells (*cancellous* tissue), in the spaces of which is red bone marrow. In the shaft of long bones is a medullary cavity containing yellow marrow. Microscopically, the bone tissue is perforated with minute (*Haversian*) canals containing blood vessels and lymphatics for the maintenance and repair of the cells. Bone is covered by a fibrous membrane—the *periosteum*—containing blood vessels and by which the bone grows in girth. *B.-graft.* Transplantation of a healthy piece of bone to replace missing or repair defective bone. *B. marrow.* Substance which fills the marrow cavities of bones. Basically there are two types, yellow and red marrow. The red marrow is responsible for producing the blood cells.

Bonney's blue (*W.F.V. Bonney,*
British gynaecologist, 1872–1953). Blue paint.

borax (*bor'-aks*). A compound of soda and boric acid. Used as a mild antiseptic and as a mouthwash.

borborygmus (*bor-bor-ig'-mus*). A rumbling sound caused by gas in the intestines.

Bordetella (*bor-det-el'-ah*). A genus of bacteria. *B. pertussis.* The causal agent of whooping cough.

Bordet–Gengou bacillus (*J.J.B.V. Bordet, Belgian bacteriologist, 1870–1961; O. Gengou, French bacteriologist, 1875–1957*). *Bordetella pertussis.*

boric acid (*bor'-ik as'-id*). A mild antiseptic.

Bornholm disease (*born'-holm diz-eez'*). An epidemic myalgia with pleural pain due to Coxsackie virus infection. It receives its name from the Danish island of Bornholm where there was an outbreak in 1930.

botulism (*bot'-u-lizm*). A rare

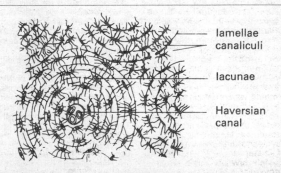

lamellae
canaliculi

lacunae

Haversian
canal

BONE

and dangerous form of food poisoning in which the central nervous system is affected by toxins produced by *Clostridium botulinum*. This is an anaerobic spore-forming organism from the soil and it survives in imperfectly canned vegetables and in meat and fish preparations, which may be otherwise normal in taste and appearance.

bougie (*boo'-je*). A flexible cylindrical instrument used to dilate a stricture, as in the oesophagus or urethra. *Medicated b.* A soluble form impregnated with a medicinal substance. Used for urethral treatment.

Bourneville's disease (*D.M. Bourneville, French neurologist, 1840–1909*). *See* Epiloia.

bovine (*bo'-vine*). Relating to the cow or ox. *B. tuberculosis.* That caused by infection from infected cow's milk, usually affecting glands and bones.

bowel (*bow'-el*). The intestine.

bow-leg (*bo'-leg*). Deformity where there is an outward curvature of one or both legs near the knee. This results in a gap between the knees on standing. Genu varum.

Bowman's capsule (*Sir W.P. Bowman, British physician, 1816–1892*). The expanded end of the kidney tubule which surrounds the glomerulus.

Boyle's anaesthetic machine (*H.E.G. Boyle, British surgeon, 1875–1941*). Apparatus by which chloroform, ether, nitrous oxide gas and now cyclopropane may be administered.

Boyle's law (*R. Boyle, British physicist, 1627–1691*). Law stating that at any determined temperature a known mass of gas varies in volume inversely as the pressure.

Bq. Abbreviation for the SI unit, the *becquerel*.

Br. Chemical symbol for *bromine*.

brace (*brase*). (1) A support used in orthopaedics to hold parts of the body in their correct positions. (2) An orthodontic appliance to correct the alignment of teeth.

brachial (*bra'-ke-al*). Relating to the arm. *B. artery.* The continuation of the axillary artery along the inner side of the upper arm. *B. plexus.* A network of nerves at the root of the neck supplying the upper limb.

brachium (*bra'-ke-um*). The arm, especially from shoulder to elbow.

brachycephaly (*brak-e-kef'-al-e*). The state of having a head shape in which the anteroposterior diameter is relatively short.

brachytherapy (*brak-e-ther'-ap-e*). Radiotherapy delivered into or adjacent to a tumour by means of an intracavitary or interstitial radioactive source. (*See also* Plesiotherapy.)

bradycardia (*brad-e-kar'-de-ah*). Abnormally low rate of heart contractions and consequent slow pulse.

bradykinin (*brad-e-ki'-nin*). Peptide formed from the degradation of protein by enzymes. It is a powerful vasodilator which also causes contraction of smooth muscle.

braille (*brale*). A method of printing developed by Louis Braille (*1809–1852*) for the blind. Letters of the alphabet are represented by patterns of raised dots. These dots are read by passing the finger tips over them.

brain (*brane*). That part of the central nervous system contained in the skull. It consists of the cerebrum, midbrain, cerebellum, medulla oblongata and pons varolii.

bran (*bran*). The husk of grain. The coarse outer coat of cereals. High in roughage and vitamins of the B complex. Frequently recommended as a dietary component both for those with alimentary disorders and for those in normal health.

branchial (*bran'-ke-al*). Relating to the clefts (branchia) that are present in the neck and pharynx in the developing embryo. Normally they disappear. *B. cyst.* A cystic swelling arising from a branchial remnant in the neck. *B. sinus* or *lateral cervical sinus.* A track leading from the posterior cervical region to open in the lower neck in front of the sternomastoid muscle.

Braun's frame (*H.F.W. Braun, German surgeon, 1862–1934*). A metal frame which incorporates one or more pulleys and is used chiefly to elevate the lower limb and to apply skeletal traction for a compound fracture of tibia and fibula.

breast (*brest*). (1) The anterior or front region of the chest. (2) The mammary gland. *B. abscess.* Formation of pus in the mammary gland. *B.bone.* The sternum. *Pigeon-b.* Prominent sternum, a deformity resulting from rickets. *B. pump.* An apparatus for removal of milk from the breast.

breech (*breech*). The buttocks. *B. presentation.* A position of the fetus in the uterus such that the buttocks present.

bregma (*breg'-mah*). The anterior fontanelle. The membranous junction between the coronal and sagittal sutures.

bridge (*brij*). In dentistry, an irremovable prosthesis carrying false teeth that bridges gaps left when natural teeth are extracted.

Bright's disease (*B. Bright, British physician, 1789–1858*). An inflammation of the kidneys. Nephritis.

brilliant green (*bril'-yant green*). An aniline dye used as an antiseptic.

British Pharmacopoeia (*brit'-ish far-mah-ko-pe'-ah*). *abbrev.* BP. List of 'official' drugs which is published by H.M. Stationary Office on behalf of the Health Minister. The drugs are listed on the recommendations of the Medicines Commission in accordance with the Medicines Act 1968.

broad ligaments (*brawd lig'-am-ents*). Folds of peritoneum extending from the uterus to the sides of the pelvis, and supporting the blood vessels to the uterus and uterine tubes.

Broca's area of speech (*P.P. Broca, French surgeon, 1824–1880*). The motor centre for speech, situated in the left cerebral hemisphere. Damage to the nerve cells contained in it can impair speech.

Brodie's abscess (*Sir B.C. Brodie, British surgeon, 1783–1862*). A chronic abscess of bone, usually the head of the tibia, caused by prolonged staphylococcal infection.

bromhidrosis (*brom-hid-ro'-sis*). Offensive and fetid sweat, especially associated with the feet.

bromide (*bro'-mide*). A compound of bromine. *Potassium b.*, *sodium b.* and *ammonium b.* can be prescribed as sedatives that are strongly depressant and cumulative in action.

bromine (*bro'-meen*). *abbrev.* Br. A poisonous, non-metallic liquid element.

bromocriptine (*bro-mo-krip'-teen*). A drug used in the treatment of parkinsonism, in cases where levodopa is not well tolerated.

bromsulphthalein (*brom-sulf-thal'-een*). A dye used in certain tests for liver function.

bronchiectasis (*brong-ke-ek'-tas-is*). Dilatation of the bronchi associated with the formation of fibrous tissue. The dilated bronchi become infected resulting in a copious secretion of pus. The symptoms include a chronic cough and purulent sputum.

bronchiole (*brong'-ke-ole*). One of the smallest of the subdivisions of the bronchi.

bronchiolitis (*brong-ke-o-li'-tis*). Inflammation of the bronchioles.

bronchitis (*brong-ki'-tis*). Inflammation of the bronchi. *Acute b.* A short-lived infection, common in young children and the elderly. It is a descending infection from the common cold, influenza, measles or other upper respiratory condition. *Chronic b.* A chronic infection, usually associated with infection of the upper respiratory tract. It may in time lead to emphysema.

bronchoadenitis (*brong'-ko-ad-en-i'-tis*). Inflammation of bronchial glands.

bronchodilator (*brong-ko-dila'-tor*). A drug that relaxes the plain muscle of the bronchi and bronchioles and so dilates them.

bronchography (*brong-kog'-raf-e*). X-ray photography of the bronchial tree after introduction of a radio-opaque medium.

bronchomycosis (*brong-ko-miko'-sis*). An industrial disease chiefly affecting agricultural workers, stablemen, etc., and due to inhalation of microfungi which infect the airpassages. Causes can be *Actinomyces* or *Aspergillus* species. Symptoms are similar to those of pulmonary tuberculosis.

bronchophony (*brong-koff'-on-e*). Resonance of the voice as heard in the chest over the bronchi on auscultation.

bronchopneumonia (*brong-ko-nu-mo'-ne-ah*). *See* Pneumonia.

bronchopulmonary (*brong-ko-pul'-mon-ar-e*). Relating to the lungs, bronchi and bronchioles.

bronchorrhoea (*brong-kor-e'-ah*). An excessive discharge of mucus from the bronchi.

bronchoscope (*brong'-ko-skope*). An instrument which enables the operator to see inside the bronchi. It can also be used to wash out the bronchi, to remove foreign bodies or to take a biopsy.

bronchoscopy (*brong-kos'-ko-pe*). Examination of the bronchi by means of a bronchoscope.

bronchospasm (*brong'-ko-spazm*). Difficulty in breathing caused by the sudden constriction of plain muscle in the walls of the bronchi. This may arise in asthma or chronic bronchitis.

bronchospirometer (*brong-ko-spi-rom'-e-ter*). An instrument used to measure the capacity of one lung or of one lobe of the lung, or of each lung separately.

bronchotracheal (*brong-ko-trak'-e-al*). Relating to both the trachea and the bronchi. *B. suction*. The removal of mucus with the aid of suction, using an electrical or foot-operated sucker.

bronchus (*brong'-kus*). *pl.* bronchi. A large air passage between the trachea and the bronchioles. The trachea itself divides into a *right* and *left principal bronchus*, and within the lungs are *lobar* and *segmental bronchi*.

brow (*brow*). The forehead. *B. presentation*. A position of the fetus such that the forehead appears at the cervix first.

brown adipose tissue (*brown ad'-ip-oze tis'-u*). Special type of adipose tissue found in the newborn infant, and which is widely distributed throughout the body. The tissue is highly vascular and owes its colour to the large number of mitochondria found in the cytoplasm of its cells. It allows the infant to increase its metabolic rate and thus its heat production when subjected to cold. At the same time the fat itself is used up.

Brown-Séquard syndrome (*C.E. Brown-Séquard, French physiologist, 1818–1894*). A condition arising when the spinal cord has been partly cut through. There is paralysis on the same side as the cut and sensory loss on the other side.

Brucella (*bru-sel'-ah*). A genus of bacteria primarily pathogenic in animals but which may affect man. *B. abortus* produces abortion in

cattle and undulant fever in man. *B. melitensis* in infected goats' milk causes brucellosis in man.

brucellosis (*bru-sel-o'-sis*). Undulant fever. An intermittent fever caused by bacteria of the genus *Brucella*. Malta fever.

Brudzinski's sign (*J. Brudzinski, Polish physician, 1874–1917*). (1) Passive flexion of one thigh causing spontaneous flexion of the opposite thigh. (2) Flexion of the neck causing bilateral flexion of the hips and knees. These signs are indicative of meningeal irritation.

bruise (*brooz*). A superficial injury to tissues produced by sudden impact in which the skin is unbroken. A contusion.

bruit (*bru'-e*). An abnormal sound or murmur heard on auscultation of the heart and large vessels.

Brunner's glands (*J.C. Brunner, Swiss anatomist, 1653–1727*). Small compound tubular glands in the mucous membrane of the duodenum.

bruxism (*bruks'-izm*). Teeth clenching, particularly during sleep. This occurs in persons under tension and may cause headaches due to muscle fatigue.

bubo (*bu'-bo*). Inflammation of the lymphatic glands of the axilla or groin. Typical of bubonic plague (*see* Plague) and venereal infections.

bubonocele (*bu-bon'-o-seel*). An inguinal hernia in the groin, resembling a bubo.

buccal (*buk'-al*). (1) Pertaining to the cheek. (2) Pertaining to the mouth.

buccinator (*buk'-sin-a-tor*). A muscle of the cheek, between the mandible and the maxilla.

Budd–Chiari syndrome (*G. Budd, British physician, 1808–1882; H. Chiari, Austrian pathologist, 1851–1916*). A condition in which thrombosis of the hepatic vein causes vomiting, jaundice, enlargement of the liver and ascites.

Buerger's disease (*L. Buerger, American physician, 1879–1943*). Thromboangeitis obliterans.

buffer (*buf'-er*). A chemical substance which, when present in a solution, will allow only a very slight change in reaction when an acid (or alkali) is added to it. Sodium bicarbonate is the chief buffer of the blood and tissue fluids.

bulbar (*bul'-bar*). Pertaining to the medulla oblongata. *B. paralysis.* See Paralysis.

bulbourethral (*bul-bo-u-re'-thral*). Relating to the bulb of the urethra (bulb of the penis). *B. glands.* Small glands opening into the male urethra. Cowper's glands.

bulimia (*bu-lim'-e-ah*). Excessive appetite.

bulla (*bul'-ah*). *pl.* bullae. A large blister.

Buller's shield (*F. Buller, Canadian ophthalmologist, 1844–1905*). A type of protection placed over one eye when the other is infected. A watch glass is placed over the eye and fixed with adhesive strapping. Now rarely used.

bumetamide (*bu-met'-am-ide*). A diuretic drug which prevents the resorption of urine from Henle's loop in the renal tubule.

bundle (*bundl*). A collection of nerve fibres all running in the same direction. *B. branch block.* The delay in conduction along either branch of the atrioventricular bundle of the

heart. The abnormality is detected by an ECG recording.

bundle of His (*L. His (Jr.), German physiologist, 1863–1934*). The band of neuro-muscular fibres which passing through the septum of the heart divides at the apex into two parts, these being distributed into the wall of the ventricles. The impulse of contraction is conducted through this structure. Atrioventricular bundle.

bunion (*bun'-yun*). A prominence of the head of the metatarsal bone at its junction with the great toe, caused by inflammation and swelling of the bursa at that joint. Usually due to shoes which distort the natural shape of the foot.

buphthalmos (*buf-thal'-mos*). A condition seen in infants where intraocular tension is raised. May be caused by failure of the iris root to separate from the cornea scleral junction or to a defect of the canal of Schlemm.

Burkitt's tumour (*D.P. Burkitt, Irish surgeon*). African lymphoma. A lymphosarcoma occurring almost exclusively in children living in low-lying moist areas of Central Africa. It is most commonly seen in the jaws.

burn (*bern*). An injury to tissues caused by: (1) physical agents, the sun, excess heat or cold, friction, nuclear radiations; (2) chemical agents, acids or caustic alkalis; (3) electrical current. Burns are described as being partial thickness (involving only the epidermis) or full thickness (involving the dermis and underlying structures). However, clinically, more emphasis is placed on the percentage of the body area affected by the burn. The treatment of shock and prevention of infection need special attention.

burr (*ber*). A bit for a surgical drill, used for cutting bone or teeth. *B. hole.* A circular hole drilled in the cranium to permit access to the brain or to release raised intercranial pressure.

bursa (*bur'-sah*). A small sac of fibrous tissue, lined with synovial membrane and containing synovial fluid. It is situated between parts that move upon one another at a joint to reduce friction.

bursitis (*bur-si'-tis*). Inflammation of a bursa. It produces pain and may impede movement of the joint. *Prepatellar b.* Housemaid's knee.

busulphan (*bu-sul'-fan*). A cytotoxic drug that depresses the bone marrow and may be used to treat myeloid leukaemia.

butobarbitone (*bu-to-bar'-bit-one*). An intermediate-acting barbiturate, formerly much used as a sedative. Now used only in severe insomnia.

buttock (*but'-ok*). Either of the two prominences formed by the flesh-covered gluteal muscles at either side of the lower spine.

by-pass (*bi'-pas*). Diversion of flow. Formation of a shunt. *Aortocoronary b.* Diversion of flow to the coronary arteries via a saphenous vein or artificial graft. *Femoropopliteal b.* Diversion of flow from the femoral to the popliteal artery to overcome an occlusion.

byssinosis (*bis-in-o'-sis*). An industrial disease caused by inhalation of cotton or linen dust in factories. A type of pneumoconiosis.

C

C. (1) Chemical symbol for *carbon.* (2) Abbreviation for *centigrade* or *Celsius.* (3) Abbreviation for the SI unit, the *coulomb.*

Ca. Chemical symbol for *calcium.*

cachectic (*kak-ek'-tik*). Pertaining to cachexia.

cachet (*kash'-a*). Two pieces of wafer, joined in the form of a capsule to contain an unpalatable medicine.

cachexia (*kak-eks'-e-ah*). A condition of extreme debility. The patient is emaciated, the skin being loose and wrinkled from rapid wasting, but shiny and tense over bone. The eyes are sunken, the skin yellowish, and there is a grey 'muddy' complexion. The mucous membranes are pale and anaemia is extreme. The condition is typical of the late stages of chronic diseases.

cadaver (*kad-av'-er*). A corpse. The dead body used for dissection.

cadmium (*kad'-me-um*). *abbrev.* Cd. A metallic element. Inhalation of fumes from the molten metal can cause lung irritation and, in the long term, renal impairment.

caecostomy (*se-kos'-tom-e*). The making of an opening into the caecum by incision through the abdominal wall.

caecum (*se'-kum*). The blind pouch forming the beginning of the large intestine. The vermiform appendix is attached to it.

caesarean section (*se-zair'-e-an sek'-shun*). Delivery of a fetus by an incision through the abdominal wall and uterus. Should not be done before the 28th week of gestation. Performed for the safety of either the mother or the infant. Tradition has it that Julius Caesar was born in this way.

caesium (*se'-ze-um*). *abbrev.* Cs. A metallic element. *C.-137.* Radioactive caesium; a fission product from uranium. Sealed in a suitable container it can be used instead of cobalt for beam therapy; or sealed in needles, tubes or applicators it can be used for local application.

caffeine (*kaf'-een*). An alkaloid of tea and coffee which acts as a nerve stimulant and diuretic. Mixed with aspirin and codeine, it is often used as an analgesic.

caisson disease (*ka'-son diz-eez'*). Decompression sickness.

calamine (*kal'-am-ine*). Preparation of zinc carbonate or zinc oxide coloured pink with ferric oxide. It is an astringent and antipruritic used in lotion or ointment form for skin diseases.

calcaneum (*kal-ka'-ne-um*). The heel bone. Calcaneus.

calcareous (*kal-kar'-e-us*). Chalky. Containing lime.

calciferol (*kal-sif'-er-ol*). The chemical name for vitamin D.

calcification (*kal-sif-ik-a'-shun*). (1) The deposit of lime in any tissue, e.g. in the formation of callus. (2) The deposit of lime salts in cartilage as part of the normal process of bone formation.

calcitonin (*kal-se-to'-nin*). Hormone produced by the thyroid gland which regulates blood calcium levels.

calcium (*kal'-se-um*). *abbrev.* Ca. A metallic element necessary for the normal development and functioning of the body. A constituent of bones and teeth. Deficiency or excess of serum calcium causes nerve and muscle dysfunctions and abnormalities in blood clotting. The correct concentration is regulated by hormones. *C. carbonate.* Chalk. *C. gluconate.* A compound that is easily absorbed and can be given by intramuscular or intravenous route to raise the blood calcium. *C. hydroxide.* Slaked lime. *C. lactate.* A compound that increases the coagulability of blood.

calculus (*kal'-ku-lus*). *pl.* calculi. A stony concretion which may be formed in any of the secreting organs of the body or their ducts. *Arthritic c.* Gouty deposits in or near joints. *Biliary c.* Gall-stone. *Coral c.* A large stone in the kidney, with branches resembling coral. *Mulberry c.* A gall-stone made of calcium

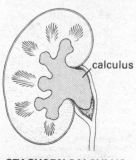

calculus

STAGHORN CALCULUS

oxalate and shaped like a mulberry. *Renal c.* One formed in the kidney. *Salivary c.* Stone in a salivary duct. *Staghorn c.* A many-branched stone sometimes found in the renal pelvis. *Urinary c.* One found anywhere in the urinary tract. *Vesical c.* Stone formed in the urinary bladder.

Caldwell–Luc operation (*G.W. Caldwell, American otolaryngologist, 1834–1918; H. Luc, French laryngologist, 1855–1925*). An antrostomy operation to drain the maxillary sinus. The incision is made above the upper canine tooth.

calibrator (*kal'-e-bra-tor*). (1) An instrument for measuring the size of openings. (2) An instrument used to dilate a tube, e.g. in urethral stricture.

caliper (*kal'-ip-er*). (1) *sing.* A two-pronged instrument that

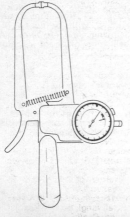

SKINFOLD CALIPERS

may be used to exert traction on a part. *Walking c.* An appliance fitted to a boot or shoe to give support to the lower limb. It may be used when the muscles are paralysed or in the repair stage of fractures. (2) *pl.* Compasses for measuring diameters and curved surfaces. *Skinfold c.* An instrument used in nutritional assessment for determining the amount of body fat. A fold of skin and subcutaneous tissue, usually over the triceps muscle, is pinched away from the underlying muscle using the thumb and forefinger.

callisthenics (*kal-is-then'-iks*). Mild gymnastics for developing the muscles and producing a graceful carriage.

callosity (*kal-os'-it-e*). The plaques of thickened skin often seen on the soles of the feet or the palms of the hand.

callous (*kal'-us*). Hard and thickened.

callus (*kal'-us*). (1) A callosity. (2) The tissue which grows round fractured ends of bone and develops into new bone to repair the injury.

Calmette–Guérin bacillus (*A.L.C. Calmette, French bacteriologist, 1863–1933; C. Guérin, French bacteriologist, b. 1872*). A deactivated tuberculosis bacillus from which the antituberculosis vaccine, BCG vaccine, is made.

calor (*kal'-or*). Heat (*Latin*). One of the signs of inflammation.

caloric (*kal-or'-ik*). Pertaining to heat or calories.

calorie (*kal'-or-e*). A unit of heat. Used to denote physiological values of various food substances, estimated according to the amount of heat they produce on being oxidized in the body. *See* Oxidation. A *Calorie* (or *kilo-calorie*) represents the heat required in raising 1 kg (1000 g or 2.2 lb) by 1°C. A *small calorie* equals the heat produced in raising 1 g of water by 1°C. In the SI system the calorie is replaced by the joule (1 Cal = 4.18 kJ).

calorific (*kal-or-if'-ik*). Heat-producing.

calorimeter (*kal-or-im'-e-ter*). An apparatus for measuring the heat that is produced or lost during a chemical or physical change.

calvaria (*kal-va'-re-ah*). The upper, dome-like part of the skull.

calvities (*kal-vish'-e-eez*). Baldness.

calx (*kalks*). Calcium oxide or lime. The basis of slaked lime, bleaching powder and quicklime.

calyx (*ka'-lix*). *pl.* calyces. Any cup-shaped vessel or part. *C. of kidney.* The cup-like terminations of the ureter in the renal pelvis surrounding the pyramids of the kidney.

camphor (*kam'-for*). A crystalline substance prepared from the camphor laurel. It is used internally as a carminative. *Camphorated oil* is 1 part camphor to 4 parts oil prepared for external application as a rubefacient.

campimetry (*kam-pim'-e-tre*). Assessment of the central part of the visual field.

canal (*kan-al'*). A tubular passage. *Alimentary c.* The passage along which the food passes on its way through the body. *Cervical c.* That through the cervix of the uterus. *Haversian c.* One of the minute channels that are present in bone. *C. of Schlemm.* That which drains the aqueous humour. *Semicircular c.* One of the three canals in the middle ear responsible for maintenance of balance.

canaliculus (*kan-al-ik'-u-lus*). *pl.* canaliculi. A small channel or canal.

cancellous (*kan-sel'-us*). Being porous or spongy. Applied to the honeycomb type of bone tissue in the ends of long bones and in flat and irregular bones. *See* Tissue.

cancer (*kan'-ser*). A general term to describe malignant growths in tissues, of which *carcinoma* is of epithelial and *sarcoma* of connective tissue origin, as in bone and muscle. A cancerous growth is one which is not encapsulated, but infiltrates into surrounding tissues, the cells of which it replaces by its own. It is spread by the lymph and blood vessels and causes metastases in other parts of the body. Death is caused by destruction of organs to a degree incompatible with life; to extreme debility and anaemia; or to haemorrhage.

cancroid (*kan'-kroid*). (1) *adj.* Resembling cancer. (2) *n.* A skin tumour of moderate degree of malignancy.

cancrum oris (*kan-krum aw'-ris*). Gangrenous stomatitis. An ulceration of the mouth, which is a rare complication of measles in debilitated children. Noma.

candela (*kan-de'-lah* or *kan'-del-ah*). (1) SI unit of luminous intensity. *abbrev.* cd. (2) A medicinal candle used in fumigation.

Candida (*kan'-did-ah*). A genus of small fungi, formerly called *Monilia. C. albicans.* The variety which causes candidiasis.

candidiasis (*kan-did-i'-as-is*).

Infection, usually superficial, by the *Candida* fungus. Occurs particularly in moist areas such as mouth, vagina, skin folds. Popularly known as thrush.

canine (*ka'-nine*). (1) *adj.* Pertaining to a dog. (2) *n.* An 'eye tooth'. There are two in each jaw between the incisors and the molars.

cannabis (*kan'-ab-is*). Marihuana,hashish. An illegal drug which may be swallowed or smoked and produces hallucinations and a temporary sense of well-being, followed by extreme lethargy.

cannula (*kan'-u-lah*). A hollow tube for insertion into the body by which fluids are introduced or removed. Usually a trocar is fitted into it to facilitate its introduction.

cantharides (*kan-thar'-id-eez*). An extract from the body of the Spanish fly, applied externally as a counter-irritant to raise a blister.

canthus (*kan'-thus*). The angle formed by the junction of the upper and lower eyelids.

capillarity (*kap-il-ar'-it-e*). The action by which a liquid will rise upwards in a fibrous substance or in a fine tube. Capillary attraction.

capillary (*kap-il'-ar-e*). (1) *adj.* Hair-like. (2) *n.* A minute vessel connecting an arteriole and a venule. (3) *n.* A minute vessel of the lymphatic system.

capitellum (*kap-it-el'-um*). Capitulum (*kap-it'-u-lum*). (1) The small rounded head at the elbow end of the humerus. (2) The bulb of a hair.

capsular (*kap'-su-lar*). Relating to a capsule. *C. ligaments.* Those which completely sur-

round a moveable joint, forming a capsule which loosely encloses the bones and is lined with synovial membrane which secretes a fluid for lubrication of the articular surfaces. Known also as *articular capsule*.

capsule (*kap'-sule*). (1) A fibrous or membranous sac enclosing an organ. (2) A small soluble case of gelatin in which a nauseous medicine may be enclosed. (3) The gelatinous envelope which surrounds and protects some bacteria.

capsulectomy (*kap-su-lek'-tom-e*). Surgical excision of a capsule.

capsulitis (*kap-su-li'-tis*). Inflammation of the capsule of a joint.

capsulotomy (*kap-su-lot'-om-e*). The incision of a capsule, particularly that of a joint or of the lens of the eye.

caput (*kap'-ut*). Head. *C. succedaneum.* A transient soft swelling on an infant's head due to pressure during labour, which disappears within the first few days of life.

carbachol (*karb'-ak-ol*). A drug related to and acting like acetylcholine, but more stable. It causes contraction of plain muscle and relaxation of the voluntary sphincter, so relieving postoperative retention of urine. Also used in the treatment of glaucoma.

carbamazepine (*kar-bam-az'-ep-een*). A drug used to control epilepsy and also in the treatment of trigeminal neuralgia.

carbaminohaemoglobin (*kar-bam'-in-o-he-mo-glo'-bin*). A compound of carbon dioxide and haemoglobin, present in the blood.

carbenicillin (*kar-ben-is-il'-in*). A synthetic penicillin which is active against a wide range of bacteria. Must be given by injection as it is poorly absorbed from the gastrointestinal tract.

carbenoxolone (*karb-en-oks'-o-lone*). An anti-inflammatory drug used in the treatment of gastric ulcers.

carbimazole (*kar-bim'-az-ol*). An antithyroid drug that is used to stabilize a patient with thyrotoxicosis.

carbo (*kar'-boh*). Charcoal. *C. ligni*. Medicinal wood charcoal. Used for the relief of digestive disorders and diarrhoea.

carbohydrate (*karb-o-hi'-drate*). That class of food represented by the starches and sugars—they are energy- and heat-producing substances.

carbolfuchsin (*karb-ol-fook'-sin*). A mixture of carbolic acid and fuchsin used for staining purposes in bacteriology.

carbolic acid (*karb-ol'-ik as'-id*). Phenol.

carbon (*kar'-bon*). abbrev. C. A non-metallic element. *C. dioxide*. A gas which, dissolved in water, forms weak carbonic acid. As a product of metabolism by the oxidation of carbon, it leaves the body by the lungs. It can be compressed till it freezes, and then forms a solid—*carbon dioxide snow*—used to destroy superficial naevi. Inhalations of the gas in a 5–7% mixture with oxygen are useful to stimulate the depth of respiration. *C. monoxide*. A colourless gas that is very poisonous. It is a major constituent of coal gas and is also usually present in the exhaust gases from petrol

and diesel engines. In poisoning there is vertigo, flushed face with very red lips, loss of consciousness, and convulsions. The blood is bright red because of the formation of carboxyhaemoglobin. *C. tetrachloride*. A powerful anthelmintic used in treating hookworm and whipworm but which in certain individuals can lead to severe necrosis of liver cells. It is also used in fire extinguishers and as a cleaning fluid.

carboxyhaemoglobin (*karboks'-e-he-mo-glo'-bin*). The combination of carbon monoxide with haemoglobin in the blood in carbon monoxide poisoning.

carbuncle (*kar'-bung-kl*). An acute staphylococcal inflammation of subcutaneous tissues, which causes local thrombosis in the veins and death of tissue. In appearance it resembles a collection of boils.

carcinogen (*kar-sin'-o-jen*). Any substance which can produce a cancer.

carcinogenic (*kar-sin-o-jen'-ik*). Pertaining to agents which produce or predispose to cancer. Crude oils are said to contain a *c. factor*.

carcinoid (*kar'-sin-oid*). A yellow, malignant tumour of the small intestine, appendix, stomach or colon. Release of substances from this tumour cause the *c. syndrome*.

carcinoma (*kar-sin-o'-mah*). A malignant growth of epithelial tissue. Microscopically the cells resemble those of the tissue in which the growth has arisen. *Adenoid c*. Adenocarcinoma. *Basal cell c*. A rodent ulcer. (*see* Ulcer). *Epithelial c*. Epithelioma. *Squamous* *cell c.* One arising from the squamous epithelium of the skin.

carcinomatosis (*kar-sin-o-mat-o'-sis*). The condition when a carcinoma has given rise to widespread metastases.

cardia (*kar'-de-ah*). The cardiac orifice of the stomach.

cardiac (*kar'-de-ak*). Pertaining to the heart. *C. arrest.* The cessation of the heart beat. *C. asthma. See* Asthma. *C. atrophy.* Fatty degeneration of the heart muscle. *C. bed.* One which can be manipulated to form a chair shape for those heart cases who are comfortable only when sitting up. *C. catheterization.* A procedure whereby a radio-opaque catheter is passed from an arm vein to the heart. Its passage through the heart can be watched on a screen. Also blood pressure readings and specimens can be taken, thus aiding diagnosis of heart abnormalities. *C. cycle.* The sequence of events lasting about 0.8 seconds during which the heart completes one contraction. *C. massage.* Rhythmic compression of the heart performed in order to re-establish circulation of the blood in cardiac arrest. *C. monitor.* Equipment used to monitor the cardiac cycle.

cardialgia (*kar-de-al'-je-ah*). Pain in the region of the heart. Cardiodynia.

cardinal (*kar'-din-al*). Of first importance. Fundamental. *C. ligaments.* Deep transverse cervical ligaments. Mackenrodt's ligaments.

cardiodynia (*kar-de-o-din'-e-ah*). Cardialgia.

cardiogenic (*kar-de-o-jen'-ik*). Originating in the heart. *C. shock.* Shock caused by disease or failure of heart action.

cardiography (*kar-de-og'-raf-e*). The recording of the force and movements of the heart.

cardiology (*kar-de-ol'-o-je*). The study of the heart—how it works, and its diseases.

cardiolysis (*kar-de-ol'-is-is*). The breaking down of adhesions between the pericardium and chest wall by operation.

cardiomyopathy (*kar-de-o-mi-op'-ath-e*). A chronic disorder of the heart muscle not resulting from atherosclerosis.

cardiopathy (*kar-de-op'-ath-e*). Any disease of the heart.

cardiopulmonary (*kar-de-o-pul'-mon-ar-e*). Relating to the heart and lungs. *C. bypass.* The use of the heart–lung machine to oxygenate and pump the blood round the body while the surgeon operates on the heart.

cardiospasm (*kar'-de-o-spazm*). Spasm of the sphincter muscle at the cardiac end of the stomach. It may result in dilatation of the oesophagus, difficulty in swallowing solids and liquids, and regurgitation of undigested food. Achalasia.

cardiotocography (*kar-de-o-to-kog'-raf-e*). The simultaneous recording of the fetal heart rate, fetal movements and the uterine contractions in order to discover possible lack of oxygen (hypoxia) to the fetus. Fetal monitoring.

cardiotomy (*kar-de-ot'-om-e*). Surgical incision into the heart or the cardia. *C. syndrome.* An inflammatory reaction following heart surgery. There is pyrexia, pericarditis, and pleural effusion.

cardiotoxic (*kar-de-o-tok'-sik*). Anything which has a deleterious or poisonous effect on the heart.

cardiovascular (*kar-de-o-vas'-ku-lar*). Concerning the heart and blood vessels. *C. system.* The heart together with the two chief networks of blood vessels, the systemic circulation and the pulmonary circulation.

cardioversion (*kar-de-o-ver'-shun*). A method of terminating abnormal heart rhythm as in atrial fibrillation by means of an electric shock.

carditis (*kar-di'-tis*). Inflammation of the heart.

caries (*kair'-re-eez*). Suppuration and subsequent decay of bone, corresponding to ulceration in soft tissues. In *caries*, the bone dissolves; in *necrosis* it separates in large pieces and is thrown off. *Dental c.* Decay of the teeth due to penetration of bacteria through the enamel to the dentine. *Spinal c.* Tuberculosis of the spine. Pott's disease.

carina (*kar'-een-ah*). A keel-like structure. Usually applied to the bifurcation of the trachea into the bronchi as the terminal cartilage is keel-shaped.

carminative (*kar'-min-at-iv*). An aromatic drug which relieves flatulence. Cloves, ginger, cardamon, and peppermint are examples.

carneous (*kar'-ne-us*). Fleshy. *C. mole.* A tumour of organized blood clot surrounding a dead fetus in the uterus. *See* Abortion.

carotene (*kar'-ot-een*). The colouring matter in carrots, tomatoes and other yellow foods and fats. It is a provitamin capable of conversion into vitamin A in the liver.

carotid (*kar-ot'-id*). The principal artery on each side of the neck. *C. bodies.* Chemoreceptors in the bifurcation of both carotid arteries that monitor the oxygen content of the blood. *C. sinuses.* Dilated portions of the internal carotids containing the baroreceptors which monitor blood pressure.

carpal (*kar'-pal*). Relating to the carpus or wrist. *C. tunnel syndrome.* Compression of the median nerve at the wrist causing numbing and tingling in the fingers.

carphology (*kar-fol'-o-je*). Constant picking at bedclothes, occurring in cases of serious illness, especially typhoid.

carpopedal (*kar-po-pe'-dal*). Relating to the wrist and foot. *C. spasm.* Spasm of the hands and feet such as occurs in tetany.

carpus (*kar'-pus*). The eight bones forming the wrist and arranged in two rows: (1) scaphoid, lunate, triquetral, pisiform, (2) trapezium, trapezoid, capitate, hamate.

carrier (*kar'-e-er*). (1) A person who harbours the micro-organisms of an infectious disease, but is not necessarily affected by it, although he may infect others. (2) One who carries and passes on a hereditary abnormality.

cartilage (*kar'-til-aje*). Gristle. A tough connective tissue of three varieties: (1) *Hyaline c.* A dense groundwork containing cartilaginous cells, forming the embryonic bones before ossification and covering the articular surfaces of bone. (2) *Fibro-c.* Cartilage in which bundles of white fibres predominate, forming the intervertebral discs and costal cartilages. (3) *Elastic c.* Cartilage containing elastic fibres and

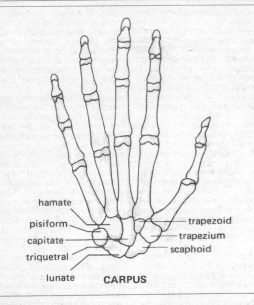

hamate
pisiform
capitate
triquetral
lunate
trapezoid
trapezium
scaphoid

CARPUS

forming the pinna of the ear, the epiglottis and part of the nasal septum.

cartilaginous (*kar-til-aj'-in-us*). Of the nature of cartilage.

caruncle (*kar-ung'-kl*). A small fleshy swelling. *Lacrimal c.* A small reddish body situated at the medial junction of the eyelids. *Urethral c.* A small fleshy growth occurring at the urinary orifice in females, and giving rise to great pain on micturition.

cascara (*kas-kar'-ah*). A laxative prepared from the bark of the Californian buckthorn. It may be prepared as an elixir or as tablets.

caseation (*ka-se-a'-shun*). De-

generation of diseased tissue into a cheesy mass.

casein (*ka'-se-in*). The chief protein of milk. It forms a curd from which cheese is made. *C. hydrolysate.* A predigested concentrated protein; a useful supplement for a high protein diet.

caseinogen (*ka-se-in'-o-jen*). A phosphate present in milk and precipitated when milk goes sour. The precursor of casein—activated by rennin.

cast (*kahst*). A piece of material thrown off in various diseases, and moulded to the shape of that part in which it has accumulated. *Renal c.* or *hyaline c.* are degenerating cells cast off into the urine in some cases of chronic kidney disease. *Plaster c.* A stiff dressing used to immobilize broken bones.

castor oil (*kah'-stor oil*). A vegetable oil. Internally it is a purgative, least nauseous when given with lemon or brandy. Externally it is protective and soothing and may be used in ointments or in eye drops.

castration (*kas-tra'-shun*). Removal of the testicles or, in a female, the ovaries.

CAT. Computerized axial tomography. *See* Tomography.

catabolism (*kat-ab'-ol-izm*). The chemical breakdown of complex substances in the body to form simpler ones, with a release of energy. *See* Metabolism.

catalase (*kat'-al-aze*). An enzyme found in body cells including red blood cells and liver cells.

catalepsy (*kat-al-ep'-se*). (1) A nervous state characterized by a trance-like sleep with passive rigidity of the muscles. During an attack the limbs will remain in any position in which they are placed. (2) A stage of hypnosis where the limbs remain rigid and in any position suggested.

catalyst (*kat'-al-ist*). A substance which hastens or brings about a chemical change without itself undergoing alteration. Enzymes act as catalysts in the process of digestion, for example.

catamenia (*kat-ah-me'-ne-ah*). Menstruation.

cataplasm (*kat'-ah-plazm*). A poultice. It acts as a counter-irritant. Materials of which it can be made are: *linseed*,

bread and *bran*. Kaolin is more frequently used.

cataplexy (*kat-ah-plek'-se*). Sudden recurrent loss of muscle power without unconsciousness, often associated with narcolepsy. It may be produced by any strong emotion.

cataract (*kat'-ar-akt*). Opacity of the crystalline lens of the eye causing partial or complete blindness. It may be congenital, or may be due to senility, injury or diabetes.

catarrh (*kat-ar'*). Simple inflammation of a mucous membrane accompanied by an excessive discharge of mucus. It is usually a chronic condition of the nose or nasopharynx with few signs of inflammation.

catatonia (*kat-ah-to'-ne-ah*). A syndrome of motor abnormalities occurring in schizophrenia, but less commonly in organic cerebral disease, characterized by stupor and the adoption of strange postures, or outbursts of excitement and hyperactivity. The patient may change suddenly from one of these states to the other.

catecholamines (*kat-e-kol-am'-eens*). A group of compounds that have the effect of sympathetic nerve stimulation. They have an aromatic and an amine portion and include dopamine, adrenaline and noradrenaline.

catgut (*kat'-gut*). A substance prepared from the intestines of sheep and used in surgery for sutures and ligatures. It becomes gradually absorbed in the body.

catharsis (*kath-ar'-sis*). (1) Purgation, e.g. of the bowels. (2) Abreaction.

cathartic (*kath-ar'-tik*). A purgative drug.

catheter (*kath'-et-er*). A fine hollow tube for removing or inserting fluid into a body cavity. Most commonly used to drain the urinary bladder through the urethra, when it is made of plastic material or rubber. *Cardiac c.* A plastic one used in investigation of heart abnormalities. *See* Cardiac. *Eustachian c.* A silver one used to open up the pharyngotympanic tube. *Self-retaining c.* A catheter made in such a way that after introduction the blind end expands so that it can remain in the bladder. Useful for continuous or intermittent drainage or where frequent specimens are required. *Ureteric c.* A fine gum-elastic catheter passed up the ureter to the renal pelvis and used to insert a dye in retrograde pyelography.

catheterization (*kath'-et-er-i-za'-shun*). The insertion of a catheter into a body cavity.

cathode (*kath'-ode*). (1) The negative electrode or pole of an electric current. (2) The negative pole of a battery. *See* Anode.

cation (*kat'-i-on*). A positively charged ion which moves towards the cathode when an electric current is passed through an electrolytic solution, e.g. hydrogen (H^+), sodium (Na^+). *See* Anion.

cauda (*kaw'-dah*). A tail-like appendage. *C. equina.* The bundle of coccygeal, sacral and lumbar nerves with which the spinal cord terminates.

caudal (*kaw'-dal*). Referring to a cauda. *C. block.* An anaesthetic agent injected into the sacral canal, so that operations may be carried out in the perineal area without a general anaesthetic.

caul (*kawl*). The amnion, which occasionally does not rupture but envelops the infant's head at birth.

causalgia (*kawz-al'-je-ah*). An intense burning pain which persists after peripheral nerve injuries.

caustic (*kaws'-tik*). A substance, usually a strong acid or alkali, capable of burning organic tissue. Silver nitrate (*lunar c.*), carbolic acid, and carbon dioxide snow are those most commonly used in surgery.

cauterization (*kaw-ter-i-za'-shun*). The destruction of tissue by burning with a cautery.

cautery (*kaw'-ter-e*). An instrument used in cauterization. *Actual c.* A red- or white-hot iron cautery. *Electric c.* A wire cautery heated to red or white heat by means of electricity. Diathermy

cavernous (*kav'-er-nus*). Having caverns or hollows. *C. breathing.* Sounds heard on auscultation over a pulmonary cavity. *C. sinus.* A venous channel lying on either side of the body of the sphenoid bone through which pass the internal carotid artery and several nerves. *C. sinus thrombosis.* A very serious complication of any infection of the face, the veins from the orbit draining into the sinus and carrying the infection into the cranium.

cavitation (*kav-it-a'-shun*). The formation of cavities, e.g. in the lung in tuberculosis.

cavity (*kav'-it-e*). A confined space or hollow with containing walls, e.g. the abdominal cavity or a decayed hollow in

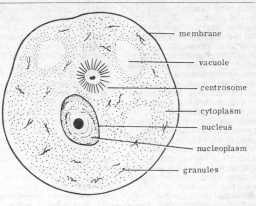

membrane
vacuole
centrosome
cytoplasm
nucleus
nucleoplasm
granules

CELL

a tooth.

Cd. Chemical symbol for *cadmium*.

cell (*sel*). A microscopic mass of protoplasm, consisting of a nucleus surrounded by cytoplasm and enclosed in a cell membrane, from which all organic tissues are constructed. Each cell can reproduce itself by mitosis.

cellulitis (*sel-u-li'-tis*). A diffuse inflammation of connective tissue, especially of subcutaneous tissue, which causes a typical brawny, oedematous appearance of the part; local abscess formation is not common.

cellulose (*sel'-u-loze*). A carbohydrate forming the covering of vegetable cells, i.e. vegetable fibres. Not digestible in the alimentary tract of man, but gives bulk, and as 'roughage' stimulates peristalsis.

Celsius scale (*A. Celsius, Swedish astronomer, 1701–1744*). A temperature scale with the melting point of ice set at 0° and the boiling point of water at 100°. The normal temperature of the human body is 36.9°C. Formerly known as the *centigrade* scale. *See* Fahrenheit.

cementum (*se-ment'-um*). Cement. Connective tissue with a bone-like structure which covers the root of a tooth and supports it within the socket.

censor (*sen'-sor*). In psychiatry, according to Freud, the psychic phenomenon which normally prevents impressions from the unconscious mind reaching the consciousness.

centigrade (*sen'-te-grade*). *See* Celsius scale.

central (*sen'-tral*). Pertaining to the centre or mid-point. *C. nervous system*. CNS. The brain and spinal cord. *C. venous pressure*. The pressure recorded by the introduction of a catheter into the right atrium, in order to monitor the condition of a patient after major operative procedures such as heart surgery.

centrifugal (*sen-trif'-u-gal*). Conveying away from a centre such as from the brain to the periphery. Efferent.

centrifuge (*sen'-tre-fuje*). An apparatus that rotates at high speed. If a test-tube, for example, is filled with a fluid such as blood or urine, and this is rotated in a centrifuge, any bacteria, cells, or other solids in it are precipitated.

centripetal (*sen-trip'-et-al*). The reverse of centrifugal. Conveying from the periphery to the centre. Afferent.

centromere (*sen'-tro-meer*). The region(s) of the chromosomes which become(s) allied with the spindle fibres at mitosis and meiosis.

centrosome (*sen'-tro-some*). A body in the cytoplasm of most animal cells, close to the nucleus. It divides during mitosis and half migrates to each daughter cell.

centrosphere (*sen'-tro-sfeer*). The cell centre, an area of clear cytoplasm near the nucleus.

cephalalgia (*kef-al-al'-je-ah*). Pain in the head.

cephalexin (*kef-al-ek'-sin*). A cephalosporin antibiotic that may be administered orally.

cephalhaematoma (*kef-al-he-mat-o'-mah*). A swelling beneath the pericranium, containing blood, which may be found on the head of the newborn infant. Caused by pressure during a long labour. Gradually reabsorbed within the first few days of life.

cephalic (*kef-al'-ik*). Relating to or situated near the head. *C. version*. The method used to convert a transverse into a head presentation to facilitate labour.

cephalocele (*kef'-al-o-seel*). Cerebral hernia. *See* Hernia.

cephalography (*kef-al-og'-raf-e*). An X-ray examination of the contours of the head.

cephalometry (*kef-al-om'-et-re*). Measurement of the fetal head by radiography. Cephalopelvimetry. *See* Pelvimetry.

cephaloridine (*kef-al-or'-id-een*). An antibiotic that is effective against a wide range of organisms.

cephalosporin (*kef-al-o-spor'-in*). Any one of a group of wide-spectrum antibiotics derived from the mould *Cephalosporium*.

cephradine (*kef'-rad-een*). A cephalosporin antibiotic similar in action to cephaloridine.

cerebellum (*ser'-e-bel'-um*). The portion of the brain below the cerebrum and above the medulla oblongata. The largest part of the hindbrain.

cerebral (*ser'-e-bral*). Relating to the cerebrum. *C. cortex*. The outer layer of the cerebrum composed of neurones. *C. haemorrhage*. Rupture of a cerebral blood vessel. Likely causes are aneurysm and hypertension. *See* Apoplexy. *C. hernia. See* Hernia. *C. irritation*. A condition of general nervous irritability and abnormality, often with photophobia, which may be an early sign of meningitis, tumour of the brain, etc. It is also associated with trauma. *C. palsy*. A condition caused by injury to the brain during or immediately after birth. Coordination of movement is affected, and may cause the child to be flaccid or athetoid, in which condition there is constant random and uncontrolled movement. *See* Spastic.

cerebration (*ser-e-bra'-shun*). Mental activity.

cerebritis (*ser-e-bri'-tis*). Inflammation of the brain.

cerebrospinal (*ser-e-bro-spi'-nal*). Relating to the brain and spinal cord. *C. fever*. A meningitis caused by the bacterium, *Neisserium meningitidis*, the meningococcus. *C. fluid*. CSF. The fluid made in the choroid plexus of the ventricles of the brain and circulating from them into the subarachnoid space around the brain and spinal cord.

cerebrovascular (*ser-e-bro-vas'-ku-lah*). Pertaining to the arteries and veins of the brain. *C. accident*. A disorder arising from an embolus, thrombus or haemorrhage in the cerebrum. *C. disease*. Any disorder of the blood vessels of the brain and its meninges.

cerebrum (*ser'-e-brum*). The largest part of the brain, occupying the greater portion of the cranium and consisting of the right and left hemispheres. The centre of the higher functions of the brain.

cerumen (*ser-u'-men*). A waxy substance secreted by the ceruminous glands of the auditory canal. Ear-wax.

cervical (*ser-vi'-kal*). Pertaining to the neck or the constricted part of an organ, e.g. uterine cervix, *C. canal*. The passage through the uterine cervix. *C. cancer*. Cancer of the uterine cervix. *C. collar*. A rigid or semi-rigid immobilizing support for the neck. *C. rib*. A short, extra rib, often bilateral, which sometimes occurs on the seventh cervical vertebra and may cause pressure on an artery or nerve. *C. smear*. A test for disorders of the cervical cells—material is scraped from the uterine cervix and examined microscopically. *C. spondylosis*. A degenerative disease of the intervertebral joints and discs of the neck. *C. vertebra*. One of the seven bones forming the neck portion of the spinal column.

cervicitis (*ser-vis-i'-tis*). Inflammation of the neck of the uterus.

cervix (*ser'-viks*). A constricted portion or neck. *C. uteri*. The neck of the uterus; it is about 2 cm long and projects into the vagina. Capable of wide dilatation during childbirth.

cestode (*ses'-tode*). Tapeworm.

cetrimide (*set'-re-mide*). Cetyltrimethylammonium bromide (CTAB). A detergent and antiseptic widely used for preoperative skin preparation and the cleansing of wounds.

cevitamic acid (*se-vit-am'-ik*

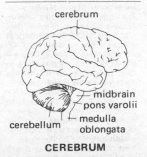

cerebrum

midbrain
pons varolii
medulla
oblongata

cerebellum

CEREBRUM

as'-id). Ascorbic acid. Vitamin C.

chafe (*chafe*). Irritation of the skin as caused by the friction between skin folds. Occurs particularly in moist areas.

chalazion (*kal-az'-e-on*). A meibomian or tarsal cyst. A swollen sebaceous gland in the eyelid. A small, hard tumour may develop.

chalicosis (*kal-ik-o'-sis*). An old term for a condition resembling silicosis, but found mainly among stone-cutters and due to the inhalation of stone dust.

chancre (*shan'-ker*). The initial lesion of syphilis developing at the site of inoculation.

chancroid (*shang'-kroid*). Soft chancre. A venereal ulceration, due to *Haemophilus ducreyi*, accompanied by inflammation and suppuration of the local glands.

charcoal (*char'-kole*). Carbon obtained by burning animal or vegetable tissue in a confined space. Activated charcoal, which has been treated to improve its adsorbency, is sometimes given in the form of biscuits or tablets, in cases of dyspepsia.

Charcot's disease or **joint** (*J.M. Charcot, French neurologist, 1825–1893*). An osteoarthritic condition of a joint, often the knee, with effusion of fluid into the joint, occurring in locomotor ataxia.

Charcot's triad. Nystagmus, intention tremor and scanning speech. A trio of signs of disseminated sclerosis.

Charnley's arthroplasty (*Sir J. Charnley, British orthopaedic surgeon, 1911–1982*). The replacement of the hip joint using a plastic acetabulum and a steel femoral head. *See*

Arthroplasty.

cheilitis (*ki-li'-tis*). Inflammation of the lip.

cheiloplasty (*ki'-lo-plas-te*). Any plastic operation on the lip.

cheilorrhaphy (*ki-lor'-af-e*). A suturing or repair of a lip.

cheiloschisis (*ki-los'-kis-is*). Hare-lip.

cheiropompholyx (*ki-ro-pom'-fo-liks*). A skin disease characterized by vesicles on the palms and soles.

cheiropractic (*ki-ro-prak'-tik*). *See* Chiropractic.

chelate (*kel'-ate*). A chemical compound in which an atom of a metal is held in a molecular ring. Chelating agents such as penicillamine are used in the treatment of metal poisoning.

chelating agent (*kel'-at-ing a'-jent*). A drug that has the power of combining with certain metals and so aiding excretion to prevent or overcome poisoning. *See* Dimercaprol *and* Penicillamine.

chemistry (*kem'-is-tre*). The science dealing with the elements and the atoms which compose them, and with the compounds that they form.

chemoreceptor (*kem-o-re-sep'-tor*). A sensory nerve ending or group of cells that are sensitive to chemical stimuli in the blood.

chemosis (*ke-mo'-sis*). Swelling of the conjunctiva, due to the presence of fluid—an oedema of the conjunctiva.

chemotaxis (*kem-o-tak'-sis*). The reaction of living cells to chemical stimuli. These are either attracted (*positive c.*) or repelled (*negative c.*) by acids, alkalis or other substances.

chemotherapy (*kem-o-ther'-ap-e*). The specific treatment of disease by the administration of chemical compounds. A term commonly applied to the sulphonamide group of drugs and to the antibiotics. Often misused to imply treatment only by the use of cytotoxic agents.

chest (*chest*). The thorax. *Barrel-c.* One more rounded than usual, with raised ribs and, usually, kyphosis. It is often present in emphysema. *Flail c.* One where part of the chest wall moves in opposition to respiration due to multiple fractures of the ribs. *C. leads.* Leads applied to the chest during the course of an electrocardiographical recording. *Pigeon-c.* A chest with the sternum protruding forward.

POSITION OF CHEST LEADS FOR ECG

Cheyne–Stokes respiration (*J. Cheyne, British physician, 1776–1836; W. Stokes, British physician, 1804–1878*). Tidal respiration. A form of irregular but rhythmic breathing with temporary cessations (apnoea). It is likely to be present in cerebral tumour, in narcotic poisoning, and in advanced cases of arteriosclerosis and uraemia.

chiasma (*ki-az'-mah*). A crossing point. *Optic c.* The crossing point of the optic nerves.

chickenpox (*chik'-en-poks*). Varicella.

chilblain (*chil'-blane*). A condition resulting from defective circulation when exposure to cold causes localized swelling and inflammation of the hands or feet, with severe itching and burning sensations.

childbirth (*chi'-ld-berth*). Parturition.

chiropody (*ki-rop'-o-de*). The study and care of the feet and the treatment of foot diseases.

chiropractic (*ki-ro-prak'-tik*). A system of treatment employing manipulation of the spine and other bony structures.

chloasma (*klo-az'-mah*). A condition in which there is brown, blotchy discolouration of the skin, appearing on the face, especially during pregnancy.

chloral (*klor'-al*). An oily liquid formed by the reaction of chlorine and alcohol. Used in the production of *c. hydrate*, a drug used as a hypnotic which is well tolerated by children and old people.

chlorambucil (*klor-am'-bu-sil*). An ankylating drug used in treating chronic leukaemia. A cytotoxic drug.

chloramphenicol (*klor-am-fen'-ik-ol*). An oral antibiotic. It gives rise to agranulocytosis and is used only for serious infectious diseases such as typhoid fever. Used in drops and ointment for eye infections.

chlordiazepoxide (*klor-di-az-e-*

poks'-ide). A drug that depresses the central nervous system and so relieves anxiety and tension.

chlorhexidine (*klor-heks'-e-deen*). An antiseptic derived from coal tar that has a wide antibacterial action and is used as a skin antiseptic and as a disinfectant solution for instruments.

chlorinated (*klor'-in-a-ted*). Containing chloride. *C. lime.* A powerful disinfectant and bleaching agent, composed of lime and chlorine.

chlorine (*klor'-een*). *abbrev.* Cl. A yellow, irritating poisonous gas. It is used in the sterilization of drinking water, and in swimming baths.

chlormethiazole (*klor-meth-i'-az-ole*). A hypnotic and sedative drug used to treat insomnia, chiefly in elderly people.

chloroacetone (*klor'-o-as'-e-tone*). Chloracetone. Tear-gas.

chlorocresol (*klor-o-kre'-sol*). A coal tar product with a bactericidal action more powerful than phenol and with a lower toxicity. Used as an antiseptic and as a preservative in injection fluids.

chloroform (*klor'-o-form*). A colourless volatile liquid administered through inhalation as a general anaesthetic. Now rarely used. *C. water.* Used in pharmacy to disguise the taste of nauseous drugs.

chloroma (*klor-o'-mah*). A tumour having a greenish colour, usually found in skull bones. It is associated with myeloid leukaemia.

chlorophyll (*klor'-o-fil*). The green pigment of plants, related chemically to the pigment in haemoglobin, which absorbs solar energy for the synthesis of complex materials from the carbon dioxide and water taken in by the plant. *See* Photosynthesis.

chloropsia (*klor-op'-se-ah*). A form of colour blindness where all objects appear to have a greenish tinge.

chloroquine (*klor'-o-kwin*). An antimalarial drug that has a strong suppressant action and is used in the treatment of amoebic hepatitis, rheumatoid arthritis and lupus erythematosus.

chlorothiazide (*klor-o-thi'-az-ide*). An oral diuretic used in the treatment of fluid retention and hypertension.

chlorotrianisene (*klor-o-tri-an'-is-een*). An oestrogen used in the treatment of menopausal symptoms and also in cancer of the prostate.

chloroxylenol (*klor-ok-zi'-len-ol*). An antiseptic which is less irritating to the skin and mucous membranes than cresol and has a powerful disinfectant action.

chlorpheniramine (*klor-fen-ir'-am-een*). An antihistamine drug used in the treatment of allergies such as hay-fever and urticaria.

chlorpromazine (*klor-pro'-maz-een*). A sedative antiemetic drug widely used to treat anxiety, agitation and vomiting, particularly in the elderly, and to control violent patients. It is also hypotensive and enhances the effect of analgesics and anaesthetics.

chlorpropamide (*klor-pro'-pam-ide*). An hypoglycaemic agent used in the treatment of mild diabetes.

chlorprothixene (*klor-pro-thiks'-een*). A tranquillizer used in the treatment of schizophrenia and other psychoneuroses and of behaviour disorders.

chlortetracycline (*klor-tet-rah-si'-kleen*). A wide-range antibiotic effective in treating many bacterial and protozoal infections.

chlorthalidone (*klor-thal'-id-one*). A diuretic used in the treatment of oedema, hypertension and diabetes.

cholaemia (*ko-le'-me-ah*). The presence of bile in the blood.

cholagogue (*ko'-lag-og*). A drug which increases the flow of bile into the duodenum.

cholangiography (*ko-lan-je-og'-raf-e*). X-ray photography of the hepatic, cystic and bile ducts after the insertion of a radio-opaque dye.

cholangitis (*ko-lan-ji'-tis*). Inflammation of the bile ducts.

cholecystectomy (*ko-le-sis-tek'-tom-e*). Excision of the gall-bladder.

cholecystitis (*ko-le-sis-ti'-tis*). Inflammation of the gall-bladder.

cholecystoduodenostomy (*ko-le-sist-o-du-o-den-os'-tom-e*). An anastomosis between the gall-bladder and the duodenum.

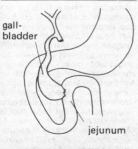

gall-bladder

jejunum

**CHOLECYSTO-
ENTEROSTOMY**

cholecystoenterostomy (*ko-le-sis-to-en-ter-os'-tom-e*). The formation of an artificial opening from the gall-bladder into the intestine. An operation performed in cases of irremovable obstruction of the bile duct.

cholecystogastrostomy (*ko-le-sis-to-gas-tros'-tom-e*). An operation by which the gall-bladder is made to open into the stomach.

cholecystography (*ko-le-sis-tog'-raf-e*). X-ray photography of the gall-bladder after administration of a radio-opaque dye.

cholecystokinin (*ko-le-sis-to-kin'-in*). A hormone released by the presence of fat in the duodenum which causes contraction of the gall-bladder.

cholecystolithiasis (*ko-le-sis-to-lith-i'-as-is*). Stones in the gall-bladder.

cholecystotomy (*ko-le-sis-tot'-om-e*). An incision into the gall-bladder usually to remove gall-stones.

choledochoduodenostomy (*ko-le-do-ko-du-o-den-os'-tom-e*). An operation in which an anastomosis is made between the common bile duct and the duodenum.

choledocholithiasis (*ko-le-do-ko-lith-i'-as-is*). The presence of stones in the bile duct.

choledocholithotomy (*ko-le-do-ko-lith-ot'-om-e*). Incision into the bile ducts to remove stones.

choledochostomy (*ko-le-do-kos'-tom-e*). Opening and draining the common bile duct.

cholelithiasis (*ko-le-lith-i'-as-is*). Presence of gall-stones in the gall-bladder or bile ducts.

cholera (*kol'-er-ah*). An acute infectious disease caused by *Vibrio cholerae* from infected food or water. It is marked by profuse diarrhoea, muscle cramp, suppression of urine and severe prostration, and is often fatal.

cholestasis (ko-le-sta'-sis). Arrest of the flow of bile due to obstruction of the bile ducts.

cholesteatoma (ko-le-ste-at-o'-mah). (1) A small tumour containing cholesterol which may occur in the middle ear. (2) A slow-growing, benign cerebral tumour.

cholesterol (ko-les'-ter-ol). A sterol found in nervous tissue, red blood corpuscles, animal fat and bile. Excess in the bile can lead to gall-stone formation.

cholesterolosis (ko-les-ter-ol-o'-sis). A chronic form of cholecystitis when the mucosa of the gall-bladder is studded with deposits of cholesterol.

cholestyramine (ko-le-sti'-ram-een). A drug which causes the excretion of bile salts by binding with them. Given to lower blood levels of cholesterol and other fats.

choline (ko'-leen). An essential amine found in the blood, cerebrospinal fluid and urine, which aids fat metabolism. Sometimes classified as a vitamin of the B complex. *C. theophyllinate.* An antispasmodic drug used in respiratory conditions.

cholinergic (ko-lin-er'-jik). Pertaining to nerves that release acetylcholine at their nerve endings as the chemical stimulator. *C. drugs.* Drugs that inhibit cholinesterase and so prevent the destruction of acetylcholine.

cholinesterase (ko-lin-est'-er-aze). An enzyme which rapid-

ly destroys acetylcholine.

choluria (ko-lu'-re-ah). The presence of bile in the urine.

chondritis (kon-dri'-tis). Inflammation of cartilage.

chondroblast (kon'-dro-blast). An embryonic cell which forms cartilage.

chondrocyte (kon'-dro-site). A mature cartilage cell.

chondrodynia (kon-dro-din-e-ah). Pain affecting a cartilage.

chondrodystrophia (kon-dro-dis-tro'-fe-ah). A congenital disorder of cartilage formation.

chondroma (kon-dro'-mah). An innocent new growth arising in cartilage.

chondromalacia (kon-dro-mal-a'-she-ah).|A|condition|of|abnormal softening of cartilage.

chondrosarcoma (kon-dro-sar-ko'-mah). A malignant new growth arising from cartilaginous tissue.

chorda (kor'-dah). A sinew or cord.

chordee (kor-de') Painful downward curvature of the erect penis caused by congenital anomaly (common in hypospadias) or urethral infection.

chorditis (kord-i'-tis). Inflammation of a vocal cord.

chordotomy (kord-ot'-om-e). An operation on the spinal cord to divide the anterolateral nerve pathways for relief of intractable pain. Cordotomy.

chorea (ko-re'-ah). A symptom of disease of the basal ganglia when the individual suffers from spasmodic involuntary movements of the face, shoulders and hips. *Huntington's c.* A rare hereditary disorder which manifests itself in early middle age. The individual also suffers from progressive dementia, which often precedes a premature death. *Sydenham's c.* St Vitus's dance. Occurs in childhood and is associated with rheumatic fever.

choreal, choreic (*ko'-re-al, ko-re'-ik*). Connected with or caused by chorea.

choreoathetosis (*ko-re-o-ath-et-o'-sis*). A nervous condition in which the jerky movements of chorea are combined with the writhing action of athetosis. Seen in some patients with cerebral lesions, most often children.

choriocarcinoma (*ko-re-o-kar-sin-o'-mah*). Chorionepithelioma.

chorion (*kor'-e-on*). The outer membrane enveloping the fetus. The placenta.

chorionepithelioma (*ko-re-on-ep-e-the-le-o'-mah*). A rare malignant growth of placental epithelium which may develop after an abortion or the evacuation of a hydatidiform mole or even in normal pregnancy. Metastases usually develop rapidly, but the disease normally carries a good prognosis following early treatment.

chorionic (*ko-re-on'-ik*). Pertaining to the chorion. *C. gonadotrophin.* Human chorionic gonadotrophin. HCG. *C. villi.* Small protrusions on the chorion from which the placenta is formed. They are in close association with the maternal blood, and, by diffusion, interchange of nutriment, oxygen, and waste matters is effected between the maternal and the fetal blood.

chorioretinitis (*ko-re-o-ret-in-i'-tis*). Choroidoretinitis.

choroid (*kor'-oid*). The pigmented and vascular coat of the eyeball, continuous with

the iris and situated between the sclera and retina. *C. plexus.* Specialized cells in the ventricles of the brain which produce cerebrospinal fluid. There is one choroid plexus in each ventricle.

choroiditis (*kor-oid-i'-tis*). Inflammation of the choroid.

choroidocyclitis (*kor-oid-o-si-kli'-tis*). Inflammation of the choroid and the ciliary body.

choroidoretinitis (*kor-oid-o-ret-in-i'-tis*). An inflammatory condition of both the choroid and retina of the eye.

Christmas disease (*krist'-mas diz-eez'*). A hereditary bleeding disease similar to haemophilia. The name is derived from that of the first patient to be studied.

chromatography (*kro-mat-og'-raf-e*). A method of chemical analysis by which substances in solution can be separated as they percolate down a column of powdered absorbent or ascend an absorbent paper by capillary traction. A definite pattern is produced and substances may be recognized by the use of appropriate colour reagents. Amino acids can be separated in this way and the antianaemic factor isolated from liver extract.

chromatolysis (*kro-mat-ol'-is-sis*). The disintegration and disappearance of the Nissl granules of a neurone if the axon is severed.

chromatometry (*kro-mat-om'-et-re*). The measurement of colour perception.

chromatopsia (*kro-mat-op'-se-ah*). Abnormal colour vision. Partial colour-blindness.

chromic acid (*kro'-mik as'-id*). A strong caustic sometimes used for the removal of warts.

chromicize (*kro'-mis-ize*). To

impregnate with chromic acid, e.g. chromicized catgut which is particularly strong and durable.

chromophil (*kro'-mo-fil*). An easily stainable cell.

chromophobe (*kro'-mo-fobe*). A cell that is not easily stained. *C. adenoma*. The commonest of the pituitary tumours giving rise to hypopituitarism.

chromosome (*kro'-mo-some*). One of the filaments into which the nucleus of a cell divides during mitosis. Each chromosome consists of hundreds of molecules of nucleoprotein called genes. Each human cell contains 46 chromosomes.

chronic (*kron'-ik*). Of long duration; the opposite of acute.

chrysarobin (*kris-ar-o'-bin*). A derivative of Goa powder, used in ointment form, especially in the treatment of psoriasis. It stains linen a yellow colour. *See* Dithranol.

Chvostek's sign (*F. Chvostek, Austrian surgeon, 1835–1884*). A spasm of the facial muscles which occurs in tetany. It can be elicited by tapping the facial nerve.

chyle (*kile*). Digested fats which, as a milky fluid, are absorbed into the lymphatic capillaries (*lacteals*) in the villi of the small intestine.

chyluria (*ki-lu'-re-ah*). The presence of chyle in the urine, giving it a milky appearance.

chyme (*kime*). The semi-liquid, acid mass of food which passes from the stomach to the intestines.

chymotrypsin (*ki-mo-trip'-sin*). An enzyme secreted by the pancreas. It is activated by trypsin and aids in the breakdown of proteins.

Ci. Abbreviation for the *curie* unit.

cicatrix (*sik'-at-riks*). The scar of a healed wound.

ciliary (*sil'-e-ar-e*). Hair-like. *C. body*. A structure just behind the corneoscleral margin composed of the ciliary muscle and processes. *C. muscle*. The circular muscle surrounding the lens of the eye. *C. processes*. The fringed part of the choroid coat arranged in a circle in front of the lens.

cilium (*sil'-e-um*). *pl.* cilia. (1) An eyelash. (2) A slender microscopic filament projecting from some epithelial cells, as in the bronchi, where cilia wave the secretion upwards.

cimetidine (*sim-et'-id-een*). A drug used in the treatment of peptic ulcers.

Cimex (*si'-meks*). A genus of blood-sucking bugs. *C. lectularius*. The common bed-bug.

cinchocaine (*sin'-ko-kane*). A local anaesthetic agent. It is applied directly to the skin.

cinchona (*sin-ko'-nah*). Peruvian bark, from which quinine is obtained.

cinchonism (*sin'-kon-izm*). Poisonous effect of cinchona and its alkaloids, i.e. tinnitus, deafness, headache, blurred vision and weakness of heart muscle. Quininism.

cine-angiocardiography (*sin-e-an-je-o-kar-de-og'-raf-e*). Angiography using a cine-camera to show the movements of the heart and blood vessels.

cine-radiography (*sin-e-ra-de-og'-raf-e*). The making of moving X-ray pictures.

cinnamon (*sin'-am-on*). An extract from the bark of an East Indian laurel, sometimes used as a digestive and carminative.

cinnarizine (*sin-ar'-iz-een*). An antihistamine drug which may also be used to treat nausea, vertigo, labyrinthine disorders and motion sickness.

circadian (*ser-ka'-de-an*). Denoting a period of 24 hours. *C. rhythm.* The rhythm of certain biological activities that take place daily.

circinate (*ser'-sin-ate*). Having a circular outline. *Tinea circinata* is ringworm.

circle of Willis (*T. Willis, British physician and anatomist, 1621–1675*). An anastomosis of arteries at the base of the brain, formed by the branches of the internal carotids and the branches of the basilar artery.

circulation (*ser-ku-la'-shun*). Movement in a circular course, as of the blood. *Collateral c.* Enlargement of small vessels establishing adequate blood supply when the main vessel to the part has been occluded. *Coronary c.* The system of vessels which supply the heart muscle itself. *Extracorporeal c.* Removal of the blood by intravenous cannulae, passing it through a machine to oxygenate it, and then pumping it back into circulation. The 'heart–lung' machine or pump respirator, used in cardiac surgery. *Lymph c.* The flow of lymph through lymph vessels and glands. *Portal c.* The passage of the blood from the alimentary tract, pancreas, and spleen, via the portal vein and its branches through the liver and into the hepatic veins. *Pulmonary c.* Passage of the blood from the right ventricle via the pulmonary artery through the lungs and back to the heart by the pulmonary veins. *Systemic c.* That of the blood throughout the body. The direction of flow is from the left atrium to the left ventricle and through the aorta with its branches and capillaries. Veins then carry it back to the right atrium, and so into the right ventricle.

circulatory (*ser-ku-la'-tor-e*). Pertaining to the circulation of blood. *C. system.* Cardiovascular system.

circumcision (*ser-kum-sizh'-un*). Excision of a circular portion of the prepuce. An operation usually performed for religious reasons, but sometimes for phimosis or paraphimosis. *Female c.* Excision of the labia minora and sometimes the clitoris, still performed ritualistically in certain countries.

circumduction (*ser-kum-duk'-shun*). Moving in a circle, e.g. the circular movement of the upper limb.

circumoral (*ser-kum-or'-al*). Around the mouth. *C. pallor.* A pale area around the mouth contrasting with the flushed cheeks, e.g. in scarlet fever.

circumvallate (*ser-kum-val'-ate*). Surrounded by a wall. *C. papilla. See* Papilla.

cirrhosis (*sir-o'-sis*). A degenerative change which can occur in any organ, but especially in the liver (*portal c.*). Fibrosis results, and this interferes with the working of the organ. In the liver it causes portal obstruction, with consequent ascites. *Alcoholic c.* Cirrhosis said to be the result of chronic alcoholism and nutritional deficiency which affects the liver. *Cardiac c.* Cirrhosis of the liver following chronic heart failure. *Post-hepatic c.* Cirrhosis of the liver following hepatitis. *Pulmonary c.* Cirrhosis of the lung tissue.

cisplatin (*sis-plat'-in*). A cytotoxic drug containing platinum which has proved useful in the treatment of ovarian carcinomas and testicular teratomas. Its use is always preceded by the administration of an antiemetic as it causes severe vomiting.

cisterna (*sis-ter'-nah*). A space or cavity containing fluid. *C. chyli.* The dilated portion of the thoracic duct containing chyle. *C. magna.* The subarachnoid space between the cerebellum and medulla oblongata.

cisternal (*sis-ter'-nal*). Concerning the cisterna. *C. puncture.* Insertion of a hollow needle into the cisterna magna to withdraw cerebrospinal fluid.

citric acid (*sit'-rik as'-id*). Acid found in the juice of lemons, limes, etc. An antiscorbutic.

Cl. Chemical symbol for *chlorine.*

clamp (*klamp*). A metal surgical instrument used to compress any part of the body, e.g. to prevent or arrest haemorrhage.

clapping (*klap'-ing*). In physiotherapy, a term used to denote rhythmic beating with cupped hands. Frequently used over the chest to aid expectoration.

claudication (*klaw-dik-a'-shun*). Lameness. *Intermittent c.* Limping, accompanied by severe pain in the legs on walking, which disappears with rest. A sign of occlusive arterial disease.

claustrophobia (*klaw-stro-fo'-be-ah*). Fear of confined spaces such as small rooms.

clavicle (*klav'-ikl*). The collarbone. A long bone, part of the shoulder girdle.

clavus (*kla'-vus*). A corn. *C. hystericus.* A pain near the midline on top of the skull associated with hysteria.

claw-foot (*klaw'-foot*). A deformity in which the longitudinal arch is abnormally raised. Pes cavus.

claw-hand (*klaw'-hand*). A deformity in which the fingers are bent and contracted, giving a claw-like appearance.

cleft (*kleft*). A fissure or longitudinal opening. *C. palate.* A congenital defect in the roof of the mouth, due to failure of the medial plates of the palate to meet. Speech is indistinct, words being slurred. Hare-lip is often present at the same time.

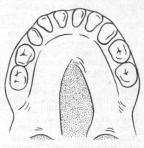

CLEFT PALATE

climacteric (*kli-mak-ter'-ik*). The period of the menopause in women. Also used to denote the decline in the sexual drive in men.

climax (*kli'-maks*). (1) The stage when a disease is at its greatest intensity. (2) The stage in sexual intercourse when orgasm occurs.

clindamycin (*klin-dah-mi'-sin*). An oral semisynthetic antibiotic used to treat serious bacterial infections.

clinic (*klin'-ik*). (1) Instruction of students at the bedside. (2) A department of a hospital devoted to the treatment of a particular type of disease.

clinical (*klin'-ik-al*). Relating to bedside observation and the treatment of patients.

clinicopathological (*klin-ik-o-path-o-loj'-ik-al*). Relating to both the symptoms and the pathology of disease.

clinicoradiological (*klin-ik-o-ra-de-o-loj'-ik-al*). Relating the bedside observations to the results of radiological investigations.

clip (*klip*). A metal device for holding the two edges of a wound together or for controlling the flow of liquid through a tube.

clitoridectomy (*klit-or-id-ek'-tom-e*). Excision of the clitoris.

clitoris (*klit'-or-is*). A small organ formed of erectile tissue, in front of the urethra in the female. The homologue of the penis.

cloaca (*klo-a'-kah*). An opening to the exterior for the purpose of discharge of waste. (1) The common intestinal and urogenital opening present in many vertebrates. (2) Opening through newly formed bone from a diseased area so that pus may escape. *See* Involucrum.

clofibrate (*klo-fi'-brate*). A drug used to lower the blood cholesterol.

clomipramine (*klo-mip'-ram-een*). An antidepressant drug used to treat patients with obsessional fears.

clonazepam (*klo-naz'-e-pam*). An anticonvulsive drug used in the treatment of severe epilepsy.

clone (*klone*). Those cells which are genetically identical to each other and have descended by asexual reproduction from the parent cell to which they are also genetically identical.

clonic (*klon'-ik*). Having the character of clonus. The second stage of a grand mal fit. *See* Epilepsy.

clonidine (*klo'-nid-een*). An antihypertensive drug which is used in lower doses to treat migraine.

clonus (*klo'-nus*). Muscle rigidity and relaxation which occurs spasmodically. *Ankle c.* Spasmodic movements of the calf muscles when the foot is suddenly pushed upwards, the leg being extended. A reaction which may be an indication of spinal cord disease.

Clostridium (*klos-trid'-e-um*). A genus of anaerobic spore-forming bacteria, found as commensals of the gut of animals and man and as saprophytes of the soil. Pathogenic species include *Cl. botulinum* (botulism), *Cl. tetani* (tetanus), *Cl. welchii* (gas gangrene).

clot (*klot*). A semi-solid mass formed in a liquid such as blood or lymph, by coagulation.

clotrimazole (*klo-tri'-maz-ole*). An antifungal drug used to treat vaginal conditions, e.g. candidiasis.

clotting (*klot'-ing*). Coagulation. The formation of a clot. *C. time.* Coagulation time. The length of time taken for shed blood to coagulate. Normally, this would be 4 to 15 minutes at 37°C.

cloxacillin (*kloks-ah-sil'-in*). An antibiotic drug effective against penicillin-resistant staphylococci.

clubbing (*klub'-ing*). Broadening and thickening of the tips of the fingers (and toes), due to bad circulation. It occurs in chronic diseases of the heart and respiratory system, such as congenital cardiac defect and tuberculosis.

clubfoot (*klub'-foot*). Talipes.

clumping (*klump'-ing*). The collecting together into clumps. The reaction of bacteria and blood cells when agglutination occurs.

Clutton's joint (*H.H. Clutton, British surgeon, 1850–1909*). A painless synovial swelling of joints, usually the knee, which may occur in congenital syphilis.

Co. Chemical symbol for *cobalt.*

coagulase (*ko-ag'-u-laze*). An enzyme formed by pathogenic staphylococci that causes coagulation of plasma. Such bacteria are termed *c. positive.*

coagulation (*ko-ag-u-la'-shun*). Clotting.

coagulum (*ko-ag'-u-lum*). The mass of fibrin and cells when blood clots, or the mass formed when other substances coagulate, e.g. milk curd.

coal tar (*cole tar*). A viscid fluid obtained by the distillation of coal, from which many germicides are derived, e.g. benzol, phenol, aniline dyes.

coarctation (*ko-ark-ta'-shun*). A condition of contraction or stricture. *C. of aorta.* Usually a congenital defect which may be incompatible with life, but in many cases a compensat-

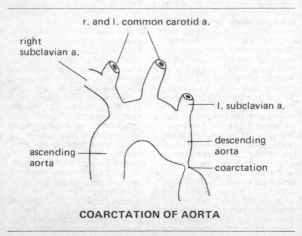

COARCTATION OF AORTA

ing collateral circulation is established. Surgical resection of the stricture may be performed.

cobalt (*ko'-bawlt*). *abbrev.* Co. A metallic element, traces of which are necessary in the diet to prevent anaemia. *Radioactive c.* Cobalt-60, used as a source of gamma irradiation in radiotherapy.

cocaine (*ko-kane'*). A colourless alkaloid obtained from cocoa leaves or prepared synthetically. Used as a local anaesthetic applied to mucous membranes for nose and throat treatments. For local anaesthesia it is increasingly being replaced by less addictive preparations like procaine, lignocaine and amethocaine.

cocainism (*ko-kane'-izm*). (1) Addiction to cocaine. (2) The condition following continued use of cocaine, when the initial stimulation and feeling of well-being is followed by mental and physical deterioration.

coccus (*kok'-us*). A bacterium of spheroidal shape.

coccydynia (*koks-e-din'-e-ah*). Persistent pain in the region of the coccyx usually following trauma.

coccygeal (*koks-ij'-e-al*). Pertaining to the coccyx.

coccygodynia (*koks-e-go-din'-e-ah*). Coccydynia.

coccyx (*koks'-iks*). The terminal bone of the spinal column, in which four rudimentary vertebrae are fused together to form a triangle.

cochlea (*kok'-le-ah*). The spiral canal of the internal ear.

codeine (*ko'-deen*). An alkaloid of opium said to be less depressant to the respiratory centre than other forms, and

particularly favoured for persistent cough. A mild analgesic and hypnotic. Also useful for stopping diarrhoea.

cod-liver oil (*kod'-liv-er oil'*). Purified oil from the liver of the codfish, particularly valuable for its vitamin A and D content.

coeliac (*se'-le-ak*). Relating to the abdomen. *C. disease.* Gluten enteropathy. A condition of early childhood, which is characterized by steatorrhoea, distended abdomen and failure to grow. The failure of carbohydrate and fat metabolism appears to be due to the gluten in wheat flour. The condition may continue into adult life. It is treated by giving a gluten-free diet. *C. plexus.* Nerve complex which supplies the abdominal organs.

co-enzyme (*ko-en'-zime*). A small non-protein molecule accessory to the larger protein enzyme and necessary for its function.

cognition (*kog-nish'-un*). Action of knowing. Cognitive function of the conscious mind in contrast to the affective (feeling) and conative (willing).

coitus (*ko'-it-us*). Sexual intercourse between male and female. *C. interruptus.* An unreliable method of birth control where the erect penis is removed from the vagina before ejaculation occurs.

colchicine (*kol'-chis-een*). A drug obtained from the seeds of *Colchicum autumnale*. Used in treating gout.

cold (*ko'-ld*). (1) *adj.* Of low temperature. (2) *n.* A viral infection affecting the membranes of the nose and throat and the bronchial tubes. *C.*

sore. Herpes simplex. *See* Herpes.

colectomy (*ko-lek'-tom-e*). The excision of a portion or all of the colon.

colic (*kol'-ik*). Severe pain due to spasmodic contraction of the involuntary muscle of tubes. *Biliary c.* Pain due to the presence of a gall-stone in a bile duct. *Intestinal c.* Severe griping spasmodic abdominal pain which may be a symptom of food poisoning or of intestinal obstruction. *Renal c.* Pain due to the presence of a stone in the ureter. *Uterine c.* Spasmodic pain originating in the uterus, as in dysmenorrhoea.

coliform (*ko'-lif-orm*). Resembling the bacillus *Escherichia coli*.

colistin (*ko'-list-in*). An oral antibiotic produced from *Bacillus polymyxa*. Used to treat gastrointestinal and other bacterial infections.

colitis (*kol-i'-tis*). Inflammation of the colon. It may be due to a specific organism, as in dysentery, but the term *ulcerative c.* denotes a chronic disease often of unknown cause in which there are attacks of diarrhoea with the passage of blood and mucus.

collagen (*kol'-aj-en*). A protein constituent of white connective tissue. *C. diseases*. Those in which there is a typical fibrinoid degeneration of collagen, e.g lupus erythematosus, rheumatoid arthritis and scleroderma.

collapse (*kol-aps'*). (1) A state of extreme prostration due to defective action of the heart, severe shock or haemorrhage. (2) Falling in of a structure. *Circulatory c.* Sudden failure of the circulation of the

blood. *C. of lung*. A condition due to alteration of air pressure between the inside of the lung and the pleural cavity. *See* Pneumothorax. *Massive c.* Collapse of one or more lobes of the lung due to blockage of a bronchus.

collar-bone (*kol'-ar-bone*). The clavicle.

collateral (*kol-at'-er-al*). Accessory to. *C. circulation*. An alternative to the direct route for the blood.

Colles's fracture (*A. Colles, Irish surgeon, 1773–1843*). Fracture of the lower end of the radius at the wrist. It is usually impacted and the styloid process of the ulna may be torn off. Typically, it produces the 'dinner fork' deformity.

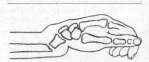

COLLES'S FRACTURE

collimator (*kol-im-a'-tor*). A device used in radiotherapy machines to help in determining the limits of the treatment field.

colloid (*kol'-oid*). A gelatinous fluid made by substances suspended in a medium but not forming a sediment. These substances will not pass through an animal membrane.

coloboma (*kol-o-bo'-mah*). A congenital fissure of the eye affecting the choroid coat and the retina.

colon (*ko'-lon*). The large intestine from the caecum to the

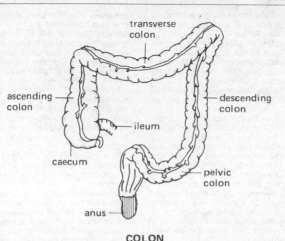

transverse colon

ascending colon

descending colon

ileum

caecum

pelvic colon

anus

COLON

rectum. *Ascending c.* That part arising to the right of the abdomen to in front of the liver. *Descending c.* That part running down from in front of the spleen to the sigmoid colon. *Giant c.* Megacolon. *Irritable c.* A nervous type associated with abdominal pain and distension. *Pelvic c., sigmoid c.* That part lying in the pelvis and connecting the descending colon with the rectum. *Transverse c.* That part lying across the upper abdomen connecting the ascending and descending portions.

colonic (*ko-lon'-ik*). Pertaining to the colon. *C. irrigation.* Colonic lavage (*see* Lavage).

colonoscope (*ko-lon'-o-skope*). A fibre-optic instrument passed through the anus, for examining the interior of the colon.

colony (*kol'-on-e*). A mass of bacteria formed by multiplication of cells when bacteria are incubated under favourable conditions.

colostomy (*ko-los'-tom-e*). The surgical formation of a temporary or permanent opening between the colon and the anterior abdominal wall.

colostrum (*kol-os'-trum*). The first fluid from the mother's breasts after childbirth. It contains more protein but less fat and sugar than true milk.

colour-blindness (*kul'-or bli'-nd-nes*). Achromatopsia.

colour index (*kul'-or in'-deks*). An index of the amount of haemoglobin in red blood cells. It is often estimated in examination of the blood, and is obtained by dividing the percentage of haemoglobin by the percentage of red cells of the norm. A normal colour index will give a value of 1. *See* Blood.

colpitis (*kol-pi'-tis*). Inflammation of the vagina.

colpocele (*kol'-po-seel*). A hernia into the vagina. Vaginocele.

colpocleisis (*kol-po-kli'-sis*). Closure of the vagina by surgical means.

colpohysterectomy (*kol-po-his-ter-ek'-tom-e*). Removal of the uterus through the vagina, usually for prolapse of uterus.

colpoperineorrhaphy (*kol-po-per-in-e-or'-af-e*). The repair by suturing of an injured vagina and torn perineum.

colpopexy (*kol'-po-peks-e*). Suture of a prolapsed vagina to the abdominal wall.

colpoplasty (*kol'-po-plas-te*). A plastic operation on the vagina.

colporrhaphy (*kol-por'-af-e*). Repair of the vagina. *Anterior c.* Repair for cystocele. *Posterior c.* Repair for rectocele.

colposcope (*kol'-po-skope*). An instrument used to study the vagina and uterine cervix. Benign and malignant changes may be seen and selective biopsy taken, so aiding early diagnosis of malignant disease.

colpotomy (*kol-pot'-om-e*). Incision of the vaginal wall.

coma (*ko'-mah*). Complete unconsciousness, in which all reflexes are absent. *Diabetic c.* Coma due to ketosis which occurs in diabetes mellitus. Treated by immediate administration of insulin and intravenous saline. *Hypoglycaemic c.* (*insulin c.*) results from too much insulin or too little food being taken. Treated by giving sugar. *Uraemic c. See* Uraemia.

comatose (*ko'-mat-oze*). In the condition of coma.

comedo (*kom'-e-do*). *Pl.* comedones. A blackhead. Formed of epithelial cells enclosing dried sebum blocking the entrance to the sebaceous gland. Common during adolescence.

commensal (*kom-en'-sal*). An organism which normally lives in or on a part of the body without detriment to it. Some are potentially pathogenic.

comminuted (*kom'-in-u-ted*). Broken into small pieces, as in a comminuted fracture. *See* Fracture.

commissure (*kom'-is-ure*). The tissue joining two similar structures, most commonly nerve fibres in the central nervous system. *C. of the vulva.* The junction between the labia majora.

communicable disease (*kom-u'-nik-abl dis-eez'*). One that can be transmitted from one person to another. An infectious or contagious disease.

commutator (*kom'-u-ta-tor*). A device by which the direction of an electrical current can be interrupted or reversed.

compatibility (*kom-pat-ib-il'-it-e*). Mutual suitability. Mixing together of two substances without chemical change or loss of power. *See* Blood grouping.

compensation (*kom-pen-sa'-shun*). (1) Making good a functional or structural defect. (2) Mental mechanism (unconscious) by which a person covers up a weakness by exaggerating a more desirable characteristic.

complement (*kom'-ple-ment*). In bacteriology, a substance present in blood which aids the destruction of bacteria invading the body. *C. fixation.* The combination of complement with antigen–antibody complex to destroy bacteria.

complementary (*kom-ple-ment'-ar-e*). Pertaining to that which completes or makes perfect. *C. feed.* Feed given to infants to supplement breast feeding when the mother has insufficient milk of her own.

complex (*kom'-pleks*). A grouping of various things, as of signs and symptoms, forming a syndrome. In psychology, a grouping of ideas of emotional origin which are completely or partially repressed in the unconscious mind. A possible cause of mental illness. *Inferiority c.* A compensation by assertiveness or aggression to cover a feeling of inadequacy. *See* Electra *and* Oedipus.

complication (*kom-plik-a'-shun*). Another disease process arising during the course of or following the primary condition.

compos mentis (*kom'-pos men'-tis*). Of sound mind (*Latin*).

compound (*kom'-pownd*). Composed of two or more parts or substances. *C. fracture.* A fracture in which a wound through to the skin has also occurred.

comprehension (*com-prehen'-shun*). Mental grasp of the meaning of a situation.

compress (*kom'-pres*). Folded material, e.g. lint, wet or dry, applied to a part of the body, for the relief of swelling and pain.

compression (*kom-presh'-un*). Pressing together. *Cerebral c.* Raised intracranial pressure due to haemorrhage, abscess,

tumour or other cause.

compulsion (*kom-pul'-shun*). An urge to perform some action that the patient recognizes to be irrational but resistance leads to mounting anxiety which is only relieved by the performance of the act. The term may also be applied to compulsive words, thoughts and fears.

conation (*ko-na'-shun*). A striving in a certain direction. *See* Cognition.

concave (*kon'-kave*). Hollowed out. The opposite of *convex.*

concept (*kon'-sept*). An image or idea held in the mind.

conception (*kon-sep'-shun*). (1) The act of becoming pregnant, by the fertilization of an ovum. (2) A concept.

concha (*kon'-shah*). A shell. Applied in anatomy to shell-like structures, e.g. *c. of the auricle* (the hollow part of the external ear).

concordant (*kon-kord'-ant*). Running a parallel course. In medicine may be applied to twins developing similar traits.

concretion (*kon-kre'-shun*). A calculus or other hardened material present within an organ such as the kidney.

concussion (*kon-kush'-un*). A violent jarring shock. *C. of the brain.* Temporary loss of consciousness produced by a fall or a blow on the head. There may be amnesia, slow respiration and a weak pulse.

condenser (*kon-den'-ser*). (1) An apparatus for collecting charges of electricity in which two conducting surfaces are separated by some insulating material, such as glass. (2) An arrangement for condensing light on to a microscope slide. (3) An apparatus by which gases may be liquefied.

conditioning (*kon-dish'-un-ing*). The process by which a response is obtained to a stimulus by repetition of a situation until it becomes automatic.

condom (*kon'-dom*). A contraceptive sheath worn by the male, affording some protection for both partners against sexually transmitted diseases.

conductor (*kon-duk'-tor*). (1) A substance through which electricity, light, heat or sound can pass. (2) Any part of the nervous system which conveys impulses.

condyle (*kon'-dile*). A rounded eminence occurring at the end of some bones, and articulating with another bone.

condyloma (*kon-di-lo'-mah*). A moist wart-like growth at the junction of skin and mucous membrane, e.g. the anal or vulval margins. The warts are infectious and are probably transmitted by sexual contact.

cone (*kone*). A solid figure with a rounded base, tapering upwards to a point. *Retinal c.* The cone-shaped end of a light-sensitive cell in the retina, used for acute vision and for distinguishing colours.

confabulation (*kon-fab-u-la'-shun*). The production of fictitious memories, and the relating of experiences which have no relation to truth, to fill in the gaps due to loss of memory. A symptom of Korsakoff's syndrome.

confection (*kon-fek'-shun*). A preparation of sugar or honey containing drugs, e.g. senna.

conflict (*kon'-flikt*). A mental state arising when two opposing wishes or impulses cause emotional tension and often cannot be resolved without repressing one of the impulses into the unconscious. Conflict situations may be associated with an anxiety neurosis.

confluent (*kon'-flu-ent*). Running together.

confusion (*kon-fu'-zhun*). A clouding of consciousness so that the capacity to think is impaired, perception is dulled and response to stimuli is less acute.

congenital (*kon-jen'-it-al*). Applied to conditions existing at or before birth but which are not necessarily hereditary. *C. dislocation of hip.* Failure in position of the head of the femur and development of the acetabulum. *C. heart disease.* Abnormalities in development or failure to adjust to extra-uterine life. *See* Fallot's tetralogy.

congestion (*kon-jest'-shun*). An abnormal accumulation of blood in any part. *Pulmonary c.* Congestion of the lung, as in pneumonia and congestive heart failure.

conization (*ko-ni-za'-shun*). Removal of a cone-shaped piece of tissue from the uterine cervix in order to treat erosion or to obtain a sample for biopsy.

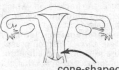

cone-shaped
area of tissue
removed

**CONIZATION OF THE
UTERINE CERVIX**

conjugate (*kon'-ju-gate*). (1) *adj.* United in pairs or couples. (2) *n.* The distance between two parts. *True c.* The distance between the symphysis pubis and the sacral prominence.

conjunctiva (*kon-junk-ti'-vah*). The mucous membrane covering the front of the eyeball and lining the eyelids.

conjunctivitis (*kon-junk-tiv-i'-tis*). Inflammation of the conjunctiva. 'Pink eye'. Ophthalmia. *Catarrhal c.* A mild form, usually due to cold or irritation. *Granular c.* Trachoma. *Phlyctenular c.* Marked by small vesicles or ulcers on the membrane. *Purulent c.* Caused by virulent organisms, with discharge of pus.

connective (*kon-ek'-tiv*). Joining together. *C. tissues.* Those that develop from the mesenchyme and are formed of a matrix containing fibres and cells. Areolar tissue, cartilage and bone are examples.

Conn's syndrome (*W.J. Conn, American physician, b. 1907*). Primary hyperaldosteronism, resulting from a tumour in the adrenal cortex. *See* Aldosteronism.

consanguinity (*kon-san-gwin'-it-e*). Blood relationship.

conscious (*kon'-shus*). The state of being awake or aware.

conservative (*kon-ser'-vat-iv*). The use of non-radical methods to restore health and preserve function.

consolidation (*kon-sol-id-a'-shun*). A state of becoming solid. *C. of lung.* In pneumococcal pneumonia the infected lobe becomes solid and congested with blood—known as red hepatization. *See* Hepatization.

constipation (*kon-stip-a'-shun*). Incomplete or infrequent action of the bowels, with consequent filling of the rectum with hard faeces. *Atonic c.* Constipation due to lack of muscle tone in the bowel wall. *Spastic c.* A form of constipation where spasm of part of the bowel wall narrows the canal.

constitutional (*kon-stit-u'-shun-al*). That which affects the whole body.

constrictor (*kon-strik'-tor*). A muscle that compresses an organ or causes a cavity to contract.

consumption (*kon-sump'-shun*). The popular name for phthisis or advanced pulmonary tuberculosis.

contact (*kon'-tact*). A person who has been exposed to a contagious disease. *C. lens.* A glass or plastic lens worn under the eyelids in the front of the eye. It may be worn for therapeutic or for cosmetic reasons.

contagion (*kon-ta'-jun*). (1) The communication of disease from one person to another by direct contact. (2) An infectious disease.

contraception (*con-trah-sep'-shun*). The prevention of conception and pregnancy.

contraceptive (*kon-trah-sep'-tiv*). An agent used to prevent conception, e.g. male sheath, cap that occludes the cervix, spermicidal pessary or cream, intrauterine device (IUD), and oral contraceptives (hormone pills).

contraction (*kon-trak'-shun*). A shortening or drawing together, especially applied to muscle action. *Braxton Hicks c.* Contractions occurring intermittently after the first trimester of pregnancy. *Uterine c.* Those occurring during labour.

contracture (*kon-trak'-chur*). Fibrosis causing permanent contraction. *Dupuytren's c.* Contraction of the palmar fascia causing permanent bending and fixation of one or more fingers. *Volkmann's ischaemic c.* Contraction resulting from impairment of the blood supply. May occur in upper or lower limbs.

contraindication (*kon-trah-in-dik-a'-shun*). Any condition that makes a particular line of treatment impracticable or undesirable.

contralateral (*kon-trah-lat'-er-al*). Occurring on the opposite side.

contrast medium (*kon'-trahst me'-de-um*). A substance used in radiography to make visible or more visible certain organs.

contrecoup (*kon-tr-koo'*). An injury occurring on the opposite side or at a distance from the site of the blow, e.g. brain damage on the opposite side of the skull to the blow.

control (*kon-trol'*). (1) Restrain or command of objects or events. (2) A standard for testing where the procedure is identical in all respects to the experiment but the factor being studied is absent. *Birth c.* Contraception.

controlled drugs (*kon-tro'-ld drugz'*). Drugs which are defined in the Misuse of Drugs Act 1971. They include those drugs which are habit-forming and certain other narcotics which have a profound effect on the central nervous system.

contusion (*kon-tu'-zhun*). A bruise.

convalescence (*kon-val-es'-ens*). Period of recovery following illness, injury or operation.

convection (*kon-vek'-shun*). A method of transmission of heat by the circulation of warmed molecules of a liquid or a gas.

conversion (*kon-ver'-shun*). In psychology, the mechanism whereby repressed mental conflicts manifest themselves by physical symptoms.

convex (*kon'-veks*). Bowing outwards. Having an outline like a segment of a sphere.

convolution (*kon-vo-lu'-shun*). A fold or coil, e.g. of the cerebrum or renal tubules.

convulsion (*kon-vul'-shun*). Spasmodic or prolonged contraction of muscle due to cerebral irritation or dysfunction. Convulsions may herald the onset of an infectious disease but may be a symptom of a more serious underlying cause. *See* Fits *and* Epilepsy.

Cooley's anaemia (*T.B. Cooley, American paediatrician, 1871 –1945*). Thalassaemia.

Coombs' test (*R.R.A. Coombs, British immunologist, b. 1921*). A quantitative test carried out to detect the presence of any antibody on the surface of the red blood cell. Used to detect rhesus incompatibility in maternal or fetal blood and in the diagnosis of haemolytic anaemia.

coordination (*ko-or-din-a'-shun*). Harmony of movement between several muscles or groups of muscle so that complicated manoeuvres can be made.

copiopia (*kop-e-o'-pe-ah*). Improper use of the eye or overwork leading to eyestrain. Copiopsia.

copper (*kop'-er*). *abbrev.* Cu. A metallic element, traces of which are present in all human tissues. *C. sulphate.* In solid form (blue stone), sometimes used as a caustic for granulating surfaces.

coprolalia (*kop-ro-la'-le-ah*). The uncontrolled use of obscene speech.

coprolith (*kop'-ro-lith*). A faecalith.

coprostasia (*kop-ro-sta'-se-ah*). The accumulation of faecal matter in the intestines, causing obstruction.

copulation (*kop-u-la'-shun*). Coitus. Sexual intercourse between male and female.

cor (*kor*). The heart (*Latin*). *C. adiposum.* Fatty degeneration of the heart. *C. pulmonale.* Heart failure secondary to disease of the lungs or pulmonary circulation.

coracoid (*kor'-ak-oid*). (1) *adj.* Shaped like a raven's beak. (2) *n.* The coracoid process of the scapula.

cord (*kord*). A long cylindrical flexible structure. *Spermatic c.* That which suspends the testicle in the scrotum, and contains the spermatic artery and vein, and vas deferens. *Spinal c.* The part of the central nervous system enclosed in the spinal column. *Umbilical c.* The connection between the fetus and the placenta, through which the fetus receives nourishment. *Vocal c's.* Folds of mucous membrane in the larynx which vibrate to produce the voice.

cordotomy (*kord-ot'-om-e*). See Chordotomy.

corium (*kor'-e-um*). The true skin. *See* Dermis.

corn (*korn*). A local hardening and thickening of the skin from pressure or friction

occurring usually on the toes. Clavus.

cornea (*kor'-ne-ah*). The transparent portion of the anterior surface of the eyeball continuous with the sclerotic coat. *Conical c.* Keratoconus.

corneal (*kor'-ne-al*). Pertaining to the cornea. *C. graft.* A means of restoring sight by grafting healthy transparent cornea from a donor in place of diseased tissue. Keratoplasty.

corneoscleral (*kor-ne-o-skler'-al*). Relating to both the cornea and sclera. *C. junction.* The point where the edge of the cornea joins the sclera. The limbus.

corneum (*kor'-ne-um*). The horny layer of the skin.

cornification (*kor-nif-ik-a'-shun*). Keratinization. The process whereby the skin becomes horny through the deposition of keratin.

cornu (*kor'-nu*). *pl.* cornua. A horn. *C. of uterus.* One of the two horn-shaped projections where the uterine tubes join the uterus at the upper pole on either side.

corona (*kor-o'-nah*). A crown or crown-like structure. *C. capitis.* The crown of the head. *C. dentis.* The crown of a tooth.

coronal (*kor'-on-al*). Relating to the crown of the head. *C. suture.* The junction of the frontal and parietal bones.

coronary (*kor'-on-ar-e*). Encircling. Crown-like. *C. arteries.* The vessels which supply the heart. *C. circulation.* See Circulation. *C. thrombosis.* See Thrombosis.

coroner (*kor'-on-er*). A medically or legally qualified person appointed to conduct inquests into the causes of sudden or unexpected deaths.

coronoid (*kor'-on-oid*). Shaped like a crow's beak. *C. process.* A bony process of the mandible or of the ulna.

corpse (*korps*). A dead body. Cadaver.

corpulent (*kor'-pu-lent*). Obese.

corpus (*kor'-pus*). *pl.* corpora. A body. *C. albicans.* The scar tissue on the surface of the ovary which replaces the corpus luteum before the recommencement of menstruation. *C. callosum.* The mass of white matter which joins the two cerebral hemispheres together. *C. cavernosum.* Either of the two columns of erectile tissue forming the body of the clitoris or the penis. *C. luteum.* The yellow body left on the surface of the ovary and formed from the remains of the Graafian follicle after the discharge of the ovum. If it retrogresses menstruation occurs, but it persists for several months if pregnancy supervenes. *C. striatum.* A mass of grey and white matter in the base of each cerebral hemisphere.

corpuscle (*kor-pus'-l*). A small protoplasmic body or cell, as of blood or connective tissue. *See* Blood.

corrective (*kor-ek'-tiv*). A corrigent. A drug which modifies the action of other drugs.

Corrigan's pulse (*Sir D.J. Corrigan, Irish physician, 1802–1880*). Water-hammer pulse. *See* Pulse.

corrosive (*kor-o'-siv*). A substance that erodes and destroys. *C. sublimate.* Mercuric chloride. An antiseptic.

cortex (*kor'-teks*). *pl.* cortices. The external layer of an organ. *Adrenal c.* The tissue surrounding the medulla or core of the adrenal gland. *Cerebral c.* The grey matter covering the two cerebral hemispheres. *Renal c.* The outer covering of the kidney.

corticospinal (*kor-tik-o-spi'-nal*). Relating to the cerebral cortex and the spinal cord. *C. tract.* The pyramidal tract. The nerve fibres making up the main pathway for rapid voluntary movement.

corticosteroid (*kor-tik-o-ster'-oid*). Any of the hormones produced by the adrenal cortex or their synthetic substitutes. Glucocorticoids are responsible for carbohydrate, fat and protein metabolism. They have powerful anti-inflammatory properties. Mineralocorticoids, e.g. aldosterone, are responsible for salt and water regulation.

corticotrophin (*kor-tik-o-tro'-fin*). ACTH. Adrenocorticotrophic hormone, secreted by the anterior lobe of the pituitary body. Stimulates the adrenal cortex to produce cortisol. If lacking, it can be given by injection.

cortisol (*kor'-tiz-ol*). The naturally occurring hormone of the adrenal cortex. Hydrocortisone.

cortisone (*kor'-tiz-one*). A naturally occurring corticosteroid. Inactive in man until converted into cortisol. *C. acetate.* A synthetic preparation with anti-inflammatory and anti-allergic properties. Used in the treatment of Addison's disease and following adrenalectomy or hypophysectomy.

Corynebacterium (*kor-i'-ne-bak-te'-re-um*). A genus of slender, rod-shaped, gram-positive and non-motile bacteria. *C. diphtheriae.* Klebs–Löffler bacillus. The causative agent of diphtheria.

coryza (*kor-i'-zah*). Cold in the head, with headache, nasal catarrh, and purulent discharge.

costal (*kos'-tal*). Relating to the ribs. *C. cartilages.* Those which connect the ribs to the sternum directly or indirectly.

costive (*kos'-tiv*). Constipated. *See* Constipation.

co-trimoxazole (*ko-tri-moks'-az-ole*). An antibiotic drug, taken orally and used mainly to treat urinary infections.

cotyledon (*kot-il-e'-don*). A cup-shaped depression. Applied to the subdivisions of the placenta.

cough (*koff*). Voluntary or reflex explosive expulsion of air from the lungs. Its purpose is usually to expel a foreign body or accumulations of mucus. *Dry c.* One where no expectoration occurs. *Wet c.* Expectoration of mucus or foreign body occurs. *Whooping c.* Infectious disease caused by *Bordetella pertussis.*

coulomb (*koo'-lom*). *abbrev.* C. SI unit of electrical charge. The electricity transferred by 1 ampere in 1 second.

counselling (*kown'-sel-ing*). A method of guidance for helping people with psychological problems where the emphasis is on the client finding his own solution.

count (*kownt*). A numerical indication. *Blood c.* Determination of the number of cells in a given amount of blood. *Differential c.* The proportion of different types of cells, usually leucocytes, in a blood sample. *Platelet c.* The number of platelets in a blood sample. *White cell c.* The total number of white cells in a blood sample.

counterextension (*kown-ter-ex-ten'-shun*). (1) The holding back of the upper fragment of

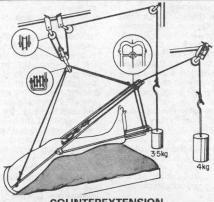

COUNTEREXTENSION

a fractured bone while the lower is pulled into position. (2) The raising of the foot of the bed in such a way that the weight of the body counteracts the pull of the extension apparatus on the lower part of the limb. Used especially for fracture of the femur.

counterirritant (*kown-ter-ir'-it-ant*). A substance which irritates the skin when applied to it, but relieves deep-seated pain.

countertraction (*kown-ter-trak'-shun*). The reduction of fractures by traction from two opposing directions at once.

counting chamber (*kown'-ting chame'-ber*). A specially designed microscope slide which is divided into 0.05 × 0.05 mm squares. It allows for the accurate counting of blood cells.

coupling (*kup'-ling*). In cardiology, the frequent occurrence of a normal heartbeat followed by an extraventricular one. May be found following digitalis overdose.

Cowper's glands (*W. Cowper, British surgeon and anatomist, 1666–1709*). Bulbourethral glands.

cowpox (*kow'-poks*). An eruption occurring on the udders of cows which is transmissible to man, and can produce immunity to smallpox. *See* Vaccinia.

coxa (*koks'-ah*). The hip joint. *C. valga.* A deformity of the hip in which there is an increase in the angle between the neck and the shaft of the femur. *C. vara.* A deformity in which the angle between the neck and the shaft of the femur is smaller than the normal.

coxalgia (*koks-al'-je-ah*). Pain in the hip joint.

Coxiella (*koks-e-el'-ah*). A genus of micro-organism similar to, but smaller than, *Rickettsia. C. burnettii.* The causative agent of Q fever.

coxitis (*koks-i'-tis*). Inflammation of the hip joint.

Coxsackie virus (*kok-sak'-e vi'-rus*). One of a group of enteroviruses that may give rise to a variety of illnesses including meningitis, pleurodynia and myocarditis.

crab louse (*krab lows*). *Phthirus pubis. See* Louse.

cramp (*kramp*). An involuntary, prolonged and painful contraction of a muscle. Associated with muscle fatigue and salt loss through dehydration.

cranial (*kra'-ne-al*). Relating to the cranium. *C. nerves.* The 12 pairs of nerves arising directly from the brain and traversing the cranium.

cranioclast (*kra'-ne-o-klast*). An instrument for crushing the head of a dead fetus to aid its delivery.

craniopharyngioma (*kra-ne-o-far-in-je-o'-mah*). A cerebral tumour arising in the craniopharyngeal pouch just above the sella turcica. It is a benign growth, but may prove fatal due to raised intracranial pressure.

craniostenosis (*kra-ne-o-sten-o'-sis*). Premature closure of the suture lines of the skull in an infant. If this leads to raised intracranial pressure surgery is indicated.

craniotabes (*kra-ne-o-ta'-beez*). A patchy thinning of the bones of the vault of the skull of an infant. Seen in rickets.

craniotomy (*kra-ne-ot'-om-e*). A surgical opening of the skull made to relieve pressure, arrest haemorrhage or remove a tumour. *Fetal c.* Craniotomy performed on a dead fetus to aid delivery.

cranium (*kra'-ne-um*). (1) The skull. (2) The bony cavity which contains the brain.

creatine (*kre'-at-een*). A nitrogenous compound present in muscle. It is also found in the urine in conditions in which muscle is rapidly broken down, e.g. acute fevers and starvation. *C. phosphate.* A high-energy phosphate store in muscle.

creatinine (*kre-at'-in-een*). A normal constituent of urine—a product of protein metabolism.

creatinuria (*kre-at-in-u'-re-ah*). Increased concentration of creatine in the urine.

creatorrhoea (*kre-at-o-re'-ah*). The presence of muscle fibres in the faeces. It occurs in certain diseases of the pancreas.

Credé's method (*K.S.F. Credé, German gynaecologist, 1819–1892*). The expulsion of the placenta by exerting pressure on the uterus through the abdominal wall.

crenation (*kre-na'-shun*). Abnormal notching of erythrocytes, which occurs when they are exposed to hypertonic solutions such as saline, or in certain diseases, or after prolonged storage of a blood specimen.

crepitation (*krep-it-a'-shun*). The grating sound caused by friction of the two ends of a fractured bone.

crepitus (*krep'-it-us*). The sound heard in the lungs through a stethoscope and produced on pressure when there is air in the subcutaneous tissues as in surgical emphysema. *See* Emphysema.

cresol (*kre'-sol*). A coal-tar phenol from which a number of commonly used disinfectants are derived.

cretinism (*kret'-in-izm*). Congenital hypothyroidism. A condition caused by lack of thyroid secretion, characterized by thickness of the neck, stunted growth, coarse facial features and impaired mental development.

cribriform (*krib'-rif-orm*). Perforated like a sieve. *C. plate.* Part of the ethmoid bone. *See* Ethmoid.

cricoid (*kri'-koid*). Ring-shaped. *C. cartilage.* The ring-shaped cartilage at the lower end of the larynx.

cri-du-chat syndrome (*kre'-doo-shah sin'-drome*). Congenital abnormalities which cause an infant to be mentally retarded and to utter a cry which sounds like the mewing of a cat.

crisis (*kri'-sis*). *pl.* crises. (1) A decisive point in acute disease; the turning-point towards either recovery or death. *See* Lysis. (2) A sudden violent attack of pain affecting certain of the viscera. *Addisonian c.* Acute onset or worsening of Addison's disease. May be due to sudden withdrawal of steroids in steroid therapy. *Dietl's c.* Severe pain in the loins, due to kinking of a ureter in the condition of 'movable kidney'. *Gastric c.* (of the stomach) and *nephralgic c.* (of the kidney) occur in tabes dorsalis. *Thyroid c.* Sudden exacerbation of symptoms in a patient with exophthalmic goitre. *See* Thyrotoxicosis.

criterion (*kri-te'-re-on*). *pl.* criteria. The basis on which a decision is made, e.g. for drug dosage, treatment plans, research trials etc.

Crohn's disease (*B.B. Crohn, American physician, b. 1884*). Regional ileitis. *See* Ileitis.

Crosby capsule (*W.H. Crosby American physician, b. 1914*). A capsule attached to the end of a flexible tube which is swallowed by the patient. When the capsule reaches the small intestine, as seen on radiological examination, a biopsy of the intestinal mucosa may be taken.

crotamiton (*kro-tam'-it-on*). An antipruritic lotion which is also used to treat scabies.

croup (*kroop*). A group of symptoms associated with inflammation and obstruction of the larynx usually occurring in young children. There is spasmodic dyspnoea, a harsh cough, and stridor.

crown (*krown*). In dentistry, that part of the tooth which appears above the gum.

crowning (*krown'-ing*). The stage in labour when the top of the infant's head becomes visible at the vulva.

cruciate (*kru'-shate*). Resembling a cross. *C. ligament. See* Ligament.

crural (*kru'-ral*). Relating to the thigh.

'crush' syndrome (*krush sin'-drome*). Severe shock with local necrosis and oedema and scanty output of urine leading to acute uraemia. Occurs when large areas of muscle tissue are damaged by crushing accidents.

crutch (*krutch*). Appliance to aid walking when the patient must not weight-bear (as in fractures of lower limbs) or when a lower limb is missing.

cryo-extractor (*kri-o-eks-trak'-*

tor). An instrument in which intense cold coagulates the lens of the eye for removal in cataract extraction.

cryosurgery (*kri-o-sur'-jer-e*). The use of extreme cold to destroy tissue.

cryotherapy (*kri-o-ther'-ap-e*). Treatment by the application of extreme cold, as in cryosurgery.

cryptogenic (*krip-to-jen'-ik*). Of unknown or obscure origin.

cryptomenorrhoea (*krip-to-men-o-re'-ah*). A condition in which menstruation occurs but the menstrual fluid fails to escape from the vagina due to an obstruction such as imperforate hymen or vaginal atresia. Haematocolpos.

cryptophthalmos (*kript-off-thal'-mos*). A covering of the eyes by a layer of skin occurring congenitally.

cryptorchidism (*kript-or'-kid-izm*). Failure of the testicles to descend into the scrotum. Cryptorchism.

crypts of Lieberkühn (*J.N. Lieberkühn, German anatomist, 1711–1756*). Glands secreting intestinal juice which are found in the mucous membrane of the small intestine.

crystalline (*kris'-tal-ine*). Having the properties of a crystal. Transparent. *C. lens.* The lens of the eye. *See* Lens.

Cs. Chemical symbol for *caesium*.

Cu. Chemical symbol for *copper*.

cubitus (*ku'-bit-us*). (1) The forearm. (2) The elbow. *C. valgus*. Deformity of the elbow where the palm of the hand is abducted and thus faces outwards. *C. varus*. Deformity where there is adduction of the forearm.

culdocentesis (kul-do-sen-te'-sis). The aspiration of fluid from the pouch of Douglas via the posterior fornix of the vagina.

culdoscope (kul'-do-skope). An instrument embodying a lighted telescope for viewing the pelvic cavity by passing it through the posterior vaginal wall.

culture (kul'-chur). In bacteriology and virology, the development of micro-organisms on artificial media.

cumulative (ku'-mu-la-tiv). Adding to. C. action. The toxic effects produced by prolonged use of a drug given in comparatively small doses. Usually occurs due to slow excretion of the drug.

cuneiform (ku'-ne-e-form). Wedge-shaped. C. bones. Three of the tarsal bones of the feet.

curare (ku-rah'-re). An extract from a South American plant used to poison the tips of arrows. Now used in surgery to produce complete muscle relaxation and thus reduce the amount of anaesthetic used. It is given intravenously as tubocurarine.

curative (ku'-rat-iv). Anything which promotes healing by overcoming disease.

curettage (ku-ret-ahzh'). Treatment by the use of a curette.

curette (ku-ret'). A spoon-shaped instrument used for the removal of unhealthy tissues by scraping. Curetting may be performed on membranous surfaces, e.g. of the uterus; on tuberculous and other chronic ulcers; or to remove dead bone.

curie (ku'-re). abbrev. Ci. A unit of radioactivity. Now replaced as an SI unit by the becquerel.

curietron (ku'-re-tron). An apparatus used for the treatment of cancer of the cervix and body of the uterus. The applicators are placed in the patient, and the radioisotope is then moved in and out of the applicators by remote control.

curvature (ker'-vat-ure). The curving of a line, whether normal or abnormal. Spinal c. Abnormal deviation of the vertebral column.

cushingoid (koosh'-ing-oid). Referring to symptoms which resemble Cushing's disease, e.g. the side-effects of steroid therapy.

Cushing's disease (H.W. Cushing, American surgeon, 1869–1939). A condition of oversecretion by the adrenal cortex due to an adenoma of the pituitary gland. Symptoms include obesity, abnormal distribution of hair, and atrophy of the genital organs.

cusp (kusp). (1) One of the projections on the crown of a tooth. (2) One of the sections of the heart valves, formed of fibrous tissue and endocardium.

cutaneous (ku-ta'-ne-us). Pertaining to the skin.

cuticle (ku'-tikl). The epidermis or external layer of skin.

cutis (ku'-tis). The skin, including both the dermis and the epidermis.

cyanide (si'-an-ide). One of the salts of hydrocyanic acid. It gives off a smell of bitter almonds and is rapidly fatal when inhaled or taken orally.

cyanocobalamin (si-an-o-ko-bal'-am-een). Vitamin B_{12}. Found in liver, eggs and fish. It may be administered by injection in the treatment of pernicious anaemia.

cyanopsia (*si-an-op'-se-ah*). Colour-blindness in which everything is seen as having a bluish tinge. Cyanopia.

cyanosis (*si-an-o'-sis*). A bluish appearance of the skin and mucous membranes, caused by imperfect oxygenation of the blood. It indicates circulatory failure and is common in respiratory diseases. It is also seen in 'blue babies'.

cycle (*si'-kl*). A series of recurring events. *Cardiac c.* The events occurring between one heart beat and the next. *Menstrual c.* The changes that occur each month in the female reproductive system.

cyclic (*si'-klik*). Pertaining to or occurring in a cycle.

cyclitis (*si-kli'-tis*). Inflammation of the ciliary body of the eye.

cyclizine (*si'-kliz-een*). An antihistamine drug and mild sedative. Useful to prevent travel sickness.

cyclobarbitone (*si-klo-bar'-bit-one*). A short-acting barbiturate drug administered orally in cases of insomnia. Prolonged use may lead to dependence.

cyclodialysis (*si-klo-di-al'-is-is*). An operation used in cases of glaucoma to improve drainage from the anterior chamber of the eye at the corneoscleral junction.

cyclodiathermy (*si-klo-di-ah-ther'-me*). A treatment for glaucoma without penetration of the eyeball. Diathermy is applied to the sclera to cause fibrosis around the ciliary body, so allowing the aqueous humour to drain away and thus reducing the pressure in the eyeball.

cyclopenthiazide (*si-klo-pen-thi'-az-ide*). An oral diuretic used in the treatment of oedema and hypertension.

cyclopentolate (*si-klo-pen'-to-late*). Eye drops that paralyse the ciliary muscles and dilate the pupils.

cyclophosphamide (*si-klo-fos'-fam-ide*). A cytotoxic drug used in the treatment of malignant tumours.

cycloplegia (*si-klo-ple'-je-ah*). Paralysis of the ciliary muscle of the eye.

cyclopropane (*si-klo-pro'-pane*). A rapid-acting gas used for general anaesthesia. It is not irritating to the respiratory tract but it is highly inflammable and is therefore potentially dangerous.

cycloserine (*si-klo-se'-rine*). An antibiotic drug used in the treatment of tuberculosis resistant to first-time treatment.

cyclothiazide (*si-klo-thi'-az-ide*). An antihypertensive agent.

cyclothymia (*si-klo-thi'-me-ah*). The alternation of mood seen in manic-depressive psychosis.

cyclotron (*si'-clo-tron*). An electromagnetic machine for imparting high velocities to atomic particles, by means of which radioactive isotopes can be prepared. Can also be employed in the treatment of malignant disease by the use of neutrons.

cyesis (*si-e'-sis*). Pregnancy. *Pseudo-c.* Signs and symptoms suggestive of pregnancy arising when no fertilization has taken place. 'Phantom pregnancy'.

cyst (*sist*). (1) A cavity or sac with epithelium, containing liquid or semi-solid matter. (2) A stage in the life-cycle of certain protozoan parasites when they acquire tough protective coats. *Branchial c.* One formed in the neck due to non-closure of the branchial cleft during development. *Chocolate c.* An ovarian cyst occurring in endometriosis. *Daughter c.* A small cyst which develops from a large one. *Dermoid c.* A congenital type containing skin, hair, teeth, etc. It is due to abnormal development of embryonic tissue. *Hydatid c.* The larval cyst stage of the tapeworm, usually found in the liver. *Meibomian c.* A swelling of a meibomian gland caused by obstruction of its duct. *Multilocular c.* A cyst that is divided into compartments or locules. *Ovarian c.* A cyst of the ovary, usually non-malignant, but sometimes becoming very large and requiring surgical removal. *Retention c.* Any cyst caused by blockage of a duct. *Sebaceous c.* A retention cyst caused by the blockage of a duct from a sebaceous gland so that the sebum collects. *Sublingual c.* A ranula. *Thyroglossal c.* One in the thyroglossal tract near the hyoid bone at the base of the tongue. *Unilocular c.* One containing only one cavity.

cystadenoma (*sist-ad-en-o'-mah*). A benign neoplasm made up of cysts containing fluid.

cystalgia (*sist-al'-je-ah*). Pain in the urinary bladder.

cystectomy (*sist-ek'-tom-e*). Complete or partial removal of the urinary bladder, with transplantation of the ureters either to an isolated loop of ileum which is brought to the surface of the abdominal wall or to the colon.

cysteine (*sis'-te-een*). A sul-phur-containing amino acid formed by the ingestion of dietary proteins.

cystic (*sist'-ik*). (1) Pertaining to a cyst. (2) Pertaining to the urinary bladder or the gallbladder. *C. fibrosis.* A congenital condition in which there is an abnormal amount of thick viscid secretion starting in the pancreas and later involving the lung with widespread bronchiectasis and emphysema.

cysticercosis (*sist-e-ser-ko'-sis*). A disease caused by infestation with the cysticercus of *Taenia solium*. The presence of this in the body causes pain and weakness, and if it reaches the brain, it may ultimately cause death.

cysticercus (*sist-e-ser'-kus*). The cystic or larval form of the tapeworm.

cystine (*sis'-teen*). An amino acid closely related to cysteine. Sometimes excreted in urine in the form of minute crystals (cystinuria).

cystinosis (*sis-tin-o'-sis*). An inherited metabolic disorder in which cystine is deposited in the tissues.

cystitis (*sist-i'-tis*). Inflammation of the urinary bladder.

cystitome (*sist'-e-tome*). A surgical knife used in cataract operations.

cystocele (*sist'-o-seel*). A herniation of the bladder into the vagina as the result of overstretching of the vaginal wall during childbirth.

cystodiathermy (*sist-o-di-ah-ther'-me*). The application of a high-frequency electric current to the bladder mucosa, usually for the removal of papilloma.

cystography (*sist-og'-raf-e*). X-ray examination of the urinary bladder after the introduction of a radio-opaque dye. *Micturating c.* Examination during the act of passing urine.

cystolithiasis (*sist-o-lith-i'-as-is*). Stone in the urinary bladder.

cystoma (*sist-o'-mah*). A tumour containing cysts. Most usual in the ovary.

cystometer (*sist-om'-e-ter*). An instrument for measuring pressure inside the urinary bladder.

cystometry (*sist-om'-et-re*). The study of pressure changes within the bladder and of variations in its capacity.

cystonephrosis (*sist-o-nef-ro'-sis*). Cystic enlargement of the kidney.

cystopexy (*sist-o-peks'-e*). An operation for stress incontinence in which the bladder neck is fastened to the fascia at the back of the symphysis pubis.

cystoscope (*sist'-o-skope*). An instrument for examining the interior of the urinary bladder.

cystostomy (*sist-os'-tom-e*). The operation of making a temporary or permanent opening into the urinary bladder.

cystotomy (*sist-ot'-om-e*). Incision of the urinary bladder for removal of calculi etc. *Suprapubic c.* Incision above the pubes.

cysto-urethroscope (*sist'-o-u-re'-thro-skope*). An instrument for examining the urethra and bladder.

cytarabine (*si-tar'-ab-een*). See Cytosine.

cytogenetics (*si-to-jen-et'-iks*). The study of cells during mitosis to examine the chromosomes and the relationship between chromo-

some abnormality and disease.

cytology (*si-tol'-o-je*). The microscopic study of the form and functions of the cells of the body. *Exfoliative c.* An aid to the early diagnosis of malignant disease. Secretions or surface cells are examined for pre-malignant changes.

cytolysin (*si-tol'-is-in*). A substance that causes cytolysis. *See* Bacteriolysin *and* Haemolysin.

cytolysis (*si-tol'-is-is*). The destruction of cells.

cytomegalovirus (*si-to-meg'-al-o-vi-rus*). A virus belonging to the herpes simplex group. It may cause symptomless infection but may lead to acute pneumonia. If contracted as an intra-uterine infection it may cause microcephaly and mental retardation.

cytoplasm (*si'-to-plazm*). The protoplasmic part of the cell surrounding the nucleus.

cytosine (*si'-to-seen*). One of the pyrimidine bases found in deoxyribonucleic acid. *See* DNA. *C. arabinoside.* An antimetabolite used in the treatment of acute leukaemia. Cytarabine.

cytotoxic (*si-to-toks'-ik*). Damaging to cell structure and division. *C. drugs.* Those that damage cells. Used to treat malignant diseases, the aim being the destruction of malignant cells with minimum harm to normal tissues.

cytotoxin (*si-to-toks'-in*). A toxin or antibody that prevents the normal function of a cell.

D

D. Abbreviation for the *dioptre* unit.

dacryoadenectomy (*dak-re-o-ad-en-ek'-tom-e*). Removal of a lacrimal gland.

dacryoadenitis (*dak-re-o-aden-i'-tis*). Inflammation of a lacrimal gland.

dacryocystitis (*dak-re-o-sist-i'-tis*). Inflammation of a lacrimal sac.

dacryocystography (*dak-re-o-sist-og'-raf-e*). X-ray examination of the lacrimal duct using a radio-opaque contrast medium.

dacryocystorrhinostomy (*dak-re-o-sis-to-ri-nos'-tom-e*). An operation to create an opening between the lacrimal sac and the nasal cavity.

dacryocystotomy (*dak-re-o-sist-ot'-om-e*). Incision of a lacrimal sac.

dacryolith (*dak'-re-o-lith*). A calculus in a lacrimal duct.

dacryoma (*dak-re-o'-mah*). A benign tumour which arises from the lacrimal epithelium.

dactyl (*dak'-til*). A finger or toe. A digit.

dactylion (*dak-til'-e-on*). Webbed fingers. *See* Syndactylism.

dactylitis (*dak-til-i'-tis*). Inflammation of a finger or toe.

dactylology (*dak-til-ol'-o-je*). Deaf and dumb language. Communication by signs made with the fingers and hands.

Dakin's solution (*H.D. Dakin, American biochemist, 1880–1952*). Sodium hypochlorite. *See* Sodium.

daltonism (*dawl'-ton-izm*). Colour-blindness. Inability to distinguish red from green.

Dalton's law (*J. Dalton, British chemist, 1766–1844*). The pressure exerted by a mixture of gases is equal to the sum of the pressures which each would exert if it alone occu-

pied the same volume at the same temperature.

danazol (*dan'-az-ol*). An anterior pituitary suppressant used in the treatment of endometriosis and metastatic breast cancer.

dandruff (*dan'-druf*). White scales shed from the scalp. If moist from serous exudate they have a greasy appearance.

danthron (*dan'-thron*). An orange-coloured laxative which sometimes turns the urine pink.

dapsone (*dap'-zone*). A sulphone drug used in the treatment of leprosy.

darwinism (*C.R. Darwin, British naturalist, 1809–1882*). The theory of the evolution of species through natural selection.

data (*dah'-tah*). *sing.* datum. A collection of facts.

daunomycin (*daw-no-mi'-sin*). A cytotoxic antibiotic. Daunorubicin.

daunorubicin (*daw-no-roo'-bi-sin*). Daunomycin.

dB. Abbreviation for *decibel.*

DDT. Dichlorodiphenyltrichloroethane. Dicophane.

deafness (*def'-nes*). The inability to hear. *Conduction* or *middle ear d.* Deafness due to the sound wave failing to reach the cochlea. *Perceptive* or *nerve d.* Deafness due to damage to the cochlea or auditory nerve.

deamination (*de-am-in-a'-shun*). A process of hydrolysis taking place in the liver by which amino acids are broken down and urea is formed.

debility (*de-bil'-it-e*). A condition of weakness and lack of physical tone.

débridement (*da-breed-mon'*). The removal of foreign substances and injured tissues from a traumatic wound. Part of the immediate treatment to promote healing.

debrisoquine (*deb-ri'-so-kween*). A powerful oral drug used in the treatment of hypertension.

decalcification (*de-kal-sif-ik-a'-shun*). Removal of calcium salts, e.g. from bone in some disorders of calcium metabolism.

decannulation (*de-kan-u-la'-shun*). The removal of a cannula, especially after tracheotomy.

decapitation (*de-kap-it-a'-shun*). The severance of the head from the body. Sometimes performed during labour where there is difficulty in delivering a dead hydrocephalic fetus.

decapsulation (*de-kaps-u-la'-shun*). Removal of a fibrous capsule. *Renal d.* The freeing and removal of the capsule of the kidney.

decerebrate (*de-ser'-e-brate*). A person with brain damage whose neurological reactions are severely impaired and where cerebral functioning has ceased.

decibel (*des'-e-bel*). *abbrev.* dB. A unit of intensity of sound, used particularly in estimating the degree of deafness.

decidua (*de-sid'-u-ah*). The thickened lining of the uterus for the reception of the fertilized ovum to protect the developing embryo. It is shed when pregnancy terminates. *D. basalis.* That part which becomes the maternal placenta. *D. capsularis.* That part which covers the embryo. *D. parietalis, d. vera.* The decidua that lines the rest of the uterine cavity. The true decidua.

deciduoma (*de-sid-u-o'-mah*). An intra-uterine tumour containing decidual cells. *D. malignum.* Chorion epithelioma.

decompensation (*de-kom-pen-sa'-shun*). Failure to compensate. In particular, failure of the heart to overcome disability or increased work load.

decomposition (*de-komp-o-zish'-un*). (1) The state of resolving into original elements, as decomposition of water into hydrogen and oxygen by electrolysis. (2) Decay or putrefaction.

decompression (*de-kom-presh'-un*). Removal of internal pressure. *Cerebral d.* A trephining operation to relieve pressure, e.g. of fluid on the brain. *D. chamber.* A compartment used to bring about a gradual lowering of atmospheric pressure to normal. *D. sickness.* Caisson disease. A condition caused by too-rapid return from high to normal pressure environments, affecting caisson workers, deep-sea divers, high-altitude fliers, etc. Symptoms include severe abdominal and joint pain, cramps, vomiting and asphyxia. Treatment is to recompress the patient urgently, and return him slowly to normal environmental pressure.

decongestive (*de-kon-jest'-iv*). An agent for relieving congestion, e.g. ephedrine.

decortication (*de-kort-ik-a'-shun*). Removal of the cortex of a structure. *D. of lung.* Removal of fibrosed pleura surrounding the lung, following chronic empyema, to allow expansion of the lung. *Renal d.* Removal of the capsule of the kidney.

decubitus (*de-ku'-bit-us*). The position assumed when lying down. *D. ulcer*. A pressure sore.

decussation (*de-kus-a'-shun*). A crossing, particularly of nerve fibres. A chiasma. *Pyramidal d.* The crossing of the pyramidal nerve fibres in the medulla oblongata.

defecation (*de-fek-a'-shun*). Evacuation of the bowels.

defence mechanism (*de-fens' mek'-an-izm*). (1) The means by which the body resists invasion by pathogenic organisms. (2) In psychiatry, the unconscious employment of psychological defences to overcome undesirable impulses.

defervescence (*de-fer-ves'-ens*). The period involved in the falling of a raised temperature to normal.

defibrillation (*de-fib-ril-a'-shun*). The restoration of normal rhythm to the heart in ventricular or atrial fibrillation.

defibrillator (*de-fib'-ril-a-tor*). An instrument by which normal rhythm is restored in ventricular or atrial fibrillation by the application of a high-voltage electric current.

defibrination (*de-fi-brin-a'-shun*). The removal of fibrin from blood plasma to prevent clotting. Used in the preparation of sera.

degeneration (*de-jen-er-a'-shun*). Deterioration in structure or function. *Adipose d.* Fatty degeneration. *Amyloid d.* The formation of a waxy starch-like substance in tissues in chronic wasting diseases. *Calcareous d.* Calcification. Calcium salts are deposited in the tissues. *Fatty d.*

The deposition of fat in the tissues. *Fibroid d.* Degeneration into fibrous tissue. *See* Fibrosis. *Senile d.* The physical and mental failings occurring in old age. *Subacute combined d. of the spinal cord.* A complication of pernicious anaemia. *See* Anaemia.

deglutition (*de-gloo-tish'-un*). The act of swallowing.

dehiscence (*de-his'-ens*). Splitting open, as of a wound.

dehydration (*de-hi-dra'-shun*). Excessive loss of fluid from the body by persistent vomiting, diarrhoea or sweating, or from the lack of intake.

déjà vu (*da'-zhah voo*). A disturbance of memory where a new experience or situation is experienced as if it had happened before.

deleterious (*de-le-te'-re-us*). Harmful; injurious.

delinquency (*de-lin'-kwen-se*). Criminal or antisocial conduct, especially among juveniles.

delirium (*de-lir'-e-um*). Mental excitement. A common condition in high fever. It is marked by an irregular expenditure of nervous energy, incoherent talk, and delusions. *D. tremens.* An acute psychosis common in chronic alcoholism, usually following abstinence from alcohol. *Traumatic d.* A possible occurrence after severe head injury. There is much confusion and disorientation.

delivery (*de-liv'-er-e*). Childbirth. Parturition. *Abdominal d.* Caesarian section. *Breech d.* Delivery of the infant in the breech position. *Premature d.* A birth after 7 months of pregnancy but before full term. *Spontaneous d.* A birth without anyone else's help.

delouse (*de-lows'*). To free from lice.

deltoid (*del'-toid*). Triangular. *D. muscle*. The triangular muscle of the shoulder arising from the clavicle and scapula, with insertion into the humerus.

delusion (*de-lu'-zhun*). A false idea or belief held by a person which cannot be corrected by reasoning. *Depressive d.* A sense of unworthiness or sinfulness. *D. of grandeur*. Erroneous belief in one's own greatness, wealth or position. *D. of persecution*. Paranoia.

dementia (*de-men'-she-ah*). A condition of permanent mental deterioration as a result of organic cerebral disease. *Arteriosclerotic d.* Dementia due to insufficient blood supply to the brain caused by arteriosclerosis. *D. paralytica*. General paralysis of the insane (GPI). *See* Paralysis. *D. praecox*. An obsolete term for schizophrenia, implying the early onset of dementia. *Presenile d.* Dementia of unknown cause occurring before the age of sixty. Characterized by cerebral atrophy and histological changes of a distinct nature. *Senile d.* Dementia occurring in old age due to cerebral atrophy.

Demodex (*de'-mo-deks*). A genus of mites parasitic in the hair follicles and in sebaceous glands, causing blackheads and sometimes dermatitis. Other species of the genus cause mange in dogs and horses.

demography (*de-mog'-raf-e*). The social study of people viewed collectively with regard to race, occupation or conditions.

demulcent (*de-mul'-sent*). An agent which soothes and allays irritation, especially of sensitive mucous membranes.

demyelination (*de-mi-el-in-a'-shun*). Destruction of the medullary or myelin sheaths of nerve fibres such as occurs in disseminated sclerosis. Demyelinization.

dendrite (*den'-drite*). One of the protoplasmic filaments of a nerve cell by which impulses are transmitted from one neurone to another. Dendron.

dendritic (*den-drit'-ik*). (1) Appertaining to a dendrite. (2) Branching. *D. ulcer*. A corneal ulcer caused by the virus of herpes simplex. It has a branching appearance as it spreads.

denervation (*de-nerv-a'-shun*). Severance or removal of the nerve supply to a part.

dengue (*deng'-ge*). A mild infectious fever lasting about seven days; occurring in the tropics and subtropics. It is caused by an arbovirus which is usually conveyed by mosquitoes. The symptoms are headache, an eruptive rash and pains in the muscles and joints, especially the knee joints.

dentalgia (*den-tal'-je-ah*). Toothache.

dentine (*den'-teen*). The calcified substance forming the bulk of a tooth between the pulp and the enamel.

dentition (*den-tish'-un*). The process of teething. *Primary d.* Cutting of the temporary or milk teeth, beginning at the age of six or seven months and continuing until the end of the second year. A full set consists of eight incisors, four canines, and eight premolars:

twenty in all. Deciduous dentition. *Secondary d.* Cutting of the permanent teeth, beginning in the sixth or seventh year, and being complete by the twelfth to fifteenth year except for the posterior molars or 'wisdom teeth'. There are thirty-two permanent teeth—eight incisors, four canines, eight premolars or bicuspids and twelve molars. Permanent dentition.

e-ri-bo-nu'-kle-ik as'-id). DNA. The nucleic acid molecule contained in the cell nucleus and consisting of long chains of atoms in a particular order. The genetic material which controls heredity.

dependence (*de-pen'-dens*). Addiction. The physical or psychological reliance on drugs. In physical dependence withdrawal of the drug causes physiological discom-

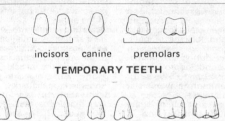

incisors   canine   premolars

TEMPORARY TEETH

incisors   canine   premolars   molars

PERMANENT TEETH

dentoid (*den'-toid*). Tooth-like.

denture (*dent'-chur*). A set of artificial teeth.

deodorant (*de-o'-dor-ant*). A substance which destroys or masks an offensive odour.

deoxycortone (*de-oks-e-kor'-tone*). A naturally occurring adrenal steroid. *D. acetate* and *d. pivalate.* Synthetic preparations used in the treatment of adrenocortical insufficiency.

deoxygenated (*de-oks'-e-jen-a-ted*). Deprived of oxygen. *D. blood.* That which has lost much of its oxygen in the tissues and is returning to the lungs for a fresh supply.

deoxyribonucleic acid (*de-oks'-*

fort with symptoms such as sweating, vomiting and tremors.

depersonalization (*de-per-son-al-i-za'-shun*). A condition in which the patient feels that his personality has changed so that he becomes an onlooker of his own actions. It may occur in almost any mental illness.

depilatory (*de-pil'-at-or-e*). An agent which will remove hair.

depolarization (*de-po-lar-i-za'-shun*). The neutralization of an electrical charge. Depolarization occurs when an impulse passes along a nerve fibre.

depressant (*de-pres'-ant*). A

drug which reduces functional activity of an organ. Anaesthetics, sedatives, tranquillizers and alcohol are depressants.

depression (de-presh'-un). (1) A hollow or indentation. (2) A lowering of psychophysical activity. A mood change is experienced as sadness, melancholy or suicidal thoughts. *Endogenous d.* Occurs sometimes without obvious cause in the course of manic-depressive psychosis. The mood change is associated with slowing of thought and action and feelings of guilt. *Involutional d.* Depression occurring during the involutional period (approximately between 45 and 65 years of age). Common in women at the menopause. *Reactive d.* Occurs as a result of some event, such as illness, loss of money, bereavement.

Derbyshire neck (dar'-be-sher nek). See Goitre.

derealization (de-re-al-i-za'-shun). Loss of a sense of reality. Surroundings and events seem unreal.

dermatitis (der-mat-i'-tis). Inflammation of the skin. *Contact d.* That arising from touching a substance to which the person is sensitive. *Exfoliative d.* Widespread scaling and itching of the skin, sometimes occurring as a reaction to treatment by certain drugs. *Industrial d., occupational d.* That caused by exposure to chemicals or other substances met with at work. *Sensitization d.* Dermatitis due to an allergic reaction. *Traumatic d.* Inflammation due to injury. *Varicose d.* Dermatitis, usually of the lower portion of the leg, due to varicosities of the smaller veins.

dermatographia (der-mat-o-graf'-e-ah). A condition in which urticarial weals occur on the skin if a blunt instrument or finger-nail is lightly drawn over it.

dermatology (der-mat-ol'-o-je). The science of skin diseases.

dermatome (der'-mat-ome). An instrument for cutting thin slices of skin for skin grafting.

dermatomycosis (der-mat-o-mi-ko'-sis). A fungal infection of the skin.

dermatomyositis (der-mat-o-mi-o-si'-tis). A collagen disease producing inflammation of the voluntary muscles with necrosis of the muscle fibres. Many sufferers have an underlying malignancy.

dermatophyte (der'-mat-o-fite). A fungus that invades the skin. There are three genera: *Epidermophyton, Microsporum,* and *Trichophyton.*

dermatosis (der-mat-o'-sis). Any skin disease, especially one which does not produce inflammation.

dermis (der'-mis). The skin, especially the layer under the epidermis.

dermoid (der'-moid). Pertaining to the skin. *D. cyst.* See Cyst.

Descemet's membrane (J. Descemet, French anatomist and surgeon, 1732–1810). The elastic membrane lining the posterior surface of the cornea.

desensitization (de-sen-sit-i-za'-shun). Hyposensitization. (1) Lessening of sensitivity to foreign protein. This process is used to prevent reaction in those likely to be susceptible, by frequent small doses of the protein. *See* Anaphylaxis. (2) In psychiatry, the treatment of phobias. The individual is gradually introduced, first in phantasy then later in reality, to the object that he fears, until gradually all fear of that object is overcome.

desiccation (*des-ik-a'-shun*). The process of drying something.

desquamation (*des-kwam-a'-shun*). The peeling of the superficial layer of the skin either in flakes or in powdery form. *Dry d.* The stage in a radiation reaction following erythema, where there is a peeling of the skin. *Moist d.* Radiation reaction where peeling of the skin is accompanied by an exudate.

detachment (*de-tach'-ment*). Separation. *D. of the retina.* Separation of the retina, or a part of it, from the choroid.

detergent (*de-ter'-jent*). A cleansing and antiseptic agent.

deterioration (*de-te-re-or-a'-shun*). Progressive impairment of function. Worsening.

detoxification (*de-toks-if-ik-a'-shun*). The process of neutralizing toxic substances. Detoxication.

detritus (*de-tri'-tus*). Debris; material which has disintegrated.

detrusor (*de-tru'-sor*). A muscle whose action is to push down. An expelling muscle.

detumescence (*de-tu-mes'-ens*). (1) The subsidence of a swelling. (2) The subsidence of an erect penis after ejaculation.

deviation (*de-ve-a'-shun*). Variation from the normal. In ophthalmology, lack of co-ordination of the two eyes.

devitalized (*de-vi'-tal-ized*). Without vitality. Used especially to describe tissues which are deprived of their nerve supply and therefore of their recuperative powers.

dexamethasone (*deks-ah-meth'-az-one*). A powerful anti-inflammatory glucocorticoid.

dexter (*deks'-ter*). Upon the right side.

dextran (*deks'-tran*). A plasma substitute formed of large glucose molecules which given intravenously increases the osmotic pressure of blood and can be used to treat shock.

dextrin (*deks'-trin*). A soluble carbohydrate which is the first product in the breakdown of starch and glycogen to sugar.

dextrocardia (*deks-tro-kar'-de-ah*). A congenital abnormality in which the heart is situated on the right side of the thorax.

dextromoramide (*deks-tro-mor'-am-ide*). A narcotic used in the treatment of chronic pain in terminal disease. A drug of addiction.

dextrose (*deks'-trose*). Grape sugar or glucose ($C_6H_{12}O_6$). The chief end-product of carbohydrate digestion. Dextrose injections in a 5% solution are used to replace fluid losses.

dhobi itch (*do'-be itch*). A term in India for ringworm of the groin (from Hindi for 'laundryman'). *See* Tinea cruris.

diabetes (*di-ah-be'-teez*). A disease characterized by excessive excretion of urine. *D. insipidus.* Diabetes marked by an increased flow of urine of low specific gravity, accompanied by great thirst. This disease, which is due to posterior pituitary dysfunction, is rare and some cases can be controlled by daily injections of pituitary extract. *D. melli-tus.* Diabetes due to deficiency or ineffectiveness of the endocrine secretion of the pancreas—*insulin*. There is polyuria and sugar is present in the urine, which makes it of high specific gravity. Other signs are lassitude and debility, loss of weight, pruritus, and a lowered resistance to infection. It is especially serious in young people. Treatment is by: (1) a properly regulated diet to maintain the nutrition of the patient; (2) keeping the blood sugar normal by injections of insulin. *Bronze d.* Haemochromatosis.

diabetic (*di-ah-bet'-ik*). Relating to diabetes.*D. coma.* The result of a severe acidosis occurring in diabetes mellitus. It is treated by immediate administration of insulin and intravenous fluids. *D. gangrene, d. retinopathy* and *d. cataract* are complications of diabetes mellitus.

diabetogenic (*di-ah-bet-o-jen'-ik*). Inducing diabetes. Some drugs or physical conditions, such as pregnancy or disease, precipitate the symptoms of diabetes in those prone to the disease.

diacetic aid (*di-ah-se'-tik as'-id*). Acetoacetic acid.

diagnosis (*di-ag-no'-sis*). Determination of the nature of a disease. *Clinical d.* Diagnosis made by the study of signs and symptoms. *Differential d.* The recognition of one disease among several presenting similar symptoms.

dialyser (*di'-al-i-zer*). (1) The membrane used in dialysis. (2) The machine or 'artificial kidney' used to remove waste products from the blood in cases of renal failure.

dialysis (*di-al'-is-is*). The process by which crystalline substances will pass through a semipermeable membrane, whereas colloids will not. In medicine this process is usually employed to remove waste and toxic products from the blood in cases of renal insufficiency. *Peritoneal d.* Use of the peritoneum as the semipermeable membrane. A dialysing solution is infused into the abdominal cavity and allowed to run out again when sufficient time has elapsed for dialysis to have occurred. Waste products are thus removed from the blood. *See* Haemodialysis.

diameter (*di-am'-e-ter*). A straight line passing through the centre of a circle to opposite points on the circumference. *Cranial d's.* Measurement of the skull, usually of the fetal head at term. If these are abnormal delivery through the vagina may not be possible. *Pelvic d's.* Measurements between the bones and joints of the pelvis made in women so as to determine whether or not the fetus can pass through at the time of childbirth.

diamorphine hydrochloride (*di-ah-mor'-feen hi-dro-klor'-ide*). A morphine derivative similar to heroin. A powerful analgesic and drug of addiction.

diapedesis (*di-ah-pe-de'-sis*). The passage of white blood cells through the walls of blood capillaries.

diaphoresis (*di-ah-for-e'-sis*). Sweating, particularly profuse sweating.

diaphoretic (*di-ah-for-et'-ik*). An agent which increases perspiration, e.g. pilocarpine.

diaphragm (*di'-ah-fram*). The muscular dome-shaped partition separating the thorax from the abdomen. *Contraceptive d.* A rubber cap which occludes the cervix.

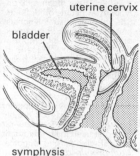

uterine cervix

bladder

symphysis pubis

CONTRACEPTIVE DIAPHRAGM

diaphragmatocele (*di-ah-fragmat'-o-seel*). A herniation of the diaphragm.

diaphysis (*di-af'-is-is*). The shaft of a long bone.

diarrhoea (*di-ar-e'-ah*). Frequent discharge of semi-solid or liquid faecal matter from the bowels. Some of the causes are: (1) incorrect diet, (2) intestinal infections, (3) poisons, (4) intestinal inflammation, (5) nervous influences. *Summer d.* Gastroenteritis of infants. *Tropical d.* Sprue.

diarthrosis (*di-ar-thro'-sis*). A freely moving articulation,

e.g. ball and socket joint. A synovial joint.

diastase (*di'-as-taze*). (1) An enzyme formed during germination of seeds, which converts starch into sugar. (2) One of the pancreatic enzymes excreted in the urine and the saliva. *D. test.* Used to estimate the excretion of diastase and therefore the pancreatic function in pancreatitis.

diastole (*di-as'-tol-e*). The resting stage of heart muscle usually applied to dilatation of the ventricles, when they fill with blood. This is followed by systole or contraction.

diastolic (*di-as-tol'-ik*). Referring to diastole. *D. murmur.* An abnormal sound produced during diastole and occurring in valvular disease of the heart.

diathermy (*di-ah-ther'-me*). Production of heat in a body tissue by a high frequency electric current. *Medical d.* Sufficient heat is used to warm the tissues but not to harm them. *Short-wave d.* Used in physiotherapy to relieve pain or treat infection. *Surgical d.* Of very high frequency; used to coagulate blood vessels or to dissect tissues. Cautery.

diathesis (*di-ath'-es-is*). A constitutional predisposition to certain diseases.

diazepam (*di-az'-e-pam*). A minor tranquillizer with muscle relaxant and anticonvulsive properties used to relieve anxiety and in the treatment of epilepsy.

diazoxide (*di-az-oks'-ide*). A vasodilator given by injection in the treatment of acute hypertension and orally in chronic hyperglycaemia.

dichloralphenazone (*di-klor-al-fen'-az-one*). A mild hypnotic and sedative drug, well suited to the elderly.

dichlorophen (*di-klor'-o-fen*). An anthelmintic, used specifically against tapeworms. No preliminary starvation is necessary and one dose can cause the worm to disintegrate.

dichlorphenamide (*di-klor-fen'-am-ide*). A diuretic used to reduce intra-ocular pressure in glaucoma.

dichotomy (*di-kot'-om-e*). Division into two parts.

dichromatic (*di-kro-mat'-ik*). Pertaining to colour-blindness when there is ability to see only two of the three primary colours.

dicophane (*di'-ko-fane*). Dichlorodiphenyltrichloroethane. Chlorophenothane. DDT. An insecticide widely used in the prevention of malaria, sandfly fever, typhus and other insect-borne diseases. Less used than formerly because of the danger of its accumulating in the body tissues.

dicrotic (*di-krot'-ik*). Having a double beat. *D. pulse.* A small wave of distension following the normal pulse beat; occurring at the closure of the aortic valve. It happens when the output from the heart is forceful and the tension of the pulse is low, as in fever.

dicyclomine (*di-si'-klo-meen*). An anticholinergic drug used in the treatment of peptic ulcer and spastic colon.

didymitis (*did-e-mi'-tis*). Orchitis. Inflammation of a testicle.

dienoestrol (*di-en-e'-strol*). A synthetic oestrogen used to treat symptoms of the menopause and to suppress lactation.

diet (*di'-et*). A regularly ordered system of nourishment, according to the requirements of the body. Hospital diets are usually graded as: (1) *full* or *ordinary d.*, (2) *light*, or *convalescent d.* (especially nutritive but easily digested foods of good calorific value), and (3) *fluid* or *milk d.*, which may mean milk only, or may include other fluids. Special diets usually consist of a reduction of, or increased quantities of, one or more of the food factors. *Diabetic d.* One which has the carbohydrate content carefully controlled. *High-calorie d.* A diet of 4000 calories (16 750 J) daily for those underweight. *Low-calorie d.* A diet reduced to 1000 calories (4200 J) daily for weight reduction. *Low-fat d.* A diet used in conditions of the gall-bladder and jaundice. *High-protein d.* One used in all cases where there has been much protein loss or excess breakdown, as in severe burns. *Low-protein d.* One suitable for cases of acute nephritis, hypertension and uraemia. *High-residue d.* One containing much roughage for the treatment of constipation. *Low-residue d.* One with a restricted fibre or roughage content suitable for inflammation of, or after operations on, the intestinal tract. *Low-salt d.* One which may consist of no table salt and salt-free cooking or may require salt-free low-salt bread and butter. Used particularly where there is tissue oedema.

dietetics (*di-et-et'-iks*). The science of regulating diet.

dietitian (*di-et-ish'-an*). One who specializes in dietetics.

diethylcarbamazine (*di-eth-il-*

kar-bam'-az-een). An anthelmintic drug used in the treatment of filariasis.

diethylpropion (*di-eth-il-pro'-pe-on*). An appetite suppressant similar in action to an emphetamine drug. Dependence can occur.

diethylstilboestrol (*di-eth-il-stil-be'-strol*). A synthetic female hormone which may be used orally or by injection to treat menopausal symptoms, or metastatic cancer of the breast and prostate. Can be used as a cream or pessary to treat vaginitis.

Dietl's crisis (*J. Dietl, Polish physician, 1804–1878*). See Crisis.

differential (*dif-er-en'-shal*). Making a difference. *D. blood count. See* Blood count. *D. diagnosis. See* Diagnosis.

differentiation (*dif-er-en-she-a'-shun*). The process in cell development whereby cells specialize and have functions which characterize them from other cells. Malignant cells are graded according to their degree of differentiation. Generally the less well-differentiated or undifferentiated tumours carry the worst prognosis.

diffuse (*dif-use'*). Scattered or widespread, as opposed to localized.

diffusion (*dif-u'-zhun*). The spontaneous mixing of molecules of liquid or gas so that they become equally distributed in the containing structure or vessel.

digestion (*di-jest'-shun*). The process performed in the alimentary system by which food is broken up for the purpose of absorption and use by the body tissues.

digit (*dij'-it*). A finger or toe.

Accessory d., supernumary d. An additional digit occurring as a congenital abnormality.

digitalis (*dij-it-a'-lis*). A group of drugs used extensively for their action on the heart. They strengthen the heartbeat and slow down the conducting power of the atrioventricular bundle, thereby enabling the ventricles to beat more effectively. Particularly valuable in treating atrial fibrillation. Prepared digitalis tablets are formed from the powdered leaves of the purple foxglove. Its chief glycosides are *digitalin* and *digitoxin. Digoxin* is the chief glycoside from the white foxglove. The effects of digitalis are cumulative, indicated by a very slow pulse and coupling of the beats.

digitalization (*dij-it-al-i-za'-shun*). The administration of large doses of digitalis within a short period of time, so that a powerful effect is produced quickly. Sometimes called *rapid* or *intensive d.*

digoxin (*dij-oks'-in*). See Digitalis.

dihydrocodeine (*di-hi-dro-ko'-deen*). A synthetic drug derived from codeine. It has greater analgesic powers but there is greater risk of addiction. Also used to suppress coughs.

dihydroergotamine (*di-hi-dro-er-got'-am-een*). A drug used in the treatment of migraine. Less effective than ergotamine, but with fewer side-effects.

dihydrotachysterol (*di-hi-dro-tak-e-ste'-rol*). A preparation closely related to vitamin D. Used in cases of vitamin D deficiency and in persistent rickets.

dilatation (*di-lat-a'-shun*). (1)

The operation of stretching a constricted passage, as in stricture of the urethra. (2) Stretching of a hollow organ. (3) Reflex widening of blood vessels to increase blood flow to an organ or tissue. Also the reflex widening of the pupil of the eye to admit more light to the retina.

dilator (*di-la'-tor*). (1) An instrument used for enlarging an opening or cavity such as the rectum, the male urethra or the cervix, by dilatation. (2) A muscle which causes dilatation. (3) A drug which causes dilatation, e.g. a vasodilator. *Hegar's d's*. A series of dilators used to widen the cervical canal prior to examination of the uterus under anaesthesia.

diluent (*dil'-u-ent*). Any agent which is used to weaken a solution. Often used to denote fluids which are mixed with powders for the purpose of injection into the body.

dimenhydrinate (*di-men-hi'-drin-ate*). An antihistamine drug, useful in preventing nausea and vomiting, particularly that associated with motion sickness.

dimercaprol (*di-mer-kap'-rol*). A drug which combines with heavy metals to form a stable compound, which is rapidly excreted. Used to treat poisoning by antimony, gold, mercury and other metals. Also called British antilewisite or BAL.

dimethylphthalate (*di-meth-il-thal'-ate*). DIMP. An insect repellent in liquid or ointment form that is effective for several hours when applied to the skin.

diodone (*di'-o-done*). A contrast medium containing iodine which is similar to iodoxyl. Used in radiology of the urinary tract.

dioptre (*di-op'-ter*). *abbrev.* D. The unit used in measuring lenses for spectacles. When parallel light enters a lens and focuses at a distance of 1 metre, the refractive power of the lens is 1 dioptre, and from this basis abnormalities are reckoned.

diphenhydramine (*di-fen-hi'-dram-een*). An antihistamine drug, used in treating allergic conditions such as hay fever and urticaria.

diphtheria (*dif-the'-re-ah*). An acute infectious disease caused by *Corynebacterium diphtheriae* (Klebs–Löffler bacillus), which most often infects the throat and tonsils, causing a greyish-white membrane to form. Powerful exotoxins are produced that cause severe toxaemia and attack the heart muscle. The disease can be prevented by using a toxoid. *D. immunization* should be carried out in infancy and booster doses given at intervals.

diphtheroid (*dif'-ther-oid*). Resembling diphtheria. A general term applied to organisms or membranes apparently similar to true diphtheria types.

Diphyllobothrium (*di-fil-o-both'-re-um*). A genus of large tapeworm. *D. latum*, the broad tapeworm, grows up to 10 m long and may infest man, following the eating of uncooked infected fish.

dipipanone (*di-pip'-an-one*). A potent analgesic used for the relief of severe pain.

diplegia (*di-ple'-je-ah*). Paralysis of similar parts on either side of the body. *Spastic d.* A congenital muscle rigidity of the lower limbs. Little's disease.

diplococcus (*dip-lo-kok'-us*). Spherical bacteria occurring in pairs. The group includes the gonococcus, the pneumococcus and the causative agent of whooping cough, *Haemophilus pertussis*.

diploë (*dip'-lo-e*). The cancellous tissue between the outer and inner surfaces of the skull.

diplopia (*di-plo'-pe-ah*). Double vision in which two images are seen in place of one, due to lack of co-ordination of the external muscles of the eye.

diprophylline (*di-pro'-fil-een*). A xanthine derivative used in the treatment of bronchospasm and left ventricular failure.

dipsomania (*dip-so-ma'-ne-ah*). A morbid craving for alcohol which occurs in bouts.

director (*di-rek'-tor*). In surgery, a grooved instrument for directing the knife during operations.

disaccharide (*di-sak'-ar-ide*). A sugar whose molecules are made up of two simple sugars or monosaccharides. *D. intolerance.* The inability to absorb disaccharides owing to an enzyme deficiency.

disarticulation (*dis-ar-tik-u-la'-shun*). Separation. Amputation at a joint.

disc (*disk*). A flattened circular structure. *Intervertebral d.* A fibrocartilaginous pad that separates the bodies of two adjacent vertebrae. *Optic d.* A white spot in the retina. It is the point of entrance of the optic nerve.

discission (*dis-izh'-un*). In cataract operations, the cut-

ting of the capsule of the lens. Also called needling. The lens is then absorbed by the surrounding ocular fluid.

discography (*dis-kog'-raf-e*). X-ray examination following the injection of a radio-opaque dye into an intervertebral disc. Degenerative changes or herniation may be seen.

discrete (*dis-kreet'*). Composed of separate parts. The opposite of confluent.

disease (*diz-eez'*). Any departure from normal health. It may be congenital (that which has been present from birth) or acquired, and it may come under one of the following headings: *Acute d.* One which has rapid onset but resolves quickly. *Autoimmune d.* One where the body tissues appear to become sensitive to themselves and start to destroy themselves. May be systemic or specific to an organ. *Chronic d.* One which has an insidious onset and is progressive. *Communicable d.* One that can be transmitted from one person to another or from an animal to a human being. *Contagious d.* One transmitted by actual physical contact with another human being or an animal suffering from that disease. *Degenerative d.* Regression of the tissues, commoner in older people. *Deficiency d.* One due to lack of vitamins or glandular secretion. *Functional d.* One which affects the working of an organ but in which no structural change can be found. *Infectious d.* Communicable disease. *Malignant d.* One which is severe, progressive and likely to prove fatal. *Metabolic d.* One in which there is improper digestion and absorption of food or improper cell function. *Neoplastic d.* One which is characterized by new growths. May be benign but usually applies to malignant disease. *Secondary d.* A condition resulting from another, e.g. bronchopneumonia consequent upon measles. (For separate diseases, see under individual names.)

disimpaction (*dis-im-pak'-shun*). Reduction of an impacted fracture.

disinfectant (*dis-in-fek'-tant*). An agent which is capable of destroying micro-organisms. Usually a germicide used to clean surgical instruments, or an antiseptic.

disinfection (*dis-in-fek'-shun*). The destruction of micro-organisms or their reduction to a level not normally harmful to health.

disinfestation (*dis-in-fest-a'-shun*). The destruction of animal parasites and pests.

dislocation (*dis-lo-ka'-shun*). The displacement of a bone from its natural position upon another at a joint. Luxation.

dismemberment (*dis-mem'-ber-ment*). The amputation of a limb or a part of a limb.

disopyramide (*di-so-pi'-ram-ide*). A drug given orally or by slow intravenous injection to treat ventricular arrhythmia.

disorder (*dis-or'-der*). Any failure of function, physical or mental.

disorientation (*dis-or-e-en-ta'-shun*). Inability to appreciate surroundings, time or personal identity.

dispensary (*dis-pen'-sar-e*). Any place where drugs are produced and supplied to patients on doctors' prescriptions.

displacement (*dis-plase'-ment*). In psychology, the replacement of one type of behaviour by another. Usually as an emotional outlet.

disposition (*dis-poz-ish'-un*). A tendency to suffer from certain diseases.

dissect (*dis-ekt'*). (1) To cut carefully in the study of anatomy. (2) During operation, to separate according to natural lines of structure.

disseminated (*dis-em'-in-a-ted*). Widely scattered or dispersed. *D. sclerosis.* Multiple sclerosis. *See* Sclerosis.

dissociation (*dis-o-she-a'-shun*). Separation. (1) The splitting up of molecules of matter into their component parts, e.g. by heat or electrolysis. (2) In psychology, the separation of ideas, emotions or experiences from the rest of the mind, giving rise to a lack of unity of which the patient is not aware.

dissonance (*dis'-on-ans*). Discord. Lack of harmony. *Cognitive d.* The inability of an individual to correlate his mental reasoning with his behaviour. Occurs when an individual acts against his will.

distal (*dis'-tal*). Situated away from the centre of the body or point of origin. The opposite of *proximal*.

Distalgesic (*dis-tal-je'-zik*). A widely used proprietary analgesic composed of dextropropoxyphene and paracetamol.

distension (*dis-ten'-shun*). Enlargement. *Abdominal d.* Enlargement of the abdomen by gas in the intestines or fluid in the abdominal cavity.

distichiasis (*dis-tik-i'-as-is*). A rare condition where there is a double row of eyelashes, the inner one causing irritation to the globe of the eye.

distillation (*dis-til-a'-shun*). Evaporation by heat of the volatile parts of a compound and subsequent condensation of the vapour.

disulfiram (*di-sul'-fir-am*). A drug used in aversion therapy in alcoholism.

dithranol (*dith'-ran-ol*). A synthetic preparation used in the treatment of psoriasis.

diuresis (*di-u-re'-sis*). Increased secretion of urine.

diuretic (*di-u-ret'-ik*). An agent which increases the flow of urine. Most such drugs act by preventing reabsorption in the renal tubule.

diurnal (*di-er'-nal*). Occurring on a daily basis.

diverticulitis (*di-ver-tik-u-li'-tis*). Inflammation of a diverticulum. It is commonest in the colon; lower abdominal pain with colic and constipation may occur and intestinal obstruction or abscesses may develop. Inflammation of Meckel's diverticulum may produce symptoms similar to appendicitis.

diverticulosis (*di-ver-tik-u-lo'-sis*). The presence of diverticula in the colon, but without any inflammation. They can be detected by X-ray after a radio-opaque meal.

diverticulum (*di-ver-tik'-u-lum*). *pl.* diverticula. A pouch or pocket in the lining of a hollow organ, as in the bladder, oesophagus or large intestine. *Meckel's d.* A small sac occurring in the ileum as a congenital abnormality.

dizziness (*diz'-e-nes*). A feeling of unsteadiness or haziness, accompanied by anxiety.

DNA. Deoxyribonucleic acid.

Döderlein's bacillus (*A.S.G.* Döderlein, German obstetrician and gynaecologist, 1860–1941*). A lactobacillus occurring normally in vaginal secretions.

dolichocephaly (*dol-ik-o-kef'-al-e*). An abnormal condition in which the anteroposterior diameter of the head is relatively long.

dolor (*dol'-or*). Pain.

dominant (*dom'-in-ant*). In genetics, the opposite of *recessive. D. gene.* One which will produce its characteristics when it is present in either a hetero- or homozygous state, i.e. it may be inherited from one parent only.

domiphen (*dom'-if-en*). An antiseptic used in tablet form for throat infections.

donor (*do'-nor*). One who gives his blood or his own organs, e.g. a kidney, or tissues to another. *Universal d.* Someone who has group O blood. *See* Blood grouping.

dopamine (*do'-pam-een*). A sympathomimetic substance allied to noradrenaline and used in the treatment of cardiogenic shock. Also occurs naturally in the adrenal medulla and the brain where it functions as a transmitter of nervous impulses.

dorsal (*dor'-sal*). Relating to the back or posterior part of an organ.

dorsiflexion (*dor-se-flek'-shun*). Bending backwards of the fingers or toes, i.e. upwards.

dorsum (*dor'-sum*). (1) The back. (2) The upper or posterior surface.

dosimeter (*do-sim'-e-ter*). An instrument that records the quantity of radiation received by X-ray operatives.

dothiepin (*do-thi'-ep-in*). A

tricyclic antidepressant and sedative drug.

douche (*doosh*). A stream of water directed to flush out a cavity of the body.

Douglas bag (*C.G. Douglas, British physiologist, 1882–1963*). A bag which is used to collect expired air when oxygen consumption has to be measured.

Douglas's pouch (*J. Douglas, British anatomist, 1675–1742*). Recto-uterine pouch. *See* Pouch.

down (*down*). The fine hair which covers the body of a fetus.

Down's syndrome (*J.L.H. Down, British physician, 1828–1896*). Mongolism.

doxorubicin (*doks-o-roo'-bis-in*). Adriamycin.

dracontiasis (*drak-on-ti'-as-is*). A tropical disease caused by infestation with the guinea worm; acquired by drinking contaminated water.

Dracunculus (*drak-ung'-ku-lus*). A genus of round worms which includes the guinea worm.

drawsheet (*draw'-sheet*). A narrow sheet placed under a patient to prevent soiling of the main sheet.

dressing (*dres'-ing*). Material applied to cover a wound or a diseased surface of the body.

drip (*drip*). A colloquial term used to denote continuous infusion of fluid (blood, saline, glucose) into the body. *Intravenous d.* Infusion into a vein.

drive (*drive*). In psychology, an urge or motivating force.

droperidol (*dro-per'-id-ol*). A major tranquillizer used to control behavioural disturbances.

droplet (*drop'-let*). A small

drop. *D. infection. See* Infection.

dropsy (*drop'-se*). A popular term used to describe excess fluid in the tissues (*oedema*) or in the peritoneal cavity (*ascites*).

drug (*drug*). Any substance used as a medicine. *D. dependence.* A possible result of taking drugs repeatedly so that the patient is unable to do without them either emotionally or physically.

Duchenne dystrophy (*G.B.A. Duchenne, French neurologist, 1806–1875*). Progressive hypertrophic muscular dystrophy occurring in childhood. *See* Dystrophy.

Ducrey's bacillus (*A. Ducrey, Italian dermatologist, 1860–1940*). *Haemophilus ducreyi,* the organism causing soft chancre. *See* Chancroid.

duct (*dukt*). A tube or channel for the passage of fluid, particularly one conveying the secretion of a gland.

ductless (*dukt'-les*). Without an excretory duct. *D. glands.* Endocrine glands. *See* Endocrine.

ductus (*duk'-tus*). A duct. *D.*

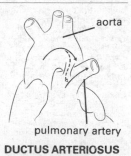

aorta

pulmonary artery

DUCTUS ARTERIOSUS

arteriosus. A passage connecting the pulmonary artery and aorta in intra-uterine life, which normally closes at birth. In some cases it remains patent, and causes a continuous cardiac murmur. The defect may close without medical intervention but an operation to close the duct has benefited many cases. *D. deferens.* Vas deferens.

dumping (*dump'-ing*). The rapid evacuation of the contents of an organ. *D. syndrome.* A feeling of fullness, weakness, sweating, dizziness and palpitations which may occur after meals following the operation of subtotal gastrectomy.

duodenal (*du-o-de'-nal*). Pertaining to the duodenum. *D. intubation.* The use of a special tube having a metal end which is passed via the mouth and stomach into the duodenum. Used for withdrawal of duodenal contents for pathological examination. *D. ulcer.* A peptic ulcer occurring in the duodenum near the pylorus.

duodenitis (*du-o-den-i'-tis*). Inflammation of the duodenum.

duodenopancreatectomy (*du-o-den-o-pan-kre-at-ek'-tom-e*). Pancreatoduodenectomy. Surgical removal of the duodenum and much of the pancreas. Usually accompanied by anastomosis of the bile ducts and the tail of the pancreas to the jejunum.

duodenostomy (*du-o-den-os'-tom-e*). The formation of an artificial opening into the duodenum, through the abdominal wall, for purposes of feeding in cases of gastric disease.

duodenum (*du-o-de'-um*). The first 20–25 cm of the small intestine, from the pyloric opening of the stomach to the jejunum. The pancreatic and common bile ducts open into it.

Dupuytren's contraction or **contracture** (*Baron G. Dupuytren, French surgeon, 1777–1835*). Contracture of the palmar fascia, causing permanent bending and fixation of one or more fingers.

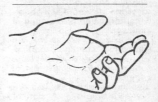

**DUPUYTREN'S
CONTRACTURE**

dura mater (*du'-rah ma'-ter*). A strong fibrous membrane, forming the outer covering of the brain and spinal cord. It lines the inner surface of the protecting bones.

dwarfism (*dworf'-izm*). Arrest of growth, e.g. due to renal rickets, cretinism or deficient pituitary function.

dynamometer (*di-nam-om'-e-ter*). An instrument by which the strength of a person's grip can be measured.

dysaesthesia (*dis-es-the'-ze-ah*). (1) Impaired sense of touch. (2) A pain arising and persisting after a normally harmless touch.

dysathrosis (*dis-ar-thro'-sis*). A deformed, dislocated or false joint.

dyschezia (*dis-ke'-ze-ah*). Difficult defecation. A form of constipation due to delay in the passage of faeces from the pelvic colon into the rectum for evacuation.

dyschondroplasia (*dis-kon-dro-pla'-ze-ah*). A condition in which cartilage is deposited in the shaft of some bones. The affected bones become shortened and deformed.

dyschromatopsia (*dis-kro-mat-op'-se-ah*). Partial loss of colour vision.

dyscoria (*dis-kor'-e-ah*). Abnormal formation of the pupil of the eye

dyscrasia (*dis-kra'-ze-ah*). An abnormal condition, particularly a disorder of development. *Blood d.* A disorder of the blood.

dysdiadochokinesis (*dis-di'-ad-o-ko-kin-e'-sis*). A sign of cerebellar disease in which the ability to perform rapid alternating movements, such as rotating the hands, is lost.

dysentery (*dis'-en-ter-e*). A tropical or subtropical infectious disease, characterized by inflammation and ulceration of the large intestine with frequent blood-stained evacuations. Specific forms are: (1) *Amoebic d.* Caused by *Entamoeba histolytica*; treated by administration of emetine, which is specific for the organism. (2) *Bacillary d.* Caused by bacteria of the genus *Shigella*; treatment is by maintenance of the salt and water intake and the giving of antibiotics.

dysfunction (*dis-funk'-shun*). Impairment of function.

dysgenesis (*dis-jen'-es-is*). Defective development.

dysgerminoma (*dis-jer-min-o'-mah*). A malignant tumour derived from germinal cells that have not been differentiated

to either sex, occurring in either the ovary or the testicle.

dyshidrosis (*dis-hi-dro'-sis*). A disturbance of the sweat mechanism, in which an itching vesicular rash may be present.

dyskinesia (*dis-kin-e'-ze-ah*). Impairment of voluntary movement.

dyslalia (*dis-la'-le-ah*). Impairment of speech, caused by a physical disorder.

dyslexia (*dis-leks'-e-ah*). Difficulty in reading or learning to read; accompanied by difficulty in writing and spelling correctly.

dysmelia (*dis-me'-le-ah*). Malformation in the development of the limbs. There may be excessive or impaired growth. *See* Amelia.

dysmenorrhoea (*dis-men-o-re'-ah*). Painful menstruation. *Primary d.* (*spasmodic*). Painful menstruation occurring without apparent cause. The onset is usually shortly following puberty and occurs with each subsequent period. May be helped by hormonal therapy. *Secondary d.* (*congestive*). Painful menstruation occurring in a woman who has previously had normal periods for some years. Often due to endometritis. The condition tends to worsen as the local congestion increases.

dysostosis (*dis-os-to'-sis*). Abnormal development of bone.

dyspareunia (*dis-par-u'-ne-ah*). Painful coitus.

dyspepsia (*dis-pep-se-ah*). Indigestion. There may be abdominal discomfort, flatulence, nausea and sometimes vomiting. *Nervous d.* Dyspepsia in which anxiety and tension aggravate the symptoms.

dysphagia (*dis-fa'-je-ah*). Difficulty in swallowing.

dysphasia (*dis-fa'-ze-ah*). Difficulty in speaking, due to a brain lesion. There is a lack of co-ordination and an inability to arrange words in their correct order.

dysplasia (*dis-pla'-ze-ah*). Abnormal development of tissue.

dyspnoea (*disp-ne'-ah*). Difficult or laboured breathing. *Expiratory d.* Difficulty in expelling air. *Inspiratory d.* Difficulty in intake of air.

dysrhythmia (*dis-rith'-me-ah*). Disturbance of a regularly occurring pattern. Often applied to an abnormality of rhythm of the brain waves as shown in an electroencephalogram.

dystaxia (*dis-taks'-e-ah*). Difficulty in controlling voluntary movements.

dystocia (*dis-to'-se-ah*). Difficult or slow labour. *Maternal d.* Difficult labour when the cause is with the mother, e.g.

contracted pelvis. *Fetal d.* Difficult labour due to abnormal size or position of the child.

dystonia (*dis-to'-ne-ah*). A lack of tonicity in a tissue, often referring to the muscles.

dystrophia (*dis-tro'-fe-ah*). Dystrophy. *D. myotonica.* A rare hereditary disease of early adult life in which there is progressive muscle wasting and gonadal atrophy.

dystrophy (*dis'-tro-fe*). A disorder of an organ or tissue caused by faulty nutrition of the affected part. Dystrophia. *Muscular d.* A group of hereditary diseases in which there is progressive muscular weakness and wasting.

dysuria (*dis-u'-re-ah*). Difficult or painful micturition.

E

ear (*e'-er*). The organ of hearing. It consists of three parts: (1) the *external e.*, made up of the expanded portion, or pinna, and the auditory canal

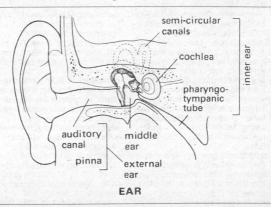

EAR

separated from the middle ear by the drum, or tympanum; (2) the *middle e.*, an irregular cavity containing three small bones of the ear (*incus, malleus* and *stapes*) which link the tympanic membrane to the internal ear. It also communicates with the pharyngotympanic tube and the mastoid cells; (3) the *internal e.*, which consists of a bony and a membranous labyrinth (the *cochlea* and *semicircular* canals).

eburnation (*e-bern-a'-shun*). Increased density of bone, following inflammation.

ecchondroma (*ek-on-dro'-mah*). A benign cartilaginous tumour arising as an outgrowth to cartilage or bone.

ecchymosis (*ek-e-mo'-sis*). A bruise. An effusion of blood under the skin causing discoloration, e.g. a black eye.

eccrine (*ek'-rine*). Secreting externally. Applied particularly to the sweat glands that are generally distributed over the body but are densest on the palms of the hands and soles of the feet. *See* Apocrine.

ECG. Electrocardiogram.

Echinococcus (*ek-in-o-kok'-us*). A genus of tapeworms. *E. granulosus* infests dogs and may also infect man if the ova are swallowed with contaminated food. The larval form develops into cysts (hydatids), which may occur in the liver, lung, brain or other organ, being carried by the blood or lymph stream from the intestine.

echocardiography (*ek-o-kar-de-og'-raf-e*). A method of studying the movements of the heart by the use of ultrasound.

echoencephalography (*ek-o-*

en-kef-al-og'-raf-e). A method of brain investigation by ultrasonic echoes.

echolalia (*ek-o-la'-le-ah*). The pathological involuntary repetition of phrases or words spoken by another person.

echophony (*e-kof'-on-e*). The echo of the voice heard in the chest on auscultation.

echopraxia (*ek-o-praks'-e-ah*). The automatic repetition by a patient of acts he has seen performed by others.

echovirus (*ek-o-vi'-rus*). One of a group of enteric *cytopathic human orphan* viruses. 'Orphan' here refers to the fact that when first isolated, it was not known which diseases were caused by the viruses, but it is now known that some of them may cause aseptic meningitis and respiratory and gastrointestinal diseases.

eclampsia (*ek-lamp'-se-ah*). A severe condition in which convulsions may occur as a result of an acute toxaemia of pregnancy.

ecmnesia (*ek-ne'-ze-ah*). A gap in memory in which recent events are forgotten.

ecology (*e-kol'-o-je*). The study of the relationship between living organisms and the environment.

écraseur (*a-krah-zer'*). An instrument having a wire loop that is tightened round the stalk of a projecting growth (e.g. a polyp) to sever it.

ecstasy (*ek'-stas-e*). A feeling of exaltation. It may be accompanied by sensory impairment and lack of activity but with an expression of rapture.

ECT. Electroconvulsive therapy.

ectasia (*ek-ta'-ze-ah*). Dilatation of a canal or organ. Ectasis. *Alveolar e.* Distension of the air sacs of the lung. *Corneal e.* Bulging and thinning of the cornea due to disease or raised intraocular pressure.

ectasis (*ek'-tas-is*). Ectasia.

ecthyma (*ek-thi'-mah*). A form of impetigo with an eruption of pustules usually with a hardened base. A pigmented scar remains after healing takes place.

ectoderm (*ek'-to-derm*). The outer germinal layer of the developing embryo from which the skin and nervous system are derived.

ectogenous (*ek-toj'-en-us*). Produced outside an organism. *See* Endogenous.

ectomorph (*ek'-to-morf*). An individual of slight build but with a large skin surface.

ectoparasite (*ek-to-par'-ah-site*). A parasite that spends all or part of its life on the external surface of its host, e.g. a louse.

ectopia (*ek-to'-pe-ah*). Displacement or abnormal position of any part. *E. cordis.* Congenital malposition of the heart outside the thoracic cavity. *E. lentis.* Abnormal position of the lens of the eye. *E. vesicae.* A congenital defect of the abdominal wall in which the bladder is exposed.

ectopic (*ek-top'-ik*). Pertaining to ectopia. Misplaced. *E. beat.* A heartbeat originating from somewhere other than the sino-atrial node. *E. gestation, e. pregnancy.* Extra-uterine pregnancy. *See* Gestation.

ectrodactylia (*ek-tro-dak-til'-e-ah*). Congenital absence of one or more fingers or toes.

ectropion (*ek-tro'-pe-on*). Eversion of an eyelid, often due to contraction of the skin or to

paralysis. It causes epiphora and hypertrophy of exposed conjunctiva and may cause corneal ulceration if the eye does not close.

eczema (*ek'-ze-mah*). An acute or chronic inflammatory condition of the skin, non-contagious although secondary infection is common. The eruption appears first as papules which become moist and finally form scabs. There is great irritation of the affected part and constitutional disturbances may also be present. Many forms are allergic in origin. *Dry e.* Eczema where the affected area is dry and scaly. *Weeping e.* Eczema in which there is a serous exudation from the affected area, which precedes drying up and healing.

eczematous (*ek-zem'-at-us*). Affected with or resembling eczema.

edentulous (*e-dent'-ul-us*). Without teeth, especially applied to the elderly.

EDTA. Ethylenediamine tetra-acetic acid. A chelating agent used in the treatment of lead poisoning. *EDTA clearance test.* A test of renal function where EDTA is labelled with radioactive chromium and injected into the patient's blood stream. Blood samples are then taken at specific intervals. The amount of EDTA remaining in the blood is an indicator of the amount excreted by glomerular filtration.

EEG. Electroencephalogram.

effector (*e-fek'-tor*). A motor or sensory nerve ending in a muscle, gland or organ.

efferent (*ef'-er-ent*). Conveying from the centre to the periphery. *E. nerves.* Motor nerves coming from the brain to supply the muscles and glands. *E. tracts*. The pathway of the motor nerves from the cerebral cortex and descending the spinal cord. *See* Afferent.

effervescent (*ef-er-ves'-ent*). Foaming or giving off gas bubbles.

effleurage (*ef'-loor-ahzh*). A form of massage which aids dispersal of oedema.

effluent (*ef'-lu-ent*). (1) *adj.* Flowing out. (2) *n.* The fluid portion of sewage. The sludge or more solid portion may have been separated from it.

effluvium (*ef-lu'-ve-um*). A subtle, usually unpleasant, odour which may be given off by a substance or person.

effort syndrome (*ef'-ort sin'-drome*). A condition characterized by breathlessness, palpitations, chest pain and fatigue, caused by an abnormal anxiety about the condition of the heart.

effusion (*e-fu'-zhun*). The escape of blood, serum or other fluid into surrounding tissues or cavities.

ego (*eg'-o*). In psychology, that part of the mind which the individual experiences as his 'self'. The ego is concerned with satisfying the unconscious primitive demands of the 'id' in a socially acceptable form.

Ehrlich's side-chain theory (*P. Ehrlich, German bacteriologist, 1854–1915*). An explanation of the phenomena of immunity, in which protoplasmic cells are said to possess certain chemical attachments or side-chains. These side-chains are capable of uniting with bacterial toxins and in so doing render them harmless.

eidetic (*i-det'-ik*). Pertaining to the ability to visualize exactly objects or events which have previously been seen. Popularly known as a photographic memory.

Eisenmenger's complex (*V. Eisenmenger, German physician, 1864–1932*). A congenital heart defect in which a ventricular septal defect is associated with increased pulmonary vascular resistance.

ejaculation (*e-jak-u-la'-shun*). The act of ejecting semen.

elastic (*e-las'-tik*). Capable of stretching. *E. bandage*. One that will stretch and will exert continuous pressure on the part bandaged. *E. stocking*. A woven rubber stocking sometimes worn for varicose veins. *E. tissue*. Connective tissue containing yellow elastic fibres.

elation (*e-la'-shun*). In psychiatry, a feeling of well-being or a state of excitement which may vary considerably in degree. It occurs in marked degree in hypomania and in intense degree in mania. *See* Euphoria.

elbow (*el'-bo*). The joint between the upper arm and the forearm. It is formed by the humerus above and the radius and ulna below.

elective (*e-lek'-tiv*). That which is chosen by the patient or physician, as opposed to emergency procedures.

Electra complex (*e-lek'-trah kom'-pleks*). The excessive attachment of a daughter for her father, with antagonism towards the mother. The female version of the Oedipus complex.

electrocardiogram (*e-lek-tro-kar'-de-o-gram*). ECG. A tracing made of the various

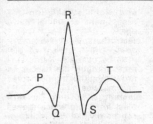

ELECTROCARDIOGRAM

phases of the heart's action by means of an electrocardiograph.

electrocardiograph (*e-lek-tro-kar'-de-o-graf*). A machine for recording the potential of electrical currents that traverse the heart muscle and initiate contraction.

electrocardiophonograph (*e-lek-tro-kar-de-o-fo'-no-graf*). An electrical machine for recording graphically the heart sounds. A phonocardiograph.

electrocautery (*e-lek-tro-kaw'-ter-e*). An instrument for the destruction of tissue by means of an electrically heated needle or wire loop.

electrocoagulation (*e-lek-tro-ko-ag-u-la'-shun*). A method of coagulation using a high-frequency current. A form of surgical diathermy.

electroconvulsive therapy (*e-lek-tro-kon-vul'-siv ther'-ap-e*). ECT. Electroplexy. The passage of an electric current through the frontal lobes of the brain, which causes a convulsion. It is used in the treatment of depression and sometimes of schizophrenia. A general anaesthetic and muscle relaxant are given prior to treatment.

electrocorticography (*e-lek-tro-kor-tik-og'-raf-e*). Electroencephalography with the electrodes applied directly to the cortex of the brain. Performed in the operating theatre to locate a small lesion, e.g. a scar.

electrode (*e-lek'-trode*). The terminal of a conducting system or cell of a battery, through which electricity is applied to the body.

electroencephalogram (*e-lek'-tro-en-kef'-al-o-gram*). EEG. A tracing of the electrical activity of the brain. Abnormal rhythm is an aid to diagnosis in epilepsy and cerebral tumour.

electroencephalograph (*e-lek'-tro-en-kef'-al-o-graf*). A machine for recording the electrical activity of the cortex of the brain. The electrodes are applied to the scalp.

electrolysis (*e-lek-trol'-is-is*). (1) Chemical decomposition by means of electricity, e.g. an electric current passed through water decomposes it into oxygen and hydrogen. (2) The destruction of tissue by means of electricity, e.g. the removal of surplus hair.

electrolyte (*e-lek'-tro-lite*). A compound which when dissolved in a solution will dissociate into ions. These ions are electrically charged particles and will thus conduct electricity. *E. balance*. The maintenance of the correct balance between the different elements in the body tissues and fluids.

electromotive force (*e-lek-tro-mo'-tiv fors*). EMF. A measure of the force needed for a current of electricity to flow from one point to another. The unit of EMF is the volt.

electromyography (*e-lek-tro-mi-og'-raf-e*). Recording of electrical currents generated in active muscle.

electron (*e-lek'-tron*). A negatively charged particle revolving round the nucleus of an atom. *See* Atom. *E. beam.* A stream of high-speed negative ions which have been accelerated by a radiotherapy machine to treat tumours near the body surface. *E. microscope.* A type of microscope employing a beam of electrons rather than a beam of light, which allows very small particles such as viruses to be identified.

electronarcosis (*e-lek-tro-nar-ko'-sis*). A state of sleep or unconsciousness induced by placing electrodes on the temple and passing an electric current through the brain. This therapy is rarely used in the West.

electro-oculography (*e-lek-tro-ok-u-log'-raf-e*). *See* Electroretinography.

electrophoresis (*e-lek-tro-fo-re'-sis*). A method of analysing the different proteins in blood serum by passing an electric current through the serum to separate the electrically charged particles. The particles gradually separate into bands due to the difference in rate of movement according to the electrical charge on the particles.

electroplexy (*e-lek'-tro-plekse*). Electroconvulsive therapy.

electroretinogram (*e-lek-tro-ret'-in-o-gram*). A record of the tracings produced by electroretinography.

electroretinography (*e-lek-tro-ret-in-og'-raf-e*). A method of examining the retina of the eye by means of electrodes and light stimulation for assessment of retinal damage.

electrotherapy (*e-lek-tro-ther'-ap-e*). The treatment of disease by passing electric currents through the tissues in order to stimulate the nerves and muscles.

element (*el'-em-ent*). The simplest form into which matter can be divided. It consists of identical atoms. Different elements combine to form compounds, e.g. iron oxide consists of the elements iron and oxygen.

elephantiasis (*el-ef-an-ti'-as-is*). A chronic disease of the lymphatics producing excessive thickening of the skin and swelling of the parts affected, usually the lower limbs. It may be due to filariasis.

elevator (*el'-e-va-tor*). An instrument used as a lever for raising bone, etc. Several types of elevator are used in dentistry. *Periosteal e.* Instrument that strips the periosteum in bone surgery.

elimination (*e-lim-in-a'-shun*). The removal of waste matter, particularly from the body. Excretion.

elixir (*e-liks'-er*). A sweetened spirituous liquid, used largely as a flavouring agent to hide the unpleasant taste of some drugs.

elliptocytosis (*e-lip-to-si-to'-sis*). An hereditary disorder where the red blood cells are elliptical in shape. Increased red cell destruction leading to anaemia occurs.

emaciation (*e-ma-she-a'-shun*). Excessive wasting of body tissues. Extreme thinness.

emanation (*em-an-a'-shun*). The act of giving out, e.g. the gamma rays from radium.

emasculation (e-mas-ku-la'-shun). The removal of the penis or testicles. Castration.

embolectomy (em-bol-ek'-tom-e). An operation to remove an embolus. It has been performed for pulmonary embolism, but more frequently for arterial emboli that are cutting off the blood supply to the limbs.

embolism (em'-bol-izm). Obstruction of a blood vessel by a travelling blood clot or particle of matter. Air e. The presence of gas or air bubbles usually sucked into the large veins from a wound in the neck or chest. Cerebral e. Obstruction of a vessel in the brain. Coronary e. The blockage of a coronary vessel with a clot. Fat e. Globules of fat released into the blood from a fractured bone. Infective e. Detached particles of infected blood clot from an area of inflammation which, obstructing small vessels, result in abscess formation, i.e. pyaemia. Pulmonary e. Blocking of the pulmonary artery or one of its branches by a detached clot, usually due to thrombosis in the femoral or iliac veins. A complication of abdominal operations, occurring about the tenth day. Smaller clots cause infarction. Retinal e. Blockage, due to air or a blood clot, of the central retinal artery, resulting in loss of vision.

embolus (em'-bo-lus). pl. emboli. A substance carried by the blood stream until it causes obstruction by blocking a blood vessel. See Embolism.

embrocation (em-bro-ka'-shun). A liquid applied to the body by rubbing to treat strains. A liniment.

embryo (em'-bre-o). The fertilized ovum in its earliest stages, i.e. until it shows human characteristics during the second month. After this it is termed a fetus.

embryology (em-bre-ol'-o-je). The study of the growth and development of the embryo from the unicellular stage until birth.

embryotomy (em-bre-ot'-om-e). The cutting-up of a fetus during a difficult birth to facilitate delivery.

emesis (em'-es-is). Vomiting.

emetic (em-et'-ik). An agent which has power to induce vomiting, e.g. salt or mustard and water by mouth, or apomorphine hypodermically.

emetine (em'-et-een). An alkaloid prepared from ipecacuanha or synthetically. Formerly much used in the treatment of amoebic dysentery.

eminence (em'-in-ens). A projection, usually rounded, from a surface, e.g. of a bone.

emission (e-mish'-un). Involuntary ejection (of semen).

emmetropia (em-e-tro'-pe-ah). Normal vision that is neither long- nor short-sighted.

emollient (e-mol'-e-ent). Any substance used to soothe or soften the skin.

emotion (e-mo'-shun). A physical and psychological excitement in response to certain stimuli, e.g. happiness and sadness.

empathy (em'-path-e). The power of projecting oneself into the feelings of another person or situation.

emphysema (em-fi-se'-mah). The abnormal presence of air in tissues or cavities of the body. *Pulmonary e.* A chronic disease of the lungs, in which there is abnormal distension of alveoli so great in some cases that intervening walls are broken down and bullae form on the lung surface. An accompaniment of chronic respiratory diseases, it causes breathlessness. *Surgical e.* The presence of air or any other gas in the subcutaneous tissues, introduced through a wound, and evidenced by crepitation on pressure. It may occur, e.g. from the lungs, owing to perforation by a fractured rib, or in tissues around a tracheostomy incision.

empirical (*em-pir'-ik-al*). Pertaining to treatment based on experience and not on scientific reasoning.

empyema (*em-pi-e'-mah*). A collection of pus in a cavity, most commonly referring to the pleural cavity.

emulsion (*e-mul'-shun*). A mixture in which an oil is suspended in water, by the addition of an emulsifying agent.

enamel (*en-am'-el*). The hard outer covering of the crown of a tooth.

enarthrosis (*en-arth-ro'-sis*). A freely moving joint, e.g. ball and socket joint.

encanthis (*en-kan'-this*). A small fleshy growth at the inner canthus of the eye which may form an abscess.

encapsulated (*en-kap'-su-la-ted*). Enclosed in a capsule.

encephalin (*en-kef'-al-in*). An opiate-like substance which is produced by the pituitary and has analgesic effects. This substance may also be produced synthetically. *See* Endorphin.

encephalitis (*en-kef-al-i'-tis*).

Inflammation of the brain. *E. lethargica* (*epidemic e.*). An inflammation of the brain due to a virus. 'Sleepy sickness'. Typical signs are increasing languor and lethargy, deepening to stupor, and accompanied by muscle weaknesses and paralyses. *Post-vaccinal e.* An occasional complication of vaccination in children.

encephalocele (*en-kef'-al-o-seel*). Herniation of the brain through the skull.

encephalography (*en-kef-al-og'-raf-e*). X-ray examination of the ventricles of the brain following the insertion of air or a gas through a lumbar or cisternal puncture.

encephaloma (*en-kef-al-o'-mah*). A tumour of the brain.

encephalomalacia (*en-kef-al-o-mal-a'-she-ah*). Softening of the brain.

encephalomyelitis (*en-kef-al-o-mi-el-i'-tis*). Inflammation of the brain and spinal cord.

encephalomyelopathy (*en-kef-al-o-mi-el-op'-ath-e*). Any disease condition of the brain and spinal cord.

encephalon (*en-kef'-al-on*). The brain.

encephalopathy (*en-kef-al-op'-ath-e*). Cerebral dysfunction. *Hepatic e.* A condition caused by liver failure, leading to dementia and then coma. *Hypertensive e.* A transient disturbance of function associated with hypertension. Disorientation, excitability, and abnormal behaviour occur, which may be reversed if the pressure is reduced. *Wernicke's e.* A complication of diseases of the gastrointestinal tract, excessive vomiting in pregnancy and chronic alcoholism; characterized by paralysis of the eye muscles, diplopia, nystagmus, ataxia and mental changes.

enchondroma (*en-kon-dro'-mah*). A benign tumour of cartilage within the shaft of the bone.

encopresis (*en-ko-pre'-sis*). Incontinence of faeces.

encyesis (*en-si-e'-sis*). A normal uterine pregnancy.

encysted (*en-sis'-ted*). Enclosed in a cyst.

endarterectomy (*end-ar-ter-ek'-tom-e*). The surgical removal of the lining of an artery, usually because of narrowing of the vessel by artheromatous plaques. *Thrombo-e.* Removal of a clot with the lining.

endarteritis (*end-ar-ter-i'-tis*). Inflammation of the innermost coat of an artery. *E. obliterans.* A type which causes collapse and obstruction in small arteries.

endemic (*en-dem'-ik*). Pertaining to a disease prevalent in a particular locality.

endemiology (*en-dem-e-ol'-o-je*). The study of all the factors pertaining to endemic disease.

endocarditis (*en-do-kar-di'-tis*). Inflammation of the endocardium. *Acute e.* Endocarditis leading to damaged heart valves; frequently caused by rheumatic fever. *Bacterial* or *malignant e.* An acute illness resulting from infection of the heart valves by bacteria, sometimes the haemolytic streptococcus. *Subacute bacterial e.* Infection of the valves by *Streptococcus viridans*.

endocardium (*en-do-kar'-de-um*). The membrane lining the heart.

endocervicitis (*en-do-ser-vis-i'-tis*). Inflammation of the membrane lining the uterine cervix.

endocrine (*en'-do-krine*). Secreting within. Applied to those glands whose secretions (*hormones*) flow directly into the blood and not outwards through a duct. The chief endocrine glands are the thyroid, parathyroids, suprarenals and pituitary. The pancreas, stomach, liver, ovaries and testicles also produce internal secretions.

endocrinology (*en-do-krin-ol'-o-je*). The science of the endocrine glands and their secretions.

endocrinopathy (*en-do-krin-op'-ath-e*). Any disease or disorder of any of the endocrine glands or their secretions.

endoderm (*en'-do-derm*). Entoderm.

endogenous (*en-doj'-en-us*). Produced within the organism. *E. depression.* One in which the disease derives from internal causes.

endolymph (*en'-do-limf*). The fluid inside the membranous labyrinth of the ear.

endolysin (*en-do-li'-sin*). A factor or enzyme present in cells that can cause dissolution of the cytoplasm.

endometriosis (*en-do-me-tre-o'-sis*). The presence of endometrium in an abnormal situation, e.g. in the ovaries, the intestines or the urinary bladder. The ectopic tissue undergoes the same hormonal changes as normal endometrium. As there is no outlet for bleeding when menstruation occurs, the woman suffers severe pain.

endometritis (*en-do-me-tri'-tis*). Inflammation of the endometrium.

endometrium (*en-do-me'-tre-*

um). The mucous membrane lining the uterus.

endomorph (*en'-do-morf*). An individual with a large, fatty trunk and small, tapering extremities.

endomyocarditis (*en-do-mi-o-kar-di'-tis*). Inflammation of the lining membrane and muscles of the heart.

endoparasite (*en-do-par'-ah-site*). A parasite that lives within the body of its host.

endophthalmitis (*end-off-thal-mi'-tis*). Inflammation of the interior of the eyeball.

endorphin (*en'-dor-fin*). A type of morphine which is produced by the body itself. Extreme fear increases the production of endorphin, resulting in analgesic effects.

endorrhachis (*en-do-rak'-is*). The spinal dura mater.

endoscope (*en'-do-skope*). An instrument used to inspect a hollow organ or cavity.

endosteitis (*end-os-te-i'-tis*). Inflammation of the endosteum.

endosteoma (*end-os-te-o'-mah*). A neoplasm in the medullary cavity of a bone.

endosteum (*end-os'-te-um*). The lining membrane of bone cavities.

endothelioma (*en-do-the-le-o'-mah*). A malignant growth originating in the endothelium.

endothelium (*en-do-the'-le-um*). The membranous lining of serous, synovial and other internal surfaces.

endotoxin (*en-do-toks'-in*). A poison produced by and retained within a bacterium, which is released only after the destruction of the bacterial cell. *See* Exotoxin.

endotracheal (*en-do-trak-e-'al*). Within the trachea. *E. tube.* A tube which is inserted into the trachea when a patient requires ventilatory support, often during general anaesthesia.

enema (*en'-em-ah*). The introduction of fluid into the rectum. *Barium e.* The injection of barium sulphate into the lower intestine for X-ray examination. *Evacuant* or *purgative e.* One to relieve constipation or to empty the bowel.

enervation (*en-er-va'-shun*). (1) General weakness and loss of strength. (2) Removal of a nerve.

engagement (*en-gaje'-ment*). In obstetrics, used to denote that the presenting part of the fetus, normally the head, has descended into the pelvic canal. Occurs in the last stage of pregnancy.

enophthalmos (*en-off-thal'-mos*). A condition in which the eyeball is abnormally sunken into its socket.

enostosis (*en-os-to'-sis*). A tumour or bony growth within the medullary cavity of a bone.

ensiform (*en'-se-form*). Xiphoid. Sword-shaped. *E. cartilage.* The lowest portion of the sternum.

Entamoeba (*en-tah-me'-bah*). A genus of protozoa, some of which are parasitic in man. *E. histolytica.* The cause of amoebic dysentery.

enteralgia (*en-ter-al'-je-ah*). Pain in the intestines. Colic.

enterectomy (*en-ter-ek'-tom-e*). Excision of a portion of the intestine.

enteric (*en-ter'-ik*). Pertaining to the intestine. *E. fever.* (1) Typhoid or paratyphoid fever. (2) Any fever of intestinal origin.

enteritis (*en-ter-i'-tis*). Inflammation of the small intestine.

Enterobacteriaceae (*en-ter-o-bak-te-re-a'-se-e*). A family of bacteria, many of which are normally found in the human intestine. Included amongst them are the genera *Escherichia*, *Klebsiella*, *Salmonella*, *Shigella* and *Proteus*.

enterobiasis (*en-ter-o-bi'-as-is*). Infestation by threadworms.

Enterobius (*en-ter-o'-be-us*). A genus of roundworms. *E. vermicularis*. The human threadworm, the commonest intestinal worm, particularly in children.

enterocele (*en'-ter-o-seel*). A hernia of the intestine.

enterocentesis (*en-ter-o-sen-te'-sis*). Puncture of the intestine to release abnormal quantities of fluid or gas.

enterococcus (*en-ter-o-kok'-us*). Any streptococcus of the human intestine. An example is *Streptococcus faecalis*, only harmful out of its normal habitat when it may cause a urinary infection or endocarditis.

enterocolitis (*en-ter-o-ko'-li-tis*). Inflammation of both the large and the small intestine.

enterokinase (*en-ter-o-ki'-naze*). An intestinal enzyme that converts trypsinogen into trypsin. Enteropeptidase.

enterolith (*en'-ter-o-lith*). A hard faecal concretion in the intestines.

enteromegaly (*en-ter-o-meg'-al-e*). Enlargement of the intestine.

enteropeptidase (*en-ter-o-pep'-tid-aze*). Enterokinase.

enteropexy (*en-ter-o-peks'-e*). The surgical fixation of a part of the intestine to the abdo-

minal wall.

enteroptosis (*en-ter-op-to'-sis*). An abnormal downward displacement of the intestines.

enterospasm (*en'-ter-o-spazm*). Intestinal colic.

enterostomy (*en-ter-os'-tom-e*). The formation of an external opening into the small intestine. It may be (1) *temporary*, to relieve obstruction, or (2) *permanent*, in the form of an ileostomy in cases of total colectomy.

enterotomy (*en-ter-ot'-om-e*). Any incision of the intestine.

enterotoxin (*en-ter-o-toks'-in*). A toxin which is produced by one of the many organisms that cause food poisoning. Such toxins frequently prove more resistant to destruction than the bacteria themselves.

enterovirus (*en-ter-o-vi'-rus*). A virus which infects the gastrointestinal tract and then attacks the central nervous system. These viruses include Coxsackie viruses, polioviruses and echoviruses.

enterozoon (*en-ter-o-zo'-on*). An animal parasite infesting the intestines.

entoderm (*en'-to-derm*). The innermost of the three germ layers of the embryo. It gives rise to the lining of most of the respiratory tract, and to the intestinal tract and its glands.

entropion (*en-tro'-pe-on*). Inversion of an eyelid, so that the lashes rub against the eyeball.

enucleation (*en-u-kle-a'-shun*). (1) The removal of a tumour or gland by shelling it out whole and free from other tissues. (2) The removal of an eye.

enuresis (*en-u-re'-sis*). Involuntary passing of urine. *E. alarm.* An apparatus used in the treatment of enuresis in children. When it occurs an alarm bell rings to waken the child. *Nocturnal e.* That occurring during sleep.

environment (*en-vi'-ron-ment*). The surroundings of an organism which influence its development and behaviour.

enzyme (*en'-zime*). A protein which will catalyse a biological reaction. *See* Catalyst.

enzymology (*en-zi-mol'-o-je*). The scientific study of enzymes and their action.

eosin (*e'-o-sin*). A red dye used to stain biological specimens. A derivative of bromine and fluorescein.

eosinophil (*e-o-sin'-o-fil*). Cell having an affinity for acid stains, e.g. some white blood cells.

eosinophilia (*e-o-sin-o-fil'-e-ah*). Excessive numbers of eosinophils present in the blood.

ependyma (*ep-en'-dim-ah*). The membrane lining the cerebral ventricles and the central canal of the spinal cord.

ependymoma (*ep-en-dim-o'-mah*). A neoplasm arising from the lining cells of the ventricles or central canal of the spinal cord. It gives rise to signs of hydrocephalus and is treated by surgery and radiotherapy.

ephedrine (*ef'-ed-reen*). A drug that relieves spasm of the bronchi, having a similar action to adrenaline, but it can be taken orally. May be used in asthma and chronic bronchitis.

ephidrosis (*ef-e-dro'-sis*). Profuse sweating. Hyperhidrosis.

epiblepharon (*ep-e-blef'-ar-on*). A congenital condition in which an excess of skin of the eyelid folds over the lid margin so that the eyelashes are pressed against the eyeball.

epicanthus (*ep-e-kan'-thus*). A fold of skin of the upper eyelid sometimes present over the inner canthus of the eye. It is congenital but, except in children suffering from Down's syndrome and in the Mongoloid races, it disappears in early childhood.

epicardium (*ep-e-kar'-de-um*). The visceral layer of the pericardium.

epicondyle (*ep-e-kon'-dile*). A protuberance on a long bone above its condyle.

epicranium (*ep-e-kra'-ne-um*). The structures that cover the cranium.

epicritic (*ep-e-krit'-ik*). Pertaining to sensory nerve fibres in the skin which give the appreciation of touch and temperature.

epidemic (*ep-e-dem'-ik*). Any disease attacking a large number of people at the same time.

epidemiology (*ep-e-de-me-ol'-o-je*). The study of the distribution of diseases.

epidermis (*ep-e-der'-mis*). The non-vascular outer layer or cuticle of the skin. It consists of layers of cells which protect the dermis.

epidermoid (*ep-e-der'-moid*). Pertaining to certain tumours which have the appearance of epidermal tissue.

Epidermophyton (*ep-e-der-mo-fi'-ton*). A genus of fungi which attacks skin and nails, but not hair. The cause of ringworm, dhobi itch and athlete's foot.

epididymis (*ep-e-did'-e-mis*).

The convoluted tube which lies above the testis and receives the ducts from that gland. It is prolonged into the vas deferens and stores and conveys the semen.

epididymitis (*ep-e-did-e-mi'-tis*). Inflammation of the epididymis.

epididymo-orchitis (*ep-e-did-e-mo-or-ki'-tis*). Inflammation of the epididymis and the testis.

epidural (*ep-e-du'-ral*). Outside the dura mater. *E. analgesia*. The injection of an analgesic solution into the space surrounding the spinal cord.

epigastrium (*ep-e-gas'-tre-um*). That region of the abdomen which is situated over the stomach.

epiglottis (*ep-e-glot'-is*). A cartilaginous structure which covers the opening from the pharynx into the larynx, and so prevents food from passing into the trachea in the act of swallowing.

epilation (*ep-il-a'-shun*). Removal of hairs with their roots. It may be effected by pulling out the hairs or by electrolysis.

epilepsy (*ep'-e-lep-se*). Convulsive attacks due to disordered electrical activity of the brain cells. In a major attack of *'grand mal'* the patient falls to the ground unconscious, following an aura or unpleasant sensation. There are first tonic and then clonic contractions, from which stage the patient passes into a deep sleep. A minor attack of *'petit mal'* is a momentary loss of consciousness only. Both these types of epilepsy are ideopathic and are not caused by any damage to the brain. *Jacksonian e*. A symptom of a cerebral

lesion. The convulsive movements are often localized and close observation of the onset and course of the attack may greatly assist diagnosis. *Temporal-lobe e*. Characterized by hallucinations of sight, hearing, taste and smell, paroxysmal disorders of memory and automatism. Caused by temporal or parietal lobe disease.

epileptiform (*ep-e-lep'-tif-orm*). Resembling an epileptic fit.

epiloia (*ep-e-loi'-ah*). Tuberous sclerosis. A congenital disorder with areas of hardening in the cerebral cortex and other organs, characterized clinically by mental deficiency and epilepsy.

epimenorrhoea (*ep-e-men-or-e'-ah*). Menstruation occurring at abnormally short intervals.

epinephrine (*ep-e-nef'-reen*). Adrenaline.

epineurium (*ep-e-nu'-re-um*). The sheath of tissue surrounding a nerve.

epiphora (*ep-if'-or-ah*). Persistent overflow of tears, often due to obstruction in the lacrimal passages or to ectropion.

epiphysis (*ep-if'-is-is*). The end of a long bone developed separately but attached by cartilage to the diaphysis (the shaft) with which it eventually unites. From the line of junction growth in length takes place.

epiplocele (*ep-ip'-lo-seel*). A hernia containing omentum.

epiploon (*ep-ip'-lo-on*). The greater omentum.

episcleritis (*ep-e-skler-i'-tis*). Inflammation of the outer coat of the eyeball. It is seen as a slightly raised bluish nodule under the conjunctiva.

episiorrhaphy (*ep-is-e-or'-af-e*). The repair of a laceration of the perineum.

episiotomy (*ep-is-e-ot'-om-e*). An incision made in the perineum when it will not stretch sufficiently during the second stage of labour.

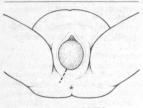

EPISIOTOMY

epispadias (*ep-e-spa'-de-as*). A malformation in which there is an abnormal opening of the urethra on to the dorsal surface of the penis. *See* Hypospadias.

epistaxis (*ep-e-staks'-is*). Bleeding from the nose.

epithelioma (*ep-e-the-le-o'-mah*). Any tumour originating in the epithelium.

epithelium (*ep-e-the'-le-um*). The surface layer of cells either of the skin or of lining tissues.

epithelization (*ep-e-the-li-za'-shun*). Development of epithelium. The final stage in the healing of a surface wound.

epizoon (*ep-e-zo'-on*). Any external animal parasite.

eponym (*ep'-on-im*). In medicine, an anatomical part, disease or structure bearing a person's name, usually that of the man who first described it.

eponymous (*ep-on'-e-mus*).

Named after a particular person.

Epstein–Barr virus (*M.A. Epstein British pathologist ; Y. Barr*). A virus which is the causative organism of infectious mononucleosis (glandular fever).

epulis (*ep-u'-lis*). A fibroid tumour of the gums.

Erb's palsy (*W.H. Erb, German physician, 1840–1921*). Paralysis of the arm, often due to birth injury causing pressure on the brachial plexus or lower cervical nerve roots.

erectile (*e-rek'-tile*). Having the power of becoming erect. *E. tissue*. Vascular tissue which, under stimulus, becomes congested and swollen, causing erection of that part. The penis consists largely of erectile tissue.

erection (*e-rek'-shun*). The enlarged and rigid state of the sexually aroused penis. The clitoris may also become erect.

erepsin (*er-ep'-sin*). The enzyme of succus entericus, secreted by the intestinal glands, which splits peptones into amino acids.

ergography (*er-gog'-raf-e*). A method of measuring the amount of work done during muscular activity.

ergometrine (*er-go-met'-reen*). An alkaloid of ergot. It stimulates contraction of the uterine muscle.

ergonomics (*er-go-nom'-iks*). The scientific study of man in relation to his work and the effective use of human energy.

ergosterol (*er-gos'-ter-ol*). A substance present in subcutaneous fat which under the influence of ultra-violet light forms vitamin D. Hence the use of artificial sunlight for rickets. Also found in plant and animal foodstuffs, which produce the vitamin when irradiated with ultra-violet light.

ergot (er'-got). A drug from a fungus which grows on rye. It causes prolonged contraction of muscle fibres, especially those of blood vessels and of the uterus. Used chiefly to contract the uterus and check haemorrhage at childbirth.

ergotamine (er-got'-am-een). An alkaloid of ergot used in the treatment of migraine.

ergotism (er'-got-izm). The effects of poisoning from ergot or of eating diseased rye, in which constriction of the arterioles may lead to gangrene.

erogenous (e-roj'-en-us). Pertaining to the arousing of erotic feelings.

erosion (e-ro'-zhun). The breaking down of tissue, usually by ulceration. Cervical e. A covering of columnar epithelium on the vaginal part of the uterine cervix, arising from erosion of the squamous epithelium which normally covers it.

erotic (e-rot'-ik). Pertaining to sexual love or desire.

eroticism (e-rot'-is-izm). A condition of morbid sexual excitement. Anal e. Sexual pleasure derived from the anus.

erotomania (e-rot-o-ma'-ne-ah). Abnormal and excessive affection for a person of the opposite sex.

eructation (e-ruk-ta'-shun). Belching. The escape of gas from the stomach through the mouth.

eruption (e-rup'-shun). A breaking out, e.g. of a skin lesion, or the cutting of teeth.

erysipelas (er-e-sip'-el-as). An acute contagious disease, caused by Streptococcus pyogenes and characterized by localized inflammation of the skin, with pain and fever. The inflammation is in the form of a raised red rash with small blebs, spreading gradually away from the centre, and having a well-defined margin. Swine e. An acute contagious disease of pigs which is transmissible to man.

erythema (er-e-the'-mah). A superficial redness of the skin. E. induratum. A manifestation of vasculitis. E. multiforme. An acute eruption of the skin, which may be due to an allergy or to drug sensitivity. E. nodosum. A painful disease in which bright red, tender nodes occur below the knee or on the forearm; it may be associated with tuberculosis. Punctate e. Erythema scarlatiniforme. An eruption mimicking scarlatina.

erythematous (er-e-the'-mat-us). Characterized by erythema.

erythrasma (er-e-thraz'-mah). A skin disease due to infection by Corynebacterium minutissimum, attacking the armpits or groins. It causes no irritation, but is contagious.

erythroblast (er-ith'-ro-blast). A nucleated cell from which an erythrocyte develops. Normally present in the blood only during the first three months of fetal development.

erythroblastosis (er-ith-ro-blas-to'-sis). The presence of erythroblasts in the blood. E. fetalis. A severe haemolytic anaemia, with an excess of erythroblasts in the newly born. Due to rhesus incompatibility between the child's and the mother's blood.

erythrocyanosis (*er-ith-ro-si-an-o'-sis*). Swelling and blueness of the legs and thighs occurring mainly in young women and during cold weather.

erythrocyte (*er-ith'-ro-site*). A mature red blood cell. The cells contain haemoglobin and serve to transport oxygen. They are developed in the red bone marrow found in the cancellous tissue of all bones. The *haemopoietic factor* vitamin B_{12} is essential for the change from megaloblast to normoblast, and iron, thyroxin, and vitamin C are

Deficiency in numbers of red blood cells.

erythrocytosis (*er-ith-ro-si-to'-sis*). Erythrocythaemia.

erythroderma (*er-ith-ro-der'-mah*). Abnormal redness of the skin, usually over a large area.

erythroedema polyneuropathy (*er-ith-re-de'-mah pol-e-nu-rop'-ath-e*). Infantile acrodynia. 'Pink' disease. *See* Acrodynia.

erythromycin (*er-ith-ro-mi'-sin*). An antibiotic drug with a wide range of activity. Mainly used for staphylococcal infections that are resistant to penicillin and for patients who cannot tolerate penicillin.

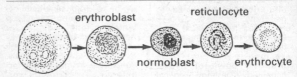

ERYTHROCYTE DEVELOPMENT IN BONE MARROW

also necessary for its perfect structure. *E. sedimentation rate*. ESR. The rate at which the cells of citrated blood form a deposit in a graduated 200 mm tube (*Westergren method*). The normal is less than 10 mm of clear plasma in 1 hour. This is much increased in severe infection and acute rheumatism.

erythrocythaemia (*er-ith-ro-si-the'-me-ah*). Increase in numbers of red blood cells due to overactivity of the bone marrow. Vazquez's disease. Polycythaemia vera.

erythrocytopenia (*er-ith-ro-si-to-pe'-ne-ah*). Erythropenia.

erythropoiesis (*er-ith-ro-poi-e'-sis*). The manufacture of red blood corpuscles.

erythropoietin (*er-ith-ro-poi'-et-in*). A hormone produced by the kidney that stimulates the production of red blood cells in the bone marrow.

erythropsia (*er-e-throp'-se-ah*). A defect of vision in which all objects appear red. Often occurs after a cataract operation.

eschar (*es'-kar*). A slough or scab which forms after the destruction of living tissue by gangrene, infection or burning.

Escherichia (*esh-er-ik'-e-ah*). A

genus of Enterobacteriaceae. *E. coli.* An organism normally present in the intestines of man and other vertebrates. Although not generally pathogenic it may set up infections of the gall-bladder, bile ducts and the urinary tract. It was formerly called *Bacillus coli.*

eserine (*es'-er-een*). Physostigmine.

Esmarch's tourniquet (*J.F.A. von Esmarch, German surgeon, 1823–1908*). A rubber bandage used in surgery to express blood from a limb and render it less vascular.

ESN. Educationally subnormal. A relatively mild degree of mental retardation.

esophoria (*e-so-for'-e-ah*). Latent convergent strabismus. The eyes turn inwards only when one is covered up.

esotropia (*es-o-tro'-pe-ah*). Convergent strabismus. One or other eye turns inwards, resulting in double vision.

ESR. Erythrocyte sedimentation rate.

essence (*es'-ens*). (1) An indispensable part of anything. (2) A volatile oil dissolved in alcohol.

essential (*e-sen'-shal*). Indispensable. *E. amino acids.* Those amino acids necessary for the maintenance of tissue growth and repair. Eight amino acids are essential for adults and ten for children. *E. fatty acids.* Unsaturated fatty acids which are necessary for body growth.

ester (*es'-ter*). A compound formed by the combination of an acid and an alcohol with the elimination of water.

esterase (*es'-ter-aze*). An enzyme that causes the hydrolysis of esters into acids and alcohol.

ethambutol (*eth-am'-bu-tol*). A drug used in the treatment of tuberculosis.

ethanol (*eth'-an-ol*). Alcohol.

ethanolamine (*eth-an-ol'-am-een*). An intravenous sclerosing agent used to inject varicose veins.

ether (*e'-ther*). A volatile liquid formerly used as a general anaesthetic agent. *Solvent e.* A skin antiseptic.

ethics (*eth'-iks*). A code of moral principles. *Nursing e.* The code governing a nurse's behaviour with her patients, their relatives and her colleagues.

ethmoid (*eth'-moid*). A sieve-like bone, separating the cavity of the nose from the cranium. The olfactory nerves pass through its perforations.

ethmoidectomy (*eth-moid-ek'-tom-e*). Surgical removal of a portion of the ethmoid bone.

ethnology (*eth-nol'-o-je*). The study of different peoples and races. Ethnics.

ethoglucid (*eth-o-glu'-sid*). An antineoplastic agent which may be used to treat bladder cancers by intravesical instillations.

ethoheptazine (*eth-o-hep'-taz-een*). An analgesic related to pethidine. It relieves pain and muscle spasm.

ethology (*e-thol'-o-je*). The study of animal behaviour.

ethopropazine (*eth-o-pro'-paz-een*). An antispasmodic drug used in the treatment of parkinsonism.

ethosuximide (*eth-o-suks'-im-ide*). An anticonvulsant used in the treatment of 'petit mal' epilepsy.

ethyl biscoumacetate (*eth'-il bis-koo-mas'-et-ate*). An anticoagulant of the coumarin group.

ethyl chloride (*eth'-il klor'-ide*). A volatile liquid used as a local anaesthetic. When sprayed on any part of the body it causes local insensitivity, through freezing.

ethylene oxide (*eth'-il-een oks'-ide*). A gas which is capable of penetrating relatively inaccessible parts of an apparatus during sterilization. It is also used for equipment which is too delicate to be sterilized by other methods.

ethyloestrenol (*eth-il-e'-strenol*). An anabolic steroid that may be used to treat severe weight loss, debility and osteoporosis.

etiolation (*e-te-o-la'-shun*). Paleness of the skin due to lack of exposure to sunlight.

etiology (*e-te-ol'-o-je*). *See* Aetiology.

eucalyptus (*u-kal-ip'-tus*). An oil derived from the leaves of the eucalyptus tree and used in the treatment of nasal catarrh.

eugenics (*u-jen'-iks*). The study of measures which may be taken to improve future generations both physically and mentally.

eugenol (*u'-jen-ol*). A local anaesthetic and antiseptic, derived from oil of cloves and cinnamon, used in dentistry.

eunuch (*u'-nuk*). A castrated male.

eupepsia (*u-pep'-se-ah*). A good digestion with normal function of the digestive juices.

euphoria (*u-for'-e-ah*). An exaggerated feeling of wellbeing often not justified by circumstances. Less than *elation*.

euplastic (*u-plas'-tik*). Capable of being transformed into healthy tissue. The term may be applied to a wound that is healing well.

eusol (*u'-sol*). A chlorine antiseptic containing hypochlorous and boric acids. The name is derived from the initials of Edinburgh University Solution of Lime.

eustachian tube (*B. Eustachio, Italian anatomist, 1520–1574*). The pharyngotympanic tube.

euthanasia (*u-than-a'-ze-ah*). The process of dying easily and painlessly. Also said of the act of aiding someone to die in this way.

euthyroidism (*u-thi'-roid-izm*). The condition of having a normally functioning thyroid gland.

eutocia (*u-to'-se-ah*). Easy, normal childbirth.

evacuant (*e-vak'-u-ant*). An aperient. Any drug or washout that empties the colon.

evacuation (*e-vak-u-a'-shun*). Emptying out, particularly the discharge of faeces from the rectum and lower bowel.

evacuator (*e-vak'-u-a-tor*). An instrument which produces evacuation, e.g. one designed to wash out small particles of stone from the bladder after these have been crushed by a lithotrite.

eventration (*e-ven-tra'-shun*). The protrusion of the intestines through the abdominal wall.

eversion (*e-ver'-shun*). Turning outwards. *E. of the eyelid.* Ectropion. The upper eyelid may be everted for examination of the eye or for the removal of a foreign body.

evisceration (*e-vis-er-a'-shun*). Removal of internal organs. *E. of eye.* Removal of the contents of the eyeball, but not the sclera. *E. of orbit.* Removal of the eye and all structures in the orbit.

evolution (*e-vol-u'-shun*). The development of living organisms which change their characteristics during succeeding generations.

evulsion (*e-vul'-shun*). Plucking out. *See* Avulsion.

Ewing's tumour (*J. Ewing, American pathologist, 1866–1943*). A form of sarcoma usually affecting the shaft of a long bone in young adults.

exacerbation (*eks-as-er-ba'-shun*). An increase in the severity of the symptoms of a disease.

exanthem (*eks-an'-them*). An infectious disease characterized by a skin rash.

exanthematous (*eks-an-them'-at-us*). Pertaining to any disease associated with a skin eruption.

excavation (*eks-kav-a'-shun*). Scooping out. **Dental e.** The removal of decay from a tooth before inserting a filling.

excipient (*ek-sip'-e-ent*). A substance that is added to a drug so that it may be made up into pills, but which has no pharmacological action itself.

excision (*ek-sizh'-un*). The cutting out of a part.

excitation (*ek-si-ta'-shun*). The act of stimulating.

excitement (*ek-site'-ment*). A physiological and emotional response to a stimulus.

excoriation (*eks-kor-e-a'-shun*). An abrasion of the skin.

excrement (*eks'-kre-ment*). Waste matter from the body.

excrescence (*eks-kres'-ens*). Abnormal outgrowth of tissue, e.g. a wart.

excreta (*eks-kre'-tah*). The natural discharges of the excretory system: faeces, urine, sweat, and sputum.

excretion (*eks-kre'-shun*). The discharge of waste from the body.

exenteration (*eks-en-ter-a'-shun*). Evisceration. The removal of an organ. Usually performed only in cases of malignant neoplasm.

exfoliation (*eks-fo-le-a'-shun*). The splitting off from the surface of dead tissue in thin flaky layers.

exhalation (*eks-hal-a'-shun*). (1) The giving off of a vapour. (2) The act of breathing out.

exhibitionism (*eks-hib-ish'-un-izm*). (1) Showing off. A desire to attract attention. (2) Exposing the genitals in order to provoke a response in one or more people.

exocrine (*eks'-o-krine*). Pertaining to those glands which discharge their secretion by means of a duct, e.g. salivary glands. *See* Endocrine.

exogenous (*eks-oj'-en-us*). Of external origin. A condition arising due to environmental factors.

exomphalos (*eks-om'-fal-os*). Umbilical hernia producing a protrusion at the navel.

exophoria (*eks-o-for'-e-ah*). A tendency of the eyes to turn outwards.

exophthalmometer (*eks-off-thal-mom'-e-ter*). An instrument for measuring the extent of protrusion of the eyeball.

exophthalmos (*eks-off-thal'-mos*). Proptosis. Protrusion of the eyeball, which may be caused by injury or disease, and is often seen in thyrotoxicosis.

exostosis (*eks-os-to'-sis*). A bony outgrowth from the surface of a bone. It may be due to chronic inflammation, constant pressure on the bone, or tumour formation.

exotic (*eks-ot'-ik*). Pertaining to a disease occurring in a region far from where it is usually found.

exotoxin (*eks-o-toks'-in*). A poison produced by a bacterial cell and released into the tissues surrounding it. *See* Endotoxin.

exotropia (*eks-o-tro'-pe-ah*). Divergent strabismus. The eyes turn outwards.

expectorant (*eks-pek'-tor-ant*). A remedy which promotes and facilitates expectoration.

expectoration (*eks-pek-tor-a'-shun*). Sputum. Secretions coughed up from the air passages. Its characteristics are a valuable aid in diagnosis and note should be taken of the quantity ejected, its colour and the amount of effort required. *Frothiness* denotes that it comes from an air-containing cavity; *fluidity* indicates oedema of the lung.

expiration (*eks-pi-ra'-shun*). (1) The act of breathing out. (2) Dying.

exploration (*eks-plor-a'-shun*). The operation of surgically investigating any part of the body.

expression (*eks-presh'-un*). (1) Pressing out. Pressure on the uterus to facilitate the expulsion of the placenta or fetus, or on the breast to obtain a flow of milk. (2) The appearance of the face as affected by emotions.

exsanguination (*eks-san-gwin-a'-shun*). The process of making bloodless.

extension (*eks-ten'-shun*). (1) The straightening out of a flexed joint such as the knee or elbow. (2) The application of traction to a fractured or dislocated limb by means of a weight.

extensor (*eks-ten'-sor*). A muscle which extends or straightens a limb.

exterior (*eks-te'-re-or*). On the outside.

exteriorize (*ex-te'-re-or-ize*). (1) To bring an organ or part of one to the outside of the body by surgery. (2) In psychology, to turn one's interests outwards.

extirpation (*eks-ter-pa'-shun*). Complete removal of an organ or tissue.

extracapsular (*eks-trah-cap-su'-lah*). Outside the capsule. May refer to a fracture occurring at the end of the bone, but outside the joint capsule, or to cataract extraction.

extracellular (*eks-trah-sel'-u-lah*). Outside the cell. *E. fluid.* Tissue fluid that surrounds the cells.

extract (*eks'-trakt*). A concentrated preparation of a drug made by extracting its soluble principles by steeping in water or alcohol and then evaporating the fluid.

extraction (*eks-trak'-shun*). The process of drawing out, as of teeth, the lens of an eye, or a baby from its mother in childbirth.

extradural (*eka-trah-du'-ral*). Outside the dura mater. *E. haemorrhage. See* Haemorrhage.

extragenital (*eks-trah-jen'-it-al*). Not related to the genitals. *E. chancre.* The primary lesion of syphilis situated elsewhere than on the genital organs. *E. syphilis.* Syphilis spread from an extragenital lesion.

extrahepatic (*eks-trah-hep-at'-ik*). Outside the liver. Relating to a condition affecting the liver in which the cause is outside the liver.

extrapleural (*eks-trah-plu'-ral*). Between the chest wall and parietal layer of the pleura. *See* Pneumothorax.

extrapyramidal (*eks-trah-pir-am'-id-al*). Outside the pyramidal (cerebrospinal) tract. *E. system*. The nerve tracts and pathways which are not within the pyramidal tracts.

extrasensory (*eks-trah-sen'-sor-e*). Outside or beyond any of the known senses. *E. perception*. ESP. Appreciation of the thoughts of others or of current or future events without any normal means of communication.

extrasystole (*eks-trah-sis'-tol-e*). Premature contraction of the atria or ventricles. *See* Systole.

extra-uterine (*eks-trah-u'-ter-ine*). Occurring outside the uterus. *E. pregnancy*. Ectopic gestation. Development of a fetus outside the uterus.

extravasation (*eks-trah-vas-a'-shun*). Effusion or escape of fluid from its normal course into surrounding tissues. *E. of blood*. A bruise. *E. of urine* into the pelvic tissues may complicate a fracture of the pelvis if the bladder is injured.

extremity (*eks-trem'-it-e*). Distal part. A hand or foot.

extrinsic (*eks-trin'-sik*). Originating externally. *E. factor*. A substance present in meat and other foodstuffs which is now considered to be cyanocobalamin (vitamin B_{12}) and which is necessary for the manufacture of red blood cells. The intrinsic factor produced in the stomach is necessary for the absorption of vitamin B_{12}. *E. muscle*. A muscle originating away from the part which it controls, such as those controlling the movements of the eye.

extroversion (*eks-tro-ver'-shun*). Turning inside out, e.g. of the uterus, as sometimes occurs after labour.

extrovert (*eks'-tro-vert*). A person who is sociable, a good mixer and interested in what goes on around him. A personality type first described by Jung. *See* Introvert.

exudation (*eks-u-da'-shun*). The slow discharge of serous fluid through the walls of the blood cells and its deposition in or on the tissues.

eye (*i*). The organ of sight. A globular structure with three

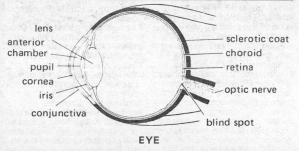

lens
anterior chamber
pupil
cornea
iris
conjunctiva

sclerotic coat
choroid
retina
optic nerve
blind spot

EYE

coats. The nerve tissue of the retina receives impressions of images via the pupil and lens. From this the optic nerve conveys the impressions to the visual area of the cerebrum.

eyelid (*i'-lid*). A protective covering of the eye, composed of muscle and dense connective tissue covered with skin, lined with conjunctiva and fringed with eyelashes. Eyelids contain the Meibomian glands.

eye-tooth (*i'-tooth*). An upper canine tooth.

F

F. (1) Abbreviation for Fahrenheit. (2) Chemical symbol for *fluorine*.

face (*fase*). The front of the head from the forehead to the chin. *F. presentation*. The appearance of the face of the fetus first at the cervix during labour.

facet (*fas'-et*). A small flat area on the surface of a bone. *F. syndrome*. A slight dislocation of the small facet joints of the vertebrae giving rise to pain and muscle spasm.

facial (*fa'-shal*). Pertaining to the face or lower anterior portion of the head. *F. nerve*. The seventh cranial nerve supplying the salivary glands and superficial face muscles. A local anaesthetic may be injected into this nerve when a general anaesthetic is contraindicated. *F. paralysis*. See Paralysis.

facies (*fa'-she-eez*). Facial expression. It often gives some indication of the patient's condition. *Abdominal f*. The face

is cold and livid, eyes and cheeks sunken, and tongue and lips dry. Seen in severe abdominal infection. *Adenoid f*. The open mouth and vacant expression associated with mouth breathing and nasal obstruction. *Hippocratic f*. The drawn, anxious expression seen in patients with extreme prostration; with pinched, pointed nostrils and cyanotic appearance of the lips and nose. *Parkinson f*. A characteristic fixed expression, due to paucity of movement of facial muscles. Characteristic of parkinsonism.

facultative (*fak'-ul-ta-tiv*). Optional. *F. bacteria*. Those which although normally *aerobes*, are also capable of being *anaerobes*. *F. parasite*. One which can live as a parasite or, in certain conditions, independently.

faecalith (*fe'-ka-lith*). A hard stony mass of faecal material which may obstruct the lumen of the appendix and be a cause of inflammation. A coprolith.

faeces (*fe'-seez*). Waste matter excreted by the bowel, consisting of indigestible cellulose, food which has escaped digestion, bacteria (living and dead), and water.

Fahrenheit scale (*G.D. Fahrenheit, German physicist, 1686–1736*). A scale of heat measurement. It registers the freezing-point of water at 32°, the normal heat of the human body at 98.4°, and the boiling-point of water at 212°.

fainting. See Syncope.

falciform (*fal'-se-form*). Sickle-shaped. *F. ligament*. A fold of peritoneum which separates the two main lobes of the liver, and connects it with the

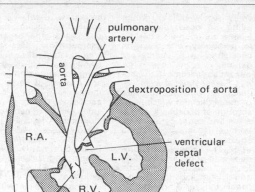

pulmonary artery

aorta

dextroposition of aorta

R.A.

ventricular septal defect

L.V.

R.V.

pulmonary valve stenosis

thickened wall of right ventricle

FALLOT'S TETRALOGY

anterior abdominal wall and the diaphragm.

fallopian tube (*G. Fallopius, Italian anatomist, 1523–1563*). Uterine tube. One of a pair of tubes about 10 to 14 cm (4 to 5½ in.) long, connecting the uterus with the ovaries. Their function is to conduct the ova from the ovaries to the interior of the uterus. An oviduct.

Fallot's tetralogy (*E.L.A. Fallot, French physician, 1850–1911*). A congenital heart disease with four characteristic defects: (a) pulmonary artery stenosis, (b) interventricular defect of the septum, (c) overriding of the aorta, i.e. opening into both right and left ventricles, (d) hypertrophy of the right ventricle.

false (*faw'-ls*). Not true. *F. pains.* Abdominal pains occurring in pregnancy which are not the real pains of labour. *F. pelvis.* The area between the brim of the true pelvis and the crest of the ilium. *F. joint.* Pseudoarthrosis. Fibrous union of a fractured bone, which gives unnatural mobility.

falx (*fal-ks*). A sickle-shaped structure. *F. cerebri.* The fold of dura mater which separates the two cerebral hemispheres.

familial (*fam-il'-e-al*). Affecting several members of one family.

family (*fam'-il-e*). (1) A group, living or dead, descended from a common ancestor. (2) In taxonomy, a subdivision consisting of a number of genera.

Fanconi's syndrome (*G. Fanconi, Swiss paediatrician, b. 1892*). An inherited disorder of metabolism in which reabsorption of phosphate, amino acids and sugar by the renal tubules is impaired. These substances then appear in the urine. The kidneys fail to produce acid urine, and resulting features are thirst, polyuria and rickets, leading to chronic renal failure. Photophobia may be present.

fang (*fang*). The root of a tooth.

fantasy (*fan'-tas-e*). Extravagant mental imagery whereby those events which are unappealing in reality are converted into an imaginary experience which is more satisfying to the individual.

faradism (*far'-ad-izm*). Electricity produced through induction by a rapidly alternating current.

faradization (*M. Faraday, British physicist, 1791–1867*). Treatment by the application of an induced or faradic current of electricity. The result is rapid and spasmodic contraction of the muscle to which it is applied.

farinaceous (*far-in-a'-shus*). Starchy or containing starch. Refers to foods such as wheat, oats, barley and rice.

farmer's lung (*far'-merz lung*). A disease occurring in those in contact with mouldy hay. It is thought to be due to a hypersensitivity, with widespread reaction in the lung tissue. It causes excessive breathlessness.

fascia (*fash'-e-ah*). A sheath of connective tissue enclosing muscles or other organs.

fasciculation (*fas-ik-u-la'-shun*). Isolated fine muscle twitching which gives a flickering appearance. It is seen in some cases of nerve impairment.

fasciculus (*fas-ik'-u-lus*). A small bundle of nerve or muscle fibres. A fascicle.

Fasciola (*fas-e-o'-lah*). A genus of flukes. *F. hepatica*. A liver fluke commonly found in sheep and occasionally in man.

fastigium (*fas-tij'-e-um*). The stage of a fever when the temperature is at its height.

fat (*fat*). Adipose tissue. The white oily portion of animal tissue. *F.-soluble vitamins.* Vitamins A, D, E, and K. *Brown f.* See Brown adipose tissue. *Wool-f.* Lanolin.

fatigue (*fat-eeg'*). A state of weariness which may range from mental disinclination for effort to profound exhaustion following great physical and mental effort. *Muscle f.* May occur during prolonged effort due to oxygen lack and accumulation of waste products.

fatty (*fat'-e*). Containing or similar to fat. *F. acid.* See Essential. *F. degeneration.* A degenerative change in tissue cells due to the invasion of fat and consequent weakening of the organ. The change occurs as a result of incorrect diet, shortage of oxygen in the tissues or excessive consumption of alcohol.

fauces (*faw'-sez*). The opening from the mouth into the pharynx. *Pillars of the f.* The two folds of muscle covered with mucous membrane which pass from the soft palate on either side of the fauces. One fold passes into the tongue, the other into the pharynx, and between them is situated the tonsil.

favism (*fa'-vizm*). An inherited allergy occurring in the Mediterranean and parts of Iran, in which certain individuals develop acute haemolysis as a result of sensitivity to certain kinds of bean, e.g. Italian lentil. They have a deficiency of glucose-6-phosphate dehydrogenase in their red blood cells.

favus (*fa'-vus*). A skin disease, rare in Britain, with formation of scabs, in appearance like a honeycomb. It usually affects the scalp and is due to a fungus infection.

Fe. Chemical symbol for *iron*.

fear (*feer*). A feeling of acute apprehension or anxiety which is normal in people exposed to external sources of danger. It may give rise to any of the following symptoms: tachycardia, pallor, faintness, sweating, tightness of the chest, irregular breathing, giddiness, dilated pupils, increased frequency of micturition, and diarrhoea. *Obsessional f.* A recurring irrational fear that is not amenable to ordinary reassurance. A phobia.

febrifuge (*feb'-re-fuje*). A drug or other treatment given to reduce fever.

febrile (*feb'-rile*). Characterized by or relating to fever. *F. convulsion.* A convulsion which occurs in childhood and is associated with pyrexia.

fecundation (*fek-un-da'-shun*). Fertilization.

feeble-mindedness (*fe-bl-mind'-ed-nes*). A mild degree of mental retardation.

feedback (*feed'-bak*). A method of control where some of the output is returned as input for monitoring purposes. Feedback mechanisms are important in the regulation of such physiological processes as hormone and enzyme reactions. *Negative f.* A rise in the output of a substance is detected and further output is thus inhibited. *Positive f.* A rise in output causes either a direct or indirect rise in the output of another substance.

felon (*fel'-on*). An abscess of the distal phalanx of a finger. A whitlow.

Felty's syndrome (*A.R. Felty, American physician, b. 1895*). A variety of rheumatoid arthritis in which the spleen is enlarged and may require removal.

femoral (*fem'-or-al*). Pertaining to the femur. *F. artery.* That of the thigh from groin to knee. *F. canal.* The opening below the inguinal ligament through which the femoral artery passes from the abdomen to the thigh. *F. thrombosis. See* Phlegmasia.

femur (*fe'-mer*). The thighbone.

fenestra (*fen-es'-trah*). A window-like opening. *F. ovalis.* The oval opening between the middle and the internal ear.

fenestration (*fen-es-tra'-shun*). An operation in which an opening is made in the bony labyrinth of the ear to assist hearing when deafness is due to otosclerosis. Now superseded by less drastic and more reliable operation.

fenfluramine (*fen-floo'-ram-een*). An amphetamine-like drug used to suppress appetite in the treatment of obesity.

fenoprofen (*fen-o-pro'-fen*). An anti-inflammatory drug used in the treatment of arthritic conditions.

ferment (1) (*fer-ment'*). v. To undergo fermentation. (2) (*fer'-ment*). n. A catalyst. A substance which can produce chemical changes in other substances, without itself undergoing change.

fermentation (*fer-men-ta'-shun*). The breaking down of carbohydrates and other organic substances by the action of an enzyme or ferment as in the production of alcohol, bread, vinegar and other food or industrial products.

ferritin (*fer'-it-in*). A complex formed of an iron and protein molecule that is one of the forms in which iron is stored in the body.

ferrous (*fer'-us*). Containing iron. *F. fumarate, f. gluconate, f. succinate* and *f. sulphate* are iron salts which are given orally to treat iron-deficiency anaemia.

ferrule (*fer'-ool*). A rubber cap used on the end of walking sticks, frames and crutches to prevent slipping.

fertilization (*fer-til-i-za'-shun*). The impregnation of the female sex cell, the ovum, by a male sex cell, a spermatozoon.

fester (*fes'-ter*). To become superficially inflamed and to suppurate.

festination (*fes-tin-a'-shun*). The involuntary acceleration of walking which occurs when the centre of gravity is displaced in Parkinson's disease. The patient totters rapidly.

fetal (*fe'-tal*). Pertaining to the fetus.

fetishism (*fet'-ish-izm*). A sex-

ual perversion in which an object is regarded with an irrational fear, or an erotic attraction which may be so strong as to replace entirely all normal types of sexual reaction.

fetor (*fe'-tor*). An offensive smell.

fetus (*fe'-tus*). The developing baby between the 8th week and the end of pregnancy.

fever (*fe'-ver*). Pyrexia. A rise in body temperature above the normal. It is often accompanied by quickened pulse and respiration, dry skin, scanty highly-coloured urine, vomiting and headache.

fibre (*fi'-ber*). A thread-like structure.

fibre-optics (*fi-ber-op'-tiks*). The transmission of light rays along flexible tubes by means of very fine glass or plastic fibres. Use is made of this in endoscopic instruments such as the gastroscope.

fibrescope (*fi'-ber-skope*). An endoscope in which fibre-optics are used.

fibrillation (*fib-ril-a'-shun*). A quivering, vibratory movement of muscle fibres. *Atrial f.* Rapid contractions of the atrium causing irregular contraction of the ventricles in both rhythm and force. *Ventricular f.* Fine rapid twitchings of the ventricles leading to circulatory arrest. Rapidly fatal unless it can be controlled.

fibrin (*fi'-brin*). An insoluble protein formed from fibrinogen in blood plasma in the process of clotting. *F. ferment*. Thrombin.

fibrinogen (*fi-brin'-o-jen*). A soluble protein which is present in blood plasma and is converted into fibrin by the action of thrombin when the blood clots.

fibrinolysin (*fi-brin-ol'-is-in*). A proteolytic enzyme that dissolves fibrin.

fibrinolysis (*fi-brin-ol'-is-is*). The dissolution of fibrin by the action of fibrinolysin. The process by which clots are removed from the circulation after healing has taken place.

fibrinopenia (*fi-brin-o-pe'-ne-ah*). A deficiency of fibrinogen in the blood. There is a tendency to bleed as the coagulation time is increased.

fibroadenoma (*fi-bro-ad-en-o'-mah*). A benign tumour of glandular and fibrous tissue. *See* Adenoma.

fibroangioma (*fi-bro-an-je-o'-mah*). A benign tumour containing both fibrous and vascular tissue.

fibroblast (*fi'-bro-blast*). A connective tissue cell.

fibrocartilage (*fi-bro-kart'-il-aje*). Cartilage with fibrous tissue in it.

fibrochondritis (*fi-bro-kon-dri'-tis*). Inflammation of fibrocartilage.

fibrocyst (*fi'-bro-sist*). A fibroma that has undergone cystic degeneration.

fibrocystic (*fi-bro-sis'-tik*). Fibrous and cystic. *F. disease of the pancreas.* An inherited disease affecting the mucus-secreting glands, the sweat glands and the pancreas. It is characterized by fatty stools and repeated lung infections. Mucoviscidosis. Cystic fibrosis.

fibroid (*fi'-broid*). (1) *adj.* Having a fibrous structure. (2) *n.* A fibroma or a fibromyoma, usually one occurring in the uterus.

fibroma (*fi-bro'-mah*). A benign tumour of connective tissue. *Cystic f.* Fibrocyst.

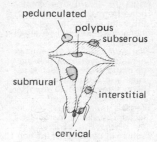

FIBROMYOMATA OF UTERUS

fibromyoma (*fi-bro-mi-o'-mah*). *pl.* fibromyomata. A tumour consisting of fibrous and muscle tissue. Frequently found in or on the uterus.

fibroplasia (*fi-bro-pla'-ze-ah*). The formation of fibrous tissue when a wound heals. *Retrolental f.* Fibrosis of the retina, leading to blindness; it occurs in new-born children who have been given too much oxygen.

fibrosarcoma (*fi-bro-sar-ko'-mah*). A malignant tumour arising in fibrous tissue.

fibrosis (*fi-bro'-sis*). Fibrous tissue formation such as occurs in scar tissue or as the result of inflammation. It is the cause of adhesions of the peritoneum or other serous membranes. *F. of lung.* Condition that may precede bronchiectasis and emphysema.

fibrositis (*fi-bro-si'-tis*). Inflammation of fibrous tissue. The term is loosely applied to pain and stiffness, particularly of the back muscles, for which no other cause can be found.

fibula (*fib'-u-lah*). The slender bone from knee to ankle, on the outer side of the leg.

filament (*fil'-am-ent*). A small thread-like structure.

Filaria (*fil-air'-e-ah*). A genus of nematode worms which may be found in the connective tissues and lymphatics, having been transmitted to man by mosquitoes.

filariasis (*fil-ar-i'-as-is*). An infection by filaria, particularly by *Wuchereria bancrofti*, resulting in blockage of the lymphatics, which causes swelling of the surrounding tissues. Elephantiasis may occur.

filiform (*fil'-e-form*). Threadlike. *F. papillae*. The fine thread-like processes that cover the anterior two-thirds of the tongue.

filtrate (*fil'-trate*). The fluid which passes through a filter.

filtration (*fil-tra'-shun*). (1) The removal of precipitate from a liquid by means of a filter. (2) The removal of rays of a certain wavelength from an electromagnetic beam. *F. angle.* The angle of the anterior chamber of the eye through which the aqueous humour drains; blockage of this channel gives rise to glaucoma.

fimbria (*fim'-bre-ah*). A fringe. *F. of the uterine tube.* The thread-like projections that surround the pelvic opening of the uterine tube.

finger (*fing'-ger*). A digit of the hand. *Clubbed f.* A broadening and thickening of the ends of the fingers, common in chronic diseases of the heart and lungs.

fission (*fish'-un*). A form of asexual reproduction by dividing into two equal parts, as in bacteria. *Binary f.* The splitting in two of the nucleus and the protoplasm of a cell, as in protozoa. *Nuclear f.* The splitting of the nucleus of an atom with the release of a great quantity of energy.

fissure (*fish'-ur*). A cleft. *Anal f.* A painful crack in the mucous membrane of the anus, generally caused by injury from hard faeces. *F. of Rolando.* A furrow in the cortex of each cerebral hemisphere dividing the sensory from the motor area. The central sulcus.

fistula (*fis'-tu-lah*). An abnormal passage connecting the cavity of one organ with another or a cavity with the surface of the body. *Anal f.* The result of an ischiorectal abscess where the channel is from the anus to the skin. *Biliary f.* A leakage of bile to the exterior, following operation on the gall-bladder or ducts. *Blind f.* One which is open at only one end. *Faecal f.* One in which the channel is from the intestine through the wound caused by an operation on the intestines when sepsis is present. *Gastrocolic f.* An opening between the colon and the stomach wall, usually the result of a carcinoma. *Rectovaginal f.* Fistula from the rectum to the vagina which may result from severe perineal tear following childbirth. *Tracheo-oesophageal f.* An opening from the windpipe into the oesophagus; usually a congenital deformity. *Vesicovaginal f.* An opening from the bladder to the vagina, either from error during operation, or from ulceration as may occur in carcinoma of the cervix.

fit (*fit*). A commonly used term for paroxysmal motor dis-

charges leading to sudden convulsive movements, as in epilepsy, eclampsia and hysteria. The term is sometimes applied to apoplexy.

fixation (*fiks-a'-shun*). The process of rendering something immovable, such as a joint or a fractured bone. In psychology, a term used to describe a failure to progress wholly or in part through the normal stages of psychological development to a fully developed personality. In ophthalmology, directing the sight straight at an object.

flaccid (*flak'-sid*). Soft, flabby. *F. paralysis. See* Paralysis.

flagellum (*flaj-el'-um*). *pl.* flagella. The whip-like protoplasmic filament by which some bacteria and protozoa move.

flap (*flap*). A mass of tissue used for grafting in plastic surgery, which is left attached to its blood supply and used to repair defects either adjacent to it or at some distance from it.

flare (*flair*). The response of the skin to an allergic or hypersensitivity reaction. Reddening of the skin that spreads outwards.

flat-foot (*flat'-foot*). A condition due to absence or sinking of the medial longitudinal arch of the foot, caused by weakening of the ligaments and tendons. Pes planus.

flatulence (*flat'-u-lens*). The presence of gas in the stomach or intestine.

flatulent (*flat'-u-lent*). Suffering from flatulence. *F. distension.* Swelling due to gas in the intestines. It is a common complication after abdominal operations and is caused by intestinal stasis.

flatus (*fla'-tus*). Gas in the stomach or intestine.

flea (*fle*). A small, wingless, blood-sucking insect parasite. The common human flea, *Pulex irritans*, rarely transmits disease. Cat and dog fleas, *Ctenocephalides*, are also relatively harmless. The rat fleas *Xenopsylla* and *Nosopsyllus* are the vectors of bubonic plague.

flexibilitas cerea (*fleks-e-bil'-it-as se'-re-ah*). Waxy flexibility in which a patient retains the posture of the body or of a limb in which it has been placed by himself or someone else. A symptom of some forms of schizophrenia.

flexion (*flek'-shun*). Bending. Moving a joint so that the two or more bones forming it draw towards each other. *Dorsi-f.* Bending the fingers or toes backwards. *Plantar f.* Bending the fingers or toes downwards.

Flexner's bacillus (*S. Flexner, American bacteriologist, 1863–1946*). One of the group of pathogenic bacteria which cause bacillary dysentery. *Shigella flexneri.*

flexor (*fleks'-or*). Any muscle causing flexion of a limb or other part of the body.

flexure (*fleks'-ure*). A bend or curve.

floaters (*flo-terz*). Opacities in the vitreous humour of the eye that move about and appear as spots before the eye. Probably degenerative deposits.

floccillation (*flok-sil-a'-shun*). Picking at the bedclothes. A phenomenon often seen in delirious patients.

flocculent (*flok'-u-lent*). Woolly or flaky. Human milk forms a flocculent curd.

flooding (*flud'-ing*). Excessive loss of blood from the uterus. It may be associated with menstruation or miscarriage.

florid (*flor'-id*). A flushed facial appearance as seen in hypertension or after consuming alcohol.

flowmeter (*flo'-me-ter*). An instrument used to measure the flow of liquids or gases.

flucloxacillin (*floo-kloks-ah-sil'-in*). An antibiotic drug used in the treatment of infection by penicillin-resistant bacteria.

fluctuation (*fluk-tu-a'-shun*). A wave-like motion felt on palpation of the abdomen. Varying from time to time.

fludrocortisone (*floo-dro-kor'-te-zone*). A synthetic corticosteroid used in the treatment of adrenal disorders.

fluke (*flook*). One of a group of parasitic flatworms (Trematoda). Different varieties may affect the blood, the intestines, the liver or the lungs.

fluorescein (*floo-or-es'-in*). A dye used to detect corneal ulcer. When it is dropped on the eye the ulcer stains green.

fluorescence (*floo-or-es'-ens*). The property of reflecting back light waves, usually of a lower frequency than that absorbed so that invisible light (e.g. ultra-violet) may become visible.

fluorescent (*floo-or-es'-ent*). Capable of producing fluorescence. *F. screen.* A screen which becomes fluorescent when exposed to X-rays.

fluoridation (*floo-or-i-da'-shun*). The adding of fluorine to water in those areas where it is lacking in order to reduce the incidence of dental caries.

fluorine (*floo'-or-een*). *abbrev.* F. An element found in the water in some localities which helps to prevent dental decay, although in excess it may produce a white mottled effect on the teeth.

fluoroscope (*floo'-or-o-skope*): A fluorescent screen which enables X-ray images to be seen without taking X-ray photographs.

fluorouracil (*floo-or-o-u'-ras-il*). An antimetabolite cytotoxic drug used particularly in the treatment of gastrointestinal tumours.

flush (*flush*). A redness of the face and neck. *Hectic f.* One occurring in conditions such as septic poisoning and pulmonary tuberculosis. *Hot f.* One occurring during the menopause accompanied by a feeling of heat.

flutter (*flut'-er*). An irregularity of the heartbeat.

flux (*fluks*). An excessive flow of any of the body secretions.

focus (*fo'-kus*). *pl.* foci. (1) The point of meeting of rays of light after passing through a lens. (2) The local seat of a disease.

focusing (*fo'-kus-ing*). The ability of the eye to alter its lens power so as to focus correctly at different distances.

folic acid (*fo'-lik as'-id*). A constituent of the vitamin B complex which influences red blood cell formation. Used in the treatment of megaloblastic anaemia. Given orally. *F. a. antagonist.* Any antimetabolite cytotoxic drug which inhibits the action of the folic acid enzyme.

folie à deux (*fo'-le ah der'*). The sharing of delusions by two people living in close contact, one of whom is usually mentally ill.

follicle (*fol'-ikl*). A very small

sac or gland. *Graafian f.* A vesicular ovarian follicle. *See* Graafian follicle. *Hair f.* The sheath in which a hair grows. *F.-stimulating hormone.* FSH. A hormone produced by the anterior pituitary gland which controls the maturation of the graafian follicles in the ovary.

follicular (*fol-ik'-u-lar*). Pertaining to a follicle. *F. conjunctivitis.* Inflammation occurring in the lower conjunctival fornix. *F. tonsillitis.* Tonsillitis arising from infection of the tonsillar follicles.

folliculitis (*fol-ik-u-li'-tis*). Inflammation of a group of follicles, usually of hair follicles in the skin.

folliculosis (*fol-ik-u-lo'-sis*). An abnormal increase in the number of lymph follicles. *Conjunctival f.* A benign non-inflammatory overgrowth of follicles of the conjunctiva of the eyelids.

fomentation (*fo-men-ta'-shun*). A poultice. The application of hot moist material to a part of the body to reduce pain and inflammation.

fomes (*fo'-meez*). *pl.* Fomites. An object which has been in contact with someone with a contagious disease and is capable of transmitting it, e.g. clothing, books and toys.

fontanelle (*fon-tan-el'*). A soft membranous space between the cranial bones of an infant. *Anterior f.* That between the parietal and frontal bones, which closes at about the age of 18 months. Rickets causes delay in this process. *Posterior f.* The junction of the occipital and parietal bones, at the sagittal suture, which closes within 3 months of birth.

food-poisoning (*food-poi'-zon-*

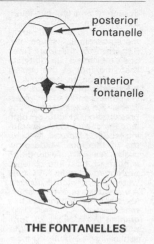

THE FONTANELLES

ing). Commonly used to indicate an acute attack of gastroenteritis after the consumption of unwholesome food. It may be due to chemical poisons such as antimony or arsenic or to poisonous fungi, but most frequently it is due to bacteria and their toxins, the commonest being: (1) the salmonella group, *Salmonella typhimurium* and *S. enteritidis*, infecting meat and fish preparations and duck eggs, (2) staphylococci, often from infected milk or synthetic cream. The excreta of rats and mice, flies or lack of care by food handlers may be the cause of an outbreak, particularly if food is allowed to stand in a warm kitchen, when the organisms can multiply. Infected food and water may also transmit dysentery and typhoid fever. *See* Botulism.

foot (*foot*). The terminal part of the lower limb. *Athlete's f.* Ringworm of the foot. Tinea pedis. *F. drop*. Inability to keep the foot at the correct angle owing to paralysis of the flexors of the ankle. Preventable condition in most cases. *F. presentation*. The presentation of one or both legs instead of the head during labour. *Madura f.* Mycetoma of the foot. Maduromycosis. *Trench f.* A condition similar to frost-bite, due to prolonged standing in cold water. *F.-and-mouth disease*. A virus disease of farm animals, transmissible to man in a mild form.

foramen (*for-a'-men*). *pl.* foramina. An opening or hole, especially in a bone. *F. magnum*. The hole in the occipital bone through which the spinal cord passes. *F. ovale*. The hole between the left and right atria in the fetus. *Obturator f.* The large hole in the innominate bone. *Optic f.* The opening in the posterior part of the orbit through which the optic nerve and the ophthalmic artery pass.

forceps (*for'-seps*). Surgical instruments used for lifting or compressing an object. *Artery f.* (*Spencer Wells f.*) compress bleeding-points during an operation. *Cheatle's f.* are lifting forceps for carrying bowls or instruments that have been sterilized. *Midwifery f.* (*obstetric f.*) are of various patterns, and are used in difficult labour to facilitate delivery. *Vulsellum f.* have claw-like ends for exerting traction.

forensic (*for-en'-sik*). Concerning the law courts. *F. medi-*

cine. The branch that is concerned with the law and has a bearing on legal problems. It includes the investigation of unexplained death or injury.

foreskin (*for'-skin*). The prepuce.

formaldehyde (*for-mal'-de-hide*). A gas used as a disinfectant, chiefly for rooms. A 40% solution in water is known as *formalin* and is used in spray form as a disinfectant.

formication (*for-mik-a'-shun*). A sensation as of insects creeping over the body.

formula (*for'-mu-lah*). (1) A prescription. (2) A detailed statement of the ingredients of a chemical compound. (3) The presentation of the molecule of a chemical compound by chemical symbols.

formulary (*for'-mu-lar-e*). A prescriber's handbook of drugs. *British National F.* One produced by the Joint Formulary Committee for easy reference for doctors and dispensers.

fornix (*for'-niks*). *pl.* fornices. An arch. *F. cerebri*. An arched structure at the back and base of the brain. *F. of the vagina*. The recesses at the top of the vagina in front (*anterior f.*), back (*posterior f.*), and sides (*lateral f.*) of the cervix uteri. *Conjunctival f.* The reflection of the conjunctiva from the eyelids on to the eyeball.

fossa (*fos'-ah*). *pl.* fossae. A small depression or pit. Usually applied to those in bones. *Cubital f.* The triangular depression at the front of the elbow. *Iliac f.* The depression on the inner surface of the iliac bone. *Pituitary f.* The depression in the sphenoid bone. *See* Sella turcica.

Fothergill's operation (*W.E. Fothergill, British gynaecologist, 1865–1926*). Amputation of the cervix, with anterior and posterior colporrhaphy for prolapse of the uterus.

fourchette (*foor-shet'*). The fold of membrane at the perineal end of the vulva.

fovea (*fo'-ve-ah*). A fossa. A small depression, particularly that of the retina. It contains a large number of cones, which give form and colour, and is therefore the area of most accurate vision.

fractionation (*frak-shun-a'-shun*). A term used in radiotherapy when the total dose to be delivered is divided into smaller portions which are given over a period of time. The rationale is that the smaller doses and time interval cause less biological damage.

fracture (*frak'-chur*). A breakage of a bone. The signs and symptoms are: pain, swelling, deformity, shortening of the limb, loss of power, abnormal mobility, and crepitus. The cause may be *direct* violence, as in a blow from a heavy object, or *indirect*, as when falling on the hand causes fracture of the clavicle or severe muscle spasm such as that of the quadriceps muscle fractures the patella. *Closed* (*simple*) f. A clean break with the skin unbroken. *Comminuted f.* The bone is broken in several places and there is splintering of the bone. *Compound* (*open*) f. There is a wound from the broken bone to the skin through which infection may enter. *Depressed f.* Of the cranium, in which part of the bone is driven inwards. *Greenstick f.* Partial break or bending in children occurring before complete ossification of bone. *Impacted f.* One end of the broken bone

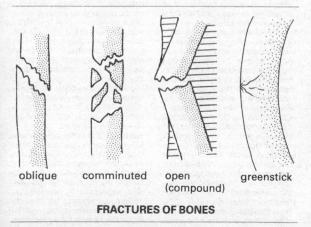

oblique   comminuted   open (compound)   greenstick

FRACTURES OF BONES

is driven into the other, causing shortening. *Intracapsular f.* The break occurs within the joint capsule, particularly that of the hip joint. *Pathological f.* Breaking occurring in diseased bones from slight injury. *Pott's f.* A fracture dislocation of the ankle involving the lower end of the fibula and sometimes the internal malleolus of the tibia. *Spontaneous f.* One that occurs as a result of little or no violence, usually of a bone weakened by disease. *F. dislocation.* One that occurs near a joint so that the fracture is combined with dislocation of that joint.

fragilitas (*fraj-il'-it-as*). Brittleness, particularly of the bones and the hair.

framboesia (*fram-be'-ze-ah*). Yaws.

frame (*frame*). A walking aid with three or four legs. *Guthrie-Smith f.* A large metal frame which fits over a treatment couch, used for attaching pulleys and strings in suspension therapy.

freckle (*frek/*). A brown pigmented spot on the skin. *Hutchinson's melanotic f.* A non-invasive malignant melanoma which occurs mainly in middle-aged women on the face. Lentigo maligna.

Freiberg's disease (*A.H. Freiberg, American surgeon, 1868–1940*). Osteochondritis of the second metatarsal bone, in which there is pain on walking and standing.

Frei test (*W.S. Frei, German dermatologist, 1885–1943*). An intradermal test to aid the diagnosis of lymphogranuloma venereum.

fremitus (*frem'-it-us*). A thrill or vibration, e.g. that produced in the chest by speaking and felt on palpation.

Frenkel's exercises (*H.S. Frenkel, German neurologist, 1860–1931*). Exercises used in the treatment of tabes dorsalis to teach muscle and joint sense.

frenotomy (*fre-not'-om-e*). The cutting of the frenulum of the tongue to cure tongue-tie.

frenulum (*fren'-u-lum*). Frenum. A fold of mucous membrane which limits the movement of an organ. *F. of the tongue.* The fold under the tongue which if too short causes difficulty in sucking and talking (tongue-tie).

freudian (*S. Freud, Austrian psychiatrist, 1856–1939*). Relating to the theories of Freud, who was the originator of psychoanalysis and the psychoanalytical theory of the cause of neurosis.

friable (*fri'-abl*). Easily crumbled.

friction (*frik'-shun*). The act of rubbing. *F. massage.* A circular or transverse pressure applied by finger-tip or thumb to a localized area. Used for the relief of pain. *F. murmur.* The grating sound heard in auscultation when two rough surfaces rub together, as in dry pleurisy.

Friedländer's bacillus (*K. Friedländer, German pathologist, 1847–1887*). The cause of a rare form of pneumonia. *Bacterium friedländeri.*

Friedreich's ataxia or **disease** (*N. Friedreich, German physician, 1825–1882*). A rare form of hereditary ataxia.

frigidity (*frij-id'-it-e*). An absence of normal sexual desire, especially in women.

Frölich's syndrome (*A. Frölich, Austrian neurologist, 1871–1953*). A group of symptoms associated with disease of the pituitary body. These are: increased adiposity, atrophy of the genital organs, and development of feminine characteristics.

frontal (*frun'-tal*). (1) Relating to the forehead. (2) Relating to the front or anterior aspect of a structure.

frost-bite (*frost'-bite*). Impairment of circulation chiefly affecting the fingers, the toes, the nose and the ears, due to exposure to severe cold. The first stage is represented by chilblains. Advanced cases show thrombosis and dry gangrene.

frozen shoulder (*fro'-zen sho'-lder*). A stiff and painful shoulder. Treatment is by stretching under anaesthesia combined with exercises. Capsulitis. The cause is unknown.

fructose (*fruk'-toze*). Fruit sugar. A monosaccharide.

frusemide (*fru'-se-mide*). A diuretic with a rapid and powerful action used in the treatment of oedema and of acute renal failure.

FSH. Follicle-stimulating hormone.

fuchsin (*fook'-zin*). A purplish-red dye used to stain bacteria in microscopy, particularly *Mycobacterium tuberculosis*.

fugue (*fu'-g*). A period of altered awareness during which a person may wander for hours or days and perform purposive actions though his memory for the period may be lost. It may follow an epileptic fit or occur in hysteria or schizophrenia.

fulguration (*ful-gu-ra'-shun*). The destruction by diathermy of papillomata (warts), particularly inside the urinary bladder.

fulminating (*ful'-min-a-ting*). Sudden in onset and rapid in course.

fumigant (*fu'-mig-ant*). A substance which produces gas for fumigation.

fumigation (*fu-mig-a'-shun*). Disinfection of a room and its contents by exposure to the fumes of a vaporized germicide.

fundus (*fun'-dus*). The base of an organ or the part farthest removed from the opening. *F. of the eye*. The posterior part of the inside of the eye as shown by the ophthalmoscope. *F. of the stomach*. That part above the cardiac orifice. *F. of the uterus*. The top of the uterus—that part farthest from the cervix.

fungate (*fun'-gate*). To grow rapidly and produce fungus-like growths. Often occurs in the late stages of malignant tumours.

fungicide (*fun'-je-side*). A preparation that destroys fungal infection.

fungiform (*fun'-je-form*). Shaped like a fungus or mushroom.

fungus (*fun'-gus*). A low form of vegetable life which includes mushrooms and moulds. Some varieties cause disease, such as actinomycosis and ringworm.

funis (*fu'-nis*). The umbilical cord.

funnel (*fun'-el*). A cone-shaped vessel, usually with a tube at its apex, used for filtering or for pouring liquids from one container to another. *F. chest*. A developmental deformity in which there is a depression in the sternum and an inward curvature of the ribs and costal cartilages.

furor (*fu-ror'*). A state of intense excitement during which violent acts may be performed. This may occur following an epileptic fit.

furuncle (*fu-run'-kl*). A boil.

furunculosis (*fu-runk-u-lo'-sis*). A staphylococcal infection represented by many, or crops of, boils.

furunculus (*fu-runk'-u-lus*). A furuncle. *F. orientalis.* A protozoal infection mainly of the tropics, which causes a chronic ulceration. Cutaneous leishmaniasis.

fusiform (*fu'-ze-form*). Shaped like a spindle.

Fusiformis (*fu-ze-for'-mis*). A genus of anaerobic bacteria, most of which are normal flora of the mouth and intestines. *F. fusiformis.* A species found with *Borrelia vincentii* in Vincent's angina.

fusion (*fu'-zhun*). (1) The union between two adjacent structures. (2) The co-ordination of separate images of the same object in the two eyes into one image.

G

g. Abbreviation for the fundamental SI unit of weight, the *gram.*

Ga. Chemical symbol for *gallium.*

Gaffky scale (*G.T.A. Gaffky, German bacteriologist, 1850–1918*). A method of sputum examination in which the tubercle bacilli present in a microscopic field are counted.

gag (*gag*). (1) An instrument placed between the teeth to keep the mouth open. (2) The reflex action which occurs when the back of the throat is stimulated.

gait (*gate*). Manner of walking. *Ataxic g.* The foot is raised high, descends suddenly, and the whole sole strikes the ground. *Cerebellar g.* A staggering walk indicative of cerebellar disease. *Four-point g.* A method which may be adopted when using sticks or crutches, which allows maximum stability. *Spastic g.* Stiff, shuffling walk, the legs being kept together.

galactagogue (*gal-akt'-ag-og*). An agent causing increased secretion of milk.

galactocele (*gal-akt'-o-seel*). (1) A cyst containing milk occurring in the breast. (2) A hydrocele containing a milky fluid.

galactorrhoea (*gal-akt-o-re'-ah*). (1) An excessive flow of milk. (2) Secretion of milk after breast-feeding has ceased.

galactosaemia (*gal-akt-o-se'-me-ah*). An inborn error of metabolism in which there is inability to convert galactose to glucose. This has proved to be one cause of retardation of mental development. If it is diagnosed early, a milk-free diet can be given with marked benefit.

galactose (*gal-akt'-oze*). Soluble sugar derived from lactose. It is converted to glucose in the liver.

galenical (*Galen (Claudius Galenus), Greek physician, c. AD 130–200*). A preparation of a crude drug of animal or vegetable, rather than mineral or chemical, origin.

gall (*gawl*). Bile, a digestive fluid secreted by the liver and stored in the gall-bladder. *G.-bladder.* The sac under the lower surface of the liver, which acts as a reservoir for bile. *G.-stone.* A concretion formed in the gall-bladder. There are three varieties: (1) cholesterol stone, usually a single large ovoid one of cholesterol, (2) pigment stones, multiple small stones occurring in haemolytic diseases, (3) mixed stones, multiple and faceted, they contain layers of cholesterol, calcium, and pigment and are associated with infection of the gall-bladder. *G.-stone colic. See* Biliary colic.

gallamine (*gal'-am-een*). A synthetic muscle relaxant, chemically related to curare but less potent and shorter acting.

gallipot (*gal'-e-pot*). A small receptacle for lotions or ointments.

gallium (*gal'-e-um*). *abbrev.* Ga. A radio-isotope used in detecting some soft tissue disorders because gallium will concentrate in malignant lymphoma, for example.

gallop rhythm (*gal'-op rithm*). Heart rhythm which may occur when there is ventricular overload. The sound is like that of horses' hooves galloping.

galvanism (*L. Galvani, Italian physician and physiologist, 1737–1798*). Electrical treatment using direct current to stimulate the muscles. *See* Faradization.

galvanocauterization (*gal'-van-o-kaw-ter-i-za'-shun*). Burning by means of a wire heated by galvanic current.

galvanofaradization (*gal'-van-o-far-ad-i-za'-shun*). The application of continuous and interrupted currents at the same time to a nerve or muscle.

galvanometer (*gal-van-om'-e-ter*). An instrument for detecting or measuring the strength of a current of electricity.

gamete (*gam'-eet*). A sex cell which combines with another to form a zygote, from which a complete organism develops. A spermatozoon or an ovum.

gametocyte (*gam-e'-to-site*). A cell that is undergoing gametogenesis.

gametogenesis (*gam-e-to-jen'-es-is*). The production of the gametes by the gonads.

gamma (*gam'-ah*). The third letter in the Greek alphabet, γ. *G.-benzene hexachloride.* A drug used as a cream or lotion or as a shampoo to treat head lice. *G. camera.* An apparatus for depicting a part of the body into which radioactive isotopes emitting gamma rays have been introduced. *G. encephalography.* A method of localizing a brain tumour by using radioactive isotopes emitting gamma rays. *G. globulins.* Plasma proteins produced by the reticulo-endothelial cells of the spleen, bone marrow and liver. They are concerned with antibody formation. *See* Globulin. *G. rays.* Electromagnetic rays of shorter wavelength and with greater penetration than X-rays, which are given off by certain radioactive substances and which are used in radiotherapy. Also used in the sterilization of articles which would be destroyed by the heat and moisture required in autoclaving.

ganglion (*gang'-gle-on*). *pl.* ganglia. (1) A collection of nerve cells and fibres, forming an independent nerve centre, as is found in the sympathetic nervous system. (2) A cystic swelling on a tendon.

ganglionectomy (*gang-gle-on-ek'-tom-e*). Excision of a ganglion.

gangrene (*gang'-green*). Death of tissue due to a failure of the supply of blood to it. *Diabetic g.* A type likely to develop in diabetic patients, due to changes in blood vessels. *Dry g.* Gangrene due to failure of arterial blood supply, e.g. from injury or ligature of main artery, frost-bite or arterial disease. The affected part is painful, pale, and later becomes discoloured and black. There is a red line of demarcation between the living and dead tissues. *Gas-g. See* Gas. *Moist g.* That caused by putrefactive changes. The part is swollen, blistered, and discoloured. There is little pain; the line of demarcation is not definite. General signs are: high fever, delirium, and all signs of blood infection. This type may result from infective thrombosis or from pressure on veins as in strangulated hernia.

Ganser state (*S.J.M. Ganser, German psychiatrist, 1853–1931*). Simulated madness. Giving approximate answers to questions which show that the correct answers are known. Hysterical pseudo-dementia.

gargle (*gar'-gl*). A disinfectant solution for washing out the throat.

gargoylism (*gar'-goil-izm*). An inherited condition in which the coarse prominent features and large head are said to resemble a gargoyle. The vision is defective and there is mental subnormality. Hurler's syndrome.

Gärtner's bacillus (*A.G. Gärtner, German bacteriologist, 1848–1934*). A species of salmonella, *S. enteritidis*.

gas (*gas*). Molecules of a substance very loosely combined—a vapour. *Laughing g.* Nitrous oxide. *Marsh g.* Methane. *Sternutatory g.* One which causes sneezing. *Tear g.* One that is irritating to the eyes and causes excessive lacrimation. *G. and air analgesia.* An authorized form of analgesia using nitrous oxide and air, by which the pains of labour are lessened without affecting uterine contractions. *G.-gangrene.* The result of infection of a wound by anaerobic organisms, especially *Clostridium welchii*, normally found in the intestine of animals and therefore likely to be present in cultivated soil, stable refuse, and road dirt.

gasserectomy (*gas-er-ek'-tom-e*). Excision of the trigeminal ganglion.

Gasser's ganglion (*J.L. Gasser, Austrian anatomist, 1723–1765*). The trigeminal ganglion. The ganglion of the sensory root of the fifth cranial nerve.

gastralgia (*gas-tral'-je-ah*). Pain in the stomach.

gastrectomy (*gas-trek'-tom-e*). Excision of a part or whole of the stomach. *Partial g.* Removal of a part, usually the distal portion of the stomach. Commonly performed in the surgical treatment of peptic ulcer. *Billroth g.* Removal of most of the lesser curvature and pyloric portion and joining of the duodenum to the refashioned stomach. This cuts down the production of secretin and acid. *Polya g.* Removal of the first part of the duodenum and the greater part of the stomach, and anas-

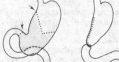

Billroth type I

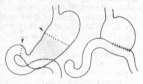

Polya type

GASTRECTOMY (PARTIAL)

tomosis of the stomach to the jejunum. The blind portion of the duodenum supplies the bile and pancreatic and duodenal secretions.

gastric (*gas'-trik*). Pertaining to the stomach. *G. juice.* The clear fluid secreted by the glands of the stomach to assist digestion. It contains an enzyme called pepsin, which acts upon proteins in the presence of weak hydrochloric acid. *G. lavage.* A treatment for some types of poisoning where the stomach contents are washed out through a stomach tube. May also be used to obtain sputum specimens from babies. *G. ulcer.* Ulceration of the gastric mucosa associated with hyperacidity and often precipitated by stress.

gastrin (*gas'-trin*). A hormone secreted by the walls of the stomach, which excites continued secretion of digestive juice whilst food is in the stomach.

gastritis (*gas-tri'-tis*). Inflammation of the lining of the stomach. *Acute g.* Severe irritation, of sudden onset, due to infected food or irritant poisons. *Chronic g.* Loss of appetite, nausea, flatulence and furred tongue, which may be due to repeated indiscretions of diet, excessive alcohol or over-smoking. Hyperchlorhydria is often present.

gastrocele (*gas'-tro-seel*). A hernia of the stomach.

gastrocnemius (*gas-trok-ne'-me-us*). The principal muscle of the calf of the leg. It flexes both the ankle and the knee.

gastrocolic (*gas-tro-kol'-ik*). Pertaining to the stomach and colon. *G. reflex.* Following a meal, increased peristalsis causes the colon to empty into the rectum. This gives rise to a desire to defecate.

gastroduodenostomy (*gas-tro-du-o-den-os'-tom-e*). A surgical anastomosis between the stomach and the duodenum.

gastroenteritis (*gas-tro-en-ter-i'-tis*). Inflammation of the stomach and intestine due to viral or bacterial infection. *Infantile g.* An acute condition of diarrhoea and vomiting producing severe dehydration. The cause may be (a) dietetic; (b) infective; (c) parenteral, when the condition is secondary to the infection elsewhere in the body, e.g. otitis media or bronchitis.

gastroenterology (*gas-tro-en-ter-ol'-o-je*). The study of diseases of the gastrointestinal tract.

gastroenteropathy (*gas-tro-en-ter-op'-ath-e*). Any disease condition affecting both the stomach and the intestine.

gastroenterostomy (*gas-tro-en-ter-os'-tom-e*). A surgical anastomosis between the stomach and small intestine. Usually performed for pyloric obstruction.

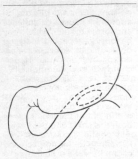

GASTROENTEROSTOMY

Gastrografin (*gas-tro-graf'-in*). A proprietary radio-opaque dye which may be introduced into the alimentary tract for the purpose of an X-ray examination.

gastrography (*gas-trog'-raf-e*). An X-ray examination using a fluorescent screen and a fluid radio-opaque dye.

gastroileac (*gas-tro-il'-e-ak*). Pertaining to the stomach and ileum. *G. reflex*. Food entering the stomach sets up powerful peristalsis in the ileum and opening of the ileocaecal valve.

gastrointestinal (*gas-tro-in-tes'-tin-al*). Pertaining to the stomach and intestine. *G. tract*. The alimentary tract.

gastrojejunostomy (*gas-tro-je-ju-nos'-tom-e*). A surgical anastomosis between the stomach and the jejunum.

gastromalacia (*gas-tro-mal-a'-se-ah*). An abnormal softening of the walls of the stomach.

gastro-oesophagostomy (*gas-tro-e-sof-ag-os'-tom-e*). A surgical anastomosis between the stomach and the oesophagus.

gastropathy (*gas-trop'-ath-e*). Any disease of the stomach.

gastroplasty (*gas'-tro-plas-te*). A surgical operation to cure any deformity or defect of the stomach.

gastroptosis (*gas-trop-to'-sis*). Downward displacement of the stomach owing to weakening of supporting ligaments or of its own musculature.

gastroscope (*gas'-tro-skope*). An instrument fitted with an electric light, which is introduced via the oesophagus to examine the interior of the stomach.

gastrostomy (*gas-tros'-tom-e*). An artificial opening through the abdominal wall into the stomach, through which a feeding tube can be passed in patients who are temporarily or permanently unable to swallow. *See* Artificial feeding.

gastrotomy (*gas-trot'-om-e*). A surgical incision of the stomach.

gastrula (*gas'-tru-lah*). An early stage in the development of the fertilized ovum.

Gaucher's disease (*P.C.E. Gaucher, French physician, 1854–1918*). A rare familial disease in which fat is deposited in the reticulo-endothelial cells causing an enlarged spleen and anaemia.

gauze (*gawz*). A thin open-meshed material used for dressing wounds.

gavage (*gav'-arzh*). Feeding by oesophageal tube. 'Forced feeding'.

Geiger counter (*H. Geiger, German physicist, 1882–1945*). An instrument for detecting and registering radioactivity. The apparatus is sensitive to the rays emitted.

gelatin (*jel'-at-in*). An albuminoid, obtained by boiling connective tissue or bone. It is used in *cooking* for the setting of jellies; in *pharmacy* for suppositories and capsules; and in *bacteriology* as a culture medium.

gene (*jeen*). One of the hereditary factors present in the chromosomes in the germ cell which help to determine the physical and mental make-up of the offspring. *Dominant g.* One that is capable of transmitting its characteristics irrespective of the genes from the other parent. *Recessive g.* One that can pass on its characteristics only if it is present with a similar recessive gene from the other parent. *See* Mendel's theory.

genetic (*jen-et'-ik*). Concerned with origin or reproduction. *G. code.* The arrangement of genetic material stored in the DNA molecule of the chromosome. *G. counselling.* Service for prospective parents who can receive advice as to the likelihood of their children being born with congenital abnormalities.

genetics (*jen-et'-iks*). The study of heredity and natural development.

genitalia (*jen-it-a'-le-ah*). The organs of reproduction.

genitourinary (*jen-it-o-u'-rin-ar-e*). Referring to both the reproductive organs and the urinary tract.

genotype (*jen'-o-tipe*). The genetic characteristics of an individual.

gentamicin (*gen-tah-mi'-sin*). An antibiotic used in the treatment of infection with a wide variety of bacteria, other than anaerobes, which do not respond to other simpler antibiotics.

gentian (*jen'-shun*). An exceedingly bitter vegetable extract. It is prescribed as a tonic and stomachic. *G. violet.* Crystal violet. Used externally as a paint, jelly or ointment in the treatment of infected wounds, burns and certain bacterial and fungoid skin infections. Used internally as an anthelmintic. Also used in microscopy as a stain.

genu (*jen'-u*). The knee. *G. valgum.* Knock-knee. *G. varum.* Bow-leg.

genupectoral (*jen'-u-pek'-tor-al*). Relating to the knee and chest. *G. position.* The knee–chest position. *See* Position.

genus (*je'-nus*). *pl.* genera. A classification of animals and plants, the species within a genus having characteristics common to themselves, but differing from those of other genera.

geriatrics (*jer-e-at'-riks*). The branch of medicine covering old age and the disorders arising from it.

germ (*jerm*). (1) A microbe. (2) That from which something may develop. A seed.

German measles (*jer'-man me-zlz*). *See* Rubella.

germicide (*jerm'-e-side*). An agent capable of destroying pathogenic micro-organisms.

germinoma (*jerm-in-o'-mah*). A neoplasm of the testis or ovum.

gerontology (*jer-on-tol'-o-je*). The study of old age and the ageing processes.

Gessel's developmental chart (*A. Gessell, American psychologist, 1880–1961*). A chart which shows the expected motor, social and psychological development of children.

gestaltism (*gest-alt'-izm*). A theory of holism in psychology which claims that ideas come as a whole and are not subdivisible.

gestation (*jes-ta'-shun*). Pregnancy. *Ectopic g.* Fetal development in some part other than the uterus—most usually the uterine tube.

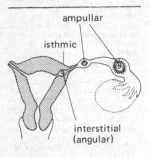

ampullar

isthmic

interstitial (angular)

ECTOPIC GESTATION

Ghon's focus (*A. Ghon, Czechoslovakian pathologist, 1866–1936*). The primary lesion of pulmonary tuberculosis, as seen on an X-ray film, after it has healed by fibrosis and calcification.

giardiasis (*A. Giard, French biologist, 1846–1908*). An infection with *Giardia lamblia*, a pear-shaped protozoon that causes a persistent mild diarrhoea. Intestinal malabsorption may also be caused, especially in children.

gibbosity (*gib-os'-it-e*). A humped back. Kyphosis.

gibbus (*gib'-us*). A hump. Applied to the prominence caused by collapse of a vertebral body and acute angling of the spinous processes.

gigantism (*ji-gant'-izm*). Abnormal growth of the body, often due to overactivity of the anterior lobe of the pituitary gland.

Gilliam's operation (*D.T. Gilliam, American gynaecologist, 1844–1923*). The correction of retroversion of the uterus by shortening the round ligaments. Ventrosuspension.

Gillies needle-holder (*Sir H.D. Gillies, British plastic surgeon, 1882–1960*). Combined scissors and fine suture needle-holder used in plastic surgery.

gingiva (*jin-ji'-vah*). The gum. Connective tissue surrounding the necks of the teeth.

gingivectomy (*jin-jiv-ek'-tom-e*). The surgical removal of the gum margins to get rid of pockets and improve the shape of the gums.

gingivitis (*jin-jiv-i'-tis*). Inflammation of the gums.

ginglymus (*jing'-gle-mus*). A hinge joint allowing movement in one plane only.

Girdlestone's operation (*G.R. Girdlestone, British surgeon, 1881–1950*). Pseudoarthrosis of hip. A false joint made by excising the head and neck of femur and part of the acetabulum, and suturing a muscle mass between the bones' ends. A treatment for osteoarthritis.

gladiolus (*glad-e-o'-lus*). The blade-like portion of the sternum.

gland (*gland*). An organ composed of cells which secrete fluid prepared from the blood, either for use in the body, or for excretion as waste material. *Ductless (endocrine) g.* One which produces an internal secretion but has no canal (duct) to carry the secretion away, e.g. the thyroid gland. *Exocrine g.* One which discharges its secretion through a duct, e.g. the parotid gland. *Lymph g. See* Lymph nodes. *Mucous g.* One which secretes mucus.

glanders (*glan'-derz*). A contagious disease of horses and asses, sometimes communicated to man, in whom it is frequently fatal.

glandular (*gland'-u-lar*). Pertaining to a gland. *G. fever.* Infectious mononucleosis. A febrile condition occurring chiefly in children and young adults. There is general enlargement and tenderness of lymph glands, especially those of the neck, axilla and groin, with leucocytosis. The cause is infection by the Epstein–Barr virus.

glans (*glanz*). An acorn-shaped body, such as the rounded end of the penis or the clitoris.

glare (*glair*). A dazzling light which causes ocular discomfort. A severe persistent headache may occur when there is strong sun or artificial light and light-reflecting surfaces. Dark glasses are preventive.

glaucoma (*glaw-ko'-mah*). Raised intra-ocular pressure. *Primary g.* One that occurs without any previous disease. It is a common cause of blindness, partial or complete, in the elderly. *Closed-angle g.* One that occurs when there is a mechanical defect in the drainage angle and may be primary or secondary. It may be *acute*, when there is pain and blurring of vision, or *chronic*, when there may be no pain, but a gradual loss of vision. *Open-angle g.* Chronic primary glaucoma in which the angle remains open but drainage becomes gradually diminished. *Secondary g.* One that occurs when some ocular disease is complicated by an increase in intra-ocular pressure.

gleet (*gleet*). Chronic gonococcal urethritis marked by a transparent mucous discharge.

glenohumeral (*glen-o-hu'-mer-al*). Referring to the shoulder joint.

glenoid (*glen'-oid*). Resembling a hollow. *G. cavity.* The socket of the shoulder joint.

glia (*gli'-ah*). Neuroglia. The connective tissue of the brain and spinal cord.

glibenclamide (*gli-ben'-klam-ide*). A drug of the sulphonylurea group used in the treatment of diabetes mellitus.

glioblastoma (*gli-o-blas-to'-mah*). A malignant glioma arising in the cerebral hemispheres.

glioma (*gli-o'-mah*). A tumour composed of neuroglia cells affecting the brain and spinal cord. The majority are malignant but seldom metastasize.

Glisson's capsule (*F. Glisson, British physician and anatomist, 1597–1677*). The connective tissue capsule of the liver which envelops the portal vein, hepatic artery and hepatic ducts.

globin (*glo'-bin*). A protein used in the formation of haemoglobin.

globulin (*glob'-u-lin*). A protein constituent of the blood (*serum globulin*) and cerebrospinal fluid. *Gamma g.* A blood fraction prepared from plasma containing antibodies which offers a temporary protection against measles, infective hepatitis and sometimes poliomyelitis and other infections.

globulinuria (*glob-u-lin-u'-re-ah*). The presence of globulin in the urine.

globus (*glo'-bus*). A ball or globe. *G. hystericus.* A symptom of hysteria when a patient feels he cannot swallow because he has a lump in his throat. *G. pallidus.* The pale medial part of the lentiform nucleus of the brain.

glomerulitis (*glo-mer-u-li'-tis*). Inflammation of the glomerulus due to a lesion, associated with the presence of kidney disease.

glomerulonephritis (*glo-mer-u-lo-nef-ri'-tis*). Acute nephritis following a streptococcal or other infection in which there is inflammation of the glomeruli of the kidneys.

glomerulosclerosis (*glo-mer-u-lo-skler-o'-sis*). Degenerative changes in the glomerular capillaries of the renal tubule leading to renal failure.

glomerulus (*glo-mer'-u-lus*). The tuft of capillaries within the nephron, which filters urine from the blood.

glossal (*glos'-al*). Relating to the tongue.

glossectomy (*glos-ek'-tom-e*). Excision of the tongue.

Glossina (*glos-i'-nah*). A genus of biting flies—the tsetse fly.

glossitis (*glos-i'-tis*). Inflammation of the tongue.

glossodynia (*glos-o-din'-e-ah*). A painful sensation in the tongue when no lesion is visible.

glossolalia (*glos-o-la'-le-ah*). Unintelligible speech. The patient speaks in an imaginary language.

glossopharyngeal (*glos-o-far-in-je'-al*). Pertaining to the tongue and pharynx. *G. nerve.* The ninth cranial nerve.

glossoplegia (*glos-o-ple'-je-ah*). Paralysis of the tongue.

glottis (*glot'-is*). The space between the vocal cords. The term is sometimes used for that part of the larynx which is associated with voice production.

glucagon (*glu'-kah-gon*). A polypeptide produced by the pancreas. It aids glycogen breakdown in the liver and raises the blood sugar level.

glucocorticoid (*glu-ko-kor'-te-koid*). An adrenal steroid which affects carbohydrate metabolism by increasing the level of blood sugar and liver glycogen.

gluconeogenesis (*glu-ko-ne-o-jen'-es-is*). The production of glucose from the non-nitrogen portion of the amino acids after deamination. It occurs in the liver and kidneys.

glucose (*glu'-koze*). Dextrose or grape-sugar found in many fruits and honey. It is the absorbable type to which carbohydrates are reduced by digestion, and is therefore found in the blood in considerable quantity. It is present in the urine of patients with untreated diabetes mellitus. *G. tolerance test.* Test in which a quantity of glucose is

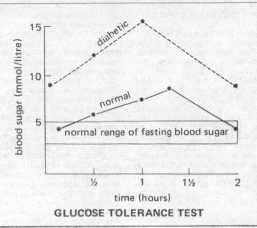

GLUCOSE TOLERANCE TEST

given and the concentration of glucose in the blood is estimated at intervals afterwards. Used mainly when diabetes mellitus is suspected. *G.-6-phosphate dehydrogenase.* A red-cell enzyme. Inherited deficiency causes a tendency to haemolytic anaemia. *See* Favism.

glutamic acid (*glu-tam'-ik as'-id*). One of the 22 amino acids formed by the digestion of dietary protein.

glutamic oxaloacetic transaminase (*glu-tam'-ik ox-al-o-as-e'-tik trans-am'-in-aze*). An enzyme found in cardiac muscle and the liver. Raised serum levels (SGOT) may indicate an acute myocardial infarction or the presence of liver disease.

glutamic pyruvic transaminase (*glu-tam'-ik pi-ru'-vik trans-am'-in-aze*). An enzyme found in the liver. Measurement of serum levels (SGPT) is used in the study and diagnosis of liver diseases.

glutaraldehyde (*glu-tar-al'-de-hide*). A solution used for tissue fixation in electron microscopy.

gluteal (*glu-te'-al*). Relating to the buttocks. *G. muscles.* Three muscles which form the fleshy part of the buttocks.

gluten (*glu'-ten*). A nitrogenous constituent of wheat and other grains. *G.-induced enteropathy.* Coeliac disease.

glutethimide (*glu-teth'-im-ide*). A hypnotic and sedative drug used in the treatment of insomnia.

glycerin (*glis'-er-een*). A colourless syrupy substance obtained from fats and fixed oils. It has a hygroscopic action. As an emollient it is an ingredient of many skin preparations. *G. suppository.* One composed of glycerine and gelatin, used as an evacuant. *G. of thymol.* An antiseptic mouth wash and gargle.

glyceryl trinitrate (*glis'-er-il tri-ni'-trate*). Nitroglycerin. Sublingual tablets that relieve anginal pain by dilating the coronary arteries.

glycine (*gli'-seen*). A non-essential amino acid.

glycogen (*gli'-ko-jen*). The form in which carbohydrate is stored in the liver and muscles. Animal starch. *G. storage disease.* Inherited disease in which there is a deficiency in the synthesis of glycogen. This accumulates in the liver causing enlargement.

glycogenesis (*gli-ko-jen'-es-is*). The process of glycogen formation from the blood glucose.

glycogenolysis (*gli-ko-jen-ol'-is-is*). The breakdown of glycogen in the body so that it may be utilized.

glycoside (*gli'-ko-side*). A crystalline body in plants which when acted on by acids or ferments produces sugar. If the sugar is glucose it may be termed a *glucoside*. See Digitalis.

glycosuria (*gli-ko-su'-re-ah*). An excess of glucose in the urine, a symptom of diabetes mellitus. *Alimentary g.* The presence of sugar in the urine after a meal rich in carbohydrate. It is transitory. *Emotional g.* Possible reaction in times of stress due to increased release of adrenaline. *Renal g.* Sugar in the urine in an otherwise healthy person, due to an unusually low renal threshold.

glycyrrhiza (*glis-e-ri'-zah*). Liquorice. Used as a flavouring in some medicines.

glymidine (*gli'-mid-een*). A drug of the sulphonylurea

group used in the treatment of diabetes mellitus.

gnathic (*nath'-ik*). Pertaining to the jaw.

gnathoplasty (*nath'-o-plas-te*). A plastic operation on the jaw.

Goa powder (*go'-ah pow'-der*). The source of chrysarobin derived from a tropical tree.

goblet cell (*gob'-let sel*). A goblet-shaped cell, found in the intestinal epithelium, which produces mucus.

goitre (*goi'-ter*). Enlargement of the thyroid gland, usually causing a marked swelling in front of the neck. It may be *endemic* and give rise to no other symptoms. Derbyshire neck is of this type. *Colloid g.* An enlarged but soft thyroid gland with no signs of hyperthyroidism. *Exophthalmic g.* Hyperthyroidism with marked protrusion of the eyeballs. Graves's disease. *Intrathoracic g.* Enlargement of the gland mainly in the thorax, so the swelling may not be easily visible. *Lymphadenoid g.* Hashimoto's disease. An enlargement in which there is infiltration by lymphocytes and deposits of lymphoid tissue. *Primary toxic g.* Signs of excess of thyroxine in the blood, where the gland has not been previously enlarged. *Secondary toxic g.* The sudden development of the signs of hyperthyroidism after previous enlargement of the gland. *Sporadic g.* A simple non-toxic enlargement. *Substernal g.* Enlargement of the gland behind the sternum so that swelling in the neck may not be apparent.

gold (*go-ld*). *abbrev.* Au. A metallic element used as an injection into a joint for reducing rheumatic inflammation.

Radioactive g. An isotope which gives off beta and gamma rays. Used in the form of small grains or seeds it may be implanted into malignant tissues. In colloidal form it may be instilled into a serous cavity to treat malignant effusions.

Golgi's apparatus or **body.** (*C. Golgi, Italian histologist, 1844–1926*). Specialized structures seen near the nucleus of a cell during microscopic examination. *Golgi's organ.* The sensory end organs in muscle tendons that are sensitive to stretch.

gonad (*gon'-ad*). A reproductive gland. The testicle or ovary.

gonadotrophic (*gon-ad-o-trof'-ik*). Having influence on the gonads. *G. hormones.* Gonadotrophin.

gonadotrophin (*gon-ad-o-trof'-in*). Any hormone that stimulates either the ovaries or the testes. These hormones are produced by the pituitary gland and include the follicle-stimulating hormone (FSH) and the luteinizing hormone (LH). *Human chorionic g.* HCG. A hormone produced by the placenta during pregnancy, the detection of which in the urine forms the basis of pregnancy tests. May also be present in the blood stream in certain malignant conditions such as teratomas. Its presence or absence in the blood is used as a tumour marker to detect response to treatment.

gonion (*go'-ne-on*). The midpoint of the mandible (lower jaw).

gonioscope (*go'-ne-o-skope*). An apparatus for examining the angle of the anterior chamber of the eye.

goniotomy (*go-ne-ot'-om-e*). An operation for congenital glaucoma.

gonococcus (*gon-o-kok'-us*). *Neisseria gonorrhoeae.* A diplococcus which causes gonorrhoea.

gonorrhoea (*gon-o-re'-ah*). A common venereal disease caused by *Neisseria gonorrhoeae* infecting the genital tract of either sex, causing a discharge and pain on micturition, although the disease is often asymptomatic in females. Spread by the blood stream, it may give rise to iritis or arthritis. Scar tissue formation may bring about urethral stricture or infertility owing to occlusion of the uterine tubes.

gonorrhoeal (*gon-o-re'-al*). Relating to gonorrhoea. *G. arthritis.* Intractable infection of joints causing great pain and disability. *G. ophthalmia.* In the newly born (*ophthalmia neonatorum*) a notifiable disease and a cause of blindness.

Goodpasture's syndrome (*E.W. Goodpasture, American pathologist, 1886–1960*). A rare haemorrhagic lung disorder associated with glomerulonephritis.

gorget (*gor'-jet*). A grooved, guiding instrument used in lithotomy.

gouge (*gowj*). A curved chisel used for scooping out diseased bone, or other hard substances.

gout (*gowt*). A metabolic disease associated with an excess of uric acid in the blood. It is characterized by painful inflammation and swelling of the smaller joints, especially those of the big toe and thumb. Inflammation is accompanied by the deposit of urates around the joints.

GPI. General paralysis of the insane. Dementia paralytica. *See* Paralysis.

graafian follicle (*R. de Graaf, Dutch physician and anatomist, 1641–1673*). A follicle which is formed in the ovary and contains an ovum. A follicle matures during each menstrual cycle, ruptures and releases the ovum which is then picked up by the fimbriated end of the uterine tube.

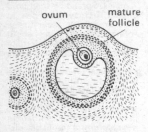

ovum   mature
            follicle

GRAAFIAN FOLLICLE

Graefe's knife (*F.W.A. von Graefe, German ophthalmologist, 1828–1870*). A narrow pointed knife used in some cataract operations.

graft (*grahft*). A portion of tissue or an organ transplanted from one part of the body to remedy a defect in a corresponding structure. *Autogenous g.* A graft taken from and given to the same individual. *Bone g.* A portion of bone transplanted to repair another bone. *Corneal g.* A portion of cornea, usually from a recently dead person, used to repair a diseased cornea. *Homogenous g.* A graft taken from one person and given to another individual of the same species. *Pedicle g.* A skin graft, one end of which remains attached to its original site until the grafting has become established.

gram (*gram*). *abbrev.* g. The fundamental SI unit of weight, equal to one thousandth of a kilogram.

Gram's stain (*H. Gram, Danish physician, 1853–1938*). A method of staining bacteria which is used to classify them into *Gram-negative* and *Gram-positive* bacteria.

grand mal (*gron mal'*). Major epilepsy. *See* Epilepsy.

granular (*gran'-u-lar*). Containing small particles. *G. casts.* The degenerated cells from the lining of renal tubules excreted in the urine in certain kidney disorders.

granulation (*gran-u-la'-shun*). (1) The division of a hard solid substance into small particles. (2) The growth of new tissue by which ulcers and wounds heal when the edges are not in apposition. It consists of new capillaries and fibroblasts which fill in the space and later form fibrous tissue. The resulting scar is liable to be hard and unsightly.

granule (*gran'-ule*). A small particle or grain.

granulocyte (*gran'-u-lo-site*). Any white blood cell containing granules, especially one containing in its cytoplasm neutrophils, basophils, or eosinophils.

granulocytopenia (*gran-u-lo-si-to-pe'-ne-ah*). A marked reduction in the number of granulocytes in the blood. The condition may precede agranulocytosis.

granulocytopoiesis (*gran-u-lo-si-to-poi-e'-sis*). The formation of granulocytes in the blood-forming bone marrow.

granuloma (*gran-u-lo'-mah*). *pl.* granulomata. A tumour composed of granulation tissue, usually due to chronic infection or invasion by a foreign body.

granulomatosis (*gran-u-lo-mat-o'-sis*). An infection producing granulomata. *Lipoid g.* Xanthomatosis. Hand–Schüller–Christian disease. *Malignant g.* Lymphadenoma. Hodgkin's disease.

granulosa cell (*gran-u-lo'-sah sel*). A type of cell present in the graafian follicle. *G. c. tumour.* A rare neoplasm of the ovary that produces excessive oestrogen.

gravel (*grav'l*). Small calculi formed in the kidneys and bladder, and sometimes excreted with the urine.

Graves's disease (*R.J. Graves, Irish physician, 1796–1853*). Exophthalmic goitre. Hyperthyroidism.

gravid (*grav'-id*). Pregnant.

gravity (*grav'-it-e*). Weight. *Specific g.* The weight of a substance compared with that of an equal volume of water.

gray (*gra*). *abbrev.* Gy. The SI unit used to denote the absorbed dose in radiation therapy.

Grenz rays (*Grenz raze*). A source of superficial X-rays that may be used to treat skin diseases.

Griffith types (*F. Griffith, British bacteriologist, d. 1941*). Types of haemolytic streptococci determined by agglutination tests.

griseofulvin (*gri-se-o-ful'-vin*). An oral antifungal antibiotic that is used in the treatment of infections of the skin, hair and nails.

guanethidine (*gwan-eth'-id-een*). A drug used in the treatment of hypertension. It is an adrenergic blocking agent.

guanine (*gwan'-een*). A purine base, one of the constituents of all nucleic acids.

gubernaculum (*gu-ber-nak'-u-lum*). A cord of fibromuscular tissue attached to the lower pole of the testis. It functions only during the descent of the testis.

Guillain–Barré syndrome (*G. Guillain, French neurologist, 1876–1961; A. Barré, French neurologist, b. 1880*). Acute infective polyneuritis. After an infection, usually respiratory, there is a general weakness or paralysis which frequently affects the respiratory muscles as well as the peripheral ones.

guillotine (*gil'-o-teen*). A surgical instrument used for excising tonsils.

guinea-worm (*gin'-e-werm*). A nematode worm, *Dracunculus medinensis*, which burrows into human tissues, particularly into the legs or feet.

gullet (*gul'-et*). The oesophagus.

gumboil (*gum'-boil*). The opening on the gum of an abscess at the root of a tooth.

gumma (*gum'-ah*). A soft, degenerating tumour characteristic of the tertiary stage of syphilis. It may occur in any organ or tissue.

gustatory (*gus'-ta-tor-e*). Relating to taste.

gut (*gut*). The intestine.

gutta (*gut'-ah*). A drop. *G. percha.* The juice of a tropical tree which, when dried, forms an elastic semi-solid substance. Used in dentistry as a root filler.

Gy. Abbreviation for the SI

unit, the *gray*.

gynaecoid (*gi'-ne-koid*). Like the female. *G. pelvis.* One with a round brim and shallow cavity suited to childbearing. A normal female pelvis.

gynaecologist (*gi-ne-kol'-o-jist*). One who specializes in the diseases of the female genital tract.

gynaecology (*gi-ne-kol'-o-je*). The science of those diseases which are peculiar to the female genital tract.

gynaecomastia (*gi-ne-ko-mas'-te-ah*). Excessive growth of the male breast.

gypsum (*jip'-sum*). Plaster of Paris (*calcium sulphate*).

gyrus (*ji'-rus*). A convolution as of the cerebral cortex.

H

H. Chemical symbol for *hydrogen*.

habit (*hab'-it*). Automatic response to a specific situation acquired as a result of repetition and learning. *Drug h.* Drug addiction. *H. training.* A method used in psychiatric nursing whereby deteriorated patients can be rehabilitated and taught personal hygiene by constant repetition and encouragement.

habitat (*hab'-it-at*). The natural surroundings of an animal or plant.

hacking (*hak'-ing*). In massage, rhythmic beating using the lateral borders of the fingers. This increases the circulation to the part being treated.

haemangioblastoma (*he-man-je-o-blas-to'-mah*). A tumour of the brain or spinal cord consisting of proliferated blood vessel cells.

haemangioma (*he-man-je-o'-mah*). A benign tumour formed by dilated blood vessels. *Strawberry h.* A birthmark, which may become very large, but frequently disappears in a few years.

haemarthrosis (*he-mar-thro'-sis*). An effusion of blood into a joint.

haematemesis (*he-mat-em'-es-is*). Vomiting of blood. If it has been in the stomach for some time and become partially digested by gastric juice, it is of a dark colour and contains particles resembling coffee grounds.

haematin (*he'-mat-in*). The iron-containing part of haemoglobin.

haematinic (*he-mat-in'-ik*). An agent which increases the amount of haemoglobin. Often used in the treatment of iron-deficiency anaemia.

haematocele (*he'-mat-o-seel*). A swelling produced by effusion of blood, e.g. in the sheath surrounding a testicle or a broad ligament.

haematocolpos (*he-mat-o-kol'-pos*). An accumulation of blood or menstrual fluid in the vagina. *See* Cryptomenorrhoea.

haematocrit (*he'-mat-o-krit*). The volume of red cells in the blood. Usually expressed as a percentage of the total blood volume.

haematology (*he-mat-ol'-o-je*). The science dealing with the nature, functions and diseases of blood.

haematoma (*he-mat-o'-mah*). A swelling containing clotted blood.

haematometra (*he-mat-o-me'-trah*). An accumulation of blood or menstrual fluid in the uterus.

haematomyelia (he-mat-o-mi-e'-le-ah). An effusion of blood into the spinal cord.

haematomyelitis (he-mat-o-mi-el-i'-tis). An effusion of blood into the spinal canal with acute inflammation of the cord.

haematosalpinx (he-mat-o-sal'-pinks). An accumulation of blood in the uterine tubes. Haemosalpinx.

haematoxylin (he-mat-oks'-il-in). A stain used in histology. It is obtained from the logwood tree.

haematuria (he-mat-u'-re-ah). The presence of blood in the urine, due to injury or disease of any of the urinary organs.

haemochromatosis (he-mo-kro-mat-o'-sis). A condition in which there is high absorption and deposition of iron leading to a high serum level, pigmentation of the skin and liver failure. Bronze diabetes.

haemoconcentration (he-mo-kon-sen-tra'-shun). A loss of circulating fluid from the blood resulting in an increase in the proportion of red blood cells to plasma. The viscosity of the blood is increased.

haemocytology (he-mo-si-tol'-o-je). The study of the cellular contents of blood.

haemocytometer (he-mo-si-tom'-e-ter). An apparatus for counting the blood corpuscles in a specific volume of blood. The cells are counted visually through a microscope. Electronic counters are now more often used.

haemodialysis (he-mo-di-al'-is-is). The removal of waste material from the blood by means of a dialyser or artificial kidney in cases of kidney failure. The apparatus is coupled to an artery and the puri-fied blood from it is returned through a vein.

haemoglobin (he-mo-glo'-bin). The complex protein molecule contained within the red blood cells which gives them their colour and by which oxygen is transported.

haemoglobinaemia (he-mo-glo-bin-e'-me-ah). The presence of haemoglobin in the blood plasma.

haemoglobinometer (he-mo-glo-bin-om'-e-ter). An instrument for estimating the haemoglobin content of the blood.

haemoglobinopathy (he-mo-glo-bin-op'-ath-e). Any one of a group of hereditary disorders, including sickle cell anaemia and thalassaemia, in which there is an abnormality in the production of haemoglobin.

haemolysin (he-mol'-is-in). A substance which destroys red blood cells. It may be an antibody, a bacterial toxin or a component of a virus.

haemolysis (he-mol'-is-is). The disintegration of red blood cells. Excessive haemolysis, which may produce anaemia, may be caused by poisoning or by bacterial infection.

haemolytic (he-mo-lit'-ik). Having the power to destroy red blood cells. *H. disease of the newborn.* A condition associated with rhesus incompatibility. *See* Rhesus factor.

haemopericardium (he-mo-per-e-kar'-de-um). The presence of blood in the pericardium, usually owing to rupture of the heart or to a knife wound.

haemophilia (he-mo-fil'-e-ah). A familial disease transmitted by females only, to their male offspring. Characterized by delayed or entire absence of clotting power of the blood due to a lack of anti-haemophilic globulin (AHG) or any of the clotting factors. Slight injuries take longer to clot. Any operation requires cover with AHF (antihaemophilic factor). All injuries or bleeds should be brought to the attention of a doctor as there is a danger of internal bleeding or damage to joints.

Haemophilus (he-mof'-il-us). A genus of gram-negative rod-like bacteria. *H. ducreyi.* The cause of soft chancre. *H. influenzae.* The cause of some respiratory infections and a secondary cause of influenza. *H. pertussis.* The cause of whooping cough. Bordet-Gengou bacillus.

haemophthalmia (he-moff-thal'-me-ah). Bleeding into the vitreous of the eye, usually the result of trauma. Haemophthalmos.

haemopneumothorax (he-mo-nu-mo-thor'-aks). The presence of blood and air in the pleural cavity, usually due to injury.

haemopoiesis (he-mo-poi-e'-sis). The formation of red blood cells which takes place normally in the bone marrow and continues throughout life. *Extramedullary h.* The formation of blood cells other than in the bone marrow, e.g. in the liver or spleen.

haemopoietic (he-mo-poi-et'-ik). Relating to red blood cell formation. *H. factors.* Those necessary for the development of red blood cells, e.g. vitamin B_{12} and folic acid.

haemoptysis (he-mop'-tis-is). The coughing up of blood from the lungs or bronchi. Being aerated, it is bright red and frothy.

haemorrhage (hem'-or-aje). An escape of blood from a ruptured blood vessel, externally or internally. *Arterial h.* Bright red blood which escapes in rhythmic spurts, corresponding to the beats of the heart. *Venous h.* Dark red blood which escapes in an even flow. Haemorrhage may also be: (a) *primary*—at the time of operation or injury; (b) *reactionary* or *recurrent*—occurring later when the blood pressure rises and a ligature slips or a vessel opens up; (c) *secondary*—as a rule about 10 days after injury, and usually due to sepsis. Special types are: *Accidental h.* Bleeding from the uterus during pregnancy. It may be *revealed* or *concealed. Antepartum h.* That which occurs before labour starts. *See* Placenta praevia. *Cerebral h. See* Apoplexy. *Concealed h.* Collection of the blood in a cavity of the body. *Extradural h.* Bleeding inside the head, but outside the dura. The result of injury to the skull causing signs of raised intracranial pressure. The cerebrospinal fluid is not blood-stained. *Intradural h.* Bleeding beneath the dura mater. It may be due to injury and causes signs of compression. The cerebrospinal fluid will be blood-stained. *Post-partum h.* That which occurs after childbirth. *Subarachnoid h.* Bleeding into the subarachnoid space. *Unavoidable h.* The bleeding that occurs in placenta praevia.

haemorrhoid (hem'-or-oid). A 'pile' or locally dilated rectal vein. Piles may be either external or internal to the anal sphincter. Pain is caused on defecation, and bleeding may occur. Acute attacks of inflammation intensify the symptoms.

haemorrhoidectomy (*hem-or-oid-ek'-tom-e*). The surgical removal of haemorrhoids.

haemosalpinx (*he-mo-sal'-pinks*). Haematosalpinx.

haemosiderosis (*he-mo-sid-er-o'-sis*). The deposition of iron in the tissues as brownish granules following excessive haemolysis of red blood cells.

haemostasis (*he-mo-sta'-sis*). The arrest of bleeding or the slowing up of blood flow in a vessel.

haemostatic (*he-mo-stat'-ik*). A drug or remedy for arresting haemorrhage. A styptic.

haemothorax (*he-mo-thor'-aks*). Blood in the thoracic cavity, e.g. from injury to soft tissues as a result of fracture of a rib.

Hageman factor (*ha'-gem-an fak'-tor*). Factor XII, which facilitates the clotting of blood (called after the first person found to be suffering from a deficiency of it).

hair (*hair*). A delicate keratinized epidermal filament growing out of the skin. The root of the hair is enclosed beneath the skin in a tubular follicle.

halazone (*hal'-az-one*). A chlorine antiseptic similar to chloramine. Used for the purification of drinking water.

half-life (*hahf'-life*). The period of time in which a radioactive isotope loses half its activity by the process of disintegration.

halibut oil (*hal'-e-but oil*). A vitamin-rich (A and D) oil derived from the liver of halibut.

halitosis (*hal-e-to'-sis*). Foul-smelling breath.

hallucination (*hal-u-sin-a'-shun*). A false perception in which the patient believes he sees, smells, hears, tastes or feels an object or person when there is no basis in the external environment for the belief.

hallucinogen (*hal-u-sin'-o-jen*). A drug that causes hallucinations, e.g. LSD and cannabis.

hallux (*hal'-uks*). The big toe. *H. valgus.* A deformity in which the big toe is bent towards the other toes. *H. varus.* A deformity in which the big toe is bent outwards away from the other toes.

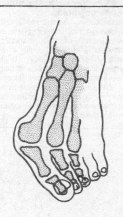

HALLUX VALGUS

halo (*ha'-lo*). The coloured ring or rings seen around lights by people with glaucoma, and also after exposure to ultra-violet light. *Glaucomatous h.* A white ring of atrophy seen round the optic disc in glaucoma.

halogen (*hal'-o-jen*). One of the non-metallic elements chlorine, iodine, bromine and fluorine.

haloperidol (*hal-o-per'-id-ol*). A sedative and tranquilizer used in the treatment of schizophrenia and other psychiatric disorders, particularly mania.

halothane (*hal'-o-thane*). A widely used anaesthetic; used as an inhalation to induce and maintain anaesthesia.

hamamelis (*ham-ah-me'-lis*). A soothing agent prepared from witch-hazel and used in suppository form in the treatment of haemorrhoids.

hamartoma (*ham-ar-to'-mah*). A benign nodule which is an overgrowth of mature tissue.

hammer (*ham'-er*). The malleus. *H.-toe.* A deformity in which the first phalanx is bent upwards, with plantar flexion of the second and third phalanx. A corn which often develops on the bend may cause much pain.

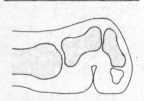

HAMMER-TOE

hamstring (*ham'-string*). The flexors of the knee joint that are situated at the back of the thigh.

hand (*hand*). The terminal part of the arm below the wrist.

Claw h. A paralytic condition in which the hand is flexed and the fingers contracted, caused by injury to nerves or muscles. *Cleft h.* A congenital deformity in which the cleft between the 3rd and 4th fingers extends into the palm. *H., foot and mouth disease.* An infectious disease caused by Coxsackie virus which results in vesicle formation on all three sites. Not the same as foot-and-mouth disease.

handicapped (*hand'-e-kapt*). Pertaining to a person with a mental or physical disability that interferes with normal living and earning capacity.

Hand–Schüller–Christian disease. (*A. Hand, American paediatrician, 1868–1949; A. Schüller, Austrian neurologist, b. 1874; H.A. Christian, American physician, 1876–1951*). A disease of the reticuloendothelial system in which granulomata containing cholesterol are formed, chiefly in the skull.

Hanot's disease (*V.-C. Hanot, French physician, 1844–1896*). A form of cirrhosis of the liver in which the fibrosis is found mainly around the ducts of the biliary system.

Hansen's disease (*G.H.A. Hansen, Norwegian physician, 1841–1912*). Leprosy. It is caused by infection by Hansen's bacillus, *Mycobacterium leprae.*

haploid (*hap'-loid*). Having one set of chromosomes after division instead of two.

hapten (*hap'-ten*). A non-protein substance which forms an antigen when combined with a body protein.

harelip (*hair'-lip*). A congenital fissure in the upper lip, often accompanied by cleft palate.

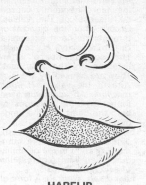

HARELIP

harness (*har'-nes*). A device used in lumbar and cervical traction. In the former, it fixes around the thorax and pelvis. In the latter, it encompasses the occipital and mandibular regions.

Harrison's groove or **sulcus** (*E. Harrison, British physician, 1789–1838*). A depression in the chest wall above the diaphragm noticed in difficult breathing, especially in children.

Harris's operation (*S. Harris, Australian surgeon, 1880–1936*). Suprapubic transvesical prostatectomy.

Hartnup disease (*hart'-nup diz-eez'*). An hereditary defect in amino acid metabolism which may produce mental retardation (named after the first person found to suffer from it).

Harvey, W. *British physician (1578–1657)*. In 1628 Harvey described his theory that blood circulates around the body. This was contained in his book *De Motu Cordis*.

Hashimoto's disease (*H. Hashimoto, Japanese surgeon, 1881–1934*). A lymphadenoid goitre caused by the formation of antibodies to thyroglobulin. It is an autoimmune condition giving rise to hypothyroidism.

hashish (*hash'-ish*). Indian hemp. *See* Cannabis.

Hassall's corpuscles (*A.H. Hassall, British chemist and physician, 1817–1894*). Small striated bodies in the thymus gland which are the remains of tissue found in the early stages of development of this gland.

haustration (*haws-tra'-shun*). A haustrum, or the process of forming one.

haustrum (*haws'-trum*). *pl.* haustra. Any one of the pouches formed by the sacculations of the colon.

haversian canal (*C. Havers, British physician and anatomist, 1650–1702*). One of the minute canals which permeate compact bone, containing blood and lymph vessels to maintain its nutrition. *See* Bone.

hay fever (*ha fe'-ver*). An acute catarrh affecting the nasal mucous membrane and the conjunctiva, and caused by hypersensitiveness to the pollen of grasses, etc. *See* Allergy.

HCG. Human chorionic gonadotrophin. *See* Gonadotrophin.

He. Chemical symbol for *helium*.

headache (*hed'-ake*). A pain felt within the head. It may arise from trauma or from mental stress, or from intracranial disorder. Migraine can produce intense headache.

Heaf test (*F.G.R. Heaf, British physician, 1894–1973*). A form of tuberculin testing. A drop of tuberculin solution on the skin is injected by means of a number of very short needles mounted on a spring-loaded device (Heaf's gun).

healing (*he'-ling*). The process of return to normal function, after a period of disease or injury. *H. by first intention* signifies union of the edges of a clean incised wound without visible granulations, and leaving only a faint linear scar. *H. by second intention* is union of the edges of an open wound by the formation of granulations which fill it in from the bottom and sides. These form fibrous tissue which contracts and causes an unsightly scar.

hearing (*heer'-ing*). The reception of sound waves and their transmission onwards to the brain in the form of nerve impulses. *H. aid.* An apparatus, now usually electronic, used to amplify sounds before they reach the inner ear.

heart (*hart*). A hollow, muscular organ which pumps the blood throughout the body, situated behind the sternum slightly towards the left side of the thorax. *Heart attack.* Myocardial infarction. *H. block.* A form of heart disease in which the passage of impulses down the bundle of His is interrupted. It may be partial, in which every second or third beat is missed, or complete, in which there is a very slow myogenic beat uninfluenced by the nervous system. *See* Stokes–Adams syndrome. *H. failure.* May be acute, as in coronary thrombosis, or chronic. *H. murmur.*

An abnormal sound heard in the heart, frequently caused by disease of the valves. Occurs when the blood flow through the heart exceeds a certain velocity. *H. sounds.* The sounds heard when listening to the heartbeat. They are caused by the closure of the valves. *H.–lung machine.* An apparatus used to perform the functions of both the heart and the lungs during heart surgery.

heartburn (*hart'-burn*). Indigestion marked by a burning sensation in the oesophagus, often with regurgitation of acid fluid. Pyrosis.

heat (*heet*). Warmth. A form of energy, which may cause an increase in temperature or a change of state, e.g. the conversion of water into steam. *Latent h.* The heat absorbed by a substance when changing its state from solid to liquid or liquid to gas. *Specific h.* The amount of heat required to raise the temperature of 1 gram of a substance by 1°C. *H. exhaustion.* Abdominal cramp, a rapid pulse, anorexia and dizziness, sometimes followed by sudden collapse, caused by loss of body fluids and salts under very hot conditions. *H.-stroke.* Sunstroke. A failure of the heat regulating mechanism of the body, with a high temperature, absence of sweating and ultimately unconsciousness. Death may follow if the condition is not treated at once. *Prickly h.* Miliaria. Heat rash. An acute itching caused by blocking of the ducts of the sweat-glands following profuse sweating.

hebephrenia (*he-be-fre'-ne-ah*). A form of schizophrenia characterized by thought disorder and emotional incongruity. Behaviour is often silly and childish. Delusions and hallucinations are common.

Heberden's nodes (*W. Heberden, British physician, 1710–1801*). Bony or cartilaginous outgrowths causing deformity of the terminal finger joints in osteoarthritis.

hebetude (*heb'-e-tude*). Emotional dullness. A common symptom in dementia and schizophrenia.

hectic (*hek'-tik*). Occurring regularly. *H. fever.* A regularly occurring increase in temperature; it is frequently observed in pulmonary tuberculosis. *H. flush.* A redness of the face accompanying a sudden rise in temperature.

hedonism (*he'-don-izm*). Excessive devotion to pleasure.

Heerfordt's syndrome (*C.F. Heerfordt, Danish ophthalmologist, b. 1871*). Uveoparotid fever. Enlargement of the parotid gland with uveitis and sometimes facial paralysis.

Hegar's dilators (*A. Hegar, German gynaecologist, 1830–1914*). A series of graduated dilators used to dilate the uterine cervix.

heliotherapy (*he-le-o-ther'-ap-e*). Treatment of disease by exposure of the body to sunlight.

helium (*he'-le-um*). abbrev. He. An inert gas sometimes used in conjunction with oxygen to facilitate respiration in obstructional types of dyspnoea and for decompressing deep-sea divers.

helix (*he'-liks*). (1) A spiral twist. Used to describe the configuration of certain molecules, e.g. deoxyribonucleic acid (DNA). (2) The outer rim of the auricle of the ear.

Heller's operation (*E. Heller, German surgeon, 1877–1964*). An operation for the relief of cardiospasm by dividing the muscle coat at the lower end of the oesophagus.

Heller's test (*J.F. Heller, Austrian physician, 1813–1871*). A test for the presence of albumin in urine, using a concentrated nitric acid.

helminthiasis (*hel-min-thi'-asis*). An infestation with worms.

helminthology (*hel-min-thol'-o-je*). The study of parasitic worms.

hemeralopia (*hem-er-al-o'-pe-ah*). Day blindness. The vision is poor in a bright light but is comparatively good when the light is dim. *See* Nyctalopia.

hemianopia (*hem-e-an-o'-pe-ah*). Partial blindness, in which the patient can see only one half of the normal field of vision. It arises from disorders of the optic tract and of the occipital lobe.

hemiballismus (*hem-e-bal-iz'-mus*). Involuntary chorea-like movements on one side of the body only.

hemicolectomy (*hem-e-ko-lek'-tom-e*). The removal of the ascending and part of the transverse colon with an ileotransverse colostomy.

hemiglossectomy (*hem-e-glos-ek'-tom-e*). Removal of approximately half the tongue.

hemiparesis (*hem-e-par-e'-sis*). Paralysis on one side of the body. Hemiplegia.

hemiplegia (*hem-e-ple'-je-ah*). Paralysis of one half of the body, usually due to cerebral disease or injury. The lesion is on the side of the brain opposite to the side paralysed.

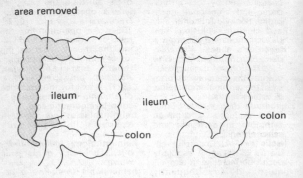

area removed

ileum

ileum

colon

colon

HEMICOLECTOMY AND TRANSVERSE ILEOCOLOSTOMY

hemisphere (*hem'-is-feer*). A half sphere. In anatomy, one of the two halves of the cerebrum or cerebellum.

hemp (*hemp*). *See* Cannabis.

henbane (*hen'-bane*). *See* Hyoscyamus.

Henle's loop (*F.G.J. Henle, German anatomist, 1809–1885*). That part of a kidney tubule that forms a loop and in which there is a movement of sodium salts between it and the tissue fluid, and a certain adjustment of osmolarity.

Henoch's purpura (*E.H. Henoch, German paediatrician, 1820–1910*). Allergic purpura. *See* Purpura.

heparin (*hep'-ar-in*). An anticoagulant formed in the liver and circulated in the blood. Injected intravenously it prevents the conversion of prothrombin into thrombin, and is used in the treatment of thrombosis.

hepatalgia (*hep-at-al'-je-ah*). Pain in the liver.

hepatectomy (*hep-at-ek'-tom-e*). Excision of a part or the whole of the liver.

hepatic (*hep-at'-ik*). Relating to the liver. *H. flexure.* The angle of the colon which is situated under the liver.

hepaticojejunostomy (*hep-at-ik-o-jej-u-nos'-tom-e*). The anastomosis of the hepatic duct to the jejunum usually following extensive excision for carcinoma of the pancreas.

hepaticostomy (*hep-at-ik-os'-tom-e*). A surgical opening into the hepatic duct.

hepatitis (*hep-at-i'-tis*). Inflammation of the liver. *Amoebic h.* Inflammation that may arise during amoebic dysentery and lead to liver abscesses. *Infective h.* Infective jaundice. Caused by a virus (A or IH) spread by faecal contamination. *Serum h.* Hepatitis occurring 1 to 6 months after parenteral infection by hepatitis B virus, usually in blood or its products. Often seen in drug addicts. Can be fatal.

hepatization (*hep-at-i-za'-shun*). The changing of lung tissue into a solid mass resembling liver which occurs in acute lobar pneumonia. *Red h.* The red solid appearance of the consolidated lung due to the invasion of the alveoli by red blood cells and fibrin. *Grey h.* The grey appearance later in the disease before resolution occurs, when white blood cells invade the area to destroy the infection.

hepatocele (*hep'-at-o-seel*). Herniation of the liver through the abdominal wall or the diaphragm.

hepatocellular (*hep-at-o-sel'-u-lah*). Referring to the cells of the liver.

hepatocirrhosis (*hep-at-o-sir-o'-sis*). Cirrhosis of the liver.

hepatogenous (*hep-at-oj'-en-us*). Arising in the liver. Applied to jaundice where the disease arises in the parenchymal cells of the liver.

hepatolenticular (*hep-at-o-len-tik'-u-lar*). Pertaining to the liver and the lentiform nucleus. *H. degeneration.* Wilson's disease. A progressive condition usually occurring between the ages of 10 and 25 years. There are tremors of the head and limbs, pigmentation of the cornea and sometimes defective twilight vision.

hepatolithiasis (*hep-at-o-lith-i'-as-is*). Calculi formation in the liver.

hepatoma (*hep-at-o'-mah*). A primary malignant tumour arising in the liver cells.

hepatomegaly (*hep-at-o-meg'-al-e*). An enlargement of the liver.

hepatosplenomegaly (*hep'-at-o-splen-o-meg'-al-e*). Enlargement of the liver and spleen, such as may be found in kala-azar.

hepatotoxic (*hep-at-o-toks'-ik*). Applied to drugs and substances that cause destruction of liver cells.

hereditary (*her-ed'-it-ar-e*). Derived from ancestry. Inherited.

heredity (*her-ed'-it-e*). The transmission of both physical and mental characteristics to the offspring from the parents. Recessive characteristics may miss one or two generations and reappear later.

Hering–Breuer reflex (*K.E.K. Hering, German physiologist, 1834–1918; J. Breuer, German physician, 1842–1925*). A reflex in which the depth of respiration is determined by the nervous impulses which affect the muscle spindles of the intercostal muscles and the diaphragm.

hermaphrodite (*her-maf'-ro-dite*). An individual whose gonads contain both testicular and ovarian tissue. These may be combined as an ovotestis or there may be a testis on one side and an ovary on the other. The external genitalia may be indeterminate or of either sex. *Pseudo-h.* One whose gonads are histologically of one sex but in whom the genitalia have the appearance of the opposite sex. *True h.* One who possesses both male and female gonads.

hernia (*her'-ne-ah*). A protrusion of any part of the internal organs through the structures enclosing them. *Cerebral h.* A protrusion of brain through an opening in the skull. *Dia-*

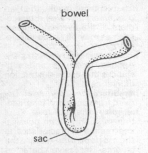

bowel

sac

STRANGULATED HERNIA

phragmatic h. and *hiatus h.* A protrusion of a part of the stomach through the oesophageal opening in the diaphragm. *Femoral h.* A loop of intestine protruding through the femoral canal. More common in females. *Incisional h.* A hernia occurring at the site of an old wound. *Inguinal h.* Protrusion of the intestine through the inguinal canal. This may be congenital or acquired, and is commoner in males. A rupture. *Irreducible h.* A hernia that cannot be replaced by manipulation. *Reducible h.* A hernia that can be returned to its normal position by manipulative measures. *Strangulated h.* A hernia of the bowel in which the neck of the sac containing the bowel is so constricted that the venous circulation is impeded, and gangrene will result if not treated promptly. *Umbilical h.* Protrusion of bowel through the umbilical ring. This may be congenital or acquired. *Vaginal h.* Rectocele or cystocele.

hernioplasty (*her'-ne-o-plaste*). A plastic repair of the abdominal wall performed after reducing a hernia.

herniorrhaphy (*her-ne-or'-af-e*). Removal of a hernial sac and repair of the abdominal wall.

herniotomy (*her-ne-ot'-om-e*). An operation to remove a hernial sac.

heroin (*her'-o-in*). A diacetate of morphine used as an analgesic. It is a strong drug of addiction and its use in medicine is now discouraged.

herpes (*her'-peez*). An inflammatory skin eruption showing small vesicles. *H. simplex.* Cold sore. An eruption that appears usually around the mouth. The vagina may also be affected. The infection tends to recur. A rare complication is encephalitis. *H. zoster.* Shingles. The eruption follows the course of a cutaneous nerve, the inflammation affecting the sensory ganglion of the nerve root just as it leaves the spinal cord. Pain can be very severe. *H. zoster ophthalmicus.* Herpes affecting the first division of the 5th cranial nerve. The forehead, face and nose are affected and the cornea also is usually involved. Neuralgic pains may be severe and vesicles may appear on the nostrils. Keratitis may occur, and the pain may persist to a lesser degree for several months.

herpesvirus (*her-peez-vi'-rus*). One of a group of DNA-containing viruses. They include the causative agents of herpes simplex, herpes zoster and chicken-pox.

Herxheimer reaction (*K. Herxheimer, German dermato-*

logist, 1861–1944). An inflammatory reaction in the tissues in cases of syphilis, which can occur on starting treatment.

Hess's operation (*C. von Hess, German ophthalmologist, b. 1863*). An operation for ptosis. The upper eyelid is sutured to the occipitofrontalis muscle above the eyebrow.

Hess's screen test (*W.R. Hess, Swiss ophthalmologist, b. 1881*). A test for paralytic squint. The degree of diplopia is recorded on a chart.

Hess's test (*A.F. Hess, American physician, b. 1875*). A test used to diagnose purpura. An inflated blood pressure cuff causes an increase in capillary pressure and rupture of the walls, causing purpuric spots to develop.

heterochromia (*het-er-o-kro'-me-ah*). A difference in colour in the irides of the two eyes or in different parts of one iris. It may be congenital or secondary due to inflammation.

heterogeneous (*het-er-o-je'-ne-us*). Composed of diverse constituents.

heterogenous (*het-er-oj'-en-us*). Derived from different sources.

heterophoria (*het-er-o-for'-e-ah*). A tendency to squint when fusion is interrupted. It occurs mainly when the person is tired or in poor health.

heteroplasty (*het'-er-o-plas-te*). A plastic operation in which the graft is obtained from an animal not of the same species. A xenograft.

heterosexual (*het-er-o-seks'-u-al*). Attracted to and desiring to establish an emotional relationship with someone of the opposite sex.

heterotropia (*het-er-o-tro'-pe-ah*). A marked deviation of the eyes. Strabismus or squint.

heterozygous (*het-er-o-zi'-gus*). Possessing dissimilar alternative genes for an inherited characteristic, one gene coming from each parent. One gene is dominant and the other is recessive.

hexachlorophane (*heks-ah-klor'-o-fane*). An antiseptic often added to soap, soap solutions, or dusting powder, which greatly reduces the bacteria on the skin. As topical preparations of it have been associated with severe neurotoxicity, they should be used with caution in neonates, and avoided on large raw areas in infancy.

hexamethonium (*heks-ah-metho'-ne-um*). A ganglionic blocking agent formerly used in the treatment of hypertension.

hexamine (*heks'-am-een*). Methenamine. A urinary antiseptic which releases formaldehyde in an acid urine.

Hg. Chemical symbol for *mercury* (hydrargyrum).

hiatus (*hi-a'-tus*). A space or opening. *H. hernia.* A protrusion of a part of the stomach through the oesophageal opening in the diaphragm.

hiccup (*hik'-up*). Hiccough. A spasmodic contraction of the diaphragm causing an abrupt inspiratory sound.

hidrosis (*hi-dro'-sis*). The excretion of sweat.

Higginson's syringe (*A. Higginson, British surgeon, b. 1808*). An india-rubber syringe with a bulb in the centre which, when compressed, forces fluid forward through the nozzle. Flow is maintained in one direction only by valves.

hilum (*hi'-lum*). Hilus. A recess

in an organ, by which blood vessels, nerves and ducts enter and leave it.

hindbrain (*hi'-nd-brane*). That part of the brain consisting of the medulla oblongata, the pons and the cerebellum.

hip (*hip*). The upper part of the thigh at its junction with the pelvis. *H. replacement.* An operation in which the head of the femur and cup of the acetabulum are replaced by a prosthesis. *See* Arthroplasty.

hippuric acid (*hip-u'-rik as'-id*). A waste product of metabolism which is excreted in the urine, particularly that of horses. It may be used in the treatment of rheumatism and also in the testing of liver function.

hippus (*hip'-us*). Alternate contraction and dilatation of the pupils. This occurs in various diseases of the nervous system, e.g. multiple sclerosis.

Hirschsprung's disease (*H. Hirschsprung, Danish physician, 1831–1916*). *See* Megacolon.

hirsute (*her'-sute*). Hairy.

hirsutism (*her'-su-tizm*). Excessive hairiness, especially in women.

hirudin (*hir-u'-din*). The active principle in the secretion of the leech and certain snake venoms which prevents clotting of blood.

Hirudo (*hir-u'-do*). A genus of leeches. *H. medicinalis.* The medical leech.

histamine (*his'-tam-een*). An enzyme that causes local vasodilatation and increased permeability of the blood vessel walls. It is readily released from body tissues and is a factor in allergy response. Injected subcutaneously, it greatly increases gastric secretion of hydrochloric acid and is used in tests of gastric function.

histidinaemia (*his-tid-in-e'-me-ah*). A rare congenital inability to metabolize histidine, causing mental retardation.

histidine (*his'-tid-een*). One of the 22 amino acids formed by the digestion of dietary protein. Histamine is derived from it.

histiocyte (*his'-te-o-site*). A stationary macrophage of connective tissue. Derived from the reticulo-endothelial cells, it acts as a scavenger, removing bacteria from the blood and tissues.

histiocytoma (*his-te-o-si-to'-mah*). A tumour containing histiocytes causing a vascular nodule.

histiocytosis (*his-te-o-si-to'-sis*). A group of diseases of bone in which granulomata appear, containing histiocytes and eosinophil cells. *See* Letterer–Siwe disease and Hand–Schüller–Christian disease.

histochemistry (*his-to-kem'-is-tre*). That branch of histology which deals with the identification of chemical compounds in the cells and tissues.

histocompatibility (*his-to-kom-pat-ib-il'-it-e*). The ability of cells to be accepted and to function in a new situation. Tissue typing reveals this and ensures a higher success rate in organ transplantation.

histogram (*his'-to-gram*). A bar-chart. Statistical values are expressed as blocks on a graph.

histology (*his-tol'-o-je*). The science dealing with the minute structure, composition and function of tissues.

histolysis (*his-tol'-is-is*). The

disintegration of tissues.

histoplasmosis (*his-to-plas-mo'-sis*). Infection caused by inhalation of the spores of a yeast-like fungus, *Histoplasma capsulatum.* Usually symptomless, the infection may progress and produce a condition resembling tuberculosis. Choroiditis and anterior uveitis may occur.

hives (*hi'-vz*). Urticaria.

Hodgkin's disease (*T. Hodgkin, British physician, 1798–1866*). Lymphadenoma. A progressive malignant condition of the reticulo-endothelial cells. There is progressive enlargement of lymph nodes and lymph tissue all over the body. Treated by radiotherapy and cytotoxic drugs. This disease has a good prognosis.

holism (*ho'-lizm*). A philosophy in which the person is considered as a functioning whole rather than as a composite of several systems.

holistic (*ho-lis'-tik*). Pertaining to holism.

holography (*hol-og'-raf-e*). A method of recording images in 3-dimensional form by using a laser beam to reflect light from an object on to photographic film.

Homans's sign (*J. Homans, American surgeon, 1877–1954*). Pain elicited in the calf when the foot is dorsiflexed. Indicative of venous thrombosis.

homatropine (*hom-at'-ro-peen*). A short-acting mydriatic used in ophthalmology to dilate the pupil and so allow a better view of the fundus of the eye.

homeopathy (*ho-me-op'-ath-e*). A system of medicine promulgated by C.F.S. Hahnemann (*German physician,*

1755–1843) and based upon the principle that 'like cures like'. Drugs are given which can produce in the patient the symptoms of the disease to be cured, but they are prescribed in very small doses.

homeostasis (*ho-me-o-sta'-sis*). Automatic self-regulation to maintain the normal or standard state of the body under variations in the environment.

homeothermic (*ho-me-o-ther'-mik*). Homothermal. Applied to warm-blooded animals, whose heat regulating mechanism maintains a constant body temperature in spite of the environment.

homicide (*hom'-is-ide*). The killing of a human being. *Culpable h.* covers murder (malice aforethought), manslaughter (without malice aforethought), causing death by reckless driving, and infanticide. *Non-culpable h.* covers justifiable homicide (e.g. lawful execution) and excusable homicide (misadventure or accident). *See* McNaghten's Rules.

homogeneous (*hom-o-je'-ne-us*). Uniform in character. Similar in nature and characteristics.

homogenize (*hom-oj'-en-ize*). To make homogeneous. To reduce to the same consistency.

homogenous (*hom-oj'-en-us*). Derived from the same source.

homogentisic acid (*hom-o-jen-tis'-ik as'-id*). Alkapton. A substance excreted in the urine where there is a congenital error of metabolism causing alkaptonuria. It is an intermediary product of tyrosine and phenylalanine metabolism.

homograft (*hom-o-graft*). A tissue or organ transplanted from one individual to another of the same species. An allograft.

homolateral (*hom-o-lat'-er-al*). On the same side. Ipsilateral.

homologous (*hom-ol'-og-us*). (1) In anatomy, having the same embryological origin although performing a different function. (2) In chemistry, possessing a similar structure. *H. chromosomes*. Those that pair during meiosis and contain an identical arrangement of genes in the DNA pattern.

homologue (*hom'-o-log*). A part or organ which has the same relative position or structure as another one.

homoplasty (*hom'-o-plas-te*). Surgical replacement of defective tissues with a homograft.

homosexual (*hom-o-seks'-u-al*). (1) *adj*. Of the same sex. (2) *n*. A person who is sexually attracted to a person of the same sex.

homosexuality (*hom-o-seks-u-al'-it-e*). The attraction for and desire to establish a sexual and/or an emotional relationship with a member of the same sex.

homozygous (*hom-o-zi'-gus*). Possessing an identical pair of genes for an inherited characteristic. *See* Heterozygous.

hookworm (*hook'-werm*). *See* Ancylostoma.

hordeolum (*hor-de-o'-lum*). A stye. Inflammation of the sebaceous glands of the eyelashes.

hormone (*hor'-mone*). A chemical substance which is generated in one organ, and carried by the blood to another in which it excites activity.

hormonotherapy (*hor-mon-o-ther'-ap-e*). Treatment by the use of hormones. Endocrinotherapy.

Horner's syndrome (*J.F. Horner, Swiss ophthalmologist, 1831–1886*). A condition in which there is a lesion on the path of sympathetic nerve fibres in the cervical region. The symptoms include enophthalmos, ptosis, a contracted pupil and a decrease in sweating.

horseshoe kidney. *See* Kidney.

Horton's syndrome (*B.T. Horton, American physician, b. 1895*). Severe headache caused by the release of histamine in the body or by its administration. Histamine cephalalgia.

host (*ho'-st*). The animal, plant or tissue on which a parasite lives and multiplies. *Definitive* or *final h.* One that harbours the parasite during its adult sexual stage. *Intermediate h.* One that shelters the parasite during a non-reproductive period.

hour-glass contraction (*ow'-er-glahs kon-trak'-shun*). A contraction near the middle of a hollow organ, such as the stomach or uterus, producing an outline resembling that shape.

housemaid's knee (*hows'-madz ne*). Prepatellar bursitis. Inflammation of the prepatellar bursa, which becomes distended with serous fluid.

humerus (*hu'-mer-us*). The bone of the upper arm.

humidifier (*hu-mid'-if-i-er*). An apparatus for maintaining the moisture in the air of a room at any given level.

humidity (*hu-mid'-it-e*). The amount of moisture in the air.

Relative h. The humidity of the atmosphere compared with what it would be if the air were saturated.

humour (*hu'-mor*). Any fluid of the body, such as lymph or blood. *Aqueous h.* The fluid filling the anterior chamber of the eye. *Crystalline h.* The lens of the eye. *Vitreous h.* The jelly-like substance which fills the chamber of the eye between the lens and the retina.

Huntington's chorea (*G.S. Huntington, American physician, 1851–1927*). A rare, degenerative inherited disorder of the brain in which there is progressive chorea and mental deterioration (dementia).

Hurler's syndrome (*G. Hurler, Austrian paediatrician*). An inherited disorder in which mental subnormality is caused by excess mucopolysaccharides being stored in the brain and reticulo-endothelial system. Gargoylism.

Hutchinson's teeth (*Sir J. Hutchinson, British surgeon, 1828–1913*). Typical notching of the borders of the permanent incisor teeth occurring in congenital syphilis.

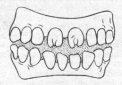

HUTCHINSON'S TEETH

hyaline (*hi'-al-een*). Resembling glass. *H. degeneration.* A form of deterioration which

occurs in tumours due to deficiency of blood supply. It precedes cystic degeneration. *H. membrane disease. See* Respiratory distress syndrome.

hyalitis (*hi-al-i'-tis*). Inflammation of the hyaloid membrane or vitreous humour in the eyeball.

hyaloid (*hi'-al-oid*). Resembling glass. Hyaline. *H. artery.* An artery running between the optic disc and the lens of the eye of a fetus. It atrophies at birth. *H. membrane.* A delicate transparent membrane surrounding the vitreous humour of the eye.

hyaluronidase (*hi-al-u-ron'-e-daze*). An enzyme which facilitates the absorption of fluids in subcutaneous tissues. It is found in the testes of mammals, and a preparation of it is used with subcutaneous and intramuscular injections to improve their distribution.

hybrid (*hi'-brid*). The offspring of distinct but related members of a species or of members of different species.

hydatid (*hi-dat'-id*). A cystic swelling containing the embryo of *Echinococcus granulosus.* It may be found in any organ of the body, e.g. in the liver. 'Daughter cysts' are produced from the original. Infection is from contaminated foods, e.g. salads. *H. disease.* The result of the presence of hydatids in the lungs, liver or brain.

hydatidiform (*hi-dat-id'-e-form*). Resembling an hydatid cyst. *H. mole. See* Mole.

hydraemia (*hi-dre'-me-ah*). An excessive quantity of water in the blood.

hydragogue (*hi'-drah-gog*). A purgative causing copious liquid evacuations, e.g. magnesium sulphate, jalap.

hydralazine (*hi-dral'-az-een*). A drug used to lower the blood pressure in the treatment of hypertension.

hydramnios (*hi-dram'-ne-os*). An excessive amount of amniotic fluid in the uterus in the later months of pregnancy.

hydrargyrism (*hi-drar'-ji-rizm*). Chronic mercurial poisoning.

hydrargyrum (*hi-drar'-ji-rum*). Mercury (*Latin*).

hydrarthrosis (*hi-drar-thro'-sis*). A collection of fluid in a joint.

hydrate (*hi'-drate*). A compound of an element with water.

hydroa (*hi-dro'-ah*). A hypersensitivity of the skin to light, resulting in the formation of a vesicular eruption on the exposed parts with intense irritation. Usually occurs in prepubescent boys.

hydrocarbon (*hi-dro-kar'-bon*). A compound of hydrogen and carbon. Fats are of this type.

hydrocele (*hi'-dro-seel*). A swelling caused by accumulation of fluid, especially in the tunica vaginalis surrounding the testicle.

hydrocephalus (*hi-dro-kef'-al-us*). 'Water on the brain'. Enlargement of the skull due to an abnormal collection of cerebrospinal fluid around the brain or in the ventricles. It may be either congenital or acquired from inflammation of the meninges during infancy. It frequently accompanies spina bifida. *See* Toxoplasmosis.

hydrochloric acid (*hi-dro-klor'-ik as'-id*). HCl. A colourless compound of hydrogen and chlorine. In 0.2% solution it is present in gastric juice and aids digestion.

hydrochlorothiazide (*hi-dro-klor-o-thi'-az-ide*). A valuable oral diuretic similar to but more potent than chlorothiazide. It is used in the treatment of oedema and hypertension.

hydrocortisone (*hi-dro-kor'-tiz-one*). Cortisol. A hormone isolated from the secretion of the adrenal cortex. It affects carbohydrate and protein metabolism and is anti-inflammatory. Used for topical application in eye, ear and skin conditions. Also used as intra-articular injection for arthritis and intravenously in status asthmaticus and in acute adrenocortical insufficiency.

hydrocyanic acid (*hi-dro-si-an'-ik as'-id*). A highly poisonous acid. In liquid or gaseous form it can be fatal within minutes. It smells of bitter almonds. Prussic acid.

hydroflumethiazide (*hi-dro-flu-meth-i'-az-ide*). An oral thiazide diuretic used in the treatment of oedema and hypertension.

hydrogen (*hi'-dro-jen*). *abbrev.* H. A combustible gas, present in nearly all organic compounds which, in combination with oxygen, forms water. *H. ion concentration.* The amount of hydrogen in a liquid, which is responsible for its acidity. The degree of acidity is expressed in pH values, and the higher the hydrogen ion concentration, the *greater* the acidity, and the *lower* the pH value. The concentration in the blood is of importance in acidosis. *H. peroxide.* H_2O_2. An antiseptic. When in contact with pus the oxygen is released and causes frothing. It also has a bleaching action. *H. sulphide.* H₂S. Sulphuretted hydrogen. A colourless gas which smells of bad eggs. Used to precipitate ferric sulphide.

hydrolysis (*hi-drol'-is-is*). The process of splitting up into smaller molecules by uniting with water.

hydrometer (*hi-drom'-e-ter*). An instrument for estimating the specific gravity of fluids, e.g. a urinometer.

hydrometra (*hi-dro-me'-trah*). A collection of watery fluid in the uterus.

hydromyelia (*hi-dro-mi-e'-le-ah*). A dilatation of the central canal of the spinal cord caused by an accumulation of cerebrospinal fluid.

hydronephrosis (*hi-dro-nef-ro'-sis*). An accumulation of urine in the pelvis of the kidney, resulting in atrophy of the kidney structure, due to an obstruction to the flow of urine from the kidney. The condition may be: (1) *congenital*, due to malformation of the kidney or ureter; or (2) *acquired*, due to an obstruction of the ureter by tumour or stone, or to back pressure from stricture of the urethra or an enlarged prostate gland.

hydropathy (*hi-drop'-ath-e*). The treatment of disease by the use of water internally and externally. Hydrotherapy.

hydropericarditis (*hi-dro-per-e-kard-i'-tis*). Inflammation of the pericardium resulting in serous fluid in the pericardial sac.

hydroperitoneum (*hi-dro-per-e-ton-e'-um*). See Ascites.

hydrophobia (*hi-dro-fo'-be-ah*). An acute infectious disease contracted by man through a bite from an animal infected with *rabies*. Caused by a virus present in the saliva. The symptoms include violent spasms of the muscles of deglutition, which are greatly aggravated by the sight of water: There are mental delusions, fever and a profuse flow of saliva. Paralysis and death occur 3 to 4 days after the symptoms appear. There is an incubation period of from 10 days to 3 months or longer, so immediate inoculation with *anti-rabies vaccine* may prevent the disease from developing.

hydropneumothorax (*hi-dro-nu-mo-thor'-aks*). The presence of fluid and air in the pleural space.

hydrops (*hi'-drops*). Dropsy. *H. abdominis.* Ascites. *H. foetalis.* Oedema of an infant suffering from haemolytic disease. *See* Haemolytic. *H. tubae.* Hydrosalpinx.

hydrorrhoea (*hi-dro-re'-ah*). A discharge of watery fluid. *H. gravidarum.* An abnormal discharge of fluid during pregnancy due to excessive mucus secretion from the endometrium.

hydrosalpinx (*hi-dro-sal'-pinks*). Distension of the uterine tubes by fluid.

hydrotherapy (*hi-dro-ther'-ap-e*). The treatment of disease by means of water.

hydrothorax (*hi-dro-thor'-aks*). Fluid in the pleural cavity due to serous effusion as in cardiac, renal and other diseases.

hydro-ureter (*hi-dro-u-re'-ter*). An accumulation of water or urine in a ureter.

hydroxyproline (*hi-droks-e-pro'-leen*). One of the 22 amino acids.

hydroxytryptamine (*hi-droks-*

e-trip'-tam-een). Serotonin.

hydroxyurea (*hi-droks-e-u-re'-ah*). An orally active cytotoxic agent used mainly in the treatment of chronic myeloid leukaemia when other agents have failed.

hygiene (*hi'-jeen*). The science of health. *Communal h.* The maintenance of the health of the community by the provision of a pure water supply, efficient sanitation, good housekeeping etc. *Industrial h.* Care of the health of workers in the industry. *Mental h.* The healthy development of the mental outlook and emotional reactions. *Oral h.* The efficient care and cleanliness of the mouth and teeth, especially important in illness. *Personal h.* Individual measures taken to preserve one's own health. *Social h.* The prevention and cure of the venereal diseases.

hygroma (*hi-gro'-mah*). A swelling caused by fluid. *Cystic h.* A cystic lymphangioma of the neck. *Subdural h.* A collection of clear fluid in the subdural space.

hygrometer (*hi-grom'-et-er*). An instrument for measuring the water vapour in the air.

hygroscopic (*hi-gro-skop'-ik*). Readily absorbing moisture. An example is *glycerin*, which is used in suppositories as a means of aiding evacuation by moistening the faeces.

hymen (*hi'-men*). A fold of mucous membrane partially closing the entrance to the vagina. *Imperforate h.* A membrane which completely occludes the vaginal orifice.

hymenectomy (*hi-men-ek'-tom-e*). The surgical removal of the hymen.

hymenotomy (*hi-men-ot'-om-e*). A surgical incision of the hymen to render the orifice larger.

hyoid (*hi'-oid*). Shaped like a U. *H. bone.* A U-shaped bone above the thyroid cartilage, to which the tongue is attached.

hyoscine (*hi'-os-een*). Scopolamine. An alkaloid obtained from solanaceous plants. It is a powerful cerebral depressant and may be used in acute mania. It diminishes glandular secretions, so it is used with papaveretum preoperatively. It is used in the treatment of gastric and duodenal ulcers and is a recognized preventive of sea-sickness.

hyoscyamus (*hi-o-si'-am-us*). Henbane. The dried leaves have an antispasmodic action which relieves the griping pain of excessive peristalsis.

hypaesthesia (*hi-pes-the'-ze-ah*). Impairment of the sense of touch.

hypalgesia (*hi-pal-je'-ze-ah*). A decrease in sensitivity to pain.

hypamnios (*hi-pam'-ne-os*). A deficiency of fluid in the amniotic sac.

hyperacidity (*hi-per-as-id'-it-e*). Excessive acidity. *Gastric h.* Hyperchlorhydria.

hyperadrenalism (*hi-per-ad-ren'-al-izm*). Overactivity of the suprarenal glands.

hyperaemia (*hi-per-e'-me-ah*). Excess of blood in any part.

hyperaesthesia (*hi-per-es-the'-ze-ah*). Excessive sensitiveness to touch or to other sensations, e.g. taste or smell.

hyperalgesia (*hi-per-al-ge'-ze-ah*). Excessive sensibility to pain.

hyperalimentation (*hi-per-al-e-men-ta'-shun*). An excess of nutrients, either ingested or administered. *Parenteral h.* Intravenous administration of carefully calculated amounts and types of nutrients. Careful monitoring of the effects of hyperalimentation are recorded. The aim is to increase weight in a patient suffering from hypercatabolism due to severe injury, burns, postoperative trauma, malignant disease, etc.

hyperasthenia (*hi-per-as-the'-ne-ah*). Extreme weakness.

hyperbaric (*hi-per-bar'-ik*). At a greater pressure than normal.

hyperbilirubinaemia (*hi-per-bil-e-ru-bin-e'-me-ah*). An excess of bilirubin in the blood.

hypercalcaemia (*hi-per-kal-se'-me-ah*). An excess of calcium in the blood. If untreated this condition leads to confusion, drowsiness and coma.

hypercalciuria (*hi-per-kal-se-u'-re-ah*). A high level of calcium in the urine leading to renal stone formation.

hypercapnia (*hi-per-kap'-ne-ah*). An increased amount of carbon dioxide in the blood causing over-stimulation of the respiratory centre. Hypercarbia.

hypercatabolism (*hi-per-kat-ab'-ol-izm*). An excessive rate of catabolism leading to wasting or destruction of a part or tissue.

hyperchloraemia (*hi-per-klor-e'-me-ah*). An excess of chloride in the blood.

hyperchlorhydria (*hi-per-klor-hi'-dre-ah*). An excess of hydrochloric acid in the gastric juice.

hyperchromic (*hi-per-kro'-mik*). Highly coloured or stained.

hypercusis (*hi-per-ku'-sis*). Excessive sensitivity to sound.

hyperdactylism (*hi-per-dak'-til-izm*). Polydactylism.

hyperdynamia (*hi-per-di-nam'-e-ah*). Excessive muscle activity. *H. uteri.* Excessive uterine contractions in labour.

hyperemesis (*hi-per-em'-es-is*). Excessive vomiting. *H. gravidarum.* Excessive and uncontrollable vomiting during pregnancy.

hyperemetic (*hi-per-em-et'-ik*). Pertaining to hyperemesis.

hyperextension (*hi-per-eks-ten'-shun*). The forcible extension of a limb beyond the normal. It is used to correct orthopaedic deformities.

hyperflexion (*hi-per-flek'-shun*). The forcible bending of a joint beyond the normal.

hyperglycaemia (*hi-per-gli-se'-me-ah*). Excess of sugar in the blood (*normal* 2.5–4.7 mmol/litre when fasting); a sign of diabetes mellitus.

hyperhidrosis (*hi-per-hi-dro'-sis*). Excessive perspiration. Hyperidrosis.

hyperinsulinism (*hi-per-in'-su-lin-izm*). (1) Excessive secretion of insulin. (2) Shock produced by an overdose of insulin.

hyperkalaemia (*hi-per-kal-e'-me-ah*). An excess of potassium in the blood. If untreated, this will lead to cardiac arrest.

hyperkeratosis (*hi-per-ker-at-o'-sis*). Hypertrophy of the horny layers of the skin.

hyperkinesis (*hi-per-ki-ne'-sis*). A condition in which there is excessive motor activity.

hyperlipaemia (*hi-per-lip-e'-me-ah*). An excess of fat or lipids in the blood.

hypermastia (*hi-per-mas'-te-ah*). (1) The presence of one or more supernumerary breasts. (2) Over-development of one or both breasts.

hypermature (*hi-per-mat-ure'*). Beyond maturity. Over-ripe, as a cataract when the lens becomes enlarged.

hypermetropia (*hi-per-met-ro'-pe-ah*). Hyperopia. Long-sightedness. The light rays entering the eye converge beyond the retina. Clear vision can be obtained by the wearing of spectacles or contact lenses.

hypermnesia (*hi-per-mne'-ze-ah*). Outstanding power of memory; may be found in infant prodigies and in some forms of mania.

hypermotility (*hi-per-mo-til'-it-e*). Excessive movement. *Gastric h.* Increased muscle action of the stomach wall, associated with increased secretion of hydrochloric acid.

hypernatraemia (*hi-per-nat-re'-me-ah*). An excess of sodium in the blood.

hypernephroma (*hi-per-nef-ro'-mah*). A malignant tumour of the kidney. Renal cell carcinoma.

hyperopia (*hi-per-o'-pe-ah*). Hypermetropia.

hyperostosis (*hi-per-os-to'-sis*). A thickening of bone. A bony outgrowth. Exostosis.

hyperparathyroidism (*hi-per-par-ah-thi'-roid-izm*). Excessive activity of the parathyroid glands, causing drainage of calcium from the bones, with consequent fragility and liability to spontaneous fracture.

hyperphagia (*hi-per-fa'-je-ah*). Over-eating.

hyperpiesis (*hi-per-pi-e'-sis*). Abnormally high blood pressure. *See* Hypertension.

hyperpituitarism (*hi-per-pit-u'-it-ar-izm*). Overactivity of the pituitary gland.

hyperplasia (*hi-per-pla'-ze-ah*). Excessive formation of normal cells in a tissue or organ, which increases in size.

hyperpnoea (*hi-per-pne'-ah*). Over-breathing. Hyperventilation. An abnormal increase in the rate and depth of breathing.

hyperpyrexia (*hi-per-pi-reks'-e-ah*). An excessively high body temperature, i.e. over 41°C.

hypersensitivity (*hi-per-sen-sit-iv'-it-e*). Abnormal sensitivity, especially to a particular antigen. The reactions include allergies (such as asthma) and anaphylaxis.

hypersplenism (*hi-per-splen'-izm*). Overactivity of an enlarged spleen resulting in the destruction of blood cells and platelets.

hypertension (*hi-per-ten'-shun*). Abnormally high arterial blood pressure. Hyperpiesis. *Essential h.* High blood pressure without demonstrable change in kidneys, blood vessels or heart. *Malignant h.* A form of hyperpiesis, which may develop at a comparatively early age, in which the prognosis is poor. *Portal h.* Raised pressure in the portal system. *Pulmonary h.* Increased pressure in the arteries of the lung, usually following emphysema or fibrosis. *Renal h.* Increased pressure in the kidney due to renal disease including stenosis of the renal artery.

hyperthermia (*hi-per-ther'-me-ah*). An exceedingly high body temperature. May be produced therapeutically to treat certain malignant diseases. *Malignant h.* A serious condition sometimes arising during general anaesthesia.

hyperthymia (*hi-per-thi'-me-ah*). Excessive emotionalism with a tendency for the individual to be impulsive.

hyperthyroidism (*hi-per-thi'-roid-izm*). Excessive activity of the thyroid gland. This affects: (1) The metabolic process, which is speeded up. The appetite is large but weight is lost. The temperature tends to be above normal, and respirations are increased. (2) The nervous system. The patient is very excitable and restless. Stimulation of the sympathetic nerves causes diarrhoea and excessive sweating. Exophthalmos may be present. The pulse is rapid and atrial fibrillation is common.

hypertonic (*hi-per-ton'-ik*). (1) Showing excessive tone or tension as in a blood vessel or muscle. (2) Describing a solution that has greater osmotic pressure than another with which it is compared. *H. saline.* A solution of sodium chloride of a strength higher than normal saline.

hypertrichosis (*hi-per-trik-o'-sis*). Excessive growth of hair on any part of the body.

hypertrophy (*hi-per'-tro-fe*). An increase in the size of a tissue or a structure caused by an increase in the *size* of the cells that compose it (as opposed to an increase in the *number* of cells). *See* Hyperplasia.

hyperuricaemia (*hi-per-u-rik-e'-me-ah*). An excess of uric acid in the blood.

hyperventilation (*hi-per-ven-til-a'-shun*). Over-breathing. Hyperpnoea.

hypervitaminosis (*hi-per-vit-am-in-o'-sis*). A condition caused by the intake of an excessive quantity of vitamins, particularly vitamins A and D.

hyphaema (*hi-fe'-mah*). Haemorrhage into the anterior chamber of the eye.

hypno-analysis (*hip-no-an-al'-is-is*). A form of psychotherapy using both psychoanalysis and hypnotism.

hypnosis (*hip-no'-sis*). An artificially induced state resembling sleep, in which there is increased suggestibility which may be used to abolish symptoms in hysterical states. It may also be favoured as a means of anaesthesia in childbirth and tooth extraction.

hypnotherapy (*hip-no-ther'-ap-e*). Treatment by hypnosis or by the induction of prolonged sleep.

hypnotic (*hip-not'-ik*). An agent which causes sleep. A soporific.

hypnotism (*hip'-not-izm*). The practice of hypnosis.

hypo-aesthesia (*hi-po-es-the'-ze-ah*). Hypaesthesia.

hypo-albuminaemia (*hi-po-al-bu-min-e'-me-ah*). A lack of serum albumin in the blood plasma, leading to oedema in the tissues.

hypo-algesia (*hi-po-al-je'-ze-ah*). Hypalgesia.

hypobaric (*hi-po-bar'-ik*). At a pressure lower than normal.

hypocalcaemia (*hi-po-kal-se'-me-ah*). A deficiency of calcium in the blood.

hypocapnia (*hi-po-kap'-ne-ah*). A deficiency of carbon dioxide in the blood.

hypochloraemia (*hi-po-klor-e'-me-ah*). A deficiency of chloride in the blood.

hypochlorhydria (*hi-po-klor-hi'-dre-ah*). A less than normal amount of hydrochloric acid in the gastric juice.

hypochondria (*hi-po-kon'-dre-ah*). A morbid preoccupation or anxiety about one's health. The sufferer feels that first one part of his body and then another part is the seat of some serious disease.

hypochondriac (*hi-po-kon'-dre-ak*). One affected by hypochondria. *H. region.* The hypochondrium.

hypochondrium (*hi-po-kon'-dre-um*). The upper region of the abdomen on each side of the epigastrium.

hypochromic (*hi-po-kro'-mik*). Deficient in pigmentation or colouring.

hypodermic (*hi-po-der'-mik*). Beneath the skin; applied to subcutaneous injections and to the syringes used for such injections.

hypofibrinogenaemia (*hi-po-fi-brin-o-jen-e'-me-ah*). A lack of fibrinogen in the blood. This may occur in severe trauma or haemorrhage or as an inherited condition.

hypogammaglobulinaemia (*hi-po-gam-ah-glob-u-lin-e'-me-ah*). A deficiency of gammaglobulin in the blood rendering the person susceptible to infection.

hypogastrium (*hi-po-gas'-tre-um*). The lower middle area of the abdomen, immediately below the umbilical region.

hypoglossal (*hi-po-glos'-al*). Under the tongue. *H. nerve.* The twelfth cranial nerve.

hypoglycaemia (*hi-po-gli-se'-me-ah*). A condition in which the blood-sugar level is less than normal. Usually arising in diabetic patients having insulin, due to too high a dose, delay in eating, or a rapid combustion of carbohydrate. *See* Hyperglycaemia.

hypohidrosis (*hi-po-hi-dro'-sis*). A lack of perspiration. Hypo-idrosis.

hypoinsulinism (*hi-po-in'-su-lin-izm*). A deficiency of in-

sulin excretion caused by pancreatic failure or incorrect treatment of diabetes mellitus.

hypokalaemia (*hi-po-kal-e'-me-ah*). A low potassium level in the blood. This is likely to be present in dehydration and with the repeated use of diuretics.

hypomania (*hi-po-ma'-ne-ah*). A degree of elation, excitement and activity higher than normal but less severe than that present in mania.

hypomastia (*hi-po-mas'-te-ah*). Underdevelopment of the breasts.

hypometropia (*hi-po-met-ro'-pe-ah*). Myopia. Short-sightedness.

hyponatraemia (*hi-po-nat-re'-me-ah*). A deficiency of sodium in the blood.

hypoparathyroidism (*hi-po-par-ah-thi'-roid-izm*). A lack of parathyroid secretion leading to a low blood calcium and tetany.

hypophysectomy (*hi-pof-is-ek'-tom-e*). Excision of the pituitary gland.

hypophysis (*hi-pof'-is-is*). An outgrowth. *H. cerebri.* The pituitary gland.

hypopiesis (*hi-po-pi-e'-sis*). Abnormally low blood pressure.

hypopituitarism (*hi-po-pit-u'-it-ar-izm*). Deficiency of secretion from the anterior lobe of the pituitary gland, causing excessive deposit of fat in children. *See* Frölich's syndrome. Dwarfism may result. In adults asthenia, drowsiness and adiposity may occur, together with an impairment of sexual activity and premature senility.

hypoplasia (*hi-po-pla'-ze-ah*). Imperfect development of a part or organ.

hypopnoea (*hi-po-pne'-ah*). Shallow breathing.

hypoproteinaemia (*hi-po-pro-tin-e'-me-ah*). A deficiency of serum proteins in the blood.

hypoprothrombinaemia (*hi-po-pro-throm-bin-e'-me-ah*). A deficiency of prothrombin in the blood leading to a tendency to bleed. *See* Haemophilia.

hypopyon (*hi-po'-pe-on*). An accumulation of pus in the anterior chamber of the eye.

hyposecretion (*hi-po-se-kre'-shun*). A deficiency in secretion from any glandular structure or secreting cells.

hyposensitivity (*hi-po-sen-sit-iv'-it-e*). A lack of sensitivity, especially to a particular allergen with which the patient may have been overdosed over a period.

hypospadias (*hi-po-spa'-de-as*). A congenital malformation in which the canal of the urethra opens upon the under surface of the penis.

hypostasis (*hi-pos'-tas-is*). (1) A sediment or deposit. (2) Congestion of blood in a part, due to slowing of the circulation.

hypostatic (*hi-po-stat'-ik*). Relating to hypostasis. *H. pneumonia*. *See* Pneumonia.

hyposthenia (*hi-po-sthe'-ne-ah*). Weakness; decreased strength.

hypotension (*hi-po-ten'-shun*). Abnormally low arterial blood pressure. Hypopiesis. *Controlled* or *induced h.* An artificially produced lowering of the blood pressure so that an operation field is rendered practically bloodless. *Orthostatic* or *postural h.* Temporary hypotension when the patient stands up, producing giddiness and sometimes a faint.

hypotensive (*hi-po-ten'-siv*). Producing a reduction in tension, especially pertaining to a drug that lowers the blood pressure.

hypothalamus (*hi-po-thal'-am-us*). Part of the brain situated at its base and concerned with temperature control, hunger, thirst and emotional changes.

hypothermia (*hi-po-ther'-me-ah*). (1) A severe reduction in the body temperature. The condition usually arises gradually and may prove fatal if untreated. It is commonest among babies and elderly people. (2) Artificial cooling of the body to reduce the oxygen requirements of the tissues. *Mild h.* A reduction of the body temperature to 34°C, which may be induced by surface cooling with cold air and is used for head injuries. *Conventional h.* A reduction to 30°C, which may be done by immersion in cold water, allowing arrest of the circulation for 9 min, without cerebral damage. Short heart operations may thus be performed. *Deep* or *profound h.* A reduction to below, often much below, 28°C. It is sometimes used in open-heart surgery in conjunction with a heart–lung machine.

hypothesis (*hi-poth'-es-is*). A theory which attempts to explain a phenomenon.

hypothrombinaemia (*hi-po-throm-bin-e'-me-ah*). A diminished amount of thrombin in the blood with a consequent tendency to bleed.

hypothyroidism (*hi-po-thi'-roid-izm*). An insufficiency of thyroid secretion. In children it may produce cretinism. In adults it leads to myxoedema.

hypotonia (*hi-po-to'-ne-ah*). (1) Deficient muscle tone. (2) Deficient tension in the eyeball.

hypotonic (*hi-po-ton'-ik*). Describing a solution that has a lower osmotic pressure than another one. *See* Hypertonic.

hypoventilation (*hi-po-ven-til-a'-shun*). Hypopnoea. Shallow breathing, usually at a very slow rate. It may cause a build-up of carbon dioxide in the blood.

hypovitaminosis (*hi-po-vit-am-in-o'-sis*). A deficiency of vitamins due to a lack of intake or an inability to absorb them.

hypovolaemia (*hi-po-vol-e'-me-ah*). A reduction in the circulating blood volume due to external loss of body fluids or to loss from the blood into the tissues, as in shock.

hypoxaemia (*hi-poks-e'-me-ah*). An insufficient oxygen content in the blood.

hypoxia (*hi-poks'-e-ah*). A diminished amount of oxygen in the tissues. *Anaemic h.* Low oxygen content due to deficiency of haemoglobin in the blood.

hystera (*his'-ter-ah*). The uterus (*Gk*).

hysteralgia (*his-ter-al'-je-ah*). Pain in the uterus.

hysterectomy (*his-ter-ek'-tom-e*). Removal of the uterus. *Abdominal h.* Removal via an abdominal incision. *Subtotal h.* Removal of the body of the uterus only. *Total h.* Removal of the body and the cervix. *Vaginal h.* Removal through the vagina. *Wertheim's h.* Additional excision of the parametrium, upper vagina and lymph glands. Radical abdominal hysterectomy.

hysteria (*his-te'-re-ah*). A psychoneurosis manifesting itself in various disorders of the mind and body. There are mental and physical symptoms, not of organic origin, produced and maintained by motives of which the patient is unconscious, but directed at some real or fancied gain to be derived from them. *Conversion h.* Hysteria which takes the form of loss of function of some part of the body. This may be loss of memory, vision or hearing, or loss of muscle power or feeling in a hand or leg. The so-called 'paralysis' or numbness does not correspond to the nerve distribution.

hysterical (*his-ter'-ikl*). Relating to hysteria.

hysterocele (*his'-ter-o-seel*). A hernia containing part of the uterus.

hysteromyoma (*his-ter-o-mi-o'-mah*). A fibromyoma of the uterus.

hysteromyomectomy (*his-ter-o-mi-o-mek'-tom-e*). Excision of a hysteromyoma.

hystero-oöphorectomy (*his'-ter-o-o-off-or-ek'-tom-e*). Excision of the uterus and the ovaries.

hysteropathy (*his-ter-op'-ath-e*). Any uterine disease.

hysteropexy (*his'-ter-o-peks-e*). Fixation of the uterus to the abdominal wall, to remedy displacement. Hysterorrhaphy. *See* Ventrofixation.

hysteroptosis (*his-ter-op-to'-sis*). Prolapse of the uterus.

hysterorrhaphy (*hister-or'-af-e*). Hysteropexy.

hysterosalpingography (*his'-ter-o-sal-ping-gog'-raf-e*). X-ray examination of the uterus and uterine tubes following the injection of a radio-opaque dye. Uterosalpingography.

hysterosalpingostomy (*his'-ter-o-sal-ping-gos'-tom-e*). The establishment of an opening between the distal portion of the uterine tube and the uterus in an effort to overcome infertility when the medial portion is occluded or excised.

hysterotomy (*his-ter-ot'-om-e*). Incision of the uterus. *See* Caesarian section.

I

I. Chemical symbol for *iodine*.

iatrogenic (*i-at-ro-jen'-ik*). Brought about by surgical or medical treatment, e.g. unwanted effects of drugs.

ibuprofen (*i-bu-pro'-fen*). An anti-inflammatory drug used in the treatment of mild rheumatic and arthritic conditions.

ice (*ise*). Water in a solid state, at or below freezing-point. *Dry i.* Carbon dioxide snow. *I. bag.* A rubber or plastic bag half-filled with pieces of ice and applied near or to a part.

ichor (*i'-kor*). A thin colourless discharge from ulcers and raw wounds.

ichthyosis (*ik-the-o'-sis*). A congenital abnormality of the skin in which there is dryness and roughness, the horny layer is thickened and large scales appear. These patients are liable to eczema and industrial dermatitis.

icterus (*ik'-ter-us*). Jaundice. *I. gravis.* A fatal form of jaundice occurring in pregnancy. Acute yellow atrophy. *I. gravis neonatorum.* Haemolytic disease of the newborn. *See* Rhesus factor.

id (*id*). The most primitive part of the personality, containing the instinctive drives, which lives in the unconscious.

idea (*i-de'-ah*). A mental image and the meaning attached to it. *Association of i's.* Ideas that recall to the mind associated objects or occasions due to some similarity or contrast. *Flight of i's.* A mode of speech in which the person passes rapidly from one idea to the next with only a slight association between them, being unable to maintain a course of thought. *I's of reference.* Thoughts based on some external circumstances that the patient thinks refer to himself when no such thing is intended. *I's of unreality.* Notions that everything has changed and that things look different and unreal or do not exist.

ideation (*i-de-a'-shun*). The formulation of ideas.

idée fixe (*e-da feeks*). A fixed idea; a delusion that impels towards some abnormal action.

identical (*i-den'-tik-al*). Exactly alike. *I. twins.* Twins developing from the same ovum.

identification (*i-den-tif-ik-a'-shun*). A mental mechanism by which an individual adopts the attitudes and ideas of another, often admired, person.

ideology (*i-de-ol'-o-je*). (1) The science of thought. (2) A philosophy.

ideomotion (*i-de-o-mo'-shun*). The association of ideas and muscle action as in involuntary acts.

ideophrenia (*i-de-o-fre'-ne-ah*). A mental disorder with perverted ideas.

idiocy (*id'-e-o-se*). Arrested development amounting to very severe mental subnormality.

The term is now obsolete.

idiopathic (*id-e-o-path'-ik*). Self-originated; applied to a condition the cause of which is not known.

idiosyncrasy (*id-e-o-sin'-kras-e*). A peculiarity of constitution or temperament. It may exist in relation to drugs, e.g. when small doses of iodine or quinine will cause symptoms of poisoning in some people; or to foods, such as when shellfish or strawberries give rise to urticaria.

idiot (*id'-e-ot*). An obsolete term for one who would now be designated severely subnormal.

idoxuridine (*i-doks-u'-rid-een*). An iodine-containing drug used to treat infections caused by herpes virus, particularly keratitis and dendritic corneal ulcer.

ileal (*i'-le-al*). Referring to the ileum. *I. conduit.* A surgical procedure in which the ureters are transplanted into the ileum, an isolated loop of which is then brought to the surface of the abdomen in order to allow the urine to drain into a bag.

ileectomy (*i-le-ek'-tom-e*). Excision of the ileum.

ileitis (*i-le-i'-tis*). Inflammation of the ileum. *Regional i.* Crohn's disease. A chronic condition of the terminal portion of the ileum in which granulation and oedema may give rise to obstruction.

ileocolitis (*i-le-o-kol-i'-tis*). Inflammation of the ileum and colon.

ileocolostomy (*i-le-o-kol-os'-tom-e*). The making of a permanent opening between the ileum and some part of the colon.

ileoproctostomy (*i-le-o-prok-tos'-tom-e*). Surgical anastomosis between the ileum and the rectum. Ileorectal anastomosis.

ileorectal (*i-le-o-rek'-tal*). Referring to the ileum and rectum. *I. anastomosis.* Ileoproctostomy.

ileosigmoidostomy (*i-le-o-sig-moid-os'-tom-e*). Surgical anastomosis between the ileum and the sigmoid flexure (pelvic colon).

ileostomy (*i-le-os'-tom-e*). An operation to make an opening through the abdominal wall

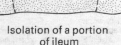
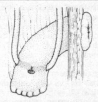

Isolation of a portion of ileum

Formation of a blind ended loop to drain urine

ILEAL CONDUIT

into the ileum. An ileal stoma is established so that the intestinal contents can be evacuated, thus by-passing the colon. (Colectomy may also be performed.) *l. bags.* Disposable bags to collect excreted matter. The bags can be adhesive or worn on a belt, and add greatly to the comfort of the patient.

ileum (*i'-le-um*). The last part of the small intestine, terminating at the caecum.

ileus (*i'-le-us*). Obstruction of the bowel. *Paralytic i.* A dynamic ileus. A condition resulting from local inflammation, the toxins of which affect the nerve supply to the bowel wall, so that intestinal stasis results. One of the effects of peritonitis. Putrefaction takes place within the bowel, the poisons are absorbed, and the patient develops all the signs of toxaemia.

iliac (*il'-e-ak*). Pertaining to the ilium. *I. artery.* The right and left arteries form the terminal branches of the abdominal aorta and supply blood to the pelvic region and the lower limbs. *I. crest.* The crest of the hip-bone. *I. fossa.* The depression on the concave surface of the iliac bone. *I. vein.* The right and left veins join to form the inferior vena cava and drain the blood from the lower limbs and pelvis.

iliacus (*il-i'-ak-us*). A muscle arising from the ilium and acting with the psoas muscle to flex the hip-joint.

iliopsoas (*il-e-o-so'-as*). A flexor muscle of the hip comprising the iliacus and the psoas.

ilium (*il'-e-um*). The haunch-bone. The upper part of the hip-bone.

illumination (*il-u-min-a'-shun*).

The amount of light intensity falling on a surface. The unit of measurement that is used is the candela. *Focal i.* Illumination by a light focused by means of a concave mirror.

illusion (*il-u'-zhun*). A mistaken perception due to a misinterpretation of a sensory stimulus; believing something to be what it is not.

image (*im'-aje*). (1) The mental recall of a former percept. (2) The optical picture transferred to the brain cells by the optic nerve.

imago (*im-a'-go*). (1) In psychology, an idea or fanciful image of the father or some other person based on fantasy or fear. (2) In zoology, an insect in its definitive, final form.

imbalance (*im-bal'-ans*). Lack of balance, e.g. of endocrine secretions, between water and electrolytes, or of muscles.

imbecile (*im'-bes-eel*). An obsolete term for a person suffering from a moderate to severe degree of subnormality.

imipramine (*i-mip'-ram-een*). A drug, chemically related to chlorpromazine, that may be effective in relieving depression. *See* Antidepressant. Also used to treat nocturnal enuresis in children.

immature (*im-at-ure'*). Unripe. Not fully developed, as a cataract when only a part of the lens is opaque.

immiscible (*im-is'-ibl*). Incapable of being mixed, e.g. oil and water.

immobilization (*im-o-bil-i-za'-shun*). Making motionless. Used in the treatment of fractures and other conditions to promote healing.

immune (*im-une'*). Protected

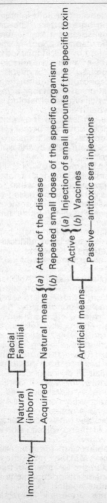

TYPES OF IMMUNITY

Immunity
- Natural (inborn)
  - Racial
  - Familial
- Acquired
  - Natural means
    - (a) Attack of the disease
    - (b) Repeated small doses of the specific organism
  - Artificial means
    - Active
      - (a) Injection of small amounts of the specific toxin
      - (b) Vaccines
    - Passive—antitoxic sera injections

against a particular infection or allergy.

immunity (*im-u'-nit-e*). The resisting power of the body to the toxins of invading microorganisms shown by the presence in the blood of neutralizing antitoxins. *Acquired i.* That which is produced naturally by (1) an attack of the disease, or (2) repeated small infections by organisms not in themselves able to produce signs of disease, but against which the body forms antibodies which accumulate in the blood. *Artificially acquired i.* is produced by (1) injections of small doses of toxins, (2) injection of vaccines (*active i.*), or (3) introduction of antitoxic sera (*passive i.*). *Natural i.* That which is inborn; can be racial or familial.

immunization (*im-u-ni-za'-shun*). The act of creating immunity by artificial means.

immunoassay (*im-u-no-as'-a*). A quantitative estimate of the proteins contained in the blood serum.

immunochemistry (*im-u-no-kem'-is-tre*). The study of the chemical aspects of immunology, particularly antigen–antibody reactions.

immunocyte (*im'-u-no-site*). A cell which is capable of producing antibodies.

immunoglobulin (*im-u-no-glob'-u-lin*). One of a group of proteins which act as antibodies. They are present in the blood plasma and serum. Abbreviated as Ig, they are divided into 5 classes with different qualities and functions.

immunology (*im-u-nol'-o-je*). The study of immunity and the body's defence mechanisms.

immunosuppressive (*im-u'-no-sup-res'-iv*). A drug such as azathioprine or antilympho-cyte immunoglobulin used to counteract the body's de-fences against infections and foreign bodies in order to pre-vent the rejection of an organ or tissue transplant.

immunotherapy (*im-u-no-ther'-ap-e*). (1) Treatment by immunization. Sometimes used in the treatment of leukaemia. (2) The estab-lishing of passive immunity.

immunotransfusion (*im-u-no-trans-fu'-zhun*). Transfusion with blood containing an anti-serum to produce immunity or treat an infection.

impaction (*im-pak'-shun*). A state of being firmly wedged. *Dental i.* The condition in which a tooth, usually a mo-lar, is unable to erupt through the gum because it is lodged in position by bone or the other teeth.

impalpable (*im-palp'-abl*). In-capable of being felt by manu-al examination. May apply to an organ or a tumour.

imperforate (*im-per'-for-ate*). Without an opening. *I. anus.* A congenital defect in which this opening is closed. *I. hy-men.* Complete closure of the vaginal opening by the hy-men. *See* Cryptomenorrhoea.

impermeable (*im-per'-me-abl*). Not permitting the passage of fluid or molecules.

impetigo (*im-pet-i'-go*). An acute contagious inflamma-tion of the skin marked by pustules and scabs; of strep-tococcal or staphylococcal origin. It occurs mainly on the face and limbs, particularly those of children. *Bullous i.* A severe form, especially if occurring in the newly born,

characterized by large blebs.

implant (*im'-plant*). Any sub-stance grafted into the tis-sues. *Hormone i.* A pellet of deoxycortone acetate or tes-tosterone, which may be im-planted subcutaneously. *In-tra-ocular lens i.* A plastic lens which may be implanted in the eye after lens extraction. *Ocular i.* An artificial eye which is inserted into the socket after enucleation of the eyeball. The muscles are su-tured to it to cause the artifi-cial eye to move normally.

implantation (*im-plant-a'-shun*). The act of planting or setting in. (1) The embedding of the fertilized ovum in the wall of the uterus. (2) The placing of a drug within the tissues. (3) The surgical intro-duction of healthy tissue to replace tissue that has been damaged.

impotence (*im'-po-tens*). In-ability in a man to carry out sexual intercourse from either psychological or physical causes.

impregnation (*im-preg-na'-shun*). Insemination. Render-ing pregnant.

impulse (*im'-puls*). A natural or instinctive tendency to action without deliberation. *Cardiac i.* The beat of the apex of the heart as felt on the chest wall. *Morbid i.* An uncontrollable desire to act rashly. *Nerve i.* The force conveyed along nerve fibres.

inaccessibility (*in-ak-ses-ib-il'-it-e*). State of unresponsive-ness characteristic of certain mental patients, e.g. schizo-phrenics.

inactivate (*in-ak'-tiv-ate*). To render inactive. To destroy the active principle bringing about change.

inanition (*in-an-ish'-un*). Wasting of the body from want of food.

inappetence (*in-ap'-et-ens*). Lack of desire or appetite, usually for food.

inarticulate (*in-ar-tik'-u-late*). (1) Without joints. (2) Unable to speak intelligibly.

incarcerated (*in-kar'-ser-a-ted*). Held fast. Applied to (1) a hernia which is immovable, and therefore only curable by operation, and (2) a pregnant uterus held under the sacral brim.

incest (*in'-sest*). Sexual intercourse between people so closely related that their marriage would be illegal.

incidence (*in'-sid-ens*). Of a particular disease, the number of cases in a specified number of persons over a given period, e.g. 3 cases in 10,000 people in 1 year.

incipient (*in-sip'-e-ent*). Beginning to exist.

incision (*in-sizh'-un*). (1) In surgery, a cut into soft tissue. (2) The act of cutting.

incisor (*in-si'-zor*). One of the four front teeth in the centre of each jaw.

inclusion (*in-klu'-zhun*). Something that is enclosed or the act of enclosing. *I. bodies.* Particles that are temporarily enclosed in the cytoplasm of a cell. For example, in trachoma virus particles can be seen in the conjunctival epithelial cells.

incoherent (*in-ko-he'-rent*). (1) Unconnected. Inconsistent. (2) Uttering speech that is disconnected and rambling.

incompatibility (*in-kom-pat-ib-il'-it-e*). The state of two or more substances being antagonistic, or destroying the efficiency of each other. Applied to mixtures of drugs, and to blood. *See* Blood grouping.

incompetence (*in-kom'-pet-ens*). Inefficiency. *Aortic i.* Failure of the aortic valves to regulate the flow of blood. *Mitral i.* Failure of the mitral valve to close properly.

incontinence (*in-kon'-tin-ens*). Inability to control natural functions or discharges. *Faecal i.* Inability to control the movements of the bowels. *Overflow i.* That from an overfull bladder, most common in elderly men with urinary obstruction. *Paralytic i.* Loss of control of anal and urethral sphincters due to injury to nerve centres. *Stress i.* That which is due to a defect in the urethral sphincters and is liable to occur when intra-abdominal pressure is increased as in coughing or lifting heavy weights; most common in women with weak pelvic muscles. *Urinary i.* Inability to control the outflow of urine.

inco-ordination (*in-ko-or-din-a'-shun*). Inability to adjust harmoniously the various muscle movements.

incrustation (*in-krus-ta'-shun*). The formation of a crust or scab on a wound.

incubation (*in-ku-ba'-shun*). The development and growth of micro-organisms and animal embryos. *I. period.* The period between the date of infection and the appearance of symptoms of an infectious disease.

incubator (*in'-ku-ba-tor*). (1) An apparatus in which prematurely born infants can be reared. (2) An apparatus used to develop bacteria at a uniform temperature suitable to their growth.

incudectomy (*in-ku-dek'-tom-e*). Surgical removal of the incus.

incus (*in'-kus*). The small anvil-shaped bone of the middle ear. The second auditory ossicle.

indican (*in'-dik-an*). A potassium salt which is excreted in the urine following the decomposition of tryptophan in the intestines.

indicanuria (*in-dik-an-u're-ah*). An excess of indican in the urine. It may be present in chronic constipation or in intestinal obstruction.

indigenous (*in-dij'-en-us*). Occurring naturally in a certain locality.

indigestion (*in-de-jes'-chun*). *See* Dyspepsia.

indole (*in'-dole*). A product of protein decomposition in the bowel. It is excreted in the faeces, and also in the urine as indican.

indolent (*in'-do-lent*). Slow growing. Reluctant to heal. Largely painless. *I. ulcer.* A chronic ulcer of the skin or mucous membrane.

indomethacin (*in-do-meth'-as-in*). An anti-inflammatory analgesic used in the treatment of arthritis and of acute attacks of gout.

induction (*in-duk'-shun*). The act of initiating something. *I. of abortion.* The intentional bringing about of an abortion. *I. of anaesthesia.* The start of the administration of a general anaesthetic. *I. of labour.* The artificial starting of the process of childbirth. *Electromagnetic i.* The production of an electric current in a body because of its nearness to an electrified (or magnetized) body.

induration (*in-du-ra'-shun*). The abnormal hardening of a tissue or organ.

industrial (*in-dus'-tre-al*). Referring to industry. *I. diseases.* Those that are caused by the nature of the work. *Prescribed i. diseases.* Those for which sickness benefit is payable, including those that are notifiable under the Factories Act.

inebriation (*in-e-bre-a'-shun*). The condition of being intoxicated by alcohol. Drunkenness.

inert (*in-ert'*). Having no action. *I. gas.* A gas which does not react with other elements, e.g. neon.

inertia (*in-er'-she-ah*). Sluggishness; inability to move except when stimulated by an external force. *Uterine i.* Lack of muscle contraction during the first and second stage of labour.

infant (*in'-fant*). A child under 1 year of age. Educationally, a child under 7 years of age. *I. feeding.* The supplying of nutrition to an infant. Breast milk is the ideal food for the baby and if breast feeding is established satisfactorily for the first few months it can aid physical and emotional development. Where it is not possible cow's milk or a dried milk preparation can be used. *I. mortality.* The liability to death of children under 1 year of age. *I.m. rate.* The number of deaths of children during the first year of life per 1000 live births.

infanticide (*in-fan'-te-side*). The killing of a child by its mother during the first year of its life.

infantile (*in'-fan-tile*). Concerning an infant. Childish. *I. paralysis.* Poliomyelitis.

infantilism (*in-fan'-til-izm*). Delayed maturity. The continuation of infantile characteristics, mental or physical, into adult life. *Coeliac i.* Failure to grow in coeliac disease. *Pancreatic i.* Lack of growth associated with fibrocystic disease of the pancreas. *Pituitary i.* Lack of growth associated with hyposecretion of the growth hormone. The result is a perfectly formed dwarf. *Renal i.* Renal osteodystrophy. Associated with disease of the kidney and upset in the calcium balance in the blood. There is dwarfism with signs of rickets.

infarct (*in'-farkt*). The wedge-shaped area of necrosis in an organ produced by the blocking of a blood vessel, usually due to an embolus. *Red i.* A haemorrhage infarct. Red blood cells infiltrate the area. *White i.* An anaemic infarct. The area is suddenly deprived of blood and is pale in colour.

infarction (*in-fark'-shun*). The formation of an infarct. *Myocardial i.* An infarct of the heart muscle following a coronary thrombosis. *Pulmonary i.* An infarct resulting from obstruction of a branch of the pulmonary artery by embolism or thrombosis.

infection (*in-fek'-shun*). Invasion of the body by organisms causing disease. *Cross i.* Hazard occurring in hospitals when infection is transmitted from one patient to another. *Droplet i.* Infection by organisms that are spread in minute particles of exhaled moisture, especially when produced by coughing or sneezing. *Mass i.* Invasion of the blood stream by large numbers of organisms. *Pyogenic i.* That caused

COMMON INFECTIOUS DISEASES

Disease	Incubation period (days)	Period of infectivity
Chicken-pox (varicella)	10–20	2–3 days before until 10 days after onset of rash
Diphtheria	2–7	Until culture of 3 consecutive nose swabs proves negative
Enteric fevers		
Typhoid	6–21	Until at least one month after onset of disease and after 6 consecutive negative stools
Paratyphoid		
Measles (morbilli)	6–12	4 days before until 4 days after onset of rash
Mumps (parotitis)	12–28	48 hours before onset until resolution of symptoms
Pertussis (whooping cough)	7–14	7 days before until 3 weeks after onset of cough
Rubella (German measles)	14–21	During incubation period until 2 days after resolution of symptoms

by pus-producing organisms. *Secondary i.* A superimposed second infection, when one is already present. *Water-borne i.* Infection by organisms that are spread by the water supply, e.g. typhoid fever.

infectious (*in-fek'-shus*). Capable of producing an infection. *I. disease.* A communicable disease. *I. hepatitis.* Infective jaundice. *See* Hepatitis. *I. mononucleosis.* Glandular fever.

infective (*in-fek'-tiv*). Of the nature of an infection. *I. exhaustive psychosis.* A psychosis developing during the course of another disease as in a severe infectious, metabolic or glandular condition. It may subside as the disease is controlled but it may require psychiatric treatment.

inferior (*in-fe'-re-or*). Lower. *I. vena cava.* The lower large vein.

inferiority (*in-fe-re-or'-it-e*). Lesser rank, stature, position or ability. *I. complex. See* Complex.

infertility (*in-fer-til'-it-e*). Inability of a woman to conceive or of a man to bring about conception.

infestation (*in-fes-ta'-shun*). Invasion by animal parasites; applied to the presence of mites, ticks or worms in or on the body, in clothing, or in a house.

infiltration (*in-fil-tra'-shun*). The entrance and diffusion of some abnormal substance, either fluid or solid, into tissues or cells. *I. analgesia.* The injection into tissues of a local analgesic solution.

inflammation (*in-flam-a'-shun*). A series of changes in tissues indicating their reaction to injury, whether mech-

anical, chemical or bacterial, so long as the injury does not cause death of the affected part. The cardinal signs are: heat, swelling, pain and redness. *Acute i.* Sudden onset of inflammation, with marked and progressive symptoms. *Catarrhal i.* Inflammation in which mucous surfaces are attacked, with stimulation of exudation. *Chronic i.* Inflammation that develops slowly. Granulation tissue forms and tends to localize the infection. *Diffuse i.* Extensive inflammation, as in nephritis and cellulitis. *Suppurative i.* That in which the formation of pus results. *Traumatic i.* That which follows an injury and is nonbacterial.

influenza (*in-flu-en'-zah*). An acute infectious disease caused by influenza virus A which causes serious epidemics, or by influenza virus B which causes minor outbreaks. There is inflammation of the upper respiratory tract causing fever, headache, pain in the back and limbs, anorexia and sometimes nausea and vomiting. The fever subsides in 2 to 3 days, leaving a feeling of lassitude and some mental depression.

infra-red (*in-frah-red'*). Pertaining to rays of a lower wavelength than those in the visible spectrum. They can produce radiant heat which is used in the treatment of rheumatic conditions. *See* Ultra-violet.

infrasonic (*in-frah-son'-ik*). Pertaining to sounds below the range of sounds that can be heard by man.

infundibulum (*in-fun-dib'-u-lum*). A funnel-shaped passage or part.

infusion (*in-fu'-zhun*). (1) The process of extracting the soluble principles of substances (especially drugs) by soaking in water. (2) The solution thus produced. (3) The slow injection of a fluid, for instance a saline solution, into a vein.

ingestion (*in-jest'-shun*). The taking in of food and drugs by mouth.

inguinal (*in'-gwin-al*). Relating to the groin. *I. canal.* The channel through the abdominal wall, above Poupart's ligament, through which the spermatic cord and vessels pass to the testis in the male, and which contains the round ligament of the uterus in the female. *I. ligament.* Poupart's ligament. That connecting the anterior superior spine of the ilium to the tubercle of the pubis.

inhalation (*in-hal-a'-shun*). The breathing into the lungs through the nose and mouth of air, gas or a vapour. Certain drugs, such as eucalyptus oil, menthol and friar's balsam, are sometimes administered by inhalation.

inhaler (*in-ha'-ler*). An apparatus used for administering an inhalation.

inherent (*in-he'-rent*). Pertaining to a characteristic that is innate or natural and essentially a part of the person.

inheritance (*in-her'-it-ans*). The acquisition of qualities and characteristics from parents and ancestors.

inhibition (*in-hib-ish'-un*). Checking or restraining. Inhibitory nerves restrain muscle action, in contrast to accelerator nerves which stimulate it. Emotionally a person may be inhibited because he has certain ideas or feelings—often unconscious—which prevent him from acting as he would wish.

injection (*in-jek'-shun*). The act of introducing a liquid into the body by means of a syringe or other instrument. Also the substance so administered. *Hypodermic i.* That made just below the skin. A subcutaneous injection. *Intramuscular i.* That made into a muscle. *Intrathecal i.* That made into the subarachnoid space of the spinal cord. *Intravenous i.* That made into a vein. *Subcutaneous i.* That made into the subcutaneous tissues. A hypodermic injection.

inlay (*in'-la*). Material inserted to replace a defect in a tissue, for example a bone graft or a filling cast in metal to fit a hole in a tooth.

innate (*in'-ate*). Inborn. Present in the individual at birth.

innervation (*in-er-va'-shun*). Nerve supply to a part.

innocent (*in'-o-sent*). As applied to a tumour, benign or non-malignant.

innocuous (*in-ok'-u-us*). Harmless.

innominate (*in-om'-in-ate*). Unnamed. *I. artery.* A branch of the aorta now termed the brachiocephalic trunk. *I. bone.* The hip-bone, formed by the union of the ilium, ischium and pubis.

inoculation (*in-ok-u-la'-shun*). The introduction through the skin of a vaccine to stimulate the production of antibodies against a disease.

inorganic (*in-or-gan'-ik*). Of neither animal nor vegetable origin.

inositol (*in-o'-sit-ol*). A form of muscle or plant carbohydrate that has the same formula as simple sugar but not its other properties. It has been used in the treatment of renal diseases and of various skin diseases, and also, combined with vitamin E, in cases of muscular dystrophy.

inotropic (in-o-trop'-ik). Affecting the force or energy of muscular contractions, particularly the heart muscle. Beta-blocking drugs are said to be inotropic.

inquest (in'-kwest). In medicine, a legal inquiry held by a coroner, with or without a jury, into the cause of sudden or unexpected death.

insanity (in-san'-it-e). An obsolete term for a state of severe mental disorder. Legally the person is not responsible for his actions and it is largely in this connection that the term is retained. For examples, see Psychosis, Mania, Schizophrenia and Paranoia.

insecticide (in-sek'-tis-ide). One of a large group of chemical compounds that kill insect pests. Some are very toxic and can cause irritability of the nervous system and gastrointestinal upsets in man and may accumulate in the body fat.

insemination (in-sem-in-a'-shun). (1) Fertilization of an ovum by a spermatozoon. (2) Introduction of semen into the vagina. Artificial i. Insemination by means other than sexual intercourse. The semen can be either the husband's (AIH) or some other donor's (AID).

insensible (in-sen'-sibl). (1) Unable to perceive with the senses. (2) Unconscious. (3) Imperceptible to the senses.

insertion (in-ser'-shun). (1) The

act of implanting. (2) Something that is implanted. (3) The attachment of a muscle to the bone which it moves.

insidious (in-sid'-e-us). Approaching by stealth. A term applied to any disease which develops imperceptibly.

insight (in'-site). Mental awareness. The capacity of an individual to estimate a situation or his own behaviour or the connection between his present attitudes and past experiences. In psychiatry, a recognition by the patient that he is ill. Insight in this connection may be complete, partial or absent, and may alter during the course of the illness.

in situ (in sit'-u). In the original position (Latin).

insolation (in-sol-a'-shun). Exposure to sun's rays.

insoluble (in-sol'-ubl). Not capable of being dissolved in a liquid.

insomnia (in-som'-ne-ah). Inability to sleep.

inspiration (in-spir-a'-shun). The act of drawing in the breath.

inspissated (in-spis'-a-ted). Thickened, through evaporation or absorption of fluid.

instillation (in-stil-a'-shun). The act of pouring a liquid into a cavity drop by drop, e.g. into the eye.

instinct (in'-stinkt). An inborn tendency to act in a certain way without the influence of reason or previous education. Herd i. The tendency to become one of a group and to conform to group standards of behaviour.

insufficiency (in-suf-ish'-ense). Inadequacy. Used to describe the failure of function of an organ such as the heart, stomach, liver or muscles.

insufflation (*in-suf-la'-shun*). The act of blowing air, gas or powder into a cavity of the body.

insulate (*in'-su-late*). To surround a heated or an electrically charged body with a non-conducting substance, so that heat or electricity cannot escape.

insulin (*in'-su-lin*). The endocrine secretion of the pancreas, which regulates sugar metabolism, and ensures complete fat combustion. A deficiency in the secretion of this hormone causes diabetes mellitus, in the treatment of which artificially produced insulin is widely used. *Globin zinc i., isophane i., protamine zinc i.* and *i. zinc suspension* are preparations in which the action is delayed and thus less frequent doses are necessary. A buffer dose of ordinary insulin may be given to tide over the period before the preferred drug comes into effect.

insulinase (*in'-su-lin-aze*). An enzyme that destroys the action of insulin.

insulinoma (*in-su-lin-o'-mah*). A benign adenoma of the islet cells of the pancreas, causing hypoglycaemia.

integument (*in-teg'-u-ment*). (1) The skin. (2) A layer of tissue covering a part or organ of the body.

intellect (*in'-tel-ekt*). The reasoning power, in contrast to the emotions or the will.

intelligence (*in-tel'-e-jens*). (1) The capacity to understand. (2) General mental ability. *I. quotient.* IQ. A measure of the mental development of a child. The ratio of the mental age to the chronological age

expressed as a percentage. *I. test.* A test designed to measure the level of intelligence, usually expressed as an IQ.

intensive (*in-ten'-siv*). Raised to a high degree. *I. care unit.* A specialized unit in which the staff are especially trained and the equipment designed to care for critically ill patients.

intention (*in-ten'-shun*). A process of healing. *Primary i.* The healing that takes place when two wound edges are drawn together and there is no infection present—as in a surgical wound. *Secondary i.* Delayed healing, which occurs by granulation, so that it is not possible to draw the two wound edges together—as in an ulcer. Infection is often superimposed.

intercellular (*in-ter-sel'-u-lar*). Between the cells of a structure. May be applied to the connective tissue or to fluid bathing the cells.

intercostal (*in-ter-kos'-tal*). Between the ribs. *I. muscles.* Muscles situated between the ribs and controlling their movements during inspiration and expiration.

intercourse (*in'-ter-kors*). Social exchange. *Sexual i.* Coitus.

intercurrent (*in-ter-kur'-ent*). Occurring at the same time. *I. infection.* One which occurs during the course of another disease in the same person.

interferon (*in-ter-fe'-ron*). A protein produced by cells infected by a virus which has an inhibitory effect on the multiplication of the invading viruses. May also have a cytotoxic effect.

interlobar (*in-ter-lo'-bar*). Between lobes.

interlobular (in-ter-lob'-u-lar). Between lobules. *l. veins.* Branches of the portal vein in the liver.

intermenstrual (in-ter-men'-stru-al). Occurring between two menstrual periods.

intermission (in-ter-mish'-un). A temporary interruption, particularly of a feverish condition.

intermittent (in-ter-mit'-ent). Occurring at intervals. *l. claudication. See* Claudication. *l. fever.* One in which the temperature drops to normal, or lower, at times. *l. positive airway pressure.* IPAP. A method of assisted ventilation, in which oxygen or air is used under pressure to inflate the lungs, when the patient is unable to breathe spontaneously.

internal (in-ter'-nal). Situated on the inside. *l. haemorrhage.* One occurring in a cavity or into the tissues. *l. secretion.* One in which the hormones pass directly into the blood stream from the secreting gland.

interphase (in'-ter-faze). The period between two cell divisions during which the chromosomes are not easily visible.

intersex (in'-ter-seks). (1) A congenital abnormality in which anatomical features of both sexes are evident. (2) A person displaying intersexuality.

intersexuality (in-ter-seks-u-al'-it-e). The condition of being between the normal male and the normal female in many respects.

interstice (in-ter'-stis). A space in a tissue or between parts of the body.

interstitial (in-ter-stish'-al). Situated within the tissue spaces or between the tissues. *l. fluid.* The fluid in which body cells are bathed. It acts as an intermediary between the cells and the blood. Extracellular fluid. *l. cell stimulating hormone.* ICSH. Luteinizing hormone. *l. keratitis. See* Keratitis. *l. nephritis.* Chronic nephritis associated with fibrosis and hypertension.

intertrigo (in-ter-tri'-go). An irritating, eczematous skin eruption caused by chafing where two moist surfaces are in close apposition.

intervertebral (in-ter-vert'-e-bral). Between the vertebrae. *l. disc.* The pad of fibrocartilage between the bodies of the vertebrae. Protrusion of the contents of the disc may give rise to sciatica by pressing on the nerve roots.

intestinal (in-tes'-tin-al). Referring to the intestine.

intestine (in-tes'-tin). That part of the alimentary canal which extends from the stomach to the anus. *Small i.* The first 6 m (20 ft) from the pylorus to the caecum, consisting of the duodenum, the jejunum and the ileum. *Large i.* The final 2 m (6 ft), consisting of the caecum, the ascending, transverse and descending colon, and the rectum.

intima (in'-tim-ah). The innermost coat of an artery or vein.

intolerance (in-tol'-er-ans). Lack of power to endure. Applied to the effect of some drugs on individuals, e.g. *iodine* and *quinine. See* Idiosyncrasy.

intoxication (in-toks-ik-a'-shun). (1) Poisoning by drugs or harmful substances. (2) A state of drunkenness induced by taking too much alcohol.

intra-abdominal (*in-trah-ab-dom'-in-al*). Within the abdomen.

intra-articular (*in-trah-ar-tik'-u-lar*). Within a joint capsule. *I-a. injection.* Injection into a joint capsule, applicable to hydrocortisone, for example.

intra-atrial (*in-trah-a'-tre-al*). Within the atrium. *I-a. thrombosis.* A blood clot formed in the atrium of the heart.

intracapsular (*in-trah-kap'-su-lar*). Within a capsule, usually of a joint. *I. extraction.* The removal of the whole lens with its capsule in the treatment of cataract. *I. fracture.* See Fracture.

intracellular (*in-trah-sel'-u-lar*). Within a cell. *I. fluid.* The water and its dissolved salts found within the cells.

intracerebral (*in-trah-ser'-e-bral*). Within the brain substance. *I. haemorrhage.* An escape of blood in the cerebrum, most often arising from the middle cerebral artery or from an aneurysm.

intracranial (*in-trah-kra'-ne-al*). Within the skull. *I. abscess.* One arising within the brain or meninges. *I. aneurysm.* Dilatation of one of the cerebral vessels. It may be congenital or acquired. *I. pressure.* The pressure within the cranium measured by lumbar puncture.

intractable (*in-trakt'-abl*). Not able to be relieved, controlled or cured.

intradermal (*in-trah-der'-mal*). Between the layers of the skin.

intradural (*in-trah-du'-ral*). Within the dura mater. *I. haemorrhage.* See Haemorrhage.

intragastric (*in-trah-gas'-trik*).

Within the stomach. *I. tube feeding.* Artificial feeding, usually by nasogastric tube.

intrahepatic (*in-trah-hep-at'-ik*). Within the liver. Referring to a condition of the liver cells or connective tissue.

intralobular (*in-trah-lob'-u-lar*). Within a lobule. *I. veins.* Veins which collect blood from within the lobules of the liver.

intramedullary (*in-trah-med-ul'-ar-e*). (1) Within the medulla oblongata. (2) Within the bone marrow. *I. nail.* A metal pin used for the internal fixation of fractures.

intramuscular (*in-trah-mus'-ku-lar*). Within muscle tissue.

intranasal (*in-trah-na'-zal*). Within the nose.

intra-ocular (*in-trah-ok'-u-lar*). Within the eyeball.

intra-orbital (*in-trah-or'-bit-al*). Within the orbit of the eye.

intra-osseous (*in-trah-os'-e-us*). Within a bone.

intraperitoneal (*in-trah-per-it-o-ne'-al*). Within the peritoneal cavity.

intrathecal (*in-trah-the'-kal*). Within the meninges of the spinal cord, usually in the subarachnoid space.

intratracheal (*in-trah-trak'-e-al*). Endotracheal. Within the trachea. *I. anaesthesia.* Inhalation anaesthesia (*see* Anaesthesia).

intra-uterine (*in-trah-u'-ter-ine*). Within the uterus. *I. contraceptive device.* A contraceptive device introduced into the uterine cavity. *I. douche.* Irrigation of the uterine cavity. A special grooved nozzle is used, so that the fluid can return and is not forced into the uterine tubes. *I. life.* Fetal development in the uterus.

intravenous (*in-trah-ve'-nus*). Within a vein. *I. pyelography.*

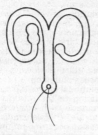

AN INTRA-UTERINE CONTRACEPTIVE DEVICE

X-ray examination of the urinary tract after the injection of a radio-opaque contrast medium into a vein.

intraventricular (*in-trah-ven-trik'-u-lah*). Within a ventricle. It may apply to a cerebral or a cardiac ventricle.

intrinsic (*in-trin'-sik*). Particular to or contained within an organ. *I. factor.* A glycoprotein contained in the gastric juices which is necessary for the absorption of the extrinsic factor (vitamin B_{12}).

introitus (*in-tro'-it-us*). An opening or entrance into a hollow organ or cavity. *I. vaginae.* The vulva.

introjection (*in-tro-jek'-shun*). A mental process by which an individual takes into himself the personal characteristics of another person, usually those of someone much loved or admired.

introspection (*in-tro-spek'-shun*). A subjective study of the mind and its processes, in which an individual studies his own reactions.

introversion (*in-tro-ver'-shun*). (1) A turning inwards within itself of a hollow organ, such as the uterus. (2) A tendency to be preoccupied with thoughts of oneself rather than of the world outside.

introvert (*in'-tro-vert*). A cool, thoughtful, reflective person who tends to be self-sufficient and is a poor mixer in society. *See* Extrovert.

intubation (*in-tu-ba'-shun*). The introduction of a tube into a part of the body, particularly into the air passages to allow air to enter the lungs.

intumescence (*in-tu-mes'-ens*). A swelling or increase in bulk, as of nasal mucous membrane in catarrh.

intussusception (*in-tus-us-ep'-shun*). A condition in which one part of the intestine becomes pushed or invaginated into another part beyond. It occurs most frequently in young children at the ileocaecal junction, and causes intestinal obstruction, with pain, vomiting, and small

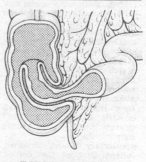

INTUSSUSCEPTION

blood-stained evacuations. Prompt surgical treatment is necessary.

inulin (*in'-u-lin*). A substance used to estimate the efficiency of renal function. It is filtered, but not re-absorbed or secreted, and its clearance rate therefore equals that of glomerular filtration.

inunction (*in-unk'-shun*). The act of rubbing an oily or fatty preparation into the skin.

invagination (*in-vaj-in-a'-shun*). (1) The folding inwards of a part, thus forming a pouch. (2) Intussusception.

invasion (*in-va'-zhun*). (1) The onset of a disease. (2) The entrance of parasites into the body of a host.

inversion (*in-ver'-shun*). A turning upside down or inside out. *Sexual i.* Homosexuality. *Uterine i.* The condition of the uterus after parturition when a part of its upper segment protrudes through the cervix.

invertase (*in-ver'-taze*). A ferment of intestinal juice which hydrolyses cane sugar.

invertebrate (*in-ver'-te-brate*). (1) *adj.* Without a spinal column. (2) *n.* An animal without a spinal column.

in vitro (*in ve'-tro*). In a glass (*Latin*). Refers to observations made outside the body. *See* In vivo.

in vivo (*in ve'-vo*). Within the living body (*Latin*). *See* In vitro.

involucrum (*in-vol-u'-krum*). New bone which forms a sheath around necrosed bone, as in chronic osteomyelitis.

involuntary (*in-vol'-un-tar-e*). Independent of the will. *I. muscle.* One that acts without conscious control, for instance the heart and stomach muscles.

involution (*in-vol-u'-shun*). (1) Turning inward; describes the contraction of the uterus after labour. The process whereby the uterus returns to its normal size. (2) Sometimes applied to the slowing down process of ageing.

involutional (*in-vol-u'-shun-al*). Relating to the retrogressive changes which occur during later life. *I. melancholia.* Depression occurring for the first time in later life and characterized by agitation and delusions of a hypochondriacal nature.

iodine (*i'-o-deen*). *abbrev.* I. A non-metallic element with a distinctive odour, obtained from seaweed. It is present in man in small quantities and a deficiency of it causes goitre. *Tincture of i.* A 2.5% spirit solution used as a skin antiseptic. *Radioactive i.* Iodine-131. A radio-opaque isotope used in the diagnosis and treatment of thyroid conditions.

iodism (*i'-o-dizm*). Poisoning from the prolonged use of iodine or iodine compounds.

iodopsin (*i-o-dop'-sin*). A violet pigment found in the retinal cones of the eye.

iodoxyl (*i-o-doks'-il*). A radio-opaque dye used in intravenous pyelography.

ion (*i'-on*). One of the components into which an electrolyte is broken up by electrolysis. *Hydrogen i. concentration.* See Hydrogen.

ionization (*i-on-i-za'-shun*). The breaking up of molecules into electrically charged particles or ions when an electric current is passed through an electrolyte solution.

iontophoresis (*i-on-to-for-e'-*

sis). The introduction through the skin of therapeutic ions by ionization.

iopanoic acid (*i-o-pan-o'-ik as'-id*). A radio-opaque dye used in X-ray examination of the gall-bladder and ducts.

iophendylate (*i-o-fen'-di-late*). A radio-opaque dye that may be used in examination of the spinal canal.

ipecacuanha (*ip-e-kak-u-an'-ah*). The dried root of a Brazilian shrub, given in small doses as an expectorant.

iproniazid (*ip-ro-ni'-az-id*). An antidepressant drug that belongs to the group of monoamine oxidase inhibitors.

ipsilateral (*ip-se-lat'-er-al*). Occurring on the same side. Applied particularly to paralysis or other symptoms occurring on the same side as the cerebral lesion causing them.

IQ. Intelligence quotient. *See* Intelligence.

Ir. Chemical symbol for *iridium*.

iridectomy (*ir-id-ek'-tom-e*). Excision of a part of the iris, usually for the treatment of glaucoma.

iridencleisis (*ir-id-en-kli'-sis*). An operation to make a drain out of a part of the iris, used in the treatment of glaucoma.

iridium (*ir-id'-e-um*). *abbrev.* Ir. A radioactive metal often used in the form of wires or hairpins to treat superficial malignancies, e.g. those of the tongue, cheek, or breast.

iridocele (*ir-id'-o-seel*). Herniation of a part of the iris, through a corneal wound.

iridocyclitis (*ir-id-o-si-kli'-tis*). Inflammation of the iris and ciliary body.

iridodialysis (*ir-id-o-di-al'-is-is*). The separation of the outer border of the iris from its ciliary attachment, often a result of trauma.

iridodonesis (*ir-id-o-do-ne'-sis*). Trembling of the iris due to lack of support from the lens in dislocation of the lens or after a cataract extraction.

iridoplegia (*ir-id-o-ple'-je-ah*). Paralysis of the iris.

iridoptosis (*ir-id-op-to'-sis*). Prolapse of the iris.

iridotomy (*ir-id-ot'-om-e*). The making of a hole in the iris to form an artificial pupil.

iris (*i'-ris*). The coloured part of the eye made of two layers of muscle, the contraction of which alters the size of the pupil and so controls the amount of light entering the eye. *I. bombé.* A bulging forward of the iris due to pressure of the aqueous humour when its passage into the anterior chamber is obstructed.

iritis (*i-ri'-tis*). Inflammation of the iris, causing pain, photophobia, contraction of the pupil and discoloration of the iris. *See* Uveitis.

iron (*i'-ern*). *abbrev.* Fe. A metallic element which is present in the body in small quantities and is essential to life. A deficiency may produce anaemia. Various preparations of it are given in tonic mixtures and for the treatment of anaemia. It causes black discoloration of the stools. *I. dextran.* A drug containing iron and dextran administered by injection intravenously in the treatment of iron-deficiency anaemia. *I. lung.* See Respirator. *I. sorbitol.* A drug containing iron and sorbitol which may be injected intramuscularly in iron-deficiency anaemia.

irradiation (*ir-a-de-a'-shun*). The treatment of disease by electromagnetic radiation.

irreducible (*ir-e-du'-sibl*). Incapable of being replaced in a normal position. Applied to a fracture or a hernia.

irrigation (*ir-ig-a'-shun*). The washing out of a cavity or wound with a stream of lotion or water.

irritable (*ir'-it-abl*). Reacting excessively to a stimulus. *I. bowel syndrome.* Mucous colitis. Spastic colon. The patient complains of disordered bowel function with abdominal pain, but no organic disease can be found.

irritant (*ir'-it-ant*). An agent causing stimulation or excitation.

irritation (*ir-it-a'-shun*). (1) A condition of undue nervous excitement, through abnormal sensitiveness. *Cerebral i.* A stage of excitement present in many brain conditions, and typical of the recovery stage of concussion. (2) Itching of the skin.

ischaemia (*is-ke'-me-ah*). A deficiency in the blood supply to a part of the body. *Myocardial i.* Ischaemia of the heart muscles, which causes angina pectoris.

ischiorectal (*is-ke-o-rek'-tal*). Concerning the ischium and the rectum. *I. abscess.* A collection of pus in the ischiorectal connective tissue. An anal fistula may result.

ischium (*is'-ke-um*). The lower posterior bone of the pelvic girdle.

Ishihara colour charts (*S. Ishihara, Japanese ophthalmologist, b. 1879*). Patterns of dots of the primary colours on similar backgrounds. The patterns can be seen by a normal-sighted person, but one who is colour-blind will only be able to identify some of them.

islet of Langerhans (*P. Langerhans, German pathologist, 1847–1888*). One of a group of cells in the pancreas that produce insulin and glucagon. Islet of the pancreas.

isocarboxazid (*i-so-kar-boks'-az-id*). A monoamine oxidase inhibitor used in the treatment of depressive illness.

isodose (*i'-so-dose*). Of equal dose. Used in radiation therapy to denote body areas receiving an equal dosage. *I. curve.* A graph which plots body areas receiving the same dose of radiation.

isograft (*i'-so-grahft*). A tissue graft from one identical twin to another.

iso-immunization (*i-so-im-u-ni-za'-shun*). The development of antibodies against an antigen derived from an individual of the same species.

isolation (*i-so-la'-shun*). The separation of a person with an infectious disease from those non-infected. *I. period.* Quarantine. The length of time during which a patient with an infectious fever is considered capable of infecting others by contact.

isoleucine (*i-so-lu'-seen*). One of the eight amino acids which are essential for health in the adult.

isometric (*i-so-met'-rik*). Having equal dimensions. *I. exercises.* The contraction and relaxation of muscles without producing movement; used to maintain muscle tone following a fracture.

isoniazid (*i-so-ni'-az-id*). INH. A drug given orally in combination with streptomycin or para-aminosalicylic acid (PAS) which is effective in treating tuberculosis.

isoprenaline (*i-so-pren'-a-leen*). A sympathomimetic drug which has an action like adrenaline and can be used to treat asthma.

isosorbide dinitrate (*i-so-sor'-bide di-ni'-trate*). A short-acting vasodilator similar in action to glyceryl trinitrate and used in the treatment of angina pectoris.

isotonic (*i-so-ton'-ik*). Having uniform tension. *I. solution* is of the same osmotic pressure as the fluid with which it is compared. Normal saline is isotonic with blood plasma.

isotope (*i'-so-tope*). One of several forms of an element with the same atomic number but different atomic weights. *Radioactive i.* An unstable isotope which decays and emits alpha, beta or gamma rays. May be ued in the diagnosis and treatment of malignant disease.

issue (*is'-u*). (1) A child. (2) A discharge of blood or pus.

itch (*itch*). (1) Scabies. (2) A skin eruption with irritation. *Baker's i.* Eczema of the hands due to the proteins of flour. *Barber's i.* Sycosis. Tinea barbae. *Dhobi i.* A form of ringworm of the groin prevalent in the tropics. Tinea cruris. *Washer-woman's i.* Eczema of the hands due to the use of soda and detergents. *I. mite.* The cause of scabies, *Sarcoptes scabiei.*

IUCD. Intra-uterine contraceptive device. A plastic or metal device which is inserted into the uterus.

IVP. Intravenous pyelography. X-ray examination of the re-nal system following the intravenous injection of a radio-opaque dye.

J

J. Abbreviation for the SI unit, the *joule.*

Jacksonian epilepsy (*J.H. Jackson, British neurologist, 1835–1911*). Focal motor epilepsy. *See* Epilepsy.

jactitation (*jak-tit-a'-shun*). The extreme restlessness of an acutely ill patient.

jargon (*jar'-gon*). (1) The terminology used and generally understood only by those who have knowledge of that speciality, e.g. medical jargon, legal jargon. (2) Gibberish talked by the insane.

jaundice (*jawn'-dis*). Icterus. A yellow discoloration of the skin and conjunctivae, due to the presence of bile pigment in the blood. It may be: (1) *Haemolytic j.*, due to excessive destruction of red blood cells, causing increase of bilirubin in the blood. The liver is not involved. *Acholuric j.* is of this type. It is characterized by increased fragility of the red blood cells. (2) *Hepatocellular j.*, in which the liver cells are damaged by either infection or drugs. (3) *Obstructive j.*, in which the bile is prevented from reaching the duodenum owing to obstruction by a gall-stone, a growth or a stricture of the common bile duct. (4) *Physiological j.* (icterus neonatorum), which occurs within the first few days of life, and is caused by the breakdown of the excessive number of red blood cells present in the newborn.

jaw (*jaw*). A bone of the face in which the teeth are embedded. *Lower j.* The mandible. *Upper j.* The two maxillae.

jejunectomy (*jej-u-nek'-tom-e*). Excision of a part or the whole of the jejunum.

jejuno-ileostomy (*jej-u'-no-i-le-os'-tom-e*). The making of an anastomosis between the jejunum and the ileum.

jejunostomy (*jej-u-nos'-tom-e*). The making of an opening into the jejunum through the abdominal wall.

jejunotomy (*jej-u-not'-om-e*). An incision into the jejunum.

jejunum (*jej-u'-num*). The portion of the small intestine from the duodenum to the ileum, about 2.4 m (8 ft) in length.

Jenner's vaccination (*E. Jenner, British physician, 1749–1823*). Arm-to-arm vaccination with fluid from the lesions of cowpox, from which modern methods of smallpox vaccination were developed.

jerk (*jerk*). A sudden muscular contraction. *Knee j.* A kicking movement produced by tapping the tendon below the patella. Used with other jerks, such as the ankle jerk, to test the nervous reflexes.

jigger (*jig'-er*). A sand flea found in the tropics which burrows into the soles of the feet and causes severe irritation.

joint (*joint*). An articulation. The point of junction of two or more bones; particularly one which permits movement of the individual bones relative to each other.

joule (*jool*). *abbrev.* J. The SI unit of energy.

judgement (*juj'-ment*). The ability of an individual to esti-

mate a situation, to arrive at reasonable conclusions, and to decide on a course of action.

jugular (*jug'-u-lar*). Relating to the neck. *J. veins.* Several veins in the neck, which drain the blood from the head.

juvenile (*joo'-ven-ile*). Relating to young people.

juxta-articular (*juks-tah-ar-tik'-u-lar*). Near a joint.

juxtaglomerular (*juks-tah-glom-er'-u-lar*). Near to a glomerulus of the kidney. *J. cells.* Specialized cells found in the kidney which appear to play an important part in the control of aldosterone release.

juxtaposition (*juks-tah-po-zish'-un*). Adjacent. Side-by-side.

K

K. Chemical symbol for *potassium.*

Kahn test (*B.L. Kahn, American bacteriologist. b. 1887*). An agglutination test for syphilis.

kala-azar (*kah-lah-ah-zar'*). Visceral leishmaniasis. A tropical disease caused by the protozoan parasite *Leishmania donovani* which is carried by the sand-fly. Symptoms include enlargement of the liver and spleen, anaemia and wasting. The disease is often fatal.

kanamycin (*kan-ah-mi'-sin*). A broad-spectrum antibiotic for use against severe infections with gram-negative organisms where penicillin is ineffective.

kaolin (*ka'-o-lin*). Powdered clay containing aluminium silicate. It is taken orally in the treatment of diarrhoea and is also used as a dusting powder and for poultices.

Kaposi's sarcoma (*M.K. Kaposi, Austrian dermatologist, 1837–1902*). A malignant disease characterized by multifocal skin eruptions, although there may be visceral foci. It usually begins on the distal parts of the extremities. There appears to be a higher incidence amongst male homosexuals.

Kaposi's spots. A serious complication of infantile eczema occurring on exposure to herpes simplex virus infection. More commonly known as Kaposi's varicelliform eruption.

karaya (*kar-i'-ah*). A gum made from certain species of *Sterculia*, a genus of tropical trees and shrubs. Used as an aid to applying ostomy bags to the skin.

karyotype (*kar'-e-o-tipe*). (1) The chromosomal constitution and arrangement of a cell of an individual. (2) The pattern which is seen when human chromosomes are photographed during metaphase. The pictures are then enlarged and paired according to the length of their short arm.

katabolism (*kat-ab'-ol-izm*). Catabolism.

Kayser–Fleischer ring (*B. Kayser, German ophthalmologist, 1869–1954; B. Fleischer, German ophthalmologist, 1848–1904*). A brownish pigmented ring seen in the cornea of patients with hepatolenticular degeneration (Wilson's disease).

Keller's operation (*W.L. Keller, American surgeon, 1874–1959*). A bone operation for correcting hallux valgus.

keloid (*ke'-loid*). Hard, whitish scar tissue in the skin, common in people with dark skins. A type occurs in a healed wound due to overgrowth of fibrous tissue, causing the scar to be raised above the skin level. They may be removed but keloids tend to re-form in the new scar.

Kennedy's syndrome (*F. Kennedy, American neurologist, 1884–1952*). Ipsilateral optic atrophy caused by a frontal lobe tumour which involves one of the optic nerves.

keratectasia (*ker-at-ek-ta'-se-ah*). Protrusion of the cornea following inflammation.

keratectomy (*ker-at-ek'-tom-e*). Excision of a portion of the cornea.

keratic (*ker-at'-ik*). (1) Horny. (2) Relating to the cornea. *K. precipitates.* Inflammatory exudates adhering to the back of the cornea. A sign of iritis and cyclitis.

keratin (*ker'-at-in*). An albuminoid substance which forms the base of all horny tissues.

keratinize (*ker-at'-in-ize*). To make or become horny.

keratitis (*ker-at-i'-tis*). Inflammation of the cornea. The causes may be physical (trauma, exposure to dust or vapours or to ultra-violet light) or to infectious conditions such as corneal and dendritic ulcers. *Interstitial k.* Deep chronic keratitis, usually arising out of congenital syphilis. *Striate k.* Inflammation that appears in lines due to the folding over of the cornea after injury or operation, particularly one for cataract.

keratocele (*ker'-at-o-seel*). Descemetocele. Protrusion of

Descemet's membrane through the base of a corneal ulcer. A horny growth of the skin.

keratoconjunctivitis (ker-at-o-kon-junk-tiv-i'-tis). Inflammation of both the cornea and the conjunctiva of the eye.

keratoconus (ker-at-o-ko'-nus). A conical cornea. A degenerative condition in which the cornea becomes thin and protruded into a cone-shape.

kerato-iritis (ker-at-o-i-ri'-tis). Inflammation of both the cornea and iris.

keratoma (ker-at-o'-mah). Keratosis.

keratomalacia (ker-at-o-mal-a'-se-ah). Ulceration and softening of the cornea, due to a deficiency of vitamin A.

keratome (ker'-at-ome). A knife with a trowel-shaped blade, for incising the cornea.

keratometer (ker-at-om'-e-ter). Ophthalmometer. An instrument by which the amount of corneal astigmatism can be measured accurately.

keratomileusis (ker-at-o-mil-u'-sis). An operation on the cornea for the correction of a high degree of myopia.

keratoplasty (ker'-at-o-plas-te). A plastic operation on the cornea, including corneal grafting.

keratoscope (ker'-at-o-skope). An instrument for examining the eye to detect keratoconus. Placido's disc.

keratosis (ker-at-o'-sis). A skin disease marked by excessive growth of the epidermis or horny tissue.

keratotomy (ker-at-ot'-om-e). Incision of the cornea.

kerion (ke'-re-on). A complication of ringworm of the scalp, with formation of pustules.

kernicterus (kern-ik'-ter-us). A complication of haemolytic jaundice of the newly born in which there is pigmentation of, and damage to, the brain cells.

Kernig's sign (V.M. Kernig, Russian physician, 1840–1917). A sign of meningitis. When the thigh is supported at right angles to the trunk, the patient is unable to straighten his leg at the knee-joint.

ketamine (ket'-am-een). A rapidly acting, non-barbiturate, general anaesthetic which is given by intramuscular or intravenous injection.

ketone (ke'-tone). An organic compound containing the carbonyl group (CO), attached to two hydrocarbon groups. Ketones are produced by the metabolization of fats.

ketonuria (ke-ton-ur'-e-ah). The presence of ketones in urine. Acetonuria.

ketosis (ke-to'-sis). The condition in which ketones are formed in excess in the body. Severe acidosis may occur.

ketosteroid (ke-to-ster'-oid). A steroid hormone which contains a ketone group attached to a carbon atom. 17-ketosteroids are excreted in the urine and formed from the adrenal corticosteroids, testosterone, and to a lesser extent from oestrogens.

kidney (kid'-ne). One of two organs situated in the lumbar region, which purify the blood and secrete urine. Artificial k. The apparatus used to remove retained waste products from the blood when kidney function is impaired. K. failure. The condition in which renal function is severely impaired and the organs are un-

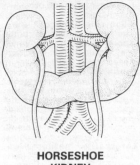

HORSESHOE KIDNEY

---

able to maintain the fluid and electrolyte balance of the body. *Granular k.* The small fibrosed kidney of chronic nephritis. *Horseshoe k.* A congenital defect producing a fusion of the two kidneys into a horseshoe shape. *Polycystic k.* A congenital bilateral condition of multiple cysts replacing kidney tissue. *K. transplant.* The surgical implantation of a kidney taken from a live donor or from one who has recently died. Used in the treatment of renal failure.

Kimmelstiel–Wilson's disease (*P. Kimmelstiel, German pathologist, 1900–1970; C. Wilson, British physician, b. 1906*). Nephrotic syndrome caused by arteriolar nephrosclerosis.

kinaesthesia (*kin-es-the'-ze-ah*). The combined sensations by which position, weight and muscular position are perceived.

kinanaesthesia (*kin-an-es-the'-ze-ah*). An inability to perceive the sensation of movements of parts of the body.

kinase (*ki'-naze*). An enzyme-activator. *See* Enterokinase *and* Thrombokinase.

kinematics (*kin-e-mat'-iks*). The science of movement, in particular that of the human body.

kineplasty (*kin-e-plas'-te*). An amputation in which the muscles and tendons in the stump are so arranged that they can control the movements of the artificial limb which is to be fitted.

kinesiology (*kin-e-ze-ol'-o-je*). The study of the mechanics of motion.

kinetic (*kin-et'-ik*). Producing or pertaining to motion.

kinetics (*kin-et'-iks*). The study of movement.

kinin (*ki'-nin*). A polypeptide which occurs naturally and is a powerful vasodilator.

Kirschner's wire (*M. Kirschner, German surgeon, 1879–1942*). A thin wire that may be passed through a bone to apply skeletal traction.

kiss of life (*kis' of life'*). The expired-air method of artificial respiration, by either mouth-to-nose or mouth-to-mouth breathing.

Klebsiella (*kleb-se-el'-ah*). A genus of bacteria. They are short bacilli, gram-negative, non-spore-forming, and encapsulated. They may cause infection of the lung, intestines and urinary tract.

Klebs–Löffler bacillus (*T.A.E. Klebs, German bacteriologist, 1834–1913; F.A.J. Löffler, German bacteriologist, 1852–1915*). *Corynebacterium diphtheriae,* the causative agent of diphtheria.

kleptomania (*klep-to-ma'-ne-ah*). An irresistible urge to steal when there is often no need and no particular desire for the objects. Often associated with depression.

Klinefelter's syndrome (*H.F. Klinefelter, American physician, b. 1912*). A congenital chromosome abnormality in which each cell has 3 sex chromosomes, XXY, rather than the usual XX or XY, making a total of 47 (normal is 46). Affected men have female breast development, small testes and are infertile.

Klippel–Feil syndrome (*M. Klippel, French neurologist, 1858–1942; A. Feil, French physician, b. 1884*). A congenital abnormality in which the neck is very short due to absence or fusion of several vertebrae in the cervical region.

Klumpke's paralysis (*A. Déjerine-Klumpke, French neurologist, 1859–1927*). A palsy affecting the hand and arm, usually caused by a birth injury to the brachial plexus.

kneading (*ne'-ding*). A method used in massage. Pétrissage.

knee (*ne*). The joint between the femur and the tibia. *K.-cap.* The patella. *K. jerk.* An upward jerk of the leg, obtained by striking the patellar tendon when the knee is passively flexed. *Housemaid's k.* Prepatellar bursitis. *Knock-k.* A condition in which the knees turn inwards towards each other. Genu valgum.

Koch's bacillus (*R. Koch, German bacteriologist, 1843–1910*). *Mycobacterium tuberculosis*, the causative organism of tuberculosis.

Köhler's disease (*A. Köhler, German physician and roentgenologist, 1874–1947*).

Osteochondritis of the navicular bone of the foot, occurring in children.

koilonychia (*koil-on-ik'-e-ah*). The development of brittle spoon-shaped nails which may occur in iron-deficiency anaemia.

Koplik's spots (*H. Koplik, American paediatrician, 1858–1927*). Small white spots that appear sometimes on the mucous membranes inside the mouth in measles on the second day of onset, before the general rash.

Korotkoff's method (*N.S. Korotkoff, Russian physician, b. 1874*). A method of finding the systolic and diastolic blood pressure by listening to the sounds produced in an artery while the pressure in a previously inflated cuff is gradually reduced.

Korsakoff's syndrome or **psychosis** (*S.S. Korsakoff, Russian neurologist, 1854–1900*). A chronic condition in which there is impaired memory, particularly for recent events, and the patient is disorientated for time and place. It may be present in psychosis of infective, toxic or metabolic origin, or in chronic alcoholism.

Krabbe's disease (*K.H. Krabbe, Danish neurologist, 1885–1961*). Mental subnormality due to degenerative disease of the white matter of the brain. Leucodystrophy.

kraurosis (*kraw-ro'-sis*). Dryness and shrinking of a part of the body. *K. vulvae.* A degenerative condition of the vulva. May be treated by giving oestrin preparations.

Krebs' cycle (*Sir H.A. Krebs, German–British biochemist, b. 1900*). A series of reactions during which the aerobic oxidation of pyruvic acid takes place. This is part of carbohydrate metabolism. *K. urea c.* The way in which urea is formed in the liver.

Kretschmer's types (*E. Kretschmer, German physician, 1888–1964*). A method of classifying potential psychopathic personalities in relation to their body shape, e.g. pyknic type is short and fat and has a tendency to manic depression; aesthetic type is tall and thin and has a tendency to schizophrenia.

Kromayer lamp (*E.L.F. Kromayer, German dermatologist, 1862–1933*). A mercury-vapour lamp used for ultra-violet radiation. It is water-cooled and is used in contact with the skin, and within cavities, using a quartz-rod applicator.

Krukenberg tumour (*G.P.H. Krukenberg, German gynaecologist, 1871–1946*). A large secondary malignant growth in an ovary. The primary one is usually in the stomach and is small.

Küntscher nail (*G. Küntscher, German orthopaedic surgeon, b. 1902*). An intramedullary nail used in treating fractures of long bones, especially the shaft of the femur.

Kupffer's cells (*K.W. won Kupffer, German anatomist, 1829 –1902*). Phagocytic reticuloendothelial cells of the liver that form bile from haemoglobin released by disintegrated erythrocytes.

kwashiorkor (*kwosh-e-or'-kor*). A condition of protein malnutrition occurring in children in underprivileged populations. Fatty infiltration of the liver arises and may cause

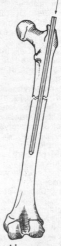

**KÜNTSCHER
INTRAMEDULLARY
NAIL**

cirrhosis.

kymograph (*ki'-mo-graf*). An apparatus consisting of a rotating drum upon which graphic records can be traced, particularly of variations in the blood pressure.

kyphoscoliosis (*ki-fo-skol-e-o'-sis*). An abnormal curvature of the spine in which there is forward and sideways displacement.

kyphosis (*ki-fo'-sis*). Posterior curvature of the spine; humpback.

L

l. Abbreviation of the fundamental SI unit, the *litre*.

labial (*la'-be-al*). Pertaining to the lips or labia.

labile (*la'-bile*). Unstable. Applied to those chemicals that are subject to change or readily altered by heat.

lability (*lab-il'-it-e*). Instability. *L. of mood.* The tendency to sudden changes of mood of short duration.

labioglossopharyngeal (*la'-be-o-glos-o-far-in-je'-al*). Concerning the lips, tongue and pharynx. *L. paralysis.* Bulbar paralysis. *See* Paralysis.

labium (*la'-be-um*). *pl.* labia. A lip. *L. majus pudendi.* The large fold of flesh surrounding the vulva. *L. minus pudendi.* The lesser fold within the labium majus.

laboratory (*lab-or'-at-or-e*). A place in which practical study of the sciences is carried out.

labour (*la'-bor*). Parturition or child-birth, which takes place in three stages: (1) dilatation of the cervix uteri, (2) passage of the child through the birth canal, and (3) expulsion of the placenta. *Induced l.* Labour brought on by artificial means before term, as in cases of contracted pelvis or if overdue. *Obstructed l.* Labour in which there is a mechanical hindrance. *Precipitate l.* Labour in which the baby is delivered extremely rapidly. *Premature l.* Labour which occurs before term. *Spurious l.* Labour pains which sometimes precede true labour pains.

labyrinth (*lab'-ir-inth*). The structures forming the internal ear, i.e. the cochlea and semicircular canals. *Bony l.* The bony canals of the internal ear. *Membranous l.* The soft structure inside the bony canals.

labyrinthectomy (*lab-ir-inth-ek'-tom-e*). Excision of the labyrinth.

labyrinthitis (*lab-ir-inth-i'-tis*). Inflammation of the labyrinth, causing vertigo.

lac (*lak*). Milk or a milk-like liquid.

laceration (*las-er-a'-shun*). A wound with torn and ragged edges—not clean cut.

lacrimal (*lak'-rim-al*). Relating

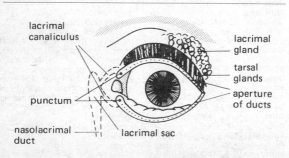

LACRIMAL APPARATUS

to tears. *L. apparatus.* The structures secreting the tears and draining the fluid from the conjunctival sac. *L. gland.* A gland that secretes tears, which drain through two small openings in the eyelids (*l. puncta*) into a pair of ducts (*l. canaliculi*) into the *lacrimal sac* and finally into the nasal cavity through the nasolacrimal duct. Situated in the outer and upper corner of the orbit.

lacrimation (*lak-rim-a'-shun*). An excessive secretion of tears.

lacrimator (*lak'-rim-a-tor*). A substance which causes excessive secretion of tears, e.g. tear-gas.

lactagogue (*lak'-tah-gog*). Galactagogue.

lactalbumin (*lak-tal'-bu-min*). An albumin of milk.

lactase (*lak'-taze*). An enzyme produced in the small intestine which converts lactose into glucose and galactose.

lactate (*lak'-tate*). A salt of lactic acid.

lactation (*lak-ta'-shun*). (1) The period during which the infant is nourished from the breast. (2) The process of milk secretion, carried on by the mammary glands.

lacteal (*lak'-te-al*). (1) *adj.* Consisting of milk. (2) *n.* A lymphatic duct in the small intestine which absorbs chyle.

lactic (*lak'-tik*). Pertaining to milk. *L. acid.* An acid formed by the fermentation of lactose or milk sugar. It is produced naturally in the body as a result of glucose metabolism. An excess of the acid accumulating in the muscles may cause cramp.

lactiferous (*lak-tif'-er-us*). Conveying or secreting milk.

lactifuge (*lak'-te-fuje*). A drug or agent which retards the secretion of milk.

Lactobacillus (*lak-to-bas-il'-us*). A genus of gram-positive rod-shaped bacteria many of which produce fermentation.

lactoflavine (*lak'-to-flav-een*). Riboflavine.

lactogenic (*lak-to-jen'-ik*). Stimulating the production of milk. *See* Luteotrophin.

lactometer (*lak-tom'-e-ter*). An instrument for measuring the specific gravity of milk.

lactose (*lak'-toze*). Milk sugar consisting of glucose and galactose.

lactosuria (*lak-to-su'-re-ah*). Lactose in the urine.

lactulose (*lak'-tu-loze*). A synthetic disaccharide which is used as a laxative. Especially useful in the treatment of hepatic encephalopathy.

lacuna (*lak-u'-nah*). *pl.* lacunae. A small cavity or depression in any part of the body.

Laënnec's disease (*R.T.H. Laënnec, French physician, 1781–1826*). The commonest type of cirrhosis of the liver, frequently attributable to high alcohol consumption.

laetrile (*la'-et-ril*). A cyanide-containing preparation obtained from peach stones. Said to be of therapeutic value in the treatment of malignant disease. It continues to be used despite lack of evidence as to its efficacy.

laevulose (*le'-vu-loze*). Fruit sugar. Fructose.

lagophthalmos (*lag-off-thal'-mos*). Failure of the eye to close.

laked (*la'-kt*). Descriptive of blood when haemoglobin has separated from the red blood cells.

laking (*la'-king*). Haemolysis of

the red blood cells. The cells swell and burst and the haemoglobin is released.

lalling (*lal'-ing*). A continuous repetitive, wordless sound as made by infants or by someone who is severely subnormal.

lambdoid (*lam'-doid*). Shaped like the Greek letter *lambda* Λ or λ. **L. suture.** The junction of the occipital bone with the parietals.

lambliasis (*lam-bli'-as-is*). Giardiasis.

lamella (*lam-el'-ah*). (1) A thin layer, membrane or plate, as of bone. (2) A thin medicated disc of gelatin used in applying drugs to the eye. The gelatin dissolves and the drugs are absorbed.

lamina (*lam'-in-ah*). A bony plate or layer.

laminectomy (*lam-in-ek'-tom-e*). Excision of the posterior arch of a vertebra, sometimes performed to relieve pressure on the spinal cord or nerves.

lanatoside (*lan-at'-o-side*). A cardiac glycoside drug similar to digitalis and used in the treatment of heart failure.

Lancefield's groups (*R.C. Lancefield, American bacteriologist, b. 1895*). Divisions of β-haemolytic streptococci, which are classified into groups A–R. Most human infections are due to group A. Other groups are mainly responsible for animal infections.

lancinating (*lan'-sin-a-ting*). Sharp, cutting. Used to describe such pains.

Landry's disease (*J.B.G. Landry, French physician, 1826–1865*). An acute ascending paralysis from the lower limbs upwards. Guillain–Barré syndrome. Acute ascending polyneuritis.

Landsteiner classification (*K. Landsteiner, Austrian biologist, 1868–1943*). A system of blood groups—the ABO system, consisting of groups A, B, AB and O.

Lange colloidal gold test (*C.F.A. Lange, German physician, b. 1883*). A test made on cerebrospinal fluid to detect syphilis, disseminated sclerosis, meningitis and other neurological conditions.

Langerhans, islet of (*P. Langerhans, German pathologist, 1847–1888*). One of a group of cells in the pancreas which produce insulin.

Langhans's cell (*T. Langhans, Swiss pathologist, 1834–1915*). A deep cell of a chorionic villus.

lanolin (*lan'-o-lin*). A fat obtained from sheep's wool, and used as a basis for ointments. Adeps lanae hydrosus.

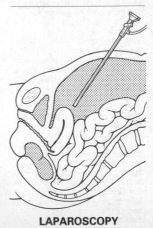

LAPAROSCOPY

lanugo (*lan-u'-go*). A fine layer of hair seen on the body of newly born infants.

laparoscopy (*lap-ar-os'-kop-e*). Viewing of the abdominal cavity by passing an endoscope through the abdominal wall.

laparotomy (*lap-ar-ot'-om-e*). Incision of the abdominal wall for exploratory purposes.

lard (*lard*). The purified internal fat of the pig; used as a basis for ointments. Adeps.

lardaceous (*lar-da'-she-us*). (1) Resembling lard. (2) Containing amyloid.

laryngeal (*lar-in'-je-al*). Pertaining to the larynx.

laryngectomy (*lar-in-jek'-tom-e*). Excision of the larynx.

laryngismus (*lar-in-jiz'-mus*). A spasmodic contraction of the larynx. *L. stridulus.* A crowing sound on inspiration following a period of apnoea due to spasmodic closure of the glottis. It occurs in children, particularly those suffering from rickets. Croup.

laryngitis (*lar-in-ji'-tis*). Inflammation of the larynx causing hoarseness or loss of voice due to acute infection or irritation by gases.

laryngologist (*lar-in-gol'-o-jist*). A specialist in diseases of the larynx.

laryngopharynx (*lar-in-go-far'-inks*). The lower part of the pharynx.

laryngoscope (*lar-in'-go-skope*). An endoscopic instrument for examining the larynx or for aiding the insertion of endotracheal tubes or the bronchoscope.

laryngospasm (*lar-in'-go-spazm*). A reflex prolonged contraction of the laryngeal muscles that is liable to occur on insertion or withdrawal of an intratracheal tube.

laryngostenosis (*lar-in-go-sten-o'-sis*). Contraction or stricture of the larynx.

laryngostomy (*lar-in-gos'-tom-e*). The making of an opening into the larynx to provide an artificial air-passage.

laryngotomy (*lar-in-got'-om-e*). An incision into the larynx to make a temporary opening in an emergency when the larynx is obstructed. Tracheostomy.

laryngotracheal (*lar-in-go-trak-e'-al*). Referring to both the larynx and trachea.

laryngotracheitis (*lar-in-go-trak-e-i'-tis*). Inflammation of both the larynx and trachea.

laryngotracheobronchitis (*lar-in-go-trak-e-o-brong-ki'-tis*). An acute viral infection of the respiratory tract which occurs particularly in young children.

larynx (*lar'-inks*). The organ of the voice, situated at the upper end of the trachea. It has a muscular and cartilaginous frame, lined with mucous membrane. Across it are spread the vocal cords of elastic tissue, and the vibrations and contractions of these produce the changes in the pitch of the voice.

laser (*la'-zer*). Light Amplification by Stimulated Emission of Radiation. An apparatus producing an extremely concentrated beam of light that can be used to cut metals. Used in the treatment of neoplasms, of detached retina, diabetic retinopathy and macular degeneration and of some skin conditions.

Lassa fever (*las'-ah fe'-ver*). A disease caused by a virus, usually seen in West Africa. The illness is severe and is likely to be fatal, particularly if contracted by Europeans. First reported from Lassa in northern Nigeria.

Lassar's paste (*G. Lassar, German dermatologist, 1849–1907*). A soothing paste used in skin diseases, containing salicylic acid, zinc oxide, starch and soft paraffin.

lassitude (*las'-it-ude*). A feeling of extreme weakness and apathy.

latent (*la'-tent*). Temporarily concealed; not manifest. *L. heat.* The heat absorbed by a substance during a change in state, e.g. from water into steam. When condensation occurs this heat is released. *L. period.* (1) The incubation period of an infectious disease. (2) The time between the application of a nerve stimulus and the reaction.

lateral (*lat'-er-al*). Situated at the side; therefore, away from the centre.

lateroversion (*lat-er-o-ver'-shun*). A turning to one side, such as may occur of the uterus.

laudanum (*law'-dan-um*). Tincture of opium; a preparation formerly used as a narcotic.

laughing gas (*lahf'-ing gas*). Nitrous oxide.

lavage (*lav-arzh'*). The washing out of a cavity. *Colonic l.* The washing out of the colon. *Gastric l.* The washing out of the stomach.

laxative (*laks'-at-iv*). A mild aperient.

lead (*led*). *abbrev.* Pb. A metallic element, many of the compounds of which are highly poisonous. *L. lotion.* Lead subacetate solution used externally on bruises. *L. poisoning.* A condition which usually occurs in children as the result of excessive lead in the atmosphere, or from chewing toys and other objects covered with paint containing lead. The symptoms and signs include malaise, diarrhoea and vomiting, and sometimes encephalitis. There is often pallor and a blue line around the gums.

Leber's disease (*T.B. Leber, German ophthalmologist, 1840–1917*). Hereditary optic atrophy.

lecithin (*les'-ith-in*). One of a group of phospholipids that are found in the cell tissues and are concerned in the metabolism of fat.

leech (*le'-tch*). *Hirudo medicinalis.* An aquatic worm which sucks blood and was formerly used to withdraw blood from patients who were thought to require bleeding.

leg (*leg*). The lower limb, from knee to ankle. *Barbados l.* Elephantiasis. *Bow l.* Genu varum. *White l.* Phlegmasia alba dolens. *Scissor l.* Condition in which the patient is cross-legged, such as occurs in cerebral diplegia.

legionnaires' disease (*le-jon-airz' diz-eez'*). A bacterial infection of the lungs. It is very contagious and symptoms include fever, pain in the muscles and across the chest, a dry cough and a partial loss of kidney function.

legumin (*leg-u'-min*). A protein of peas, beans, and all pulses.

leiomyoma (*li-o-mi-o'-mah*). A benign muscle tumour (fibroid) found in the uterus and also in the stomach and on the outer surfaces of the limbs.

leimyosarcoma (*li-o-mi-o-sar-ko'-mah*). A malignant muscle tumour.

Leishman–Donovan bodies

(*Sir W.B. Leishman, British pathologist, 1865–1926; C. Donovan, Irish physician, 1863–1951*). The intracellular forms of *Leishmania donovani*, the parasite producing kala-azar. These bodies occur in the spleen and liver of patients.

Leishmania (*leesh-ma'-ne-ah*). A genus of parasitic protozoa having flagella which infect the blood of man and are the cause of leishmaniasis.

leishmaniasis (*leesh-man-i-i'-as-is*). A group of diseases caused by one of the protozoan *Leishmania* parasites. *See* Kala-azar.

Lembert's suture (*A. Lembert, French surgeon, 1802–1851*). A series of stitches used for wounds of the intestine. So arranged that the edges are turned inwards and the peritoneal surfaces are in contact.

lens (*lenz*). (1) A piece of glass or other material shaped to transmit light rays in a particular direction. (2) The transparent crystalline body situated behind the pupil of the eye. It serves as a refractive medium for rays of light. *Contact l.* A thin sheet of glass or plastic moulded to fit directly over the cornea. Worn instead of spectacles.

lenticonus (*len-te-ko'-nus*). Excessive curvature of the front surface of the lens of the eye causing myopia and distorted vision. It is usually congenital.

lentigo (*len-ti'-go*). A brownish or yellowish spot on the skin. A freckle. *L. maligna.* Hutchinson's melanotic freckle. *See* Freckle.

leontiasis (*le-on-ti'-as-is*). An osseous deformity of the face which produces a lion-like appearance. It occurs sometimes in leprosy and rarely in osteitis deformans.

lepidosis (*lep-id-o'-sis*). Any scaly eruption of the skin.

leprosy (*lep'-ro-se*). Hansen's disease. An incurable, chronic infection of the skin, mucous membrane and nerves with *Mycobacterium leprae.* It is predominantly a tropical disease which is transmitted by direct contact. There is an insidious onset of symptoms, mainly involving the skin and nerves, after an incubation period of between one and thirty years. The disease can be classified into three types: (1) *Lepromatous*, which is a steadily progressive form, often resulting in paralysis, disfigurement and deformity. This form is often complicated by tuberculosis. (2) *Tuberculoid*, which is often self-limiting and generally runs a more benign course. (3) *Indeterminate*, in which there are skin symptoms representative of both lepromatous and tuberculoid forms. Leprosy can be controlled by the use of sulphone drugs.

leptomeningitis (*lep-to-men-in-ji'-tis*). Inflammation of the pia mater and arachnoid membranes of the brain and spinal cord.

Leptospira (*lep-to-spi'-rah*). A genus of spirochaetes. *L. icterohaemorrhagiae.* The cause of spirochaetal jaundice (Weil's disease).

leptospirosis (*lep-to-spi-ro'-sis*). A group of diseases caused by *Leptospira* infection, including Weil's disease.

Leriche's syndrome (*R. Leriche, French surgeon, 1879–1955*). A condition in which atherosclerosis of peripheral arteries is accompanied by obstruction of the lower end of the aorta.

lesbianism (*lez'-be-an-izm*). Sexual attraction of one woman to another. Female homosexuality.

lesion (*le'-zhun*). An injury, wound, or morbid structural change in an organ. Used as a general term for some local disease condition.

lethargy (*leth'-ar-je*). A condition of drowsiness or stupor which cannot be overcome by the will.

Letterer–Siwe disease (*E. Letterer, German physician, b. 1895; S.A. Siwe, German physician, b. 1897*). Reticuloendotheliosis. A disease occurring in young children in which histiocytic granules appear and the spleen and liver become enlarged, as do the lymph glands. The disease runs a rapid and fatal course.

leucine (*lu'-seen*). An essential amino acid. It may be excreted in the urine from excessive endogenous breakdown of protein, as in acute atrophy of the liver.

leucocyte (*lu'-ko-site*). A white blood corpuscle. There are three types: (a) *granular* (polymorphonuclear cells) formed in bone marrow, consisting of neutrophils, eosinophils and basophils; (b) *lymphocytes* (formed in the lymph glands); and (c) *monocytes.* Normal leucocyte count is as follows:

Type of leucocyte	No. of cells per litre
Neutrophils	$2.5–7.4 \times 10^9$
Lymphocytes	$1.5–3.5 \times 10^9$
Monocytes	$2–8 \times 10^9$
Eosinophils	$4–44 \times 10^9$
Basophils	$0–1 \times 10^9$

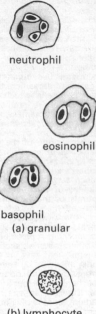

neutrophil

eosinophil

basophil
(a) granular

(b) lymphocyte

(c) monocyte

LEUCOCYTES

leucocytolysis (*lu-ko-si-tol'-is-is*). Destruction of white blood cells.

leucocytopoiesis (*lu-ko-si-to-poi-e'-sis*). Leucopoiesis.

leucocytosis (*lu-ko-si-to'-sis*). An increase in the number of leucocytes in the blood.

leucoderma (*lu-ko-der'-mah*). An absence of pigment in patches or bands, producing abnormal whiteness of the skin. Vitiligo.

leucodystrophy (*lu-ko-dis'-tro-fe*). A degenerative disorder of the brain which starts during the first few months of life and leads to mental, visual and motor deterioration.

leucoma (*lu-ko'-mah*). A white spot on the cornea, usually following an injury to the eye.

leuconychia (*lu-ko-nik'-e-ah*). White patches on the nails due to air underneath.

leucopenia (*lu-ko-pe'-ne-ah*). A decreased number of white cells, usually granulocytes, in the blood.

leucophoresis (*lu-ko-for-e'-sis*). Withdrawal of blood for the selective removal of leucocytes. The remaining blood is re-transfused.

leucoplakia (*lu-ko-pla'-ke-ah*). A chronic inflammation, characterized by white thickened patches on the mucous membranes, particularly of the tongue, gums and inside of the cheeks. *L. vulvae*. Thickening of the mucous membrane of the labia with the appearance of scattered white patches.

leucopoiesis (*lu-ko-poi-e'-sis*). The formation of white blood cells. Leucocytopoiesis.

leucorrhoea (*lu-kor-e'-ah*). A thick whitish discharge from the vagina, which may be caused by an infection.

leucotomy (*lu-kot'-om-e*). An operation in which the white nerve fibres within the brain are severed. It is used to treat severe anxiety neurosis, deep depression and other conditions of strong emotional tension. It may considerably relieve symptoms of worry, tension, and fear but there may also be changes in personality, such as lack of initiative and perseverance. The process is irreversible.

leukaemia (*lu-ke'-me-ah*). A generic name for a group of malignant diseases of the bone marrow and blood-forming organs. Individual diseases are classified according to the line of cells involved and the state of maturity of the cells, e.g. acute forms involve primitive or blast cells, whereas in chronic forms the cells are more differentiated. In each case the immature cell line proliferates at the cost of other cell lines, causing anaemia, susceptibility to infection and bruising or bleeding. The common forms involve lymphocytes, monocytes or granulocytes.

levator (*lev-a'-tor*). A muscle which raises a structure or organ of the body.

levodopa (*le-vo-do'-pah*). L-dopa. A synthetic drug used in the treatment of parkinsonism.

levorphanol (*lev-or'-fan-ol*). An analgesic somewhat resembling morphine in its action and addiction potentialities. It is used to relieve severe pain.

Li. Chemical symbol for *lithium*.

libido (*lib-e'-do*). (1) The vital force or impulse which brings about purposeful action. (2) Sexual drive. In Freudian psychoanalysis, the motive force of all human beings.

lichen (*li'-ken*). A group of inflammatory affections of the skin, in which the lesions consist of papular eruptions. *L. planus.* Raised flat patches of dull, reddish-purple colour, with smooth or scaly surface.

lichenification (*li-ken-if-ik-a'-shun*). The stage of an eruption when it resembles lichen.

lichenoid (*li'-ken-oid*). A rash that resembles lichen.

lid (*lid*). Eyelid. *Granular l.* Trachoma. *L. lag.* Jerky movement of the upper lid when it is being lowered. A sign of exophthalmic goitre (thyrotoxicosis).

lie (*li*). A position or direction. *L. of fetus.* The position of the fetus in the uterus. The normal lie is longitudinal.

Lieberkühn's glands (*J. N. Lieberkühn, German anatomist, 1711–1756*). Tubular glands of the small intestine.

lien (*li'-en*). The spleen.

lienculus (*li-en'-ku-lus*). An accessory spleen.

lienitis (*li-en-i'-tis*). Inflammation of the spleen. Splenitis.

lienorenal (*li-en-o-re'-nal*). Relating to the spleen and kidneys. Splenorenal. Splenonephric.

lientery (*li'-en-ter-e*). Diarrhoea consisting mainly of undigested food.

lienunculus (*li-en-un'-ku-lus*). A detached portion of spleen which is functioning on its own.

ligament (*lig'-am-ent*). (1) A band of fibrous tissue connecting bones forming a joint. (2) A layer or layers of peritoneum connecting one abdominal organ to another or to the abdominal wall. *Annular l.* The ring-like band which fixes the head of the radius to the

ulna. *Cruciate l.* Crossed ligaments within the knee-joint. *Inguinal l.* That between the pubic bone and anterior iliac crest. *Round l.* For example, one of the two anterior ligaments *of the uterus,* passing through the inguinal canal and ending in the labia majora. There are also round ligaments *of the femur* and *of the liver.*

ligation (*lig-a'-shun*). The application of a ligature.

ligature (*lig'-at-chur*). A thread of silk, catgut or other material used for tying round a blood vessel to stop it bleeding.

light (*lite*). Electromagnetic waves which stimulate the retina of the eye. *L. adaptation.* The changes that take place in the eye when the intensity of the light increases or decreases. *L. coagulation.* A method of treating retinal detachment by directing a beam of strong light from a carbon arc through the pupil to the affected area.

lightening (*li'-ten-ing*). The relief experienced in pregnancy, 2 to 3 weeks before labour, when the uterus sinks into the pelvis and ceases to press on the diaphragm.

lignocaine (*lig'-no-kane*). A local anaesthetic administered by injection and by surface application. Also used intravenously in cases of cardiac arrhythmia, especially myocardial infarction.

limbus (*lim'-bus*). An edge or border. *Corneal l.* The border where the cornea joins the sclera.

lime (*lime*). (1) A citrus fruit resembling a small lemon. (2) Calcium oxide, the salts of which help to form bone.

Quicklime. *Chlorinated l.* Bleaching powder. *Slaked l.* Calcium hydroxide. *L. water.* Calcium hydroxide solution. Given to counteract acidity.

liminal (*lim'-in-al*). Pertaining to the threshold of perception.

lincomycin (*lin-ko-mi'-sin*). An antibiotic derived from the *Streptomyces* genus. Used in the treatment of streptococcal bone and joint infections, including osteomyelitis.

linctus (*link'-tus*). A thick syrup given to soothe and allay coughing.

linea (*lin'-e-ah*). A line. *L. alba.* The tendinous area in the centre of the abdominal wall into which the transversalis and part of the oblique muscles are inserted. *L. albicantes.* White streaks that appear on the abdomen when it is distended by pregnancy or a tumour. *L. aspera.* The rough ridge on the back of the femur into which muscles are inserted. *L. nigra.* The pigmented line which often appears in pregnancy on the abdomen between the umbilicus and the pubis.

linear (*lin'-e-ar*). Pertaining to line. *L. accelerator.* A megavoltage machine for accelerating electrons so that powerful X-rays are given off for use in the treatment of deep-seated tumours.

lingual (*ling'-gwal*). Pertaining to the tongue.

lingula (*ling'-u-lah*). A tongue-like structure such as the projection of lung tissue from the left upper lobe.

liniment (*lin'-im-ent*). A liquid to be applied externally by rubbing on to the skin.

linseed (*lin'-seed*). Seed of the common flax, which contains an oil with a demulcent action.

liothyronine (*li-o-thi'-ro-neen*). A preparation of thyroid hormone used in the treatment of hypothyroidism where rapid results are desired.

lipaemia (*lip-e'-me-ah*). The presence of excess fat in the blood. Sometimes a feature of diabetes. *L. retinalis.* Condition in which the retinal blood vessels appear to be filled with milk due to the presence of an excess of fat in the blood.

lipase (*lip'-aze*). Steapsin. The fat-splitting ferment of pancreatic juice.

lipid (*lip'-id*). One of a group of fatty substances that are insoluble in water but soluble in alcohol or chloroform. They form an important part of the diet and are normally present in the body tissues.

lipochondrodystrophy (*lip-o-kon-dro-dis'-tro-fe*). A congenital condition affecting the metabolism of fat and producing bone deformities, dwarfism, facial abnormalities and mental retardation. Hurler's syndrome.

lipodystrophy (*lip-o-dis'-tro-fe*). A disorder of fat metabolism. *Progressive l.* A rare condition occurring mainly in females in which there is progressive loss of fat over the upper half of the body.

lipoidosis (*lip-oid-o'-sis*). A group of diseases in which there is an error in lipoid metabolism producing reticuloendothelial hyperplasia. Xanthomata are common.

lipolysis (*lip-ol'-is-is*). The breakdown of fats by the action of bile salts and enzymes to a fine emulsion and fatty acids.

lipoma (*lip-o'-mah*). A benign

tumour composed of fatty tissue, arising in any part of the body, and developing in connective tissue. *Diffuse l.* A tumour of fat in an irregular mass, without a capsule, occurring above the pelvis.

lipoprotein (*lip-o-pro'-teen*). One of a group of fatty proteins that are present in blood plasma.

liposarcoma (*lip-o-sar-ko'-mah*). A malignant tumour of the fat cells.

lipuria (*lip-u'-re-ah*). The presence of fat in urine.

liquefaction (*lik-we-fak'-shun*). Reduction to liquid form.

liquor (*lik'-er;* Latin *li'-kwor*). A watery fluid. A solution. *L. amnii.* The fluid in which the fetus floats. Amniotic fluid.

Lister, J. (*British surgeon, 1827 –1912*). The inventor of the antiseptic technique (in 1867) which prepared the way for modern surgery.

lithagogue (*lith'-ag-og*). A drug which helps to expel calculi.

lithiasis (*lith-i'-as-is*). The formation of calculi. *Conjunctival l.* The formation of small white chalky areas on the inner surface of the eyelids.

lithium (*lith'-e-um*). *abbrev.* Li. An alkaline metallic element. *L. carbonate.* A drug used in the treatment of manic-depressive illness.

litholapaxy (*lith-o-lap-aks'-e*). The removal of fragments of a calculus from the bladder after lithotripsy.

lithonephrotomy (*lith-o-nef-rot'-om-e*). Incision into the kidney to remove a stone. Nephrolithotomy.

lithopaedion (*lith-o-pe'-de-on*). A dead fetus that has been retained and has become calcified.

lithosis (*lith-o'-sis*). Pneumoconiosis resulting from inhalation of particles of silica, etc., into the lungs.

lithotome (*lith'-o-tome*). A knife used in lithotomy.

lithotomy (*lith-ot'-om-e*). Incision into the bladder for the removal of calculi.

lithotripsy (*lith'-o-trip-se*). The crushing of calculi in the bladder. Lithotrity.

lithotrite (*lith'-o-trite*). An instrument used for lithotripsy.

lithuresis (*lith-u-re'-sis*). Passage of small calculi or gravel in the urine.

litmus (*lit'-mus*). A blue pigment obtained from lichen and used for testing the reaction of fluids. *Blue l.* is turned red by an acid. *Red l.* is turned blue by an alkali.

litre (*le'-ter*). *abbrev.* l. The SI unit of capacity. One cubic metre.

Little's disease (*W.J. Little, British surgeon, 1810–1894*). Spastic diplegia. A congenital muscle rigidity of the lower limbs, causing 'scissor leg' deformity.

liver (*liv'-er*). The large gland situated in the right upper area of the abdominal cavity. Its chief functions are: (1) the secretion of bile, (2) the maintenance of the composition of the blood, and (3) the regulation of metabolic processes. *Cirrhotic l.* Fibrotic changes which occur in the liver as the result of chronic inflammation. *Hobnail l.* One affected by atrophic cirrhosis. *Nutmeg l.* A mottled condition, typical of the effect of congestive heart failure.

livid (*liv'-id*). Descriptive of the bluish-grey discoloration of the skin produced by congestion of blood.

LOA. Left occipito-anterior. Refers to a possible position of the fetus in the uterus.

lobar (*lo'-bar*). Relating to a lobe.

lobe (*lobe*). A section of an organ, separated from neighbouring parts by fissures. The liver, lungs and brain are divided into lobes.

lobectomy (*lo-bek'-tom-e*). Removal of a lobe, e.g. of the lung.

lobotomy (*lo-bot'-om-e*). An operation in which the nerve fibres in the prefrontal area of the brain are severed to effect a change of behaviour. Leucotomy.

lobular (*lob'-u-lar*). Relating to a lobule.

lobule (*lob'-ule*). A small lobe, particularly one making up a larger lobe.

localize (*lo'-kal-ize*). (1) To limit the spread, e.g. of disease or infection, to a certain area. (2) To determine the site of a lesion.

lochia (*lo'-ke-ah*). The discharge of blood and tissue debris from the uterus following childbirth and lasting for several weeks. *L. alba.* The final pale discharge. *L. rubra.* The earlier discharge first containing bright blood and later dark blood. *L. serosa.* A thin brown discharge which occurs after the discharge of lochia rubra.

lochiometra (*lo-ke-o-me'-trah*). The retention of lochia in the uterus, causing its distension.

lock-jaw (*lok'-jaw*). Tetanus.

locomotor (*lo-ko-mo'-tor*). Pertaining to movement from one place to another. *L. ataxia.* Tabes dorsalis. *See* Ataxia.

loculated (*lok'-u-la-ted*). Divided into small locules or cavities.

loculus (*lok'-u-lus*). A small

cystic cavity, one of a number.

logopaedics (*log-o-pe'-diks*). The study and treatment of speech defects.

logorrhoea (*log-o-re'-ah*). Excessive and often unintelligible volubility.

loiasis (*lo-i'-as-is*). Infestation of the conjunctiva and eyelids with a parasite worm, *Loa loa.* A tropical condition.

loin (*loin*). The area of the back between the thorax and the pelvis.

long-acting (*long-ak'-ting*). Of great duration. Used to differentiate certain varieties of drug, especially sedative drugs. *L. thyroid stimulator.* LATS. A substance found in the plasma of some patients with thyrotoxicosis. Thought to be formed as the result of an auto-immune reaction.

long-sight (*long-site*). Hypermetropia.

loop (*loop*). A complete bend in a cord or tube. *Ileal l. See* Ileal conduit. *Platinum l.* A platinum wire in a handle used for transferring bacteriological material. It is always flamed to red heat before and after use.

LOP. Left occipitoposterior. Refers to a possible position of the fetus in the uterus.

lorazepam (*lor-az'-e-pam*). A minor tranquillizer used to treat anxiety and insomnia.

lordosis (*lor-do'-sis*). A form of spinal curvature in which there is an abnormal forward curve of the lumbar spine.

lotion (*lo'-shun*). A medicinal solution for external application to the body. Lotions usually have a soothing or antiseptic effect. *Calamine l.* A soothing mixture containing calamine and zinc oxide. *Evaporating l.* A dilute alcoholic solution applied to bruises. *Lead l.* A weak solution of lead acetate used for sprains and bruises where the skin is unbroken.

loupe (*loop*). A magnifying lens which may be used in eye examination.

louse (*lows*). *pl.* lice. A general term covering a number of small insects which are parasitic to man and to other mammals and birds. Three varieties are parasitic to man: (1) *Pediculus capitis*, the head louse; (2) *Pediculus corporis*, the body louse; and (3) *Phthirus pubis*, which infects the coarse hair on the body, and also the eyebrows. Diseases known to be transmitted by lice are typhus fever, relapsing fever and trench fever.

lozenge (*loz'-enj*). A medicated tablet with sugar basis, used to treat mouth and throat conditions.

LSD. *See* Lysergide.

lubb-dupp (*lub-dup'*). Representation of the sounds heard through the stethoscope when listening to the normal heart—*lubb* when the atrioventricular valves shut, and *dupp* when the semilunar valves meet each other.

lucid (*lu'-sid*). Clear, particularly of the mind. *L. interval.* Period of clear thinking that may occur in cerebral injury between two periods of unconsciousness or as a sane interval in a mental disorder.

Ludwig's angina (*W.F. von Ludwig, German surgeon, 1790–1865*). *See* Angina.

lues (*lu'-eez*). Syphilis.

Lugol's solution (*J.G.A. Lugol, French physician, 1786–1851*). A preparation of iodine and potassium iodide. It is best given in milk and is fre-

quently used in the treatment of toxic goitre.

lumbago (*lum-ba'-go*). Pain in the lower part of the back. It may be caused by muscular strain or by a prolapsed intervertebral disc ('slipped disc').

lumbar (*lum'-bar*). Pertaining to the loins. *L. puncture.* Insertion of a trocar and cannula into the spinal canal in the lower back, and withdrawal of cerebrospinal fluid for diagnostic purposes.

lumbosacral (*lum-bo-sa'-kral*). Relating to both the lumbar vertebrae and the sacrum. *L. support.* A corset aimed at both supporting and restricting movement in that region. *L. vertebra.* One of the five vertebrae in the lower back lying between the thoracic vertebrae and the sacrum.

Lumbricus (*lum'-brik-us*). (1) A genus of annelids, including the earthworm (2) *Ascaris lumbricoides.* A species of nematode which is parasitic in the intestine of man.

lumen (*lu'-men*). The space inside a tube.

lunacy (*lu'-nas-e*). A term formerly applied to insanity.

lunatic (*lu'-nat-ik*). Obsolete term for one suffering from a psychopathic disease.

lung (*lung*). One of a pair of conical organs of the respiratory system, consisting of an arrangement of air tubes terminating in air vesicles (*alveoli*) and filling almost the whole of the thorax. The right lung has three lobes and the left lung two. They are connected with the air by means of the bronchi and trachea.

lunula (*lu'-nu-lah*). The white semicircle near the root of each nail.

lupus (*lu'-pus*). A chronic skin

disease, having many manifestations. *L. erythematosus.* An inflammatory disease affecting both the internal organs and the skin which finally produces a round plaque-like area of hyperkeratosis. It is thought to be due to an auto-immune reaction to sunlight, infection or other unknown cause. *L. vulgaris.* A tuberculous disease of the skin producing brownish nodules, frequently on the nose or cheek, and severe scarring.

luteinizing hormone (*lu'-te-in-i-zing hor'-mone*). LH. One of three hormones produced by the anterior pituitary gland which control the activity of the gonads.

luteotrophin (*lu-te-o-trof'-in*). An anterior pituitary hormone which stimulates the formation of the corpus luteum and the production of milk. Prolactin.

luxation (*luks-a'-shun*). The dislocation of a joint. *L. of the lens.* Displacement of the lens of the eye into the anterior chamber or posteriorly into the vitreous.

lying (*li'-ing*). Making an untruthful statement. *Pathological l.* A disorder of conduct which may occur as a symptom in behaviour disorders of children or in certain mental disorders such as addiction or psychopathic personality.

lying-in (*li'-ing in*). A term formerly used to denote the puerperium.

lymph (*limf*). The fluid from the blood which has transuded through capillary walls to supply nutriment to tissue cells. It is collected by lymph vessels which ultimately return it to the blood. *L. nodes*

or *glands.* Structures placed along the course of lymph vessels, through which the lymph passes and is filtered of foreign substances, e.g. bacteria. These nodes also make lymphocytes. *Plastic l.* An inflammatory exudate which tends to cause adhesion between structures and so limit the spread of infection. *Vaccine l.* A lymph preparation obtained from calves or other animals and used for vaccination against smallpox.

lymphadenectomy (*limf-aden-ek'-tom-e*). Excision of a lymph gland or nodes.

lymphadenitis (*limf-ad-en-i'-tis*). Inflammation of a lymph gland.

lymphadenoma (*limf-ad-en-o'-mah*). Lymphoma. *Multiple l.* Hodgkin's disease.

lymphadenopathy (*limf-ad-en-op'-ath-e*). Any disease condition of the lymph nodes.

lymphangiectasis (*limf-an-je-ek'-tas-is*). Dilatation of the lymph vessels due to some obstruction of the lymph flow. It may be congenital.

lymphangiography (*limf-an-je-og'-raf-e*). X-ray examination of lymph vessels following the insertion of a radio-opaque dye.

lymphangioma (*limf-an-je-o'-mah*). A swelling composed of dilated lymph vessels.

lymphangioplasty (*limf-an-je-o-plas'-te*). Any plastic operation which aims at making an artificial lymph drainage.

lymphangitis (*limf-an-ji'-tis*). Inflammation of lymph vessels, manifested by red lines on the skin over them. It occurs in cases of severe infection through the skin.

lymphatic (*limf-at'-ik*). Referring to lymph. *L. system.* The system of vessels and glands through which the lymph is returned to the circulation. The vessels end in the thoracic duct and the right lymphatic duct.

lymphoblast (*limf'-o-blast*). An early developmental cell that will mature into a lymphocyte.

lymphocyte (*limf'-o-site*). A white blood cell formed in the lymphoid tissue. Lymphocytes produce immune bodies to overcome and protect against infection.

lymphocythaemia (*limf-o-si-the'-me-ah*). An excessive number of lymphocytes in the blood. Lymphocytosis.

lymphocytopenia (*limf-o-si-to-pe'-ne-ah*). Absence or scarcity of lymphocytes in the blood. Lymphopenia.

lymphocytosis (*limf-o-si-to'-sis*). Lymphocythaemia.

lymphoedema (*limf-e-de'-mah*). A condition in which the intercellular spaces contain an abnormal amount of lymph due to obstruction of the lymph drainage.

lymphogranuloma (*limf-o-gran-u-lo'-mah*). Hodgkin's disease. *L. venereum.* A sexually transmitted disease due to a virus, primarily a tropical condition.

lymphoid (*limf'-oid*). Relating to the lymph.

lymphoma (*limf-o'-mah*). Lymphadenoma. Used to denote any malignant condition of the lymphoid tissue. Generally these diseases are classified as either Hodgkin's or non-Hodgkin's lymphomas. *Burkitt's l.* A type of lymphoma found predominantly in East Africa and affecting the jaws of children.

lymphopenia (*limf-o-pe'-ne-ah*). Lymphocytopenia.

lymphopoesis (*limf-o-poi-e'-sis*). The production of lymphocytes. Occurs chiefly in the bone marrow, lymph nodes, thymus, spleen and gut wall.

lymphorrhagia (*limf-o-raj'-e-ah*). The escape of lymph from a ruptured lymphatic vessel. Lymphorrhoea.

lymphosarcoma (*limf-o'-sar-ko'-mah*). A term formerly used to denote a malignant lymphoma—with the exception of Hodgkin's disease.

lynoestrenol (*lin-e'-stren-ol*). A synthetic drug similar in action to progesterone, used chiefly in oral contraceptives.

lyophilization (*li-off-il-i-za'-shun*). A method of preserving biological substances in a stable state by freeze-drying. It may be used for plasma, sera, bacteria, viruses and tissues.

lysergide (*li-ser'-jide*). Lysergic acid diethylamide. LSD. A psychotomimetic drug that can cause visual hallucinations and increased auditory acuity but may prove very disrupting to the personality and affect mental ability.

lysin (*li'-sin*). A specific antibody present in the blood that can destroy cells. *See* Bacteriolysin.

lysine (*li'-seen*). One of the 22 amino acids formed by the digestion of dietary protein. It is essential for normal health.

lysis (*li'-sis*). (1) The gradual decline of a disease, especially of a fever. The temperature falls gradually, as in typhoid. (*See* Crisis.) (2) The destruction of cells.

lysosome (*li'-so-some*). A particle found in the cytoplasm of cells which causes the breakdown of metabolic substances and foreign particles (e.g. bacteria) within the cell.

lysozyme (*li'-so-zime*). An enzyme present in tears, nasal mucus and saliva that can kill most bacteria coming into contact with it.

M

m. (1) Abbreviation for the fundamental SI unit of length, the *metre*. (2) Abbreviation for *misce* (mix).

M. Abbreviation for *molar*.

McArdle's disease (*B. McArdle, British biochemist*). Myopathy resulting from the congenital absence in voluntary muscle of the enzyme phosphorylase.

McBurney's point (*C. McBurney, American surgeon, 1845–1913*). The spot midway between the *anterior iliac spine* and the *umbilicus* where pain is felt on pressure if the appendix is inflamed.

maceration (*mas-er-a'-shun*). Softening of a solid by soaking it in liquid. *Neonatal m.* The natural softening of a dead fetus in the uterus.

Mackenrodt's ligaments (*A.K. Mackenrodt, German gynaecologist, 1959–1925*). The transverse or cardinal ligaments that support the uterus in the pelvic cavity.

McNaghten's Rules on Insanity at Law. The rules which define the factors on which a defence to a charge of murder on grounds of insanity may be established. These were evolved after Sir Robert Peel's Secretary was killed by McNaghten in 1843. He was suffering from delusions and the judge ordered that he be

found not guilty. The Homicide Act 1957 provided for a defence based on 'diminished responsibility', i.e. the accused was suffering from such abnormality of mind as to impair his mental responsibility for his actions.

macrocephalic (*mak-ro-kef-al'-ik*). Possessing an abnormally large head.

macrocheilia (*mak-ro-ki'-le-ah*). A congenital condition in which there is excessive development of the lips.

macrocyte (*mak'-ro-site*). An abnormally large red corpuscle found in the blood in some forms of anaemia.

macrocythaemia (*mak-ro-si-the'-me-ah*). The presence of abnormally large red cells in the blood. Macrocytosis.

macrodactylism (*mak-ro-dak'-til-izm*). Abnormal enlargement of one or more of the fingers or toes.

macroglossia (*mak-ro-glos'-e-ah*). Abnormal enlargement of the tongue.

macromastia (*mak-ro-mas'-te-ah*). Abnormal increase in the size of the breast.

macromelia (*mak-ro-me'-le-ah*). Abnormal enlargement of one or more of the hands or legs.

macrophage (*mak'-ro-fage*). A large reticulo-endothelial cell which has the power to ingest cell debris and bacteria. It is present in connective tissue, especially when there is inflammation.

macrophthalmia (*mak-roff-thal'-me-ah*). A congenital condition of abnormally large eyes.

macroscopic (*mak-ro-skop'-ik*). Discernible with the naked eye. The opposite of *microscopic*.

macrostomia (*mak-ro-sto'-me-ah*). An abnormal development of the mouth in which the mandibular and maxillary processes do not fuse and the mouth is excessively wide.

macula (*mak'-u-lah*). *pl.* maculae. A spot or discoloured area of the skin, not raised above the surface. A macule. *M. corneae*. A small area of opacity in the cornea, seen through an ophthalmoscope as a deeper red. *M. lutea*. The yellow central area of the retina, where vision is clearest.

maculopapular (*mak-u-lo-pap'-u-lar*). Displaying both maculae and papules. *M. eruption*. A rash comprised of both, as in measles.

Maddox rod test (*E.E. Maddox, British ophthalmologist, 1860–1933*). A test for muscle balance of the eyes using a lens comprised of red glass cylinders. *M. wing test*. A method of measuring the amount of heterophoria.

Madura foot (*mad-u'-rah foot*). Mycetoma of the foot.

Madurella (*mad-u-rel'-ah*). A genus of fungi causing mycetoma.

maduromycosis (*mad-u-ro-mi-ko'-sis*). A chronic disease caused by *Madurella mycetoma*. The commonest form is Madura foot.

Magendie's foramen (*F. Magendie, French physiologist, 1783–1855*). Aperture in the roof of the fourth ventricle of the brain through which cerebrospinal fluid passes into the subarachnoid space.

magnesium (*mag-ne'-ze-um*). *abbrev.* Mg. A bluish-white metallic element. It occurs widely in mineral sources and is present in some of the body tissues. *M. sulphate*. A saline purgative. Epsom salts. *M. trisilicate*. An antacid powder taken after food for dyspepsia and peptic ulceration. *M. carbonate* and *M. hydroxide*. Neutralizing antacids used in hyperacidity.

magnet (*mag'-net*). In ophthalmology, an instrument used for removing metallic foreign bodies that have penetrated the eye.

main (*mahn*). Hand (*Fr.*). *M. en griffe*. A claw-like deformity of the hand.

mal (*mal*). Disease (*Fr.*). *M. de mer*. Sea-sickness. *Grand m.*, *petit m.* Forms of epilepsy.

malabsorption (*mal-ab-sorp'-shun*). Inability of the small intestine to absorb certain substances. It may be the cause of a deficiency disease due to the lack of an essential factor.

malacia (*mal-a'-se-ah*). Softening of tissues. *Osteo-m.* Softening of bone tissue. *Kerato-m.* Softening of the cornea.

maladjustment (*mal-ad-just'-ment*). In psychiatry, a failure to adjust to the environment.

malaise (*mal-aze'*). A feeling of general discomfort and illness.

malar (*ma'-lar*). Relating to the cheek or cheek-bone.

malaria (*mal-air'-e-ah*). A febrile disease caused by a parasite of the genus *Plasmodium* introduced into the blood by mosquitoes of the genus *Anopheles*. The attacks are periodic every 48 to 72 hours according to the type of plasmodium. A typical malarial paroxysm consists of three stages: (1) the shivering fit, (2) high fever, and (3) the sweating stage.

malario-therapy (*mal-air-e-o-*

ther'-ap-e). Form of cure in which a hyperpyrexia is induced by infecting a patient with malaria. Sometimes used in the treatment of neurosyphilis.

malaxation (*mal-aks-a'-shun*). A kneading movement in massage. Pétrissage.

malformation (*mal-form-a'-shun*). Deformity. A structural defect.

malignant (*mal-ig'-nant*). A term applied to any disease of a virulent and fatal nature. *M. pustule*. Anthrax. *M. endocarditis. See* Endocarditis. *M. exophthalmos*. A condition seen in thyrotoxicosis where there is raised intraocular pressure causing pain and the threat of damage to the optic nerve. *M. growth* or *tumour*. A tumour which has the properties of anaplasia, invasion and metastazisation. *M. hypertension. See* Hypertension.

malingering (*mal-ing'-ger-ing*). Shamming illness.

malleolus (*mal-e-o'-lus*). One of the two protuberances on either side of the ankle joint. *Lateral m*. That on the outer surface at the lower end of the fibula. *Medial m*. That on the inner surface at the lower end of the tibia.

malleus (*mal'-e-us*). The hammer-shaped bone in the middle ear.

malnutrition (*mal-nu-trish'-un*). The condition in which nutrition is defective in quantity or quality.

malocclusion (*mal-o-klu'-zhun*). An abnormality of dental development which causes overlapping of the bite.

malpighian body (*M. Malpighi, Italian anatomist, physician and physiologist, 1628–1694*).

The glomerulus and Bowman's capsule of the kidney.

malposition (*mal-po-zi'-shun*). An abnormal position of any part of the body.

malpractice (*mal-prak'-tis*). Failure to maintain accepted ethical standards. Professional misconduct.

malpresentation (*mal-prez-en-ta'-shun*). Any abnormal position of the fetus at birth, which renders delivery difficult or impossible.

malt (*mawlt*). Grain which has been soaked, made to germinate, and dried. It is used as a nutrient in wasting diseases. *M. sugar*. Maltose.

Malta fever (*mawl'-tah fe'-ver*). Brucellosis. Undulant fever.

maltase (*mawl'-taze*). A sugar-splitting enzyme which converts maltose to glucose. Present in pancreatic and intestinal juice.

maltose (*mawl'-toze*). The sugar formed by the action of digestive enzymes on starch.

malunion (*mal-u'-ne-on*). Faulty repair of a fracture.

mamilla (*mam-il'-ah*). A nipple.

mamma (*mam'-ah*). A breast. A milk-secreting gland.

mammary (*mam'-ar-e*). Relating to the breasts.

mammography (*mam-og'-raf-e*). Radiographic or infra-red examination of the breast to detect abnormalities.

mammoplasty (*mam'-o-plas-te*). A plastic operation to reduce the size of abnormally large, pendulous breasts or augment the size of very small breasts.

mammothermography (*mam-o-therm-og'-raf-e*). An examination of the breast that depends on the more active cells producing heat that can be shown on a thermograph, and may indicate abnormalities of the breast tissue.

mandible (*man'-dibl*). The lower jaw-bone.

manganese (*man'-gan-eez*). *abbrev.* Mn. A grey-white metallic element, from the salts of which the permanganates are formed.

mania (*ma'-ne-ah*). Elevation of the mood accompanied by acceleration of thought and action and often by delusions of grandeur.

maniac (*ma'-ne-ak*). Colloquial term for one suffering from a violent or extreme form of insanity.

manic (*man'-ik*). Pertaining to mania. *M.-depressive psychosis.* A mental illness characterized by mania or endogenous depression. The attacks may alternate between mania and depression or the patient may just have recurrent attacks of mania or depression.

manipulation (*man-ip-u-la'-shun*). Use of the hands to produce a desired movement, such as in reducing a fracture or a hernia or changing the position of the fetus. A skilfully applied forced movement upon a joint in order to relocate the joint or increase its range of movements by tearing adhesions round it.

mannerism (*man'-er-izm*). A small action performed without thought, which is characteristic of the individual. Mannerisms assume psychiatric significance when they become exaggerated or excessive and are associated with emotional stress.

mannitol (*man'-it-ol*). A synthetic carbohydrate given intravenously to reduce intracranial pressure by its diuretic action.

manometer (*man-om'-e-ter*). An instrument for measuring the pressure of liquids or gases.

Mantoux test (*C. Mantoux, French physician, 1877–1947*). An intradermal injection of a small amount of tuberculin to determine susceptibility to tuberculosis. If positive, a weal develops in 24 to 48 hours.

manubrium (*man-u'-bre-um*). The upper part of the sternum to which the clavicle is attached.

MAOI. *See* Monoamine oxidase.

maple syrup urine disease (*ma'-pul sir'-up u'-rin diz-eez'*). An inborn error of metabolism in which there is an excess in the urine of certain amino acids. The urine smells like maple syrup and there is mental subnormality, spasticity and convulsions.

marasmus (*mar-az'-mus*). Severe and chronic malnutrition producing a gradual wasting of the tissues, owing to insufficient or unassimilated food, occurring especially in infants. It is not always possible to discover the cause.

marble bone disease (*marbl' bone diz-eez'*). A condition in which there is increased density of bone, which is visible on X-ray. Albers–Schönberg's disease. Osteopetrosis.

Marburg virus (*mar'-berg vi'-rus*). A virus found in Africa which may be transmitted to man from green monkeys. The resulting illness is severe and likely to be fatal, particularly if contracted by Europeans. An outbreak occurred among laboratory workers in Marburg, Germany, in 1967.

Marfan's syndrome (*B.J.A. Marfan, French paediatrician, 1858–1942*). A hereditary disorder in which there is excessive height with very long digits, a high arched palate, hypertonus, and cardiac lesions, the most common of which is atrial septal defect. There is often partial dislocation, usually bilateral, of the lens of the eyes.

marihuana (*mar-e-hwah'-nah*). *Cannabis indica*. Indian hemp or hashish. *See* Cannabis.

marrow (*mar'-o*). (1) The substance contained in the middle of long bones and in the cancellous tissue of all bones. *Red m.* That found in all cancellous tissue at birth. Blood cells are made in it. *Yellow m.* The fatty substance contained in the centre of long bones in later life. *M. puncture.* Investigatory procedure in which marrow cells are aspirated from the sternum or iliac crest. (2) *Spinal m.* The spinal cord.

masculinization (*mas-ku-lin-i-za'-shun*). The development in a woman of male secondary sexual characteristics.

masochism (*mas'-o-kizm*). A sexual perversion in which pleasure is derived from suffering mental or physical pain.

massage (*mas-ahzh'*). A method of rubbing, kneading, and manipulating the body to stimulate circulation, improve metabolism and break down adhesions. *External cardiac m.* The application of rhythmic pressure to the lower sternum to cause expulsion of blood from the ventricles and restart circulation in cases of sudden heart failure.

masseter (*mas-e'-ter*). The muscle of the cheek chiefly concerned in mastication.

masseur (*mas-ur'*). A man who performs massage.

masseuse (*mas-urz'*). A woman who performs massage.

mastalgia (*mast-al'-je-ah*). Pain in the breast.

mastatrophia (*mast-a-tro'-fe-ah*). Atrophy of the breast.

mast cell (*mast sel*). A large connective tissue cell found in many body tissues including the heart, liver and lungs. Most cells contain granules which release heparin, serotonin and histamine in response to inflammation or allergy.

mastectomy (*mas-tek'-tom-e*). Amputation of the breast. *Radical m.* Removal of the breast, axillary lymph glands and the pectoral muscle.

mastication (*mas-tik-a'-shun*). The act of chewing food.

mastitis (*mas-ti'-tis*). Inflammation of the breast, usually due to bacterial infection.

mastodynia (*mas-to-din'-e-ah*). Pain in the breasts, which frequently occurs during the premenstrual phase.

mastoid (*mas'-toid*). Breast-shaped. *M. antrum.* The cavity in the mastoid process which communicates with the middle ear, and contains air. *M. cells.* Hollow spaces in the mastoid bone. *M. operation.* Drainage of mastoid cells when infection spreads from the middle ear. *M. process.* The breast-shaped prominence on the temporal bone which projects downwards behind the ear and into which the sternocleidomastoid muscle is inserted.

mastoidectomy (*mas-toid-ek'-tom-e*). Removal of diseased bone and drainage of the mastoid antrum in severe purulent mastoiditis.

mastoiditis (*mas-toid-i'-tis*). Inflammation of the mastoid antrum and cells.

mastoidotomy (*mas-toid-ot'-om-e*). Surgical opening of the mastoid antrum.

masturbation (*mas-ter-ba'-shun*). The production of sexual excitement by friction of the genitals.

materia medica (*mat-e'-re-ah med'-ik-ah*). The science of the source and preparation of drugs used in medicine.

maternal (*mat-ern'-al*). Pertaining to the mother. *M. mortality rate.* The number of deaths in childbirth per 1000 births.

matrix (*ma'-triks*). (1) That tissue in which cells are embedded. (2) The uterus or womb.

matter (*mat'-er*). Substance. *Grey m.* A collection of nerve cells or non-medullated nerve fibres. *White m.* Medullated nerve fibres massed together, as in the brain.

maturation (*mat-u-ra'-shun*). Ripening or developing.

maxilla (*maks-il'-ah*). *pl.* maxillae. One of the pair of bones forming the upper jaw and carrying the upper teeth.

maxillary (*maks-il'-ar-e*). Pertaining to the upper jaw bones.

maxillectomy (*maks-il-ek'-tom-e*). Surgical removal of a maxilla.

MCHC. Mean corpuscular haemoglobin concentration.

MCV. Mean corpuscular volume.

measles (*meez'-lz*). Morbilli. Rubeola. An acute infectious disease of childhood caused by a virus spread by droplets. Onset is catarrhal before the rash appears at the 4th day.

Koplik's spots are diagnostic earlier. Secondary infection may give rise to the serious complications of otitis media or bronchopneumonia. The severity of the attack may be lessened by giving gamma-globulin between the 5th and 9th days following contact. Vaccination provides a high degree of immunity. *German m. See* Rubella.

meatus (*me-a'-tus*). An opening or passage. *Auditory m.* The opening leading into the auditory canal. *Urethral m.* The opening of the urethra to the exterior.

mecamylamine (*mek-am-il'-am-een*). A ganglion-blocking drug which, given by mouth, causes a marked fall in blood pressure. Used in treating arterial hypertension.

mechanotherapy (*mek-an-o-ther'-ap-e*). The use of mechanical equipment to treat injury or disease.

Meckel's diverticulum (*J.F. Meckel, German anatomist and surgeon, 1781–1833*). The remains of a passage which, in the embryo, connected the yolk sac and intestine, evident as an enclosed sac or tube in the region of the ileum.

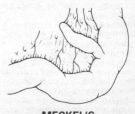

MECKEL'S DIVERTICULUM

meconium (*me-ko'-ne-um*). The first intestinal discharges of a newly born child. Dark green in colour and consisting of epithelial cells, mucus and bile. *M. ileus.* Intestinal obstruction due to blockage of the bowel by a plug of meconium in a neonate with cystic fibrosis.

median (*me'-de-an*). (1) *adj.* Placed in the centre. (2) *n.* In a series of values, the value middle in *position.*

mediastinum (*me-de-as-ti'-num*). The space in the middle of the thorax, between the two pleurae.

medical (*med'-ik-al*). Pertaining to medicine. *M. jurisprudence.* Medical science as applied to aid the law, e.g. in case of death by poisoning, violence, etc. *M. social worker.* A trained hospital worker who looks after the patients' social welfare.

medicament (*med-ik'-am-ent*). Any medicinal substance used in treatment.

medicated (*med'-ik-a-ted*). Impregnated with a medicinal substance.

medication (*med-ik-a'-shun*). (1) A substance administered to a patient for therapeutic purposes. (2) The treatment of a patient by means of drugs.

medicinal (*med-is'-in-al*). (1) Having therapeutic qualities. (2) Pertaining to a medicine.

medicine (*med'-is-in*). (1) A drug or preparation given for the cure of disease. (2) The science of healing by use of internal remedies. *Forensic m.* Medical jurisprudence. *Industrial m.* That concerned with the prevention and treatment of diseases due to manufacturing processes. *Preventive m.* Medical measures taken to prevent disease, e.g. spread of infection. *Proprietary m.* A drug commercially produced and patented as suitable for use in the treatment of diseases. *Psychosomatic m.* The study of the relationship of physical and mental illness. *Social m.* The study of the influences of environment and economic conditions on physical and mental illnesses.

medicochirurgical (*med-ik-o-ki-rur'-jik-al*). Applying to both medicine and surgery.

medico-legal (*med-ik-o-le'-gal*). Relating to forensic medicine.

medico-social (*med-ik-o-so'-shal*). Applying to both medicine and the social factors involved.

medium (*me'-de-um*). In bacteriology, a preparation for the culture of micro-organisms. *Contrast m.* A substance used in radiography to make visible structures which could not otherwise be seen.

medroxyprogesterone (*med-roks-e-pro-jes'-ter-one*). A synthetic female sex hormone used to treat menstrual disorders. Used in combination with oestrogen as a contraceptive.

medulla (*med-ul'-ah*). (1) Bone marrow. (2) The innermost part of an organ, particularly the kidneys, lymph glands and suprarenal glands. *M. oblongata.* That portion of the spinal cord which is contained inside the cranium. In it are the nerve centres which govern respiration, the action of the heart, etc.

medullary (*med-ul'-ar-e*). Pertaining to the marrow or a medulla. *M. cavity.* The hollow in the centre of long bones.

medullated (*med'-ul-a-ted*). Having a myelin covering. *M. nerve fibre.* One enclosed in a myelin sheath.

medulloblastoma (*med-ul-o-blast-o'-mah*). A rapidly growing tumour of neuro-epithelial origin occurring in childhood and appearing near the fourth ventricle of the brain. The tumour is highly radiosensitive.

mefenamic acid (*mef-en-am'-ik as'-id*). An analgesic and antipyretic drug used in the treatment of mild to moderate pain.

megacolon (*meg-ah-ko'-lon*). Extreme dilatation and hypertrophy of the large intestine. When the condition is congenital it is known as Hirschsprung's disease.

megaduodenum (*meg-ah-du-o-de'-num*). A gross enlargement of the duodenum.

megakaryocyte (*meg-ah-kar'-e-o-site*). A large cell of the bone marrow, responsible for blood platelet formation.

megaloblast (*meg'-al-o-blast*). An abnormally large nucleated cell from which mature red blood cells are derived.

megalocephaly (*meg-al-o-kef'-al-e*). (1) Abnormal largeness of the head. (2) Leontiasis ossea.

megalomania (*meg-al-o-ma'-ne-ah*). Delusions of grandeur or self-importance.

mega-ureter (*meg-ah-u-re'-ter*). Dilatation of the ureter.

megrim (*me'-grim*). Migraine.

meibomian glands (*H. Meibom, German anatomist, 1638–1700*). Small sebaceous glands situated beneath the conjunctiva of the eyelid. Tarsal glands. *M. cyst.* A small

swelling of the gland caused by obstruction of its duct. If untreated, it may become infected. A chalazion.

meibomianitis (*mi-bo-me-an-i'-tis*). A bilateral chronic inflammation of the meibomian glands.

Meigs's syndrome (*J.V. Meigs, American surgeon, 1892–1963*). A fibroma or benign solid tumour of the ovary causing ascites and pleural effusion.

meiosis (*mi-o'-sis*). (1) A stage of reduction cell division when the chromosomes are halved in number ready for union at fertilization. (2) Contraction of the pupil of the eye. Miosis.

Meissner's plexus (*G. Meissner, German anatomist and physiologist, 1829–1905*). The submucous plexus. A network of autonomic nerve fibres in the wall of the intestines.

melaena (*mel-e'-nah*). The discharge of black faeces stained with blood which has undergone change after haemorrhage into the alimentary tract.

melancholia (*mel-an-ko'-le-ah*). A state of extreme depression. *See* Depression.

melanin (*mel'-an-in*). A dark pigment found in the hair, the choroid coat of the eye, the skin and in melanotic tumours.

melanism (*mel'-an-izm*). A condition marked by an abnormal deposit of dark pigment in the skin or other tissue. Melanosis.

melanocyte (*mel'-an-o-site*). A cell responsible for the formation of the skin pigment melanin. *M.-stimulating hormone.* MSH. Hormone produced in the pituitary gland which stimulates the formation of melanin, causing the skin to darken.

melanoderma (*mel-an-o-der'-mah*). A patchy pigmentation of the skin.

melanoma (*mel-an-o'-mah*). A malignant tumour arising in any pigment-containing tissues, especially the skin and the eye. *Amelanotic m.* An unpigmented malignant melanoma. *Juvenile m.* A benign lesion which usually occurs on the face before puberty. May be mistaken for a malignant melanoma.

melanosis (*mel-an-o'-sis*). *See* Melanism.

melanotic (*mel-an-ot'-ik*). Pertaining to melanosis. *M. sarcoma. See* Sarcoma.

melanuria (*mel-an-u'-re-ah*). The presence of black pigment in the urine. Occurs in melanotic sarcoma and porphyria.

melasma (*mel-az'-mah*). Dark discoloration of the skin. Chloasma.

melomelus (*mel-om'-el-us*). A fetus with normal limbs and additional rudimentary limbs.

melphalan (*mel'-fal-an*). A cytotoxic drug which is particularly useful in the treatment of multiple myeloma.

membrane (*mem'-brane*). A thin elastic tissue covering the surface of certain organs and lining the cavities of the body. *Basement m.* The delicate layer of cells beneath the surface cells of mucous membrane. *Mucous m.* A membrane that secretes mucus and lines all cavities connected directly or indirectly with the skin. *Serous m.* Membrane lining the abdominal cavity and thorax and covering most of the organs within.

menaphthone (*men-af'-thone*). A synthetic preparation of vitamin K. Menadione.

menarche (*men-ar'-ke*). The first appearance of menstruation.

Mendelson's syndrome (*C.L. Mendelson, American obstetrician*). A condition in which there is severe oedema and spasm of the bronchioles due to the inhalation of acid gastric contents.

Mendel's theory (*G.J. Mendel, Austrian monk, 1822–1884*). A theory that the offspring do not inherit the characteristics of the parents in equal proportion, but that some characteristics are *dominant* while others are *recessive,* and that the dominant ones are transmitted from parents to children in full measure.

Menière's disease or **syndrome** (*P. Menière, French physician, 1799–1862*). A disease of the inner ear causing attacks of vertigo and tinnitus with progressive deafness.

meningeal (*men-in-je'-al*). Relating to the meninges.

meninges (*men-in'-jeez*). The membranes covering the brain and spinal cord. There are three: the dura mater (outer), arachnoid mater (middle) and pia mater (inner).

meningioma (*men-in-je-o'-mah*). A slow-growing, usually benign tumour developing from the arachnoid and pia mater.

meningism (*men'-in-jizm*). A condition in which there are signs of cerebral irritation similar to meningitis but where no causative organism can be isolated.

meningitis (*men-in-ji'-tis*). Inflammation of the meninges due to viral or bacterial infection. *Meningococcal m.* Cerebrospinal fever. An epidemic form with a rapid onset caused by infection by *Neisseria meningitidis. Tuberculous m.* Inflammation of tuberculous origin. Once always fatal, it now responds to medical treatment.

meningocele (*men-ing'-go-seel*). A protrusion of the meninges through the skull or spinal column, appearing as a cyst filled with cerebrospinal fluid. *See* Spina bifida.

meningococcus (*men-ing-go-kok'-us*). *Neisseria meningitidis.* A diplococcus, the micro-organism of cerebrospinal meningitis.

meningoencephalitis (*mening-go-en-kef-al-i'-tis*). Inflammation of the brain and meninges.

meningomyelocele (*men-ing-go-mi'-el-o-seel*). A protrusion of the spinal cord and meninges through a defect in the vertebral column. Myelomeningocele. *See* Spina bifida.

meniscectomy (*men-is-ek'-tom-e*). Surgical removal of a cartilage in a knee-joint.

meniscus (*men-is'-kus*). (1) The convex or concave surface of a liquid as observed in its container. (2) A lens having one convex and one concave surface. (3) A semilunar cartilage of the knee-joint.

menopause (*men'-o-pawz*). The normal cessation of menstruation, usually occurring between the 45th and 50th year of life. Ovulation ceases and there is an associated hormonal imbalance which may cause symptoms such as night sweats, hot flushes and irritability. *Artificial m.* An in-duced cessation by surgery or by irradiation.

menorrhagia (*men-or-aj'-e-ah*). An excessive flow of the menses. Menorrhoea.

menses (*men'-seez*). The discharge from the uterus during menstruation.

menstrual (*men'-stru-al*). Relating to the menses. *M. cycle.* The monthly cycle commencing with the first day of menstruation, when the endometrium is shed, through a process of repair and hypertrophy till the next period. It is governed by the anterior pituitary gland and the ovarian hormones, oestrogens, and progesterone.

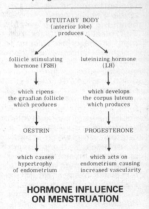

HORMONE INFLUENCE ON MENSTRUATION

menstruation (*men-stru-a'-shun*). The monthly discharge of blood and endometrium from the uterus, starting at the age of puberty and lasting until the menopause. *Vicarious m.* Discharge of blood at the time of menstruation from some organ other than the uterus, e.g. epistaxis, which is not uncommon.

mental (*men'-tal*). (1) Pertaining to the mind. *M. age.* The measurement of the intelligence level of an individual in terms of the average chronological age of children showing the same mental standard, as measured by a scale of mental tests. *M. disorder.* A term defined by the Mental Health Act 1983 to cover all forms of mental illness and disability, including mental impairment and psychopathic disorder. *M. handicap.* Arrested or incomplete development of mind in which the patient does not require compulsory detention. *M. illness.* A term used to describe a number of disorders of the mind which affect the emotions, perceptions, reasoning or memory of the individual, e.g. psychoses and neuroses. *M. impairment.* Arrested or incomplete development of mind associated with abnormally aggressive or socially irresponsible conduct. If the patient is considered treatable, he may be compulsorily admitted to hospital. *M. mechanism.* Any unconscious process which protects the individual against outside threats or internal anxiety-arousing impulses by distorting reality in some way. *M. subnormality.* A condition of arrested or incomplete development of the mind. The term has been superseded by mental handicap and mental impairment. *M. Health Review Tribunal.* A board to whom persons detained under compulsory admission orders or taken into guardianship have the right of appeal at stated intervals. *M. Health Welfare Officer.* A social worker who carries out the requirements of the Mental Health Act. (2) Pertaining to the chin.

mentha (*men'-thah*). Mint. *M. piperata.* Peppermint oil.

menthol (*men'-thol*). A crystalline substance derived from oil of peppermint and used in neuralgia and rhinitis, as a local anodyne and antiseptic.

mepacrine (*mep'-ah-kreen*). A synthetic drug used as an antimalarial agent and in the treatment of giardiasis.

mephenesin (*mef-en'-ez-in*). A muscle relaxant used in the treatment of parkinsonism, chorea and athetosis.

mephitic (*mef-it'-ik*). Producing an offensive smell.

meprobamate (*mep-ro-bam'-ate*). A tranquillizer used in the treatment of nervous anxiety.

mepyramine (*mep-ir'-am-een*). An antihistamine drug used in the treatment of allergic reactions.

mercaptopurine (*mer-kap-to-pu'-reen*). A drug which prevents nucleic acid synthesis and may be used in the treatment of some types of leukaemia.

mercurialism (*mer-ku'-re-al-izm*). Chronic poisoning due to absorption of mercury.

mercury (*mer'-ku-re*). *abbrev.* Hg. Quicksilver. A heavy liquid metallic element, the salts of which are used occasionally as antiseptics and disinfectants. *M.-vapour lamp.* One in which air is exhausted from the tube and replaced by mercury vapour, through which passes a strong electric current, resulting in a powerful ultra-violet light. Quartz glass permits the ultra-violet rays to pass through.

mersalyl (*mer'-sal-il*). A mercurial diuretic which prevents reabsorption of water in the renal tubules, so reducing oedema in heart failure and renal insufficiency.

mesarteritis (*mes-ar-ter-i'-tis*). Inflammation of the middle coat of an artery.

mescaline (*mes'-kal-een*). An alkaloid drug which produces intoxication and hallucinations. It is a drug of addiction.

mesencephalon (*mes-en-kef'-al-on*). The middle brain.

mesenchyme (*mes'-en-kime*). In the embryo, the connective tissue developed from the mesoderm.

mesenteric (*mes-en-ter'-ik*). Pertaining to the mesentery.

mesentery (*mes'-en-ter-e*). A fold of the peritoneum which connects the intestine to the posterior abdominal wall.

mesmerism (*F.A. Mesmer, Austrian physician, 1734–1815*). Hypnotism.

mesocolon (*mes-o-ko'-lon*). A fold of the peritoneum which connects the colon with the posterior abdominal wall.

mesoderm (*mes'-o-derm*). The middle of the three primary layers of cells in the embryo from which the connective tissues develop.

mesometrium (*mes-o-me'-tre-um*). The broad ligament connecting the uterus with the abdominal wall.

mesomorph (*mes'-o-morf*). A stocky individual of medium height with well developed muscles.

mesonephros (*mes-o-nef'-ros*). Woolfian body. One of two small organs in the embryo representing the primitive kidneys.

mesosalpinx (*mes-o-sal'-pinks*). That part of the broad ligament which surrounds the uterine tubes.

mesothelioma (*mes-o-the-le-o'-mah*). A rapidly growing tumour of the pleura, peritoneum or pericardium which may be seen in patients with asbestosis. However, this tumour may also occur in people who have no history of exposure to asbestos.

mesovarium (*mes-o-var'-e-um*). A fold of peritoneum connecting the ovary to the broad ligament.

messenger RNA (*mes'-en-jer*). mRNA. The ribonucleic acid which acts as a template for the linking of amino acids during the formation of protein in the cells.

mestranol (*mes'-tran-ol*). A synthetic oestrogen commonly used in combination with a progesterone in contraceptive pills.

metabolic (*met-ah-bol'-ik*). Referring to metabolism.

metabolism (*met-ab'-ol-izm*). The use of foods by the body following digestion, absorption and circulation to the body cells. Ingested foods are used both as an energy source and, after being broken down chemically during digestion, as basic materials for making complex chemical compounds required by the body. *Catabolism* covers all reactions which release energy from foods. *Anabolism* covers all reactions which use foods as basic materials for making complex chemical compounds.

metabolite (*met-ab'-o-lite*). Any product or substance taking part in metabolism. *Essential m.* A substance that is necessary for normal metabolism, e.g. a vitamin.

metacarpal (*met-ah-kar'-pal*). One of the five bones of the hand which join the fingers to the wrist.

metacarpophalangeal (*met-ah-kar-po-fal-an'-je-al*). Relating to the metacarpal bones and the phalanges.

metacarpus (*met-ah-kar'-pus*). The five bones of the hand uniting the carpus with the phalanges of the fingers.

metamorphosis (*met-ah-mor-fo'-sis*). A structural change or transformation.

metaphase (*met'-ah-faze*). The second stage of mitosis or cell division.

metaphysis (*met-af'-is-is*). The junction of the epiphysis with the diaphysis in a long bone.

metaplasia (*met-ah-pla'-ze-ah*). Abnormal change in the structure of a tissue. May be indicative of malignant change.

metastasis (*me-tas'-tas-is*). The transfer of a disease from one part of the body to another, through the blood vessels, via the lymph channels or across the body cavities. (1) Secondary deposits may occur from a primary malignant growth. (2) Septic infection may arise in other organs from some original focus.

metatarsal (*met-ah-tar'-sal*). One of the five bones of the foot which join the tarsus to the toes.

metatarsalgia (*met-ah-tar-sal'-je-ah*). Pain in the metatarsal bones.

metatarsus (*met-ah-tar'-sus*). The five bones of the foot uniting the tarsus with the

phalanges of the toes.

Metazoa (*met-ah-zo'-ah*). All multi-cellular animals, i.e. all animals except the Protozoa.

meteorism (*me'-te-or-izm*). Distension of the intestines with gas. Tympanites.

methadone (*meth'-ad-one*). A powerful analgesic with no sedative action. Similar in action to morphine, it is used to relieve pain in terminal illness. Amidone.

methaemalbumin (*met-he-mal-bu'-min*). A compound of haem with plasma albumin found in the blood in some types of anaemia.

methaemoglobin (*met-he-mo-glo'-bin*). An altered form of haemoglobin found in the blood and usually produced by the action of a drug on the red blood corpuscles. Commonly caused by phenacetin and other aniline derivatives.

methaemoglobinaemia (*met-he-mo-glo-bin-e'-me-ah*). Cyanosis and inability of the red blood cells to transport oxygen due to the presence of methaemoglobin.

methandienone (*meth-an-di'-en-one*). An anabolic steroid used to build up body tissues in wasting diseases.

methane (*me'-thane*). Marsh gas. An important constituent of coal gas.

methanol (*meth'-an-ol*). Methyl alcohol.

methicillin (*meth-is-il'-in*). A form of penicillin that is resistant to staphylococcal penicillinase.

methimazole (*meth-im'-az-ole*). A powerful drug used in the treatment of thyrotoxicosis.

methionine (*meth-i'-o-neen*). An essential amino acid containing sulphur; it is necessary for fat metabolism.

methohexitone (*meth-o-heks'-it-one*). A barbiturate anaesthetic agent. Given intravenously it has a quick recovery time.

methotrexate (*meth-o-treks'-ate*). A cytotoxic drug that antagonizes folic acid and prevents cell formation. It is used to treat various types of malignant disease.

methyl alcohol (*meth'-il al'-ko-hol*). Wood alcohol. Methanol. A poisonous form of alcohol which can damage the eyes and cause blindness. It can also cause acidosis.

methylamphetamine (*meth-il-am-fet'-am-een*). A synthetic drug which stimulates the central nervous system and raises the blood pressure. Its usage can be habit forming.

methylated spirit (*meth'-il-a-ted spir'-it*). A mixture of 95% ethyl alcohol and 5% methyl alcohol. An industrial spirit which, taken as a drink, is poisonous.

methylcellulose (*meth-il-sel'-u-loze*). A bulk-forming drug used as a laxative and to control diarrhoea.

methyldopa (*meth-il-do'-pah*). A hypotensive drug whose action is increased if used with thiazide diuretics. Used to treat hypertension.

methylene blue (*meth'-il-een bloo*). An aniline dye. Used to test renal function and to stain bacterial cells for microscopic examination.

methylpentynol (*meth-il-pen'-tin-ol*). A sedative and tranquillizing drug which allays apprehension and may be used before operation or other procedures that might cause the patient discomfort.

methylphenidate (*meth-il-fen'-e-date*). An antidepressant drug that stimulates the central nervous system.

methyl salicylate (*meth'-il sal-is'-il-ate*). A compound used externally for rheumatic pains, lumbago, etc. Oil of wintergreen.

metoclopramide (*met-o-klo'-pram-ide*). A drug which speeds up gastric action and is used to treat nausea, heartburn and vomiting.

metra (*me'-trah*). The uterus.

metralgia (*me-tral'-je-ah*). Pain in the uterus.

metre (*me'-ter*). *abbrev.* m. The fundamental SI unit of length.

metritis (*me-tri'-tis*). Inflammation of the uterus.

metrocolpocele (*me-tro-kol'-po-seel*). The protrusion of the uterus into the vagina, the wall of the latter being pushed forward also.

metrodynia (*me-tro-din'-e-ah*). Pain in the uterus.

metronidazole (*me-tron-id'-azole*). A drug that is effective in overcoming *Trichomonas* infection of the genital tract of both sexes. Also used in the treatment of giardiasis, of acute amoebic dysentery and of infection by anaerobic bacteria.

metropathia (*me-tro-path'-e-ah*). Any disorder affecting the uterus. Metropathy. *M. haemorrhagica.* Excessive loss of blood from the uterus due to disease. Uterine haemorrhage.

metroptosis (*me-trop-to'-sis*). Prolapse of the uterus.

metrorrhagia (*me-tror-aj'-e-ah*). Irregular bleeding from the uterus not associated with menstruation.

metrostaxis (*me-tro-staks'-is*). Persistent slight haemorrhage from the uterus.

Mg. Chemical symbol for *magnesium*.

Michel's suture clips (*G. Michel, French surgeon, 1875 –1937*). Small metal clips used for suturing wounds.

microbe (*mi'-krobe*). A minute living organism, especially one causing disease. A microorganism.

microbiology (*mi-kro-bi-ol'-o-je*). The study of microorganisms and their effect on living cells.

microcephalic (*mi-kro-kef-al'-ik*). Having an abnormally small head.

Micrococcus (*mi-kro-kok'-us*). A genus of bacteria, each of which has a spherical shape. They occur in pairs or in groups and are gram-positive.

microcornea (*mi-kro-kor'-ne-ah*). A condition in which the cornea is smaller than normal, producing hypermetropia and sometimes causing glaucoma.

microcythaemia (*mi-kro-si-the'-me-ah*). The presence of abnormally small red cells in the blood. Microcytosis.

microdissection (*mi-kro-dis-ek'-shun*). The dissection of minute structures with the aid of a microscope.

micrognathia (*mi-kro-nath'-e-ah*). Failure of development of the lower jaw, causing a receding chin.

microgram (*mi'-kro-gram*). *abbrev.* μg. One millionth of a gram.

micrograph (*mi'-kro-graf*). A photograph taken through a microscope. *Electron m.* A photograph taken through an electron microscope.

micromastia (*mi-kro-mas'-te-ah*). The condition of exceptional smallness of the breasts.

micrometer (*mi-krom'-e-ter*). An instrument for the precise measurement of small objects.

micron (*mi'-kron*). *abbrev.* μm. One millionth of a metre, i.e. a micrometre.

micro-organism (*mi-kro-or'-gan-izm*). A minute animal or vegetable, particularly a virus, a bacterium, a fungus, a rickettsia or a protozoon.

microphage (*mi'-kro-faje*). A minute phagocyte.

microphthalmos (*mi-kroff-thal'-mos*). A condition in which one or both eyes are smaller than normal. Their function may or may not be impaired.

micropsia (*mi-krop'-ze-ah*). A condition in which objects appear abnormally small.

microscope (*mi'-kro-skope*). An instrument which produces a greatly enlarged image of objects that are normally invisible to the human eye. *Electron m.* A microscope in which a beam of electrons is used instead of a light beam, allowing magnification of as much as 500,000 diameters.

microscopic (*mi-kro-skop'-ik*). Visible only by means of the microscope.

Microsporum (*mi-kro-spor'-um*). A genus of fungi. The cause of some skin diseases, especially ringworm.

microsurgery (*mi-kro-ser'-jer-e*). The carrying out of surgical procedures using a microscope and miniature instruments.

microtome (*mi'-kro-tome*). An instrument for cutting exceedingly thin sections for examination through a microscope.

micturition (*mik-tu-rish'-un*). The act of passing urine.

midbrain (*mid'-brane*). That portion of the brain which connects the cerebrum with the pons and cerebellum. The mesencephalon.

midriff (*mid'-rif*). The diaphragm.

midwife (*mid'-wife*). A person who has been trained and has qualified to attend women in labour.

midwifery (*mid-wif'-er-e*). Obstetrics.

migraine (*me'-grane*). Paroxysmal attacks of severe headache, often with nausea, vomiting and visual disturbance.

milestone (*mile'-stone*). One of the 'norms' against which the motor, social and psychological development of a child is measured.

miliaria (*mil-e-a'-re-ah*). Prickly heat, an acute itching eruption common among white people in tropical and subtropical areas.

miliary (*mil'-e-ar-e*). Resembling millet seed. *M. tuberculosis.* See Tuberculosis.

milk (*milk*). The secretion of mammary glands.

Composition of milk (%):

	Cows' milk	Human milk
Protein	3.5	2.0
Fats	3.5	3.5
Carbo-hydrates	4.0	6.0
Mineral salts	0.7	0.2
Water	88.0	88.0

The milk now generally supplied throughout the United Kingdom is known as *certified milk*. It may be: (1) *tuberculin tested milk*, from herds regularly tested and shown to be free from tuberculosis; (2) *pasteurized milk*, which has been heated to 72°C and then cooled; and (3) *sterilized milk*, which has been heated to and kept for 15 minutes at 100°C. *M. sugar.* Lactose, a disaccharide present in the milk of all mammals. *M. teeth.* The first set of teeth. *Witch's m.* Milk secreted from the breasts of a newborn child.

Miller–Abbott tube (*T.G. Miller, American physician, b. 1886; W.O. Abbott, American physician, 1902–1943*). A double-channel intestinal tube for treating obstruction—especially that due to *paralytic ileus* of the small intestine. It has an inflatable balloon at its distal end.

milliampere (*mil-e-am'-pair*). *abbrev.* mA. One thousandth of an ampere.

milliequivalent (*mil-e-ek-wiv'-al-ent*). *abbrev.* mEq *or* m-equiv. The amount of a substance that balances or is equivalent in combining power to 1 mg of hydrogen. A method of assessing the body's acid–base balance or needs during electrolyte upset.

milligram (*mil'-e-gram*). *abbrev.* mg. One thousandth of a gram.

millilitre (*mil'-e-le-ter*). *abbrev.* ml. One thousandth of a litre (one cubic centimetre).

millimetre (*mil'-e-me-ter*). *abbrev.* mm. One thousandth of a metre.

Milroy's disease (*W.F. Milroy, American physician, 1855–1942*). A disease in which there is a congenital obstruction of the lymph channels in the legs.

mineralocorticoid (*min-er-al-o-kor'-te-koid*). A hormone produced by the adrenal cortex. Its function is to maintain the salt and water balance in the body.

miosis (*mi-o'-sis*). Contraction of the pupil of the eye, as in reaction to a bright light. Meiosis.

miotic (*mi-ot'-ik*). A drug which causes contraction of the pupil.

miscarriage (*mis-kar'-ij*). Abortion. The expulsion of the fetus before the 28th week of pregnancy, i.e. before it is legally viable.

miscegenation (*mis-ej-en-a'-shun*). Marriage or breeding between different races.

misogynist (*mis-oj'-in-ist*). A man who has a hatred of women.

mite (*mite*). A minute animal, frequently parasitic on man and animals, and causing various forms of dermatitis.

mithramycin (*mith-rah-mi'-sin*). An antitumour antibiotic which is particularly helpful in the treatment of hypercalcaemia.

mitochondrion (*mi-to-kon'-dre-on*). *pl.* mitochondria. A body which occurs in the cytoplasm of cells and is concerned with energy production and the oxidation of food.

mitosis (*mi-to'-sis*). A method of multiplication of cells by a specific process of division.

mitral (*mi'-tral*). Shaped like a mitre. *M. incompetence.* The result of a defective mitral valve, when there is a back flow or regurgitation following closure of the valve. *M. stenosis.* The formation of fibrous tissue, causing a narrowing of the valve; usually due to rheumatic heart disease and endocarditis. *M. valve.* The bicuspid valve between the left atrium and left ventricle of the heart. *M. valvotomy.* An operation for overcoming stenosis by dividing the fibrous tissue to free the cusps.

mittelschmerz (*mit'-el-shmertz*). Pain occurring in the period between the menses, accompanying ovulation.

Mn. Chemical symbol for *manganese*.

mobilization (*mo-bil-i-za'-shun*). The bringing back into mobility of a limb by carefully applied pressure on a joint.

modiolus (*mo-de'-o-lus*). The central pillar of the cochlea of the inner ear around which the bony labyrinth winds.

molar (*mo'-lar*). (1) *n.* A back tooth used for grinding. There are three on either side of each jaw, making twelve in all (only eight in children). (2) *adj.* In chemistry, referring to moles. *M. solution.* One containing 1 mole of dissolved substance per litre.

molarity (*mo-lar'-it-e*). The concentration of a fluid expressed in moles.

mole (*mole*). (1) The molecular weight of a substance expressed in grams. (2) A pigmented naevus or dark-coloured growth on the skin. Moles are of various sizes, and are sometimes covered with hair. (3) A uterine tumour. *Carneous m.* An organized blood clot surrounding a shrivelled fetus in the uterus. *Hydatidiform m.* (*vesicular m.*). A condition in pregnancy in which the chorionic villi of the placenta degenerate into clusters of cysts like hydatids. Malignant growth is very likely to follow if any remnants are left in the uterus. *See* Chorion epithelioma.

molecular (*mol-ek'-u-lar*). Pertaining to or composed of molecules. *M. weight.* The weight of a molecule of a substance compared with that of an atom of carbon.

molecule (*mol'-e-kule*). The chemical combination of two or more atoms which form a specific chemical substance, e.g. H_2O (water). The smallest amount of a substance that can exist independently.

molluscum (*mol-us'-kum*). A skin disease characterized by the development of soft round tumours. *M. contagiosum.* A benign tumour arising in the epidermis caused by a virus, transmitted by direct contact or fomites.

monarticular (*mon-ar-tik'-u-lah*). Referring to one joint only.

Mönckeberg's sclerosis (*J.G. Mönckeberg, German pathologist, 1877–1925*). Extensive degeneration of the arteries, with atrophy and calcareous deposits in the middle muscle coats. Mainly affects small and middle sized arteries.

mongolism (*mon'-gol-izm*). Down's syndrome. A type of congenital mental subnormality. Associated with an extra chromosome. There is retarded mental and physical growth with characteristic facial appearance somewhat resembling that of the Mongolian races.

Monilia (*mon-il'-e-ah*). Former name for the genus of fungi now known as *Candida*.

monitoring (*mon'-it-or-ing*). Recording. *Patient m.* The use of electrodes or transducers attached to the patient so that information such as temperature, pulse, respiration, and blood pressure can be seen

on a screen or automatically recorded. Much used in Intensive Care Units.

monoamine oxidase (*mon-o-am'-een oks'-e-daze*). An enzyme that breaks down noradrenaline and serotonin in the body. *M. o. inhibitor.* MAOI. A drug that prevents the breakdown of serotonin and leads to an increase in mental and physical activity.

monochromatism (*mon-o-kro'-mat-izm*). Colourblindness. The patient sees all colours as black, grey or white.

monoclonal (*mon-o-klo'-nal*). Derived from a single cell. *M. antibodies.* Antibodies derived from a single clone of cells. All the antibody molecules are identical and will react with the same antigenic site.

monocular (*mon-ok'-u-lar*). Pertaining to, or affecting, one eye only.

monocyte (*mon'-o-site*). A white blood cell having one nucleus, derived from the reticular cells, and having a phagocytic action.

monocytosis (*mon-o-si-to'-sis*). Mononucleosis.

mononucleosis (*mon-o-nu-kle-o'-sis*). An excessive number of monocytes in the blood. Monocytosis. *Infective m.* An infectious disease due to the Epstein-Barr virus. Glandular fever.

monophasia (*mon-o-fa'-ze-ah*). Aphasia in which speech is limited to one word or phrase.

monoplegia (*mon-o-ple'-je-ah*). Paralysis of one limb or of a single muscle or a group of muscles.

monorchid (*mon-or'-kid*). An individual with only one testicle in the scrotum.

monosaccharide (*mon-o-sak'-ar-ide*). A simple sugar. The end result of carbohydrate digestion. Examples are glucose, fructose and galactose.

monosomy (*mon-o-so'-me*). A congenital defect in the number of human chromosomes. There is one less than the normal 46.

Monro's foramen (*A. Monro, British anatomist and surgeon, 1733–1817*). The communication between the lateral and third ventricles of the brain.

mons (*monz*). A prominence or mound. *M. pubis* or *m. veneris*. The eminence, consisting of a pad of fat, which lies over the pubic symphysis in the female.

monster (*mon'-ster*). A grossly malformed fetus.

Montgomery's glands or **tubercles** (*W.F. Montgomery, Irish obstetrician, 1797–1859*). Sebaceous glands around the nipple, which grow larger during pregnancy.

mood (*mood*). Emotional reaction. Variations in mood are natural, but in certain psychiatric conditions there is severe depression in some cases and wild excitement in others, or alternations between both.

moon face (*moon fase*). One of the features occurring in Cushing's syndrome and as a result of prolonged treatment with steroid drugs.

Mooren's ulcer (*A. Mooren, German ophthalmologist, 1829–1899*). A rare basal cell carcinoma of the cornea. The cause is unknown.

morbid (*mor'-bid*). Diseased, or relating to an abnormal or disordered condition.

morbidity (*mor-bid'-it-e*). The state of being diseased. *M. rate.* A figure that shows the susceptibility of a population to a certain disease. Usually shown statistically as the number of cases which occur annually per thousand or other unit of population.

morbilli (*mor-bil'-e*). Measles.

morbilliform (*mor-bil'-e-form*). Resembling measles.

morbus (*mor'-bus*). A disease. *M. caducus.* Epilepsy. *M. cordis.* Heart disease. *M. coxarius.* Coccydynia. *M. maculosus neonatorum.* Haemorrhagic disease of the newborn.

Morgagni, hydatid of (*G.B. Morgagni, Italian anatomist and pathologist, 1682–1771*). A small congenital cyst which may be present at the fimbriated end of the uterine tube in the female and in the epididymis in the male.

moribund (*mor'-ib-und*). In a dying condition.

Morison's pouch (*J.B. Morison, British surgeon, 1853–1939*). A fold of the peritoneum below the liver.

morning sickness (*mor'-ning sik'-nes*). Nausea and vomiting which occurs in early pregnancy.

moron (*mor'-on*). An obsolete term for a person suffering from a mild degree of mental subnormality.

Moro reflex (*E. Moro, German paediatrician, 1874–1951*). The reaction to loud noise or sudden movement which should be present in the newborn. Startle reflex.

morphine (*mor'-feen*). The principal alkaloid obtained from opium, and given mainly to relieve severe pain. It is a drug of addiction. Morphia.

morphology (*mor-fol'-o-je*). The study of the structure of organisms.

mortality (*mor-tal'-it-e*). The state of being liable to die. *M. rate.* The number of deaths per 1000 occurring annually from a certain disease or condition.

mortification (*mor-tif-ik-a'-shun*). Gangrene or death of tissue. Necrosis.

morula (*mor'-u-lah*). An early stage of development of the ovum when it is a solid mass of cells.

mosaic (*mo-za'-ik*). An individual who has cells of varying genetic composition.

motile (*mo'-tile*). Capable of movement.

motility (*mo-til'-it-e*). The ability of something to move spontaneously.

motion (*mo'-shun*). (1) The process of moving. (2) Evacuation of the bowels. Defecation. *M. sickness.* Sickness occurring as the result of travel by land, sea or air. Appears to be caused by excessive stimulation of the vestibular apparatus within the inner ear.

motivate (*mo'-tiv-ate*). To provide an incentive or purpose for a course of action.

motivation (*mo-tiv-a'-shun*). The reason or reasons, conscious or unconscious, behind a particular attitude or behaviour.

motive (*mo'-tiv*). The incentive that determines a course of action or its direction.

motor (*mo'-tor*). Something that causes movement. *M. end-plate.* The nuclei and cytoplasm of muscle fibres at the termination of motor nerves. *M. nerve.* One of the nerves which convey an impulse from a nerve centre to a muscle or gland to promote activity. *M. neuron disease.* A disease in which there is progressive degeneration of the anterior cells in the spinal cord, the motor nuclei of cranial nerves and the corticospinal tracts. The cause is unknown.

mould (*mo-ld*). (1) A species of fungus. (2) The plastic shell used to immobilize a part of the body, usually the head, during radiotherapy.

moulding (*mo'-ld-ing*). The alteration in shape of the infant's head as it is forced through the maternal passages during labour.

mountain sickness (*mown'-tain sik'-nes*). Dyspnoea, headache, rapid pulse and vomiting, which occur on sudden change to the rarefied air of high altitudes.

mouth (*mowth*). An opening, particularly the external opening in the face of the alimentary canal. *M.-wash.* A solution for rinsing the mouth.

mucilage (*mu'-sil-aj*). A solution of gum and water used in pharmacy when administering insoluble substances.

mucin (*mu'-sin*). The chief constituent of mucus.

mucocele (*mu'-ko-seel*). A mucous tumour. *M. of the gall-bladder* occurs if a stone obstructs the cystic duct. *Lacrimal m.* A distension of the lacrimal sac caused by a blockage of the nasolacrimal duct.

mucocutaneous (*mu-ko-ku-ta'-ne-us*). Pertaining to mucous membrane and skin.

mucoid (*mu'-koid*). Resembling mucus.

mucolytic (*mu-ko-lit'-ik*). A drug that has a mucous softening effect and so re-

mucopurulent (*mu-ko-pu'-ru-lent*). Containing mucus and pus.

mucosa (*mu-ko'-sah*). Mucous membrane.

mucous (*mu'-kus*). Pertaining to or secreting mucus. *M. membrane.* A membrane that secretes mucus and lines many of the body cavities, particularly those of the respiratory and alimentary tracts.

mucoviscidosis (*mu-ko-vis-id-o'-sis*). Fibrocystic disease of the pancreas. *See* Fibrocystic.

mucus (*mu'-kus*). The viscous secretion of mucous membrane.

müllerian duct (*J.P. Müller, German physiologist, 1801–1858*). One of a pair of ducts in the female fetus that develops into the uterine tube, uterus and vagina. Paramesonephric duct.

multicellular (*mul-te-sel'-u-lar*). Consisting of many cells.

multigravida (*mul-te-grav'-id-ah*). A pregnant woman who has had two or more pregnancies.

multilocular (*mul-te-lok'-u-lah*). Having many locules. *M. cyst.* A cyst, usually in the ovary, containing many compartments.

multinuclear (*mul-te-nu'-kle-ah*). Possessing many nuclei.

multipara (*mul-tip'-ar-ah*). A woman who has had two or more children.

multiple (*mul'-tipl*). Of diseases, one affecting many parts of the body. *M. myeloma.* Malignant disease of the plasma cells which invade the bone marrow and suppress its functioning. *M. sclerosis.* *See* Sclerosis.

mumps (*mumps*). Epidemic parotitis. A contagious disease common amongst children, and characterized by inflammation and swelling of the parotid glands. The symptoms are fever, and a painful swelling in front of the ears, making mastication difficult.

Munchausen's syndrome (*Baron von Munchausen, 16th Century German traveller noted for his lying tales*). A mental condition in which the patient goes from hospital to hospital seeking treatment for imaginary diseases.

murmur (*mer'-mer*). A sound, heard on auscultation, usually originating in the cardiovascular system. *Aortic m.* One indicating disease of the aortic valve. *Diastolic m.* One heard after the second heart sound. *Friction m.* One present when two inflamed surfaces of serous membrane rub on each other. *Mitral m.* A sign of incompetence of the mitral valve. *Systolic m.* One heard during systole.

Murphy's sign (*J.B. Murphy, American surgeon, 1857–1916*). A sign denoting inflammation of the gallbladder. Continuous pressure over the organ will cause the patient to 'catch' his breath at the zenith of inspiration.

Musca (*mus'-kah*). A genus of flies. *M. domestica.* The common house fly.

muscae volitantes (*mus'-ke vol-e-tan'-tes*). Floating bodies in the vitreous humour which can be seen through an ophthalmoscope and are visible to the patient as black spots floating before the eyes. They do not obscure the sight.

muscarine (*mus'-kar-een*). A poisonous alkaloid found in certain fungi, and causing muscle paralysis.

muscle (*mus'-l*). Strong tissue composed of fibres which have the power of contraction, and thus produce movements of the body. *Cardiac m.* Muscle composed of partially striped interlocking cells. Not under the control of the will. *Striped* or *striated m.* Voluntary muscle. Transverse bands across the fibres give the characteristic appearance. It is under the control of the will. *Smooth* or *non-striated m.* Involuntary muscle of spindle-shaped cells, e.g. that of the intestinal wall. Contracts independently of the will. *M. relaxant.* One of a group of drugs used to reduce muscular spasm and also to relax the muscles during surgery.

muscular (*mus'-ku-lar*). (1) Pertaining to muscle. (2) Well provided with strong muscles. *M. dystrophy.* One of a number of inherited diseases in which there is progressive muscle wasting. *See* Duchenne dystrophy.

musculocutaneous (*mus-ku-lo-ku-ta'-ne-us*). Referring to the muscles and the skin. *M. nerve.* One of the nerves which supply the muscles and the skin of the arms and legs.

musculoskeletal (*mus-ku-lo-skel'-et-al*). Referring to both the osseus and muscular systems.

mustine hydrochloride (*mus'-teen hi-dro-klor'-ide*). Nitrogen mustard. A cytotoxic drug which may be given intravenously for malignant disease of lymph glands and reticulo-endothelial cells, such as Hodgkin's disease.

mutant (*mu'-tant*). A gene in which mutation has occurred.

mutation (*mu-ta'-shun*). A chemical change in the genes of a cell causing it to show a new characteristic. Some produce evolutional changes, others disease.

mute (*mute*). Without the power of speech. Dumb. *Deaf m.* One who cannot speak because he cannot hear.

mutilation (*mu-til-a'-shun*). Deliberate infliction of bodily injury.

myalgia (*mi-al'-je-ah*). Pain in the muscles.

myasthenia (*mi-as-the'-ne-ah*). Muscle weakness. *M. gravis.* An extreme form of muscle weakness which is progressive. There is a rapid onset of fatigue, thought to be due to the too rapid destruction of acetylcholine at the neuro-muscular junction. Commonly affected muscles are those of vision, speaking, chewing and swallowing. Neostigmine injections may be useful. Thymectomy has been curative in some cases.

mycetoma (*mi-se-to'-mah*). A chronic fungus infection of the tissues both external and internal, but most commonly affecting the hands and feet. There is swelling and the formation of sinuses. Madura foot.

Mycobacterium (*mi-ko-bak-te'-re-um*). A genus of slender, rod-shaped, acid-fast, gram-positive bacteria. *M. leprae.* The causative organism of leprosy. *M. tuberculosis.* The cause of tuberculosis.

mycology (*mi-kol'-o-je*). The study of fungi.

mycosis (*mi-ko'-sis*). Any disease which is caused by a fungus. *M. fungoides.* A rare malignant lymphoreticular neoplasm of the skin which later progresses to the lymph nodes and viscera.

mydriasis (*mid-ri'-as-is*). Abnormal dilatation of the pupil of the eye. It is usually caused by injury to the pupil sphincter or by the use of mydriatic drugs.

mydriatic (*mid-re-at'-ik*). Any drug which causes mydriasis. They are used in examination of the eye and in the treatment of inflammatory conditions.

myectomy (*mi-ek'-tom-e*). Excision of a portion of muscle.

myelin (*mi'-el-in*). The fatty covering of medullated nerve fibres.

myelitis (*mi-el-i'-tis*). (1) Inflammation of the spinal cord, causing pain in the back and sometimes numbness and paralysis of the legs and the lower part of the trunk. (2) Inflammation of the bone marrow. Osteomyelitis.

myeloblast (*mi'-el-o-blast*). A primitive cell in the bone marrow from which develop the granular leucocytes.

myelocyte (*mi'-el-o-site*). A cell of the bone marrow, derived from a myeloblast.

myelography (*mi-el-og'-raf-e*). X-ray examination of the spinal cord following the insertion of a radio-opaque substance into the subarachnoid space by means of lumbar puncture.

myeloid (*mi'-el-oid*). Resembling bone marrow or referring to the spinal cord. *M. leukaemia.* A malignant disease in which there is excessive production of leucocytes in the bone marrow.

myeloma (*mi-el-o'-mah*). A malignant tumour in the medullary cavity of bone.

myelomatosis (*mi-el-o-mat-o'-*

sis). A malignant disease of the bone marrow, in which multiple myeloma are present.

myelomeningocele (*mi-el-o-men-ing'-go-seel*). Meningomyelocele.

myelopathy (*mi-el-op'-ath-e*). A disease affecting the spinal cord.

myocardial (*mi-o-kar'-de-al*). Pertaining to the myocardium. *M. infarction.* Necrosis of a part of the myocardium, usually following a coronary thrombosis. Ventricular fibrillation may occur, followed by death.

myocarditis (*mi-o-kar-di'-tis*). Inflammation of the myocardium.

myocardium (*mi-o-kar'-de-um*). The muscle tissue of the heart.

myocele (*mi'-o-seel*). Protrusion of muscle through a rupture of its sheath.

myoclonus (*mi-o-klo'-nus*). A spasmodic contraction of the muscles.

myofibrosis (*mi-o-fi-bro'-sis*). A degenerative condition in which there is some replacement of muscle tissue by fibrous tissue.

myogenic (*mi-o-jen'-ik*). Originating in muscle tissue.

myoglobin (*mi-o-glo'-bin*). Myohaemoglobin.

myohaemoglobin (*mi-o-he-mo-glo'-bin*). A substance resembling haemoglobin, which is present in muscle cells. It is a pigment and is responsible for the colour of muscle. It acts as an oxygen store. Myoglobin.

myohaemoglobinuria (*mi-o-he-mo-glo-bin-u'-re-ah*). The presence of myohaemoglobin in the urine.

myoma (*mi-o'-mah*). A benign

tumour of muscle tissue. *See* Fibromyoma.

myomectomy (*mi-o-mek'-tom-e*). Removal of a myoma—usually referring to a uterine fibroma.

myometritis (*mi-o-me-tri'-tis*). Inflammation of the myometrium.

myometrium (*mi-o-me'-tre-um*). The muscular tissue of the uterus.

myoneural (*mi-o-nu'-ral*). Relating to both muscle and nerve. *M. junction*. The point at which nerve endings terminate in a muscle. Neuromuscular junction.

myopathy (*mi-op'-ath-e*). Any disease of the muscles. Muscular dystrophy is one of a group of inherited myopathies in which there is wasting and weakness of the muscles.

myopia (*mi-o'-pe-ah*). Shortsightedness. The light rays focus in front of the retina and a biconcave lens is needed to focus them correctly.

myoplasty (*mi'-o-plas-te*). Any operation in which muscle is detached and utilized, as may be done to correct deformities.

myosarcoma (*mi-o-sar-ko'-mah*). A sarcomatous tumour of muscle.

myosin (*mi'-o-sin*). Muscle protein.

myositis (*mi-o-si'-tis*). Inflammation of a muscle. *M. ossificans*. A condition in which bone cells deposited in muscle continue to grow and cause hard lumps. It may occur after fractures.

myotomy (*mi-ot'-om-e*). The division or dissection of a muscle.

myotonia (*mi-o-to'-ne-ah*). Lack of muscle tone. *M. con-genita*. An hereditary disease in which the muscle action has a prolonged contraction phase and slow relaxation.

myringa (*mir-ing'-gah*). The ear drum or tympanic membrane.

myringitis (*mir-in-ji'-tis*). Inflammation of the tympanic membrane.

myringoplasty (*mir-ing'-go-plas-te*). A plastic operation to repair the tympanic membrane. Tympanoplasty.

myringotome (*mir-ing'-go-tome*). An instrument for puncturing the tympanic membrane in myringotomy.

myringotomy (*mir-ing-got'-om-e*). Incision of the tympanic membrane to drain fluid from an infected middle ear.

myxoedema (*miks-e-de'-mah*). A condition caused by hypothyroidism which is marked by mucoid infiltration of the skin. There is oedematous swelling of the face, limbs, and hands; dry and rough skin; loss of hair; slow pulse; subnormal temperature; slowed metabolism; and mental dullness. *Congenital m.* Cretinism.

myxoma (*miks-o'-mah*). A benign mucous tumour of connective tissue.

myxosarcoma (*miks-o-sar-ko'-mah*). A sarcoma containing mucoid tissue.

myxovirus (*miks-o-vi'-rus*). The group name of a number of related viruses, including the causal viruses of influenza, para-influenza, mumps and Newcastle disease (of fowls).

N

N. (1) Chemical symbol for *nitrogen.* (2) Abbreviation for the SI unit, the *newton.*

Na. Chemical symbol for *sodium*.

Naboth's follicle or cyst (*(M. Naboth, German anatomist, 1675–1721)*. Cystic swelling of a cervical gland, the duct of which has become blocked by regenerating squamous epithelium.

naevus (*ne'-vus*). A birthmark; a circumscribed area of pigmentation of the skin due to dilated blood vessels. A haemangioma. *N. flammeus.* A flat bluish-red area usually on the neck or face; popularly known as 'port-wine stain'. *N. pilosus.* A hairy naevus. *Spider n.* A small red area surrounded by dilated capillaries. *Strawberry n.* A raised tumour-like structure of connective tissue containing spaces filled with blood.

Naffziger's operation (*H.C. Naffziger, American surgeon, 1884–1961*). Incision of the orbit transfrontally to reduce orbital pressure in exophthalmos.

nail (*nale*). The keratinized portion of epidermis covering the dorsal extremity of the fingers and toes. *N. bed.* The skin underlying a nail. *Hang-n.* A strip of epidermis hanging at one side or at the root of a nail. *Ingrowing n.* A condition in which the flesh overhangs the edge of the nail, a sharp corner of which may pierce the skin, causing a wound which may become septic. *Spoon n.* A nail with a depression in the centre and raised edges. Koilonychia.

nalidixic acid (*nal-e-diks'-ik as'-id*). An antibacterial agent used in the treatment of urinary infections.

nalorphine (*nal-or'-feen*). An antidote for morphine, pethi-dine and methadone overdosage.

nandrolone (*nan'-dro-lone*). An anabolic steroid that promotes protein metabolism and skeletal growth.

nanogram (*nan'-o-gram*). *abbrev.* ng. One thousand millionth of a gram.

nanometre (*nan'-o-me-ter*). *abbrev.* nm. One thousand millionth of a metre. One thousandth of a micron.

nape (*nape*). The back of the neck.

napkin rash (*nap'-kin rash*). An erythematous rash which may occur in infants in the napkin area. Often caused by the passage of frequent loose stools containing fatty acids which cause breakdown of urea in the urine, producing ammonia which burns the skin.

narcissism (*nar-sis'-izm*). (From the Greek legend of Narcissus.) The stage of infant development when the child is mainly interested in himself and his own bodily needs. In adults it may be a symptom of mental disorder.

narcoanalysis (*nar-ko-an-al'-is-is*). A form of psychotherapy in which an injection of a narcotic drug produces a drowsy, relaxed state during which a patient will talk more freely, and in this way much repressed material may be brought to consciousness.

narcolepsy (*nar'-ko-lep-se*). A condition in which there is an uncontrollable desire for sleep.

narcosis (*nar-ko'-sis*). A state of unconsciousness produced by a narcotic drug. *Basal n.* A state of unconsciousness produced prior to surgical anaesthesia.

narcosynthesis (*nar-ko-sin'-thes-is*). The inducement of an hypnotic state by means of drugs. An aid to psychotherapy.

narcotic (*nar-kot'-ik*). A drug that produces narcosis or unnatural sleep.

nares (*nar'-eez*). *sing.* naris. The nostrils. *Posterior n.* The opening of the nares into the nasopharynx.

nasal (*na'-zal*). Pertaining to the nose.

nascent (*nas'-ent*). (1) At the time of birth. (2) Incipient.

nasogastric (*na-zo-gas'-trik*). Referring to the nose and stomach. *N. tube.* One passed into the stomach via the nose.

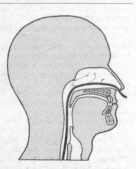

POSITION OF NASOGASTRIC TUBE

nasolacrimal (*na-zo-lak'-rim-al*). Concerning both the nose and lacrimal apparatus. *N. duct.* The duct draining the tears from the inner aspect of the eye to the inferior meatus of the nose.

nasopharynx (*na-zo-far'-inks*). The upper part of the pharynx; that above the soft palate.

nasosinusitis (*na-zo-si-nu-si'-tis*). Inflammation of the nose and adjacent sinuses.

nates (*na'-teez*). The buttocks.

naturopathy (*na-cher-op'-ath-e*). A method of treatment using no surgery or drugs, but only natural substances such as herbs, sunlight, fresh air and unadulterated foodstuffs.

nausea (*naw'-se-ah*). A sensation of sickness with an inclination to vomit.

navel (*na'-vel*). The umbilicus.

navicular (*nav-ik'-u-lah*). Boat-shaped. *N. bone.* One of the tarsal bones of the foot.

nebula (*neb'-u-lah*). A slight opacity or cloudiness of the cornea, caused by injury or by corneal ulceration.

nebulizer (*neb'-u-li-zer*). An apparatus for reducing a liquid to a fine spray. An atomizer.

neck (*nek*). (1) The narrow part of an organ or bone. (2) The part of the body which connects the head and the trunk. *Derbyshire n.* Simple goitre. *Wry n.* Torticollis.

necrobiosis (*nek-ro-bi-o'-sis*). Localized death of a part as a result of degeneration.

necrophilia (*nek-ro-fil'-e-ah*). (1) Sexual pleasure in the presence of a corpse. (2) Sexual intercourse with a corpse. Necrophilism.

necropsy (*nek-rop'-se*). Autopsy. A post-mortem examination of a body.

necrosis (*nek-ro'-sis*). Death of a portion of tissue.

necrospermia (*nek-ro-sper'-me-ah*). The presence of dead spermatozoa in the semen.

necrotomy (*ne-krot'-om-e*). An

operation to remove a dead piece of bone.

needling (*need'-ling*). Discission; the operation for cataract of lacerating and splitting up the lens so that it may be absorbed.

negative (*neg'-at-iv*). The opposite of positive. The absence of some quality or substance. *N. pole*. The cathode. That which attracts positively charged bodies and repels negatively charged bodies.

negativism (*neg'-at-iv-izm*). A symptom of mental illness in which the patient does the opposite of what is required of him and so presents an uncooperative attitude. Common in schizophrenia.

Neisseria (*ni-seer'-e-ah*). A genus of paired, spherical, gram-negative bacteria. *N. gonorrhoeae*. The causative organism of gonorrhoea. *N. meningitidis*. The cause of meningococcal meningitis.

Nematoda (*nem-at-o'-dah*). A phylum of worms, including the *Ascaris* or roundworm and the *Enterobius* or threadworm.

neo-arthrosis (*ne-o-ar-thro'-sis*). An artificial joint.

neocerebellum (*ne-o-ser-e-bel'-um*). The middle lobe of the cerebellum.

neocortex (*ne-o-kor'-teks*). The cerebral cortex excluding the hippocampal formation and piriform area.

neoglycogenesis (*ne-o-gli-ko-jen'-es-is*). The formation of liver glycogen from non-carbohydrate sources. Glyconeogenesis.

neologism (*ne-ol'-o-jizm*). The formation of new words, either completely new ones or ones formed by contraction of two separate words. This is done particularly by schizophrenic patients.

neomycin (*ne-o-mi'-cin*). An antibiotic drug used against a wide range of bacteria, frequently those affecting the skin or the eyes. Also given orally to sterilize the bowel before surgery.

neonatal (*ne-o-na'-tal*). Referring to the first month of life. *N. mortality rate*. The number of deaths during this period per 1000 live births.

neonate (*ne'-o-nate*). Newborn; specifically, pertaining to a baby under one month old.

neoplasm (*ne'-o-plazm*). A morbid new growth. A tumour. It may be benign or malignant.

neostigmine (*ne-o-stig'-meen*). A synthetic preparation akin to physostigmine used in the treatment of myasthenia gravis and as an antidote to some muscle-relaxant drugs, and as eye drops in the treatment of glaucoma.

nephralgia (*nef-ral'-je-ah*). Pain in the kidney of neuralgic type.

nephralgic (*nef-ral'-jik*). Relating to pain arising from the kidney. *N. crises*. Spasms of pain in the lumbar region in tabes dorsalis.

nephrectomy (*nef-rek'-tom-e*). Excision of a kidney.

nephritis (*nef-ri'-tis*). Inflammation of the kidneys (Bright's disease). A non-specific term used to describe a wide variety of diseases of the kidney.

nephroblastoma (*nef-ro-blas-to'-mah*). Wilms's tumour. A malignant tumour of the kidney which occurs only in young children.

nephrocalcinosis (*nef-ro-kal-*

sin-o'-sis). A condition in which there is deposition of calcium in the renal tubules resulting in calculi formation and renal insufficiency. A complication of hyperparathyroidism.

nephrocapsulectomy (*nef-ro-kap-su-lek'-tom-e*). Operation for removal of the capsule of the kidney.

nephrocele (*nef'-ro-seel*). Hernia of the kidney.

nephrolith (*nef'-ro-lith*). Stone in the kidney; renal calculus.

nephrolithiasis (*nef-ro-lith-i'-as-is*). The presence of a calculus or of gravel in the kidney.

nephrolithotomy (*nef-ro-lith-ot'-o-me*). Removal of a renal calculus by incising the kidney.

nephroma (*nef-ro'-mah*). Tumour of the kidney.

nephron (*nef'-ron*). The functional unit of the kidney, comprising Bowman's capsule, the proximal and distal tubules, the loop of Henle and the collecting duct.

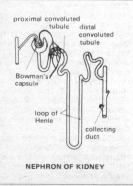

proximal convoluted tubule

distal convoluted tubule

Bowman's capsule

loop of Henle

collecting duct

NEPHRON OF KIDNEY

nephropathy (*nef-rop'-ath-e*). Any disease condition of the kidney.

nephropexy (*nef'-ro-pek-se*). The fixation of a floating (mobile) kidney, usually by sutures to neighbouring muscle.

nephroptosis (*nef-rop-to'-sis*). Downward displacement, or undue mobility, of a kidney.

nephropyeloplasty (*nef-ro-pi'-el-o-plast-te*). A plastic operation on the pelvis of the kidney performed in cases of hydronephrosis.

nephropyosis (*nef-ro-pi-o'-sis*). Suppuration in the kidney.

nephrosclerosis (*nef-ro-skler-o'-sis*). Constriction of the arterioles of the kidney. Seen in benign and malignant hypertension and in arteriosclerosis in old age.

nephrosis (*nef-ro'-sis*). Any disease of the kidney, especially that which is characterized by oedema, albuminuria and a low plasma albumin. Caused by non-inflammatory degenerative lesions of the tubules.

nephrostomy (*nef-ros'-tom-e*). Drainage of a kidney by passing a catheter at operation through the kidney.

nephrotic (*nef-rot'-ik*). Referring to or caused by nephrosis. *N. syndrome.* A clinical syndrome in which there are albuminuria, low plasma protein, and gross oedema. Due to increased capillary permeability in the glomeruli. It may occur as a result of acute glomerulonephritis—in subacute nephritis, diabetes mellitus, amyloid disease, systemic lupus erythematosus and renal vein thrombosis.

nephrotomy (*nef-rot'-om-e*). Incision of the kidney.

nephrotoxic (nef-ro-toks'-ik). Poisonous or destructive to the cells of the kidney.

nephro-ureterectomy (nef-ro-u-re-ter-ek'-tom-e). Surgical removal of the kidney and the ureter.

nerve (nerv). A bundle of conducting fibres enclosed in a sheath called the epineurium. Its function is to transmit impulses between any part of the body and a nerve centre. *Motor* (efferent) *n.* One that conveys impulses causing activity from a nerve centre to a muscle or gland. *Sensory* (afferent) *n.* One that conveys sensation from an area to a nerve centre. *N. block.* A method of producing regional anaesthesia by injecting a local anaesthetic into the nerves supplying the area to be operated on. *N. fibre.* The prolongation of the nerve cell, which conveys impulses. Each fibre has a sheath. Medullated nerve fibres have an insulating myelin sheath. *N. gas.* A gas that interferes with the functioning of the nerves and muscles. Such gases may cause death from respiratory paralysis and some of them act through the skin and cannot be avoided by the use of gas-masks.

nervous (ner'-vus). (1) Pertaining to, or composed of, nerves. (2) Apprehensive.

nervousness (ner'-vus-nes). Excitability of the nervous system, characterized by a state of mental and physical unrest.

nettle-rash (netl'-rash). An allergic skin condition. Urticaria.

Nettleship's dilator (E. Nettleship, British ophthalmologist, 1845–1913). An instrument for dilating the lacrimal puncta.

neural (nu'-ral). Pertaining to the nerves. *N. arch.* The bony arch on each vertebra which encloses the spinal cord.

neuralgia (nu-ral'-je-ah). A sharp stabbing pain, usually along the course of a nerve owing to neuritis or functional disturbance.

neurapraxia (nu-rap-raks'-e-ah). An injury to a nerve resulting in temporary loss of function and paralysis. It is usually caused by compression of the nerve, and there is no lasting damage.

neurasthenia (nu-ras-the'-ne-ah). A neurosis in which there is much mental and physical fatigue, inability to concentrate, loss of appetite, and a failure of memory.

neurectomy (nu-rek'-tom-e). Excision of part of a nerve.

neurilemma (nu-re-lem'-ah). The membranous sheath surrounding a nerve fibre.

neurinoma (nu-rin-o'-mah). A benign tumour arising in the neurilemma of a nerve fibre.

neuritis (nu-ri'-tis). Inflammation of a nerve with pain, tenderness, and loss of function. *Multiple n.* That involving several nerves. Polyneuritis. *Nutritional* (alcoholic) *n.* That which may be caused by alcoholism or lack of vitamin B complex. *Optic n.* That affecting the optic disc or nerve. *Peripheral n.* That involving the terminations of nerves. *Sciatic n.* Sciatica. *Tabetic n.* A type occurring in tabes dorsalis. *Traumatic n.* That which results from an injury to a nerve.

neuroanatomy (nu-ro-an-at'-om-e). The study of the structure of the nervous system.

neuroblast (*nu'-ro-blast*). An embryonic nerve cell.

neuroblastoma (*nu-ro-blas-to'-mah*). A malignant tumour of immature nerve cells, most often arising in the very young.

neurodermatitis (*nu-ro-der-mat-i'-tis*). A localized prurigo of somatic and psychogenic origin. It irritates, and rubbing causes thickening and pigmentation of the skin.

neuro-epithelioma (*nu-ro-ep-e-the-le-o'-mah*). A malignant tumour of the retina of the eye, which may spread into the brain.

neurofibroma (*nu-ro-fi-bro'-mah*). A benign tumour of nerve and fibrous tissue.

neurofibromatosis (*nu-ro-fi-bro-mat-o'-sis*). Von Recklinghausen's disease. A generalized hereditary disease in which there are numerous tumours of the skin and nervous system.

neurogenic (*nu-ro-jen'-ik*). Derived from or caused by nerve stimulation. *N. bladder.* A disorder ofthe urinary bladder caused by a lin othe nervous system. *N. shock.* Shock originating in the nervous system.

neuroglia (*nu-rog'-le-ah*). The special form of connective tissue supporting nerve tissues.

neurohypophysis (*nu-ro-hi-pof'-is-is*). The posterior lobe of the pituitary gland.

neuroleptic (*nu-ro-lep'-tik*). A drug which acts on the nervous system.

neurologist (*nu-rol'-o-jist*). One who is an expert in the treatment of diseases of the nervous system.

neurology (*nu-rol'-o-je*). The scientific study of the nervous system.

neuroma (*nu-ro'-mah*). A tumour consisting of nervous tissue.

neuromuscular (*nu-ro-mus'-ku-lah*). Appertaining to nerves and muscles. *N. junction.* The small gap between the end of the motor nerve and the motor end-plate of the muscle fibre supplied. This gap is bridged by the release of acetylcholine whenever a nerve impulse arrives.

neuromyelitis (*nu-ro-mi-el-i'-tis*). Neuritis associated with myelitis. It is a condition akin to multiple sclerosis. *N. optica.* A disease in which there is bilateral optic neuritis and paraplegia.

neuron (*nu'-ron*). A nerve cell. *Lower motor n.* The anterior horn cell and its neuron which conveys impulses to the appropriate muscles. *Upper motor n.* That in which the cell is in the cerebral cortex and the fibres conduct impulses to associated cells in the spinal cord.

neuroparalysis (*nu-ro-par-al'-is-is*). Paralysis caused by a disorder of the nerve controlling the affected muscle.

neuropathy (*nu-rop'-ath-e*). A disease process of nerve degeneration and loss of function. *Diabetic n.* That associated with diabetes. *Ischaemic n.* That caused by a lack of blood supply.

neuroplasty (*nu'-ro-plas-te*). The surgical repair of a damaged nerve.

neurorrhaphy (*nu-ror'-af-e*). The operation of suturing a divided nerve.

neurosis (*nu-ro'-sis*). A mental disorder, which does not affect the whole personality, characterized by exaggerated anxiety and tension. *Anxiety* *n.* Persistent anxiety and the accompanying symptoms of fear, rapid pulse, sweating, trembling, loss of appetite and insomnia. *Obsessive-compulsive n.* One characterized by compulsions and obsessional rumination.

neurosurgery (*nu-ro-ser'-jer-e*). That branch of surgery dealing with the brain, spinal cord and nerves.

neurosyphilis (*nu-ro-sif'-il-is*). A manifestation of third stage syphilis in which the nervous system is involved. The three commonest forms are: (1) meningovascular syphilis, affecting the blood vessels to the meninges, (2) tabes dorsalis (*see* Ataxia), and (3) general paralysis of the insane.

neurotic (*nu-rot'-ik*). A loosely applied adjective denoting association with neurosis.

neurotmesis (*nu-rot-me'-sis*). Degeneration of a nerve due to severance.

neurotomy (*nu-rot'-om-e*). The surgical division of a nerve.

neurotoxic (*nu-ro-toks'-ik*). Poisonous or destructive to nervous tissue.

neurotransmitter (*nu-ro-trans-mit'-er*). A chemical released from nerve endings to produce activity in other nerves.

neurotripsy (*nu-ro-trip'-se*). The surgical bruising or crushing of a nerve.

neurotropic (*nu-ro-trop'-ik*). Having an affinity for nerve tissue. *N. viruses.* Those that particularly attack the nervous system.

neutral (*nu'-tral*). (1) In chemistry, neither acid nor alkaline. (2) Producing no electrical charge.

neutron (*nu'-tron*). An electrically neutral particle forming a part of an atom. *N. beam.* A high-speed beam used in radiotherapy on oxygen-deficient tumours which are insensitive to X- and gamma-radiation.

neutropenia (*nu-tro-pe'-ne-ah*). A decrease in the number of neutrophils in the blood.

neutrophil (*nu'-tro-fil*). A polymorphonuclear leucocyte which has a neutral reaction to acid and alkaline dyes.

newton (*nu'-ton*). *abbrev.* N. The SI unit of force.

niacin (*ni'-as-in*). Nicotinic acid.

nicotine (*nik'-o-teen*). A poisonous alkaloid in tobacco.

nicotinic acid (*nik-o-tin'-ik as'-id*). Niacin. A water-soluble vitamin in the B complex. A deficiency of this vitamin causes pellagra.

nictitation (*nik-tit-a'-shun*). The act of winking.

nidation (*ni-da'-shun*). Implantation.

nidus (*ni'-dus*). (1) A nest. (2) A place in which an organism finds conditions suitable for its growth and development. (3) The focus of an infection.

Niemann–Pick disease (*A. Niemann, German paediatrician, 1880–1921; F. Pick, German physician, 1868–1935*). A rare inherited disease in which there is lipoid storage abnormality and widespread deposition of lecithin in the tissues. Mental retardation is usual.

night-blindness (*nite-blind'-nes*). Nyctalopia. Difficulty in seeing in the dark. This may be a congenital defect or be caused by a vitamin A deficiency. Also occurs as a result of retinal degeneration.

night-sweat (*nite'-swet*). Profuse perspiration during sleep, especially typical of tuberculosis.

night-terror (*nite-ter'-or*). An unpleasant experience in which the subject, usually a young child, screams in his sleep and seems terrified. On waking he is unable to remember the cause of his fear.

nihilism (*ni'-hil-izm*). In psychiatry, a term used to describe feelings of not existing and hopelessness, that all is lost or destroyed.

nikethamide (*nik-eth'-am-ide*). A cardiac and respiratory stimulant given intravenously in cases of extreme respiratory failure.

nipple (*nipl*). The small conical projection at the tip of the breast, through which, in the female, milk can be withdrawn. *Depressed n.* One that does not protrude. This should be drawn out during pregnancy, so that later the infant can suck. *Retracted n.* One that is drawn inwards. It may be a sign of cancer of the breast.

Nissl granules (*F. Nissl, German neuropathologist, 1860–1919*). RNA-containing units found in the cytoplasm of cells. Probably associated with protein synthesis.

nit (*nit*). The egg of the head louse attached to the hair near the scalp.

nitrazepam (*ni-traz'-e-pam*). A hypnotic and sedative drug used to treat insomnia with early morning wakening.

nitrofurantoin (*ni-tro-fu-ranto'-in*). A urinary antiseptic which is bactericidal and is effective against a wide range of organisms.

nitrofurazone (*ni-tro-fu'-razone*). An antibacterial agent used chiefly as ear drops in the treatment of otitis externa.

nitrogen (*ni'-tro-jen*). *abbrev.* N. A gaseous element. Air is largely composed of nitrogen, and it is one of the essential constituents of all protein foods.

nitroglycerin (*ni-tro-glis'-er-een*). Glyceryl trinitrate. A drug which causes dilatation of the coronary arteries. In angina pectoris a tablet should be dissolved sublingually before exertion.

nitrous oxide (*ni'-trus oks'-ide*). N_2O. Laughing-gas. A general anaesthetic ensuring a brief spell of unconsciousness, and used largely for dental operations.

noci-association (*no-se-as-o-se-a'-shun*). The discharge of nervous energy which occurs unconsciously in trauma, as in surgical shock. *See* Anoci-association.

noctambulation (*nokt-am-bu-la'-shun*). Sleep-walking. Somnambulism.

nocturia (*nok-tu'-re-ah*). The production of large quantities of urine at night.

nocturnal (*nok-ter'-nal*). Referring to the night. *N. enuresis.* Bed wetting. Incontinence of urine during sleep.

node (*node*). A swelling or protuberance. *Atrioventricular n.* The specialized tissue between the right atrium and the ventricle, at the point where the coronary vein enters the atrium, from which is initiated the impulse of contraction down the atrioventricular bundle. *Sino-atrial n.* The pacemaker of the heart. The specialized neuromuscular tissue at the junction of the superior vena cava and the right atrium, which, stimulated by the right vagus nerve, controls the rhythm of contraction in the heart. *N. of Ranvier.* A constriction occurring at intervals in a nerve fibre to enable the neurilemma with its blood supply to reach and nourish the axon of the nerve.

nodule (*nod'-ule*). A small swelling or protuberance.

noma (*no'-mah*). A gangrenous condition of the mouth. Cancrum oris.

nomenclature (*no-men'-klatchur*). The terminology of a science; a classified system of names.

non compos mentis (*non kom'-pos men'-tis*). (Latin). Applied to a person whose mental state is such that he is unable to manage his own affairs.

non-conductor (*non-kon-duk'-tor*). A substance that does not readily transmit electricity, light, heat or sound.

non-specific (*non-spes-if'-ik*). Applied to a disease or drug which is not activated by any particular micro-organism. *N. urethritis.* A urethritis which may be venereal in origin, but is not caused by a gonococcus. It may be caused by a virus.

non-union (*non-u'-ne-on*). In a fracture, failure of the two pieces of bone to unite.

noradrenaline (*nor-ad-ren'-al-een*). Norepinephrine. A hormone present in extracts of the suprarenal medulla and at synapses in the peripheral sympathetic nervous system. It causes vasoconstriction and raises both the systolic and the diastolic blood pressure.

norepinephrine (*nor-ep-e-nef'-reen*). Noradrenaline.

norethandrolone (*nor-eth-an'-dro-lone*). An anabolic steroid that aids in the utilization of

protein. May be used to treat severe wasting and in osteoporosis.

norethisterone (*nor-eth-is'-ter-one*). An anabolic steroid similar in action to progesterone. Used in the treatment of amenorrhoea. Also used in the combined contraceptive pill.

normal (*nor'-mal*). Conforming to a standard; regular or usual. *N. flora.* Bacteria which normally live on body tissues and have a beneficial effect. *N. saline.* Isotonic solution of sodium chloride. Physiological solution.

normoblast (*nor'-mo-blast*). A nucleated precursor red blood cell in bone marrow. *See* Erythrocyte.

normochromic (*nor-mo-kro'-mik*). Normal in colour. Applied to the blood when the haemoglobin level is within normal limits.

normocyte (*nor'-mo-site*). A red blood cell that is normal in size, shape and colour.

normoglycaemia (*nor-mo-gli-se'-me-ah*). Normal blood sugar level.

normotension (*nor-mo-ten'-shun*). Normal tone, tension or pressure. Usually used in relation to blood pressure.

nortriptyline (*nor-trip'-til-een*). A tricyclic antidepressant drug used for the relief of all types of depression.

nose (*noze*). The organ of smell and the airway for respiration.

nosology (*nos-ol'-o-je*). The scientific classification of diseases.

nostalgia (*nos-tal'-je-ah*). Home-sickness.

nostril (*nos'-tril*). One of the anterior orifices of the nose.

notifiable (*no-te-fi'-abl*). Applied to such diseases as must be reported to the health authorities. These include measles, scarlet fever, typhus and typhoid fever, cholera, diphtheria, tuberculosis, dysentery and food poisoning.

novobiocin (*nov-o-bi'-o-sin*). A wide-range oral antibiotic that is effective against staphylococcal infections resistant to other antibiotics and against some *Proteus* organisms.

noxious (*nok'-she-us*). Harmful. The term may be applied to drugs or other substances liable to cause injury.

nucha (*nu'-kah*). The nape of the neck.

nuclear (*nu'-kle-ar*). Pertaining to a nucleus.

nuclease (*nu'-kle-aze*). An enzyme which breaks down the nucleic acids.

nucleic acids (*nu'-kle-ik as-idz*). Deoxyribonucleic acid (DNA) and ribonucleic acid (RNA), both of which are found in cell nuclei, and RNA in the cytoplasm also. They are composed of series of nucleotides.

nucleolus (*nu-kle'-o-lus*). A small dense body in the cell nucleus which contains ribonucleic acid. It disappears during mitosis.

nucleoprotein (*nu-kle-o-pro'-teen*). A compound of nucleic acid and protein.

nucleotide (*nu'-kle-o-tide*). A compound formed from pentose sugar, phosphoric acid and a nitrogen-containing base (a purine or a pyrimidine).

nucleus (*nu'-kle-us*). (1) The essential part of a cell, governing nutrition and reproduction, its division being essential for the formation of new cells. (2) The positively-charged centre portion of an atom. (3) A group of nerve cells in the central nervous system. *Caudate n.* and *lenticular n.* Part of the basal ganglia. *N. pulposus.* The jelly-like centre of an intervertebral disc.

nullipara (*nul-ip'-ar-ah*). A woman who has never given birth to a child.

nutation (*nu-ta'-shun*). Uncontrollable nodding of the head.

nutrient (*nu'-tre-ent*). Food. Any substance that nourishes.

nutrition (*nu-trish'-un*). The process by which food is assimilated into the body in order to nourish it.

nutritional (*nu-trish'-un-al*). Relating to the process of nutrition. *N. disease.* One that is due to the continued absence of a necessary food factor.

nux (*nuks*). A nut. *N. vomica.* The seed of an East Indian tree, from which strychnine is derived.

nyctalgia (*nik-tal'-je-ah*). Pain occurring during the night.

nyctalopia (*nik-tal-o'-pe-ah*). Night-blindness.

nycturia (*nik-tu'-re-ah*). Incontinence of urine at night. Nocturnal enuresis.

nymph (*nimf*). The larval form of certain insects.

nympha (*nim'-fah*). *pl.* nymphae. One of the two labia minora. *See* Labium.

nymphomania (*nim-fo-ma'-ne-ah*). Excessive sexual desire in a woman.

nystagmus (*nis-tag'-mus*). An involuntary rapid movement of the eyeball. It may be hereditary or result from disease of the semicircular canals or of the central nervous system. It can occur from visual defect or be associated with other muscle spasms. *Miner's n.* An occupational disease of coal-miners.

nystatin (*ni'-stat-in*). An antibiotic drug effective against fungi. Used in the treatment of candidiasis and of fungal infections of the ear.

O

O. Chemical symbol for *oxygen*.

obese (*o-bees'*). Very fat. Corpulent.

obesity (*u-be'-sit-e*). Corpulence; excessive development of fat throughout the body.

objective (*ob-jek'-tiv*). (1) *n.* In microscopy, the lens nearest the object being looked at. (2) *n.* A purpose. A desired end result. (3) *adj.* Concerning matters outside oneself. *O. signs.* Signs which the observer notes, as distinct from symptoms of which the patient complains (*subjective*).

oblique (*o-bleek'*). Slanting. *O. muscles.* (1) A pair of muscles, the inferior and the superior, which turn the eye upwards and downwards and inwards and outwards. (2) Muscles found in the wall of the abdomen.

obsession (*ob-sesh'-un*). An idea which persistently recurs to an individual although he resists it and regards it as being senseless. A compulsive thought. *See* Compulsion.

obstetrician (*ob-stet-rish'-un*). One who is trained and specializes in obstetrics.

obstetrics (*ob-stet'-riks*). The branch of medicine and surgery dealing with pregnancy, labour and the puerperium.

obturator (*ob'-tu-ra-tor*). That which closes an opening. *O. foramen.* The large hole in the hip-bone closed by fascia and muscle.

obtusion (*ob-tu'-zhun*). Weakening or blunting of normal sensations, a condition produced by certain diseases.

occipital (*ok-sip'-it-al*). Relating to the occiput. *O. bone.* The bone forming the back and part of the base of the skull.

occipito-anterior (*ok-sip'-it-o-an-te'-re-or*). Referring to the position of the child's head when it is to the front of the pelvis when it comes through the birth canal. *Occipito-posterior* is the reverse position.

occiput (*ok'-sip-ut*). The back of the head.

occlusion (*ok-lu'-zhun*). Closure, applied particularly to alignment of the teeth in the jaws. *Coronary o.* Obstruction of the lumen of a coronary artery. *O. of the eye.* Covering a good eye to improve the visual acuity of the other, lazy eye. *O. of the pupil.* Occlusio pupillae. Obstruction of the pupil, which may be congenital or occur in iridocyclitis or after injury.

occult (*ok-ult'*). Hidden, concealed. *O. blood.* Blood excreted in the stools in such a small quantity as to require chemical tests to detect it.

occupational (*ok-u-pa'-shun-al*). Relating to work and working conditions. *O. disease.* One likely to occur among workers in certain trades. An industrial disease. *O. therapy. See* Therapy.

ocular (*ok'-u-lar*). Relating to the eye. *O. myopathy.* A gradual bilateral loss of mobility of the eyes. *O.*

myositis. Inflammation of the orbital muscles.

oculentum (*ok-u-len'-tum*). An eye ointment.

oculist (*ok'-u-list*). An ophthalmologist.

oculogyric (*ok-u-lo-ji'-rik*). Causing movements of the eyeballs. *O. crisis*. Involuntary, violent movements of the eye, usually upwards.

oculomotor (*ok-u-lo-mo'-tor*). Relating to movements of the eye. *O. nerves*. The third pair of cranial nerves, which control the eye muscles.

Oddi, sphincter of (*R. Oddi, 19th century Italian surgeon*). The muscular sphincter situated at the junction of the common bile duct and the pancreatic duct.

odontalgia (*o-don-tal'-je-ah*). Toothache.

odontoid (*o-don'-toid*). Resembling a tooth. *O. process*. A toothlike projection from the axis vertebra upon which the head rotates.

odontolith (*o-don'-to-lith*). Tartar, the calcareous matter deposited upon teeth.

odontology (*o-don-tol'-o-je*). The science of treating teeth. Dentistry.

odontoma (*o-don-to'-mah*). A tumour of tooth structures.

odontoprisis (*o-don-to-pri'-sis*). Grinding of the teeth.

oedema (*e-de'-mah*). An excessive amount of fluid in the body tissues. If the finger is pressed upon an affected part, the surface pits and regains slowly its original contour. *Cardiac o*. That due to heart failure. *Famine o*. That due to protein deficiency. *Lymphatic o*. That due to blockage of the lymph vessels. *Pulmonary o*. Effusion of fluid into the alveoli and tissues between them. A serious cause of cyanosis. *Renal o*. That occurring in acute nephritis.

Oedipus complex (*e'-dip-us kom'-pleks*) (from character in Greek mythology). The suppressed sexual desire of a son for his mother, with hostility towards his father. It is a normal stage in the early development of the child, but may become fixed if the child cannot solve the conflict during his early years or during adolescence.

oesophageal (*e-sof-ah-je'-al*). Pertaining to the oesophagus. *O. atresia*. A congenital abnormality in which the oesophagus is not continuous between the pharynx and the stomach. May be associated with a fistula into the trachea. *O. varices*. Varicose veins of the lower oesophagus secondary to portal hypertension.

oesophagectasis (*e-sof-ah-jekt'-as-is*). Dilatation of the oesophagus.

oesophagitis (*e-sof-ah-ji'-tis*). Inflammation of the oesophagus. *Reflux o*. That caused by regurgitation of acid stomach contents through the cardiac sphincter.

oesophagocele (*e-sof'-ag-o-seel*). A protrusion of the mucous lining through a tear in the muscular wall of the oesophagus.

oesophagojejunostomy (*e-sof-ag-o-je-ju-nos'-tom-e*). The operation to create an anastomosis of the jejunum with the oesophagus following a total gastrectomy.

oesophagoscope (*e-sof'-ag-o-skope*). An instrument for viewing the inside of the oesophagus.

oesophagoscopy (*e-sof-ag-os'-*

ko-pe). An examination carried out with an oesophagoscope.

oesophagostomy (*e-sof-ag-os'-tom-e).* The making of an artificial opening into the oesophagus.

oesophagotomy (*e-sof-ag-ot'-om-e).* Surgical incision of the oesophagus.

oesophagus (*e-sof'-ag-us).* The canal which extends from the pharynx to the stomach. It is about 23 cm (9 in.) long. The gullet.

oestradiol (*e-strad'-e-ol).* The chief naturally occurring female sex hormone produced by the ovary. Prepared synthetically, it is now used to treat menopausal conditions and amenorrhoea.

oestrogen (*e'-stro-jen).* One of several steroid hormones including oestradiol, all of which have similar functions. Although they are largely produced in the ovary, they can also be extracted from the placenta, the adrenal cortex, and the testis. They control female sexual development.

ohm (*ome).* abbrev. Ω. The SI unit of electrical resistance.

ointment (*oint'-ment).* An external application with a greasy base in which the remedy is incorporated.

olecranon (*o-lek'-ran-on).* The curved process of the ulna which forms the point of the elbow.

oleum (*o'-le-um).* An oil.

olfactory (*ol-fak'-tor-e).* Relating to the sense of smell. *O. nerves.* The first pair of cranial nerves; those of smell.

oligaemia (*ol-ig-e'-me-ah).* A deficiency in the volume of blood.

oligocythaemia (*ol-ig-o-si-the'-me-ah).* A cell deficiency in the blood.

oligodendroglioma (*ol-ig-o-den-dro-gli-o'-mah).* A central nervous system tumour of the glial tissue.

oligohydramnios (*ol-ig-o-hi-dram'-ne-os).* A deficiency in the amount of amniotic fluid.

oligomenorrhoea (*ol-ig-o-men-or-e'-ah).* (1) A diminished flow at the menstrual period. (2) Infrequent occurrence of menstruation.

oligophrenia (*ol-ig-o-fre'-ne-ah).* Mental subnormality.

oligospermia (*ol-ig-o-sper'-me-ah).* A diminished output of spermatozoa.

oliguria (*ol-ig-u'-re-ah).* A deficient secretion of urine.

olivary (*ol'-iv-ar-e).* Like an olive in shape. *O. body.* A mass of grey matter situated behind the anterior pyramid of the medulla oblongata.

omentectomy (*o-ment-ek'-tom-e).* The surgical removal of all or part of the omentum.

omentopexy (*o-ment'-o-peks-e).* The surgical fixation of the omentum to some other tissue, usually the abdominal wall. *Cardio-o.* Attachment of the omentum to the heart to establish a collateral circulation when there is coronary occlusion.

omentum (*o-ment'-um).* A fold of peritoneum joining the stomach to other abdominal organs. *Greater o.* The fold reflected from the greater curvature of the stomach and lying in front of the intestines. *Lesser o.* The fold reflected from the lesser curvature and attaching the stomach to the under surface of the liver.

omphalitis (*om-fal-i'-tis).* Inflammation of the umbilicus.

omphalocele (*om'-fal-o-seel).* An umbilical hernia.

omphàloproptosis (*om-fal-o-prop-to'-sis*). Excessive protrusion of the umbilicus.

omphalus (*om'-fal-us*). The umbilicus.

Onchocerca (*on-ko-ser'-kah*). A genus of filarial worms, found in tropical parts of Africa and America, which may give rise to skin and subcutaneous lesions and attack the eye.

onchocerciasis (*on-ko-ser-ki'-as-is*). A tropical skin disease caused by infestation with *Onchocerca*.

oncogenesis (*on-ko-jen'-es-is*). The causation and formation of tumours.

oncogenic (*on-ko-jen'-ik*). Giving rise to tumour formation.

oncology (*on-kol'-o-je*). The scientific study of tumours.

oncometer (*on-kom'-e-ter*). An instrument for measuring the size of the spleen, kidneys and other organs. *See* Plethysmography.

onychia (*on-ik'-e-ah*). Inflammation of the matrix of a nail, with suppuration, which may cause the nail to fall off.

onychogryphosis (*on-ik-o-grifo'-sis*). Enlargement of the nails, with excessive curvature, most commonly affecting the big toes.

onycholysis (*on-ik-ol'-is-is*). Loosening or separation of a nail from its bed.

onychomycosis (*on-ik-o-miko'-sis*). Infection of the nails by a fungus.

onychosis (*on-ik-o'-sis*). A disease or deformity of the nails or of a nail.

oöcyte (*o'-o-site*). The immature egg cell or ovum in the ovary.

oögenesis (*o-o-jen'-es-is*). The development and production of the ovum.

oöphoralgia (*o-off-or-al'-je-ah*). Pain in an ovary.

oöphorectomy (*o-off-or-ek'-tom-e*). Excision of an ovary. Ovariectomy.

oöphoritis (*o-off-or-i'-tis*). Inflammation of an ovary.

oöphorocystectomy (*o-off-or-o-sist-ek'-tom-e*). Surgical removal of an ovarian cyst.

oöphorocystosis (*o-off-or-o-sist-o'-sis*). The development of one or more ovarian cysts.

oöphoron (*o-off'-or-on*). An ovary.

oöphoropexy (*o-off'-or-o-pek-se*). The surgical fixation of a displaced ovary to the pelvic wall.

oöphorosalpingectomy (*o-off-or-o-sal-pin-jek'-tom-e*). Removal of an ovary and its associated uterine tube.

opacity (*o-pas'-it-e*). Cloudiness, lack of transparency. Opacities occur in the lens of an eye when a cataract is forming. They also occur in the vitreous humour and appear as floating objects.

operant conditioning (*op'-er-ant con-dish'-un-ing*). A form of behaviour therapy in which a reward is given when the subject performs the action required of him. The reward serves to encourage repetition of the action.

operation (*op-er-a'-shun*). A surgical procedure in which instruments or hands are used by the operator. *Avascular o.* One in which there is little or no bleeding, achieved by applying a tourniquet or by the use of drugs causing hypotension. *Magnet o.* The removal of a foreign body from the eye by means of a magnet. *Major o.* One which entails a risk to life. *Minor o.* One in which there is minimal risk to life. *Palliative o.* One that relieves symptoms, but does not cure.

ophthalmia (off-thal'-me-ah). Inflammation of the eye, involving especially the conjunctiva. *Gonorrhoeal o.* or *o. neonatorum.* A serious infection of infants, usually caused by a gonococcus. *Granular o.* An acute and purulent form when there is a gritty feeling on moving the eyelids. Trachoma. *Phlyctenular o. See* Conjunctivitis.

ophthalmic (off-thal'-mik). Relating to the eye.

ophthalmitis (off-thal-mi'-tis). Inflammation of the eyeball. *Sympathetic o.* A serious complication in a sound eye following a perforating wound in the other.

ophthalmologist (off-thal-mol'-oj-ist). A specialist in diseases of the eye.

ophthalmology (off-thal-mol'-o-je). The study of the eye and its diseases.

ophthalmometer (off-thal-mom'-e-ter). An instrument for accurately measuring corneal astigmatism. A keratometer.

ophthalmoplegia (off-thal-mo-ple'-je-ah). Paralysis of the muscles of the eye.

ophthalmoscope (off-thal'-mo-skope). An instrument fitted with a light and lenses by which the interior of the eye can be illuminated and examined.

ophthalmotomy (off-thal-mot'-om-e). Incision of the eyeball.

ophthalmotonometer (off-thal'-mo-to-nom'-e-ter). An instrument for measuring the intra-ocular tension of the eye. A tonometer.

opiate (o'-pe-ate). Any medicine containing opium.

opisthotonos (o-pis-thot'-on-os). A muscle spasm causing the back to be arched and the head retracted, with great rigidity of the muscles of the neck and back. This condition may be present in acute cases of meningitis, tetanus, and strychnine poisoning.

opium (o'-pe-um). A drug derived from dried poppy-juice and used as a narcotic. It produces deep sleep, slows the pulse and respiration, contracts the pupils and checks all secretions of the body except sweat. It is a highly addictive drug. Opium derivatives include apomorphine, codeine, morphine and papaverine.

opponens (op-o'-nens). Opposing. A term applied to certain muscles controlling the movements of the fingers. *O. pollicis.* A muscle that adducts the thumb so that it and the little finger can be brought together.

opsonic index (op-son'-ik in'-deks). A measurement of the bactericidal power of the phagocytes in the blood of an individual.

opsonin (op'-son-in). An antibody present in the blood which renders bacteria more easily destroyed by the phagocytes. Each kind of bacteria has its specific opsonin.

optic (op'-tik). Relating to vision. *O. atrophy.* Degeneration of the optic nerve. *O. chiasma.* The crossing of the fibres of the optic nerves at the base of the brain. *O. disc.* The point where the optic nerve enters the eyeball. *O. foramen.* The opening in the posterior part of the orbit through which pass the optic nerve and the ophthalmic artery. *O. nerve.* A bundle of

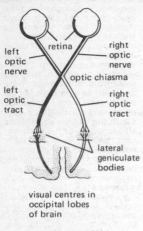

left optic nerve — retina

right optic nerve

optic chiasma

left optic tract

right optic tract

lateral geniculate bodies

visual centres in occipital lobes of brain

OPTIC CHIASMA

nerve fibres running from the optic chiasma in the brain to the optic disc on the eyeball.

optical (*op'-tik-al*). Pertaining to sight. *O. density*. The refractive power of the transparent tissues through which light rays pass, changing the direction of the ray.

optician (*op-tish'-an*). One who makes and fits spectacles. *Ophthalmic o.* An optician who tests people's eyes. An optometrist.

optimum (*op'-tim-um*). The best and most favourable.

optometry (*op-tom'-et-re*). The measuring of visual acuity and the fitting of glasses to correct visual defects.

ora (*o'-rah*). A margin. *O. serrata*. The jagged edge of the retina.

oral (*or'-al*). (1) Relating to the mouth. (2) Spoken. (3) Of medicines, taken by mouth. *O. contraceptive*. A hormone preparation taken by women to inhibit conception. *O. eroticism*. Oral gratification which the infant gains from sucking and exploring objects with his mouth. It is still in evidence in later life in the pleasure derived from eating, gum-chewing, smoking and kissing.

orbicular (*or-bik'-u-lar*). Circular.

orbit (*or'-bit*). (1) The bony cavity containing the eyeball. (2) The path of an object moving around another object.

orchidalgia (*or-kid-al'-je-ah*). Pain in a testicle.

orchidectomy (*or-kid-ek'-tom-e*). Excision of a testicle. *Bilateral o.* The operation of castration.

orchidopexy (*or'-kid-o-pek-se*). An operation to free an undescended testicle and place it in the scrotum.

orchi-epididymitis (*or-ke-ep-e-did-e-mi'-tis*). Inflammation of a testicle and its epididymis.

orchis (*or'-kis*). A testicle.

orchitis (*or-ki'-tis*). Inflammation of a testicle.

orf (*orf*). A virus infection transmitted from sheep to man. It may give rise to a boil-like lesion on the hands of meat handlers.

organ (*or'-gan*). A part of the body designed to perform a particular function.

organelle (*or-gan-el'*). A structure within a cell which has specialized functions, e.g. nucleus, endoplasmic reticulum, mitochondrion, etc.

organic (*or-gan'-ik*). (1) Pertaining to the organs. *O. disease*. Disease of an organ, accompanied by structural changes.

(2) Pertaining to chemicals containing carbon.

organism (*or'-gan-izm*). An individual living being, animal or vegetable.

orgasm (*or'-gazm*). The climax of sexual excitement.

orientation (*or-e-en-ta'-shun*). A sense of direction. (1) The ability of a person to estimate his position in regard to time, place and persons. (2) The imparting of relevant information at the onset of a course or conference so that its content and objects may be understood.

orifice (*or'-if-is*). Any opening in the body.

origin (*or'-ij-in*). In anatomy: (1) the point of attachment of a muscle; (2) the point at which a nerve or a blood vessel branches from the main stem.

ornithosis (*or-nith-o'-sis*). A virus disease of birds, usually pigeons, which may be transmitted to man in a form resembling bronchopneumonia.

oropharynx (*or-o-far'-inks*). The lower portion of the pharynx behind the mouth and above the oesophagus and larynx.

orphenadrine (*or-fen'-ad-reen*). A drug used to treat parkinsonism, especially when accompanied by depression.

orthodontics (*or-tho-don'-tiks*). Dentistry which deals with the prevention and correction of malocclusion and irregularities of the teeth.

orthopaedics (*or-tho-pe'-diks*). The science dealing with deformities, injuries and diseases of the bones and joints.

orthopnoea (*or-thop-ne'-ah*). Difficulty in breathing unless in an upright position, e.g. sitting up in bed.

orthoptics (*or-thop'-tiks*). The practice of treating by nonsurgical methods (usually eye exercises) abnormalities of vision such as strabismus (squint).

orthoptist (*or-thop'-tist*). One who specializes in the treatment of squints by ocular exercises.

orthostatic (*or-tho-stat'-ik*). Pertaining to or caused by standing erect. *O. albuminuria.* See Albuminuria. *O. hypotension.* Low blood pressure, occurring when someone stands up.

Ortolani's sign (*M. Ortolani, Italian orthopaedic surgeon*). A test performed soon after birth to detect possible congenital dislocation of the hip. A 'click' is felt on reversing the movements of abduction and rotation of the hip while the child is lying with knees flexed.

os (*os*). (1) A bone. *O. calcis.* The heel-bone or calcaneum. (2) A mouth or opening. *External o.* The opening of the cervix into the vagina. *Internal o.* The junction of the cervical canal and body of the uterus.

oscheocele (*os'-ke-o-seel*). A scrotal hernia or swelling.

oscillation (*os-il-a'-shun*). (1) A backwards and forwards motion. (2) Vibration.

oscilloscope (*os-il'-o-skope*). An apparatus using a cathode-ray tube to depict visibly data fed into it electronically, e.g. the way in which the heart is performing.

Osgood–Schlatter disease (*R.B. Osgood, American orthopaedic surgeon, 1873– 1956; C. Schlatter, Swiss surgeon, 1864–1934*).

Osteochondritis of the tibial tuberosity.

Osler's nodes (*Sir W. Osler, Canadian physician, 1849–1919*). Small painful swellings which occur in or beneath the skin, especially of the extremities in subacute bacterial endocarditis, caused by minute emboli. They usually disappear in 1–3 days.

osmoreceptor (*oz-mo-re-sep'-tor*). One of a group of specialized nerve cells which monitor the osmotic pressure of the blood and the extracellular fluid. Impulses from these receptors are relayed to the hypothalamus.

osmosis (*oz-mo'-sis*). The passage of fluid from a low concentration solution to one of a higher concentration through a semi-permeable membrane.

osmotic (*oz-mot'-ik*). Pertaining to osmosis. *O. pressure.* The pressure exerted by large molecules in the blood, e.g. albumin and globulin proteins, which draws fluid into the blood stream from the surrounding tissues.

osseous (*os'-e-us*). Bony.

ossicle (*os'-ikl*). A small bone. *Auditory o.* One of the three bones in the middle ear: the malleus, incus, and stapes.

ossification (*os-if-ik-a'-shun*). The process by which bone is developed. Osteogenesis.

ostalgia (*os-tal'-je-ah*). Pain in a bone.

osteitis (*os-te-i'-tis*). Inflammation of bone. *O. deformans.* See Paget's disease. *O. fibrosa cystica* or *parathyroid o.* Defects of ossification, with fibrous tissue production, leading to weakening and deformity. It affects children chiefly, and is associated with parathyroid tumour, removal

of which checks it. *See* von Recklinghausen's disease.

osteo-arthritis (*os-te-o-ar-thri'-tis*). A degenerative disease in which there is destruction of articular cartilage and bony outgrowths at the edges of joints. A painful disease of the elderly, occurring in the larger joints where most weight is carried. Osteo-arthrosis.

osteo-arthrotomy (*os-te-o-ar-throt'-om-e*). Surgical excision of the jointed end of a bone.

osteoblast (*os'-te-o-blast*). A cell which develops into an osteocyte and turns into bone.

osteochondritis (*os-te-o-kon-dri'-tis*). Inflammation of bone and cartilage, particularly a degenerative disease of an epiphysis causing pain and deformity. *O. of the hip.* Perthes' disease. *O. of the tarsal scaphoid bone.* Köhler's disease. *O. of the tibial tuberosity.* Osgood–Schlatter disease.

osteochondroma (*os-te-o-kon-dro'-mah*). A tumour consisting of both bone and cartilage.

osteoclasis (*os-te-o-kla'-sis*). (1) The surgical fracture of bones to correct a deformity such as bow-leg. (2) The restructuring of bone by osteoclasts during growth or the repair of damaged bone.

osteoclast (*os'-te-o-klast*). (1) A large cell that breaks down and absorbs bone and callus. (2) An instrument designed for surgical fracture of bone.

osteocyte (*os'-te-o-site*). A bone cell.

osteodystrophy (*os-te-o-dis'-tro-fe*). A metabolic disease of bone.

osteo-ectomy (*os-te-o-ek'-*

tom-e). Surgical excision of bone.

osteogenesis (*os-te-o-jen'-es-is*). The formation of bone. *O. imperfecta.* A congenital disorder of the bones, which are very brittle and fracture easily. Fragilitas osseum.

osteogenic (*os-te-o-jen'-ik*). Originating in or derived from bone. *O. sarcoma.* A malignant growth of bone.

osteoma (*os-te-o'-mah*). A benign tumour arising from bone.

osteomalacia (*os-te-o-mal-a'-she-ah*). A disease characterized by painful softening of bones. Due to vitamin D deficiency.

osteomyelitis (*os-te-o-mi-el-i'-tis*). Inflammation of the bone marrow due to infection. *Acute o.* Type that commonly occurs in children due to a blood-borne bacterial infection. The vascular edge of the epiphyseal cartilage is first attacked. *Chronic o.* Type that may result from an acute attack or from an open fracture.

osteopath (*os'-te-o-path*). One who practises osteopathy.

osteopathy (*os-te-op'-ath-e*). (1) Any bone disease. (2) A system of treatment of disease by bone manipulation.

osteoperiostitis (*os'-te-o-per-e-os-ti'-tis*). Inflammation of bone and periosteum.

osteopetrosis (*os-te-o-pet-ro'-sis*). A rare congenital disease in which the bones become abnormally dense. Albers–Schönberg disease.

osteophony (*os-te-off'-on-e*). Conduction of sound by bone.

osteophyte (*os'-te-o-fite*). A small outgrowth of bone.

osteoplasty (*os'-te-o-plas-te*). A plastic operation on bone.

osteoporosis (*os-te-o-por-o'-sis*). Rarefaction of bone, seen most commonly in elderly people. The bones are lacking in mineral salts due to deficiency of bony matrix. This may be due to protein or hormone insufficiency.

osteosarcoma (*os-te-o-sar-ko'-mah*). An osteogenic sarcoma. A malignant bone tumour.

osteosclerosis (*os-te-o-skler-o'-sis*). An increase in density and a hardening of bone. *O. congenita.* Achondroplasia. *O. fragilis.* Osteopetrosis.

osteotome (*os'-te-o-tome*). A surgical chisel for cutting bone.

osteotomy (*os-te-ot'-om-e*). The cutting into or through a bone, sometimes performed to correct deformity. *O. of hip.* A method of treating osteoarthritis by cutting the bone and altering the line of weight-bearing.

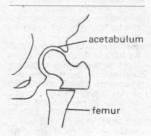

acetabulum

femur

OSTEOTOMY OF HIP

ostium (*os'-te-um*). A mouth. *Abdominal o.* The opening at the end of the uterine tube into the peritoneal cavity.

otalgia (*o-tal'-je-ah*). Ear-ache.

otic (*o'-tik*). Relating to the ear.

otitis (*o-ti'-tis*). Inflammation of the ear. *O. externa.* Inflammation of the outer passage of the ear. *O. interna.* Labyrinthitis. Inflammation of the inner ear. *O. media.* Inflammation of the middle ear.

otolaryngology (*o-to-lar-ing-gol'-o-je*). The scientific study of the ear and the larynx and the diseases affecting them.

otolith (*o'-to-lith*). (1) A calculus in the middle ear. (2) One of a number of small calcareous concretions of the inner ear, at the base of semicircular canals.

otology (*o-tol'-o-je*). The scientific study of the ear and its diseases.

otomycosis (*o-to-mi-ko'-sis*). A fungal infection of the auditory canal.

otoplasty (*o'-to-plas-te*). Plastic surgery of the outer ear.

otorhinolaryngology (*o-to-ri-no-lar-ing-gol'-o-je*). The scientific study of diseases of the ear, nose and throat.

otorrhoea (*o-tor-e'-ah*). Discharge from the ear, especially of pus.

otosclerosis (*o-to-skler-o'-sis*). An hereditary disorder where there is thickening and ossification of the tissues and ligaments that convey the sound waves to the internal ear. The stapes become fixed in the fenestra ovalis (oval window), causing deafness.

otoscope (*o'-to-skope*). An auriscope. An instrument for examining the ear.

otoscopy (*o-tos'-ko-pe*). An examination of the tympanic membrane and auditory canal by means of an otoscope.

ototoxic (*o-to-toks'-ik*). Anything which has a deleterious effect on the eighth cranial nerve or on the organs of hearing.

ovarian (*o-vair'-e-an*). Relating to an ovary. *O. cyst.* A tumour of the ovary containing fluid.

ovariectomy (*o-vair-e-ek'-tom-e*). Oöphorectomy. Excision of an ovary.

ovariotomy (*o-vair-e-ot'-om-e*). (1) Surgical removal of an ovary. (2) Excision of an ovarian tumour.

ovaritis (*o-var-i'-tis*). Oöphoritis. Inflammation of an ovary.

ovary (*o'-var-e*). One of a pair of glandular organs in the female pelvis. They produce ova which pass through the uterine tubes into the uterus, and steroid hormones which control the menstrual cycle.

overbite (*o'-ver-bite*). An overlapping of the lower teeth by the upper teeth.

over-compensation (*o-ver-kom-pen-sa'-shun*). A mental mechanism by which a person tries to assert himself by aggressive behaviour or by talking or acting 'big' to compensate for a feeling of inadequacy.

overdosage (*o-ver-do'-saje*). The toxic effects resulting from too high a blood level of a drug. This may be from too large or repeated doses or from the cumulative effect of the drug.

oviduct (*o'-ve-dukt*). A uterine tube.

ovotestis (*o-vo-tes'-tis*). A gonad containing both ovarian and testicular tissue.

ovulation (*ov-u-la'-shun*). The process of rupture of the mature graafian follicle when the ovum is shed from the ovary.

ovum (*o'-vum*). *pl.* ova. An egg. The reproductive cell of the female.

oxidization (*oks-e-di-za'-shun*). Oxidation. The process by which combustion occurs and breaking up of matter takes place; e.g. oxidation of carbohydrates gives carbon dioxide and water:

$$C_6H_{12}O_6 + 6O_2 = 6CO_2 + 6H_2O$$

oximeter (*oks-im'-e-ter*). A photoelectric cell used to determine the oxygen saturation of blood. *Ear o.* One attached to the ear by which the oxygen content of blood flowing through the ear can be measured.

oxprenolol (*oks-pren'-o-lol*). A beta-blocking drug used in the treatment of angina, hypertension and cardiac arrhythmias.

oxygen (*oks'-e-jen*). abbrev. O. A colourless, odourless gas constituting one-fifth of the atmosphere. It is stored in cylinders at high pressure or as liquid oxygen. It is used medicinally to enrich the air when either respiration or circulation is impaired.

oxygenation (*oks-e-jen-a'-shun*). Saturation with oxygen; a process which occurs in the lungs to the haemoglobin of blood, which is saturated with oxygen to form oxyhaemoglobin.

oxygenator (*oks'-e-jen-a-tor*). A machine through which the blood is passed to oxygenate it during open heart surgery. *Pump o.* A machine which pumps oxygenated blood through the body during heart surgery.

oxyhaemoglobin (*oks-e-he-mo-glo'-bin*). Haemoglobin which has been oxygenated, as in arterial blood.

oxyntic (*oks-in'-tik*). Acid forming. *O. cell.* A parietal cell of the gastric glands which sec-

retes hydrochloric acid.

oxypertine (*oks-e-per'-teen*). An antipsychotic tranquillizing drug used in the treatment of schizophrenia and related psychoses, and of mania and hyperactivity.

oxytetracycline (*oks-e-tet-rah-si'-kleen*). A broad-spectrum antibiotic, chiefly used against infections caused by chlamydia, rickettsia and brucella.

oxytocic (*oks-e-to'-sik*). Any drug which stimulates uterine contractions and may be used to hasten delivery.

oxytocin (*oks-e-to'-sin*). A pituitary hormone which stimulates uterine contractions and the ejection of milk. Synthetically prepared, it is used to induce labour and to control post-partum haemorrhage.

oxyuriasis (*oks-e-u-ri'-as-is*). Infestation by thread worms of the genus *Enterobius*.

ozaena (*o-ze'-nah*). Atrophic rhinitis. A condition of the nose in which there is loss and shrinkage of the ciliated mucous membrane and of the turbinate bones. There may be an offensive nasal discharge.

ozone (*o'-zone*). An intensified form of oxygen containing three O atoms to the molecule (i.e. O_3), and often discharged by electrical machines such as X-ray apparatuses. In medicine it is employed as an antiseptic and oxidizing agent.

P

P. Chemical symbol for *phosphorus*.
Pa. Abbreviation for the SI unit, the *pascal*.

pace-maker (*pase'-ma-ker*). The sino-atrial node. *See* Node. *Artificial p.* An electrically operated mechanical device which stimulates the myocardium to contract. It consists of an energy source, usually batteries, and electrical circuitry connected to an electrode which is in direct contact with the myocardium. Pace-makers may be temporary or permanent. Temporary ones usually have an external energy source whereas permanent ones have a subcutaneously implanted one. The rate the pace-maker delivers pulses may be either fixed or on demand. *Fixed* pacing means that pulses are delivered to the heart at a predetermined rate irrespective of any cardiac activity. A *demand* pace-maker is programmed to deliver pulses only in the absence of spontaneous cardiac activity. The need for replacement batteries is usually indicated when the rate of the pulse slows by five beats or more.

pachydactyly (*pak-e-dak'-til-e*). Abnormal thickening of the fingers or toes.

pachydermia (*pak-e-der'-me-ah*). An abnormal thickening of the skin. *P. laryngis.* A chronic hypertrophy of the vocal cords.

pachyonychia (*pak-e-on-ik'-e-ah*). Abnormal thickening of the nails.

pachysomia (*pak-e-so'-me-ah*). Abnormal thickening of parts of the body, as in acromegaly.

Pacini's corpuscles (*F. Pacini, Italian anatomist, 1812–1883*). Specialized end-organs, situated in the subcutaneous tissue of the extremities and near joints, which react to firm pressure.

pack (*pak*). A pad or plug of cotton wool or gauze which can be placed in an orifice.

pad (*pad*). A soft cushion of cotton wool or other material used to protect a part of the body from injury or to absorb bleeding or other discharge.

paediatrician (*pe-de-at-rish'-an*). A specialist in the diseases of children.

paediatrics (*pe-de-at'-riks*). The branch of medicine dealing with the care and development of children and with the treatment of diseases that affect them.

paedophilia (*pe-do-fil'-e-ah*). A sexual attraction towards young children.

Paget's disease (*Sir J. Paget, British surgeon, 1814–1899*). (1) A chronic disease of bone in which overactivity of the osteoblasts and osteoclasts leads to dense bone formation with areas of rarefaction. Osteitis deformans. (2) An inflammation of the nipple caused by cancer of the milk ducts of the breast..

palate (*pal'-at*). The roof of the mouth. *Artificial p.* A plate made to close a cleft palate. *Cleft p.* A congenital deformity where there is lack of fusion of the two bones forming the palate. *Hard p.* The bony part at the front. *Soft p.* A fold of mucous membrane that continues from the hard palate to the uvula.

palatine bone (*pal'-at-ine bone*). One of a pair of bones which form a part of the nasal cavity and the hard palate.

palatoplasty (*pal'-at-o-plas-te*). Plastic surgery of the roof of the mouth.

palatoplegia (*pal-at-o-ple'-je-ah*). Paralysis of the soft palate.

palliative (*pal'-e-at-iv*). Treatment which relieves, but does not cure, disease.

pallidectomy (*pal-id-ekt'-tom-e*). An operation performed to decrease the activity of the globus pallidus, the medial part of the lentiform nucleus in the base of the cerebrum. It has brought about a marked improvement in severely agitated cases of parkinsonism.

pallor (*pal'-or*). Abnormal paleness of the skin.

palmar (*pal'-mar*). Relating to the palm of the hand. *P. fascia*. The arrangement of tendons in the palm of the hand. *Deep* and *superficial p. arches*. The chief arterial blood supply to the hand formed by the junction of the ulnar and radial arteries.

palpation (*pal-pa'-shun*). The examination of the organs by touch or pressure of the hand over the part.

palpebral (*pal'-pe-bral*). Referring to the eyelids. *P. ligaments*. A band of ligaments which stretches from the junction of the upper and lower lid to the orbital bones, both medially and laterally.

palpitation (*pal-pit-a'-shun*). Rapid and forceful contraction of the heart of which the patient is conscious.

palsy (*pawl'-ze*). Paralysis. *Bell's p*. Paralysis of the facial muscles on one side, supplied by the seventh cranial nerve. *Crutch p*. Paralysis due to pressure of a crutch on the radial nerve and a cause of 'dropped wrist'. *Erb's p*. Paralysis of one arm due to a birth injury to the brachial plexus. *Shaking p*. Parkinsonism. Paralysis agitans.

panacea (*pan-a-se'-ah*). An alleged cure for all diseases.

panarthritis (*pan-ar-thri'-tis*). Inflammation of all the joints or of all the structures of a joint.

pancarditis (*pan-kar-di'-tis*). Inflammation of all the structures of the heart, such as may occur in rheumatic fever and in virus infections.

Pancoast's tumour (*H.K. Pancoast, American radiologist, 1875–1939*). Pain, wasting and weakness of the arm which occur as secondary features of carcinoma of the bronchus due to neurological involvement. The tumour is at the apex of the lung.

pancreas (*pan'-kre-as*). An elongated, racemose gland about 15 cm (6 in.) long, lying behind the stomach, with its head in the curve of the duodenum, and its tail in contact with the spleen. It secretes a digestive fluid (*pancreatic juice*) containing ferments which act on all classes of foods. The fluid enters the duodenum by the pancreatic duct which joins the common bile duct. The pancreas also secretes the hormones insulin and glucagon.

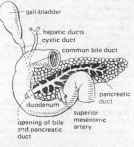

gall-bladder

hepatic ducts
cystic duct
common bile duct
pancreatic duct
duodenum
superior mesenteric artery
opening of bile and pancreatic duct

PANCREAS

pancreatectomy (*pan-kre-at-ek'-tom-e*). Surgical excision of the whole or a part of the pancreas.

pancreatin (*pan'-kre-at-in*). An extract from the pancreas containing the digestive enzymes. Used to treat deficiency as in fibrocystic disease of the pancreas and after pancreatectomy.

pancreatitis (*pan-kre-at-i'-tis*). Inflammation of the pancreas. *Acute p.* A severe condition in which the patient experiences sudden pain in the upper abdomen and back. The patient often becomes severely shocked. *Chronic p.* Chronic inflammation occurring after acute attacks. Pancreatic failure leading to diabetes mellitus may ensue. This condition is sometimes associated with chronic alcohol dependency.

pancreatolith (*pan-kre-at'-o-lith*). A stone (calculus) in the pancreas.

pancytopenia (*pan-si-to-pe'-ne-ah*). A reduction in number of all types of blood cell due to failure of bone marrow formation.

pandemic (*pan-dem'-ik*). An epidemic spreading over a wide area, sometimes all over the world.

panhypopituitarism (*pan-hi-po-pit-u'-it-ar-izm*). Simmond's disease. A deficiency of all the hormones produced by the anterior pituitary gland.

panhysterectomy (*pan-his-ter-ek'-tom-e*). Surgical removal of the whole of the uterus.

panic (*pan'-ik*). An unreasoning and overwhelming fear or terror. It may occur in anxiety states and acute schizophrenia.

panleucopenia (*pan-lu-ko-pe'-ne-ah*). A deficiency of all the white blood cells.

panmyelopathy (*pan-mi-el-op'-ath-e*). A disease affecting all the cells formed in the bone marrow.

panniculitis (*pan-ik-u-li'-tis*). Inflammation of the subcutaneous fat causing tender nodules on the abdomen and thorax and on the thighs.

panniculus (*pan-ik'-u-lus*). A sheet of membrane. *P. adiposus.* The fatty layer beneath the skin.

pannus (*pan'-us*). Increased vascularity of the cornea leading to granulation tissue formation and impaired vision. It occurs after inflammation of the cornea.

panophthalmia (*pan-off-thal'-me-ah*). Panophthalmitis. Inflammation of all the tissues of the eyeball.

panosteitis (*pan-os-te-i'-tis*). Inflammation of all the structures of a bone.

panotitis (*pan-o-ti'-tis*). Inflammation of all parts of the ear.

pansystolic murmur (*pan-sis-tol'-ik mer'-mer*). A heart murmur heard throughout the time when the heart is in systole. *See* Murmur.

pantothenic acid (*pan-to-then'-ik as'-id*). One of the vitamins in the B complex.

Papanicolaou test (*G.N. Papanicolaou, Greek physician, anatomist and cytologist, 1883–1962*). A smear test to detect diseases of the uterine cervix and endometrium.

papaveretum (*pap-av-er-e'-tum*). A preparation of the alkaloids of opium with an action similar to morphine. It is used to counteract severe pain.

papilla (*pap-il'-ah*). *pl.* papillae.

A small nipple-shaped protuberance. *Circumvallate p.* One surrounded by a ridge. A number are found at the back of the tongue arranged in a V-shape, and containing taste buds. *Filiform p.* One of the fine, slender filaments on the main part of the tongue which give it its velvety appearance. *Fungiform p.* A mushroom-shaped papilla of the tongue. *Optic p.* The optic disc, where the optic nerve leaves the eyeball. *Tactile p.* A projection on the true skin which contains nerve endings responsible for relaying sensations of pressure to the brain. A touch corpuscle.

papillary (*pap'-il-ar-e*). Composed of or pertaining to papillae.

papillitis (*pap-il-i'-tis*). Inflammation of the optic disc.

papilloedema (*pap-il-e-de'-mah*). Oedematous swelling of the optic disc indicating increase of intracranial pressure.

papilloma (*pap-il-o'-mah*). A benign growth of epithelial tissue, e.g. a wart.

papillomatosis (*pap-il-o-mato'-sis*). The occurrence of multiple papillomas.

papovavirus (*pap-o'-vah-virus*). A family of DNA-producing viruses which cause tumours, usually benign, such as warts.

papular (*pap'-u-lah*). Referring to papules.

papule (*pap'-ule*). A pimple, or small solid elevation of the skin.

papulopustular (*pap-u-lo-pus'-tu-lar*). Descriptive of skin eruptions of both papules and pustules.

papulosquamous (*pap-u-lo-skwa'-mus*). Descriptive of skin eruptions which are both papular and scaly. They include such conditions as lichen planus, pityriasis and psoriasis.

para-aminobenzoic acid (*par-ah-am-in-o-ben-zo'-ik as'-id*). A member of the B group of vitamins. It is used in creams and lotions to prevent sunburn.

para-aminosalicylic acid (*par-ah-am-in-o-sal-is-il'-ik as'-id*). PAS. An acid, the salts of which are used together with other drugs, usually isoniazid (INH) or streptomycin, in the treatment of tuberculosis.

paracentesis (*par-ah-sen-te'-sis*). Puncture of the wall of a cavity with a hollow needle in order to draw off excess fluid or to obtain diagnostic material.

paracetamol (*par-ah-set'-am-ol*). A mild analgesic drug used to treat headaches, toothache and rheumatic pains, and also to treat pyrexia.

parachlorometacresol (*par-ah-klor-o-met-ah-kre'-sol*). Chlorocresol. A coal-tar antiseptic preparation.

parachlorometaxylenol (*par-ah-klor-o-met-ah-zi'-len-ol*). Chloroxylenol. A powerful antiseptic used chiefly as a skin disinfectant.

paracusis (*par-ah-ku'-sis*). A perverted sense of hearing. *P. of Willis.* An improvement in hearing when surrounded by noise.

paraesthesia (*par-es-the'-ze-ah*). An abnormal tingling sensation. 'Pins and needles'.

paraffin (*par'-af-in*). Any saturated hydrocarbon obtained from petroleum. *P. wax.* A hard paraffin that can be used for wax treatment for chronic inflammation of joints. *Liquid p.* A mineral oil which is used as a laxative. *Soft p.* Petroleum jelly. Used as a barrier agent to protect the skin.

paraformaldehyde (*par-ah-for-mal'-de-hide*). Paraform. A preparation of formaldehyde used as an antiseptic and also for fumigating rooms.

Paragonimus (*par-ah-gon'-im-us*). A genus of trematode parasites. The flukes infest the lungs and are found mainly in tropical countries.

paraldehyde (*par-al'-de-hide*). A drug used in the treatment of status epilepticus. *See* Status.

paralysis (*par-al'-is-is*). Loss of the power of movement of any part, as the result of interference with the nerve supply. *P. agitans.* Parkinsonism. *Bulbar p.* (*Labioglossopharyngeal p.*). Paralysis due to changes in the motor centre of the medulla oblongata. It affects the muscles of the mouth, tongue, and pharynx. *Diphtheritic p.* A complication of diphtheria, the soft palate being first affected. *Facial p.* (*Bell's palsy*). Paralysis that affects the muscles of the face and is due to injury to or inflammation of the facial nerve. *Flaccid p.* Loss of tone and absence of reflexes in the paralysed muscles. *General p. of the insane.* GPI. Paralytic dementia occurring in the late stages of syphilis. *Infantile p.* A former term for acute anterior poliomyelitis (*see* Poliomyelitis). *Spastic p.* Paralysis characterized by rigidity of affected muscles.

paralytic (*par-ah-lit'-ik*). Affected by or relating to paralysis. *P. ileus.* Obstruction of the ileum due to absence of peristalsis in a portion of the intestine.

paramedian (*par-ah-me'-de-an*). Situated on the side of the median line.

paramedical (*par-ah-med'-ik-al*). Having some association with the science or practice of medicine. The paramedical services include occupational and speech therapy, physiotherapy, radiography and medical social work.

parametritis (*par-ah-me-tri'-tis*). Inflammation of the parametrium; pelvic cellulitis.

parametrium (*par-ah-me'-tre-um*). The connective tissue surrounding the uterus.

paramnesia (*par-am-ne'-ze-ah*). A defect of memory in which there is a false recollection. The patient may fill in the forgotten period with imaginary events which he describes in great detail.

paramyotonia congenita (*par-ah-mi-o-to'-ne-ah kon-jen'-it-ah*). A rare congenital condition in which a prolonged muscle contraction develops when the patient is exposed to cold.

paranoia (*par-ah-noi'-ah*). A mental disorder characterized by delusions of grandeur or persecution which may be fully systematized in logical form, with the personality remaining fairly well preserved.

paranoid (*par'-ah-noid*). Resembling paranoia. Refers to a condition that can occur in many forms of mental disease. Delusions of persecution are a marked feature. *P. schizophrenia. See* Schizophrenia.

paranormal (*par-ah-nor'-mal*). Pertaining to phenomena lying outside the range of current scientific knowledge, e.g.

extra-sensory perception.

paraparesis (*par-ah-par-e'-sis*). An incomplete paralysis affecting the lower limbs.

paraphasia (*par-ah-fa'-ze-ah*). A speech disorder involving the substitution of a similar sound or word for that intended, thereby producing a nonsensical utterance.

paraphimosis (*par-ah-fi-mo'-sis*). Retraction of the prepuce behind the glans penis, with inability to replace it, resulting in a painful constriction.

paraphrenia (*par-ah-fre'-ne-ah*). Schizophrenia occurring for the first time in later life and not accompanied by deterioration of the personality.

paraplegia (*par-ah-ple'-je-ah*). Paralysis of the lower extremities and lower trunk. All parts below the point of lesion in the spinal cord are affected. It may be of sudden onset from injury to the cord or may develop slowly as the result of disease.

parasite (*par'-ah-site*). Any animal or vegetable organism living upon or within another, from which it derives its nourishment.

parasiticide (*par-ah-sit'-is-ide*). A drug which kills parasites.

parasympathetic system (*par-ah-sim-path-et'-ik sis'-tem*). The craniosacral part of the autonomic nervous system.

parasympatholytic (*par-ah-sim-path-o-lit'-ik*). Anticholinergic. An agent that opposes the effects of the parasympathetic nervous system.

parathormone (*par-ah-thor'-mone*). The endocrine secretion of the parathyroid glands.

parathyroid gland (*par-ah-thi'-roid gland*). One of four small endocrine glands—two of which are associated with each lobe of the thyroid gland, and sometimes embedded in it. The secretion from these has some control over calcium metabolism, and lack of it is a cause of tetany.

parathyroidectomy (*par-ah-thi-roid-ek'-tom-e*). The surgical removal of parathyroid glands.

paratyphoid fever (*par-ah-ti'-foid fe'-ver*). A disease resembling typhoid, but usually of a milder nature. It is caused by a bacterium, *Salmonella paratyphi A, B* or *C*. In preventive inoculation, TAB vaccine prepared from typhoid and paratyphoid A and B bacilli, may be given, or a vaccine to which paratyphoid C has been added.

parencephalous (*par-en-kef'-al-us*). Having a congenital malformation of the brain.

parenchyma (*par-en-ki'-mah*). The essential active cells of an organ as distinguished from vascular and connective tissue.

parenteral (*par-en'-ter-al*). Apart from the alimentary canal. Applied to the introduction into the body of drugs or fluids by routes other than the mouth or rectum, for instance intravenously or subcutaneously.

paresis (*par-e'-sis*). Partial paralysis.

paries (*par'-e-eez*). *pl.* parietes. The wall of a cavity.

parietal (*par-i'-et-al*). Relating to the walls of any cavity. *P. bones.* The two bones forming part of the roof and sides of the skull. *P. cells.* The oxyntic cells in the gastric mucosa that secrete hydrochloric acid. *P. pleura.* The pleura attached to the chest wall.

Parinaud's oculogranular syn-

drome (*H. Parinaud, French ophthalmologist, 1844–1905*). A chronic granulomatous conjunctivitis with regional lymphadenitis and pyrexia.

parity (*par'-it-e*). In medicine, the condition of a woman with regard to the number of children which have been born live to her.

parkinsonism (*par'-kin-son-izm*). Paralysis agitans. Parkinson's disease. A degenerative disease of middle and old age manifesting as a tremor, starting in one hand and later affecting the other limbs, accompanied by a shuffling gait and a mask-like expression. The symptoms may also occur following an attack of encephalitis lethargica.

Parkinson's disease (*J. Parkinson, British physician, 1755–1824*). Parkinsonism.

paronychia (*par-on-ik'-e-ah*). An abscess near the fingernail; a whitlow or felon. *P. tendinosa.* A pyogenic infection that involves the tendon sheath.

parosmia (*par-oz'-me-ah*). A disordered sense of smell.

parotid (*par-ot'-id*). Situated near the ear. *P. glands.* Two salivary glands, one in front of each ear.

parotitis (*par-o-ti'-tis*). Inflammation of a parotid gland. Caused usually by ascending infection via its duct, when hygiene of the mouth is neglected or when the natural secretions are lessened, especially in severe illness or following operation. *Epidemic p.* Mumps.

parous (*par'-us*). Having borne one or more children.

paroxysm (*par'-oks-izm*). (1) A sudden attack or recurrence of a symptom of a disease. (2) A convulsion.

paroxysmal (*par-oks-iz'-mal*). *Ocurring in paroxysms. P. cardiac dyspnoea.* Cardiac asthma. Recurrent attacks of dyspnoea associated with pulmonary oedema and left-sided heart failure. *P. tachycardia.* Recurrent attacks of rapid heart beats that may occur without heart disease.

parrot disease (*par'-ot diz-eez'*). See Psittacosis.

parthenogenesis (*par-then-o-jen'-es-is*). Asexual reproduction by means of an egg which has not been fertilized.

particle (*par'-tikl*). A minute piece of substance.

parturient (*par-tu'-re-ent*). Giving birth; relating to childbirth.

parturition (*par-tu-rish'-un*). The act of giving birth to a child.

Parvobacteriaceae (*par-vo-bak-te-re-a'-se-e*). A family of bacteria which include the genera *Brucella, Haemophilus* and *Pasteurella.*

pascal (*pas'-kal*). *abbrev.* Pa. The SI unit of pressure.

Paschen bodies (*E. Paschen, German pathologist, 1860–1936*). Small granules demonstrable in the fluid of the vesicles of smallpox.

passive (*pas'-iv*). Not active. *P. immunity.* See Immunity. *P. movements.* In massage, manipulation by a physiotherapist without the help of the patient.

passivity (*pas-iv'-it-e*). In psychiatry, a delusional feeling that a person is under some outside control and must therefore be inactive.

Pasteur, L. (*French chemist and bacteriologist, 1833–1895*). Founder of the science of microbiology and developer of the technique of vaccination.

Pasteurella (*pas-tur-el'-ah*). A genus of short gram-negative bacilli. *P. pestis.* The causative organism of plague transmitted by rat fleas to man.

pasteurization (*pas-tur-i-za'-shun*). The process of checking fermentation in milk and other fluids by heating them to a temperature of 72°C for 15—20 seconds or 63°C for 30 minutes and then rapidly cooling. This kills most pathogenic bacteria.

patch test (*pach test*). A test of skin sensitivity in which a number of possible allergens are applied to the skin under a plaster. The causal agent of the allergy will produce an inflammation.

patella (*pat-el'-ah*). The small, circular, sesamoid bone forming the knee-cap.

patellar (*pat-el'-ar*). Belonging to the patella. *P. reflex.* A knee jerk obtained by tapping the tendon below the patella.

patellectomy (*pat-el-ek'-tom-e*). Excision of the patella.

patent (*pa'-tent*). Open. *P. ductus arteriosus.* Failure of the ductus arteriosus to close, causing a shunt of blood from the aorta into the pulmonary artery and producing a continuous heart murmur.

pathogen (*path'-o-jen*). A parasitic micro-organism such as a virus or a bacterium which can cause disease.

pathogenicity (*path-o-jen-is'-it-e*). The ability of a micro-organism to cause disease.

pathognomonic (*path-og-no-mon'-ik*). Specifically characteristic of a disease. A sign or symptom by which a pathological condition can positively be identified.

pathological (*path-o-loj'-ik-al*). (1) Pertaining to pathology. (2) Causing or arising from disease. *P. fracture.* A fracture occurring in diseased bone where there has been little or no external trauma.

pathology (*path-ol'-o-je*). The branch of medicine treating of disease, and the changes in structure and function which it causes.

pathophobia (*path-o-fo'-be-ah*). An exaggerated dread of disease.

Paul—Bunnell test (*J.R. Paul, American physician b. 1893; W.W. Bunnell, American physician, b. 1902*). An agglutination test which, if positive, confirms the diagnosis of glandular fever.

Pavlov's method (*I.P. Pavlov, Russian physiologist, 1849—1936*). A method for the study of the conditioned reflexes. Pavlov noticed that his experimental dogs salivated in anticipation of food when they heard a bell ring.

peau d'orange (*po dor-ahnj'*). A dimpled appearance of the overlying skin. Blockage of the skin lymphatics causes dimpling of the hair follicle openings which resembles orange skin.

pecten (*pek'-ten*). (1) The middle third of the anal canal. (2) A ridge on the pubic crest to which the inguinal ligament is attached.

pectoral (*pek'-tor-al*). Relating to the chest. *P. muscles.* Two pairs of muscles, pectoralis major and pectoralis minor, which control the movements of the shoulder and upper arm.

pectus (*pek'-tus*). The chest.

pedicle (*ped'-ikl*). The stem or neck of a tumour. *P. graft.* A

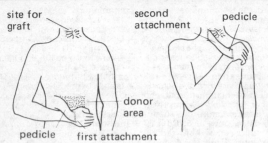

site for graft · second attachment · pedicle · donor area · pedicle · first attachment

PEDICLE GRAFT

tissue graft that is partially detached and inserted in its new position while temporarily still obtaining its blood supply from the original source.

pediculosis (*ped-ik-u-lo'-sis*). The condition of being infested with lice.

Pediculus (*ped-ik'-u-lus*). A genus of lice, small parasites infesting the skin and hairy parts of the body. *P. capitis.* The head louse. *P. corporis.* The body or clothes louse. It can transmit typhus and relapsing fever.

peduncle (*ped-ung'-kl*). A narrow part of a structure acting as a support. *Cerebellar p.* One of the collections of nerve fibres connecting the cerebellum with the medulla oblongata.

Pel–Ebstein syndrome (*P.K. Pel, Dutch physician, 1852– 1919; W. Ebstein, German physician, 1836–1912*). A recurrent pyrexia having a cycle of 15 to 21 days which occurs in cases of lymphadenoma.

pellagra (*pel-ag'-rah*). A deficiency disease due to lack of vitamin B (nicotinic acid). It is characterized by debility, digestive disorders and erythema with exfoliation of the skin.

pellicle (*pel'-ikl*). (1) A scum on the surface of a liquid. (2) A thin skin or membrane.

pelvic (*pel'-vik*). Pertaining to the pelvis. *P. exenteration.* Removal of all the pelvic organs. *P. girdle.* The ring of bone to which the lower limbs are jointed. It consists of the two hip-bones and the sacrum and coccyx.

pelvimetry (*pel-vim'-et-re*). Measurement of the pelvis. *X-ray p.* is used to measure the internal pelvic diameters, and late in pregnancy these can be assessed in relation to the fetal head.

pelvirectal (*pel-ve-rek'-tal*). Pertaining to the flexure where the pelvic colon joins the rectum at an acute angle.

pelvis (*pel'-vis*). A basin-shaped cavity. *Bony p.* The pelvic girdle formed of the hip-bones and the sacrum and coccyx. *Contracted p.* Narrowing of the diameter of the pelvis. *See* Conjugate. It may be of the *true* conjugate or the *diagonal.* Effective antenatal care will recognize this condition, and caesarian section is often necessary to ensure live birth. The deformity may be the result of rickets. *False p.* The part formed by the concavity of the iliac bones above the ileopectineal line. *Renal p.* The dilatation of the ureter, which by enclosing the hilus surrounds the pyramids of the kidney substance. *True p.* The basin-like cavity below the false pelvis, its upper limit being the pelvic brim.

pemphigoid (*pem'-fig-oid*). (1) Resembling pemphigus. (2) A bullous disease of the elderly with the blisters arising beneath the epidermis. The skin and the mucosa are affected, and sometimes the conjunctiva.

pemphigus (*pem'-fig-us*). Any one of a number of acute or chronic skin diseases characterized by an eruption of large blisters.

pendulous (*pen'-du-lus*). Hanging down. *P. abdomen.* The hanging down of the abdomen over the pelvis, due to weakness and laxity of the abdominal muscles. In pregnancy it causes the uterus to fall forwards.

penicillamine (*pen-e-sil'-am-een*). A chelating agent that is used in copper and lead poisoning to aid excretion of the metal and in the treatment of hepatolenticular degeneration (Wilson's disease). Also used in the treatment of severe rheumatoid arthritis.

penicillin (*pen-e-sil'-in*). An antibiotic cultured from certain moulds of the genus *Penicillium notatum.* The drug is used in various forms to treat a wide variety of bacterial infections. Discovered by Fleming in 1929, it

was first used therapeutically in 1941. Varieties of the drug include: benethamine penicillin, benzylpenicillin, benzathine penicillin, procaine penicillin, cloxacillin, ampicillin and amoxycillin.

penicillinase (*pen-e-sil'-in-aze*). An enzyme that inactivates penicillin. Many bacteria, particularly staphylococci, produce this enzyme.

Penicillium (*pen-e-sil'-e-um*). A genus of mould-like fungi from some of which the penicillins are derived. Some species are pathogenic to man.

penis (*pe'-nis*). The male organ of copulation and of urination.

pentagastrin (*pen-tah-gas'-trin*). A synthetic hormone with a similar structure to gastrin. It has largely replaced histamine in gastric secretion tests as it has no apparent side effects.

pentazocine (*pent-az'-o-seen*). An analgesic similar to morphine and used in the treatment of moderate to severe pain.

pentobarbitone (*pen-to-barb'-it-one*). A basal narcotic of the barbiturate group used in the treatment of severe insomnia.

pepsin (*pep'-sin*). An enzyme found in gastric juice. It partially digests proteins in an acid solution.

pepsinogen (*pep-sin'-o-jen*). The precursor of pepsin, activated by hydrochloric acid.

peptic (*pep'-tik*). Relating to pepsin or to the action of the gastric juices in promoting digestion. *P. ulcer.* An ulcer, usually in the stomach or the duodenum, caused by an excess of acid in the gastric juices.

peptone (*pep'-tone*). A substance produced by the action of pepsin on protein.

peptonuria (*pep-ton-u'-re-ah*). Presence of peptones in urine.

percept or **perception** (*per'-sept, per-sep'-shun*). An awareness and understanding of an impression that has been presented to the senses. The mental process by which we perceive.

percussion (*per-kush'-un*). A method of diagnosis by tapping with the fingers or with a light hammer upon any part of the body. Information can thus be gained as to the condition of underlying organs.

percutaneous (*per-ku-ta'-ne-us*). Through the skin, particularly in relation to ointments that are applied to unbroken skin.

perforation (*per-for-a'-shun*). A hole through the whole thickness of a wall of a cavity or organ.

perfusion (*per-fu'-zhun*). The passage of liquid through a tissue or an organ, particularly the passage of blood through the lung tissue.

perianal (*per-e-a'-nal*). Surrounding or located around the anus. *P. abscess*. A small subcutaneous pocket of pus near the anal margin.

periarteritis (*per-e-ar-ter-i'-tis*). Inflammation of the outer coat and surrounding tissues of an artery.

periarthritis (*per-e-ar-thri'tis*) Inflammation of the tissues surrounding a joint.

pericardiectomy (*per-e-kar-de-ek'-tom-e*). Surgical removal of the pericardium. Pericardectomy. Used in the treatment of chronic constrictive pericarditis.

pericardiocentesis (*per-e-kar-de-o-sen-te'-sis*). Drainage of fluid from the pericardium.

pericardiotomy (*per-e-kar-de-ot'-om-e*). Surgical incision of the pericardium. Pericardotomy.

pericarditis (*per-e-kar-di'-tis*). Inflammation of the pericardium. *Adhesive p.* The presence of adhesions between the two layers of pericardium owing to a thick fibrinous exudate. *Bacterial p.* Inflammation of the pericardium due to a bacterial infection. *Chronic constrictive p.* Thickening and sometimes calcification of the pericardium, which inhibits the action of the heart. *Rheumatic p.* Pericarditis due to rheumatic fever.

pericardium (*per-e-kar'-de-um*). The smooth membranous sac enveloping the heart, consisting of an outer fibrous and an inner serous coat. The sac contains a small amount of serous fluid.

perichondritis (*per-e-kon-dri'-tis*). Inflammation of the perichondrium.

perichondrium (*per-e-kon'-dre-um*). The membrane covering cartilaginous surfaces.

pericolpitis (*per-e-kol-pi'-tis*). Inflammation of the tissues around the vagina.

pericranium (*per-e-kra'-ne-um*). The periosteum of the cranial bones.

pericystitls (*per-e-sis-ti'-tis*). Inflammation of the tissues surrounding the bladder.

perihepatitis (*per-e-hep-at-i'-tis*). Inflammation of the peritoneum covering the liver.

perilymph (*per'-e-limf*). The fluid which separates the bony and the membranous labyrinths of the ear.

perimeter (*per-im'-e-ter*). (1) The line marking the boundary of any area or geometrical figure; the circumference. (2)

An instrument for measuring the field of vision.

perimetritis (*per-e-me-tri'-tis*). Inflammation of the perimetrium.

perimetrium (*per-e-me'-tre-um*). The peritoneal covering of the uterus.

perimetry (*per-im'-et-re*). The process of determining the visual fields.

perinatal (*per-e-na'-tal*). Pertaining to the period around the time of birth and including the pre- and postnatal periods. *P. respiratory distress syndrome. See* Respiratory. *P. mortality rate.* The number of deaths per 1000 live births that occur between the 28th week of pregnancy and the 4th week after the birth.

perineal (*per-e-ne'-al*). Relating to the perineum.

perineorrhaphy (*per-e-ne-or'-af-e*). Suture of the perineum to repair a laceration caused during childbirth.

perinephritis (*per-e-nef-ri'-tis*). Inflammation of the perinephrium.

perinephrium (*per-e-nef'-re-um*). The tissue surrounding the kidney.

perineum (*per-e-ne'-um*). The tissues between the anus and external genitals. *Lacerated p.* A torn perineum, which may result from childbirth, but is often forestalled by performing an episiotomy. Treatment is by perineorrhaphy.

periodic syndrome (*pe-re-od'-ik sin'-drome*). Recurrent head, limb or abdominal pains in children for which no organic cause can be found. It often leads to migraine in adult life.

periodontitis (*per-e-o-don-ti'-tis*). Inflammation of the periodontium.

periodontium (*per-e-o-don'-te-um*). The connective tissue between the teeth and their bony sockets.

periosteal (*per-e-os'-te-al*). Pertaining to or composed of periosteum. *P. elevator.* An instrument for separating the periosteum from the bone.

periosteotome (*per-e-os'-te-o-tome*). An instrument for incising the periosteum and separating it from the bone.

periosteum (*per-e-os'-te-um*). The fibrous membrane covering the surface of bone. It consists of two layers, the inner or *osteogenic*, which is closely adherent, and which forms new cells (by which the bone grows in girth), and in close contact with it the *fibrous* layer richly supplied with blood vessels.

periostitis (*per-e-os-ti'-tis*). Inflammation of the periosteum.

peripheral (*per-if'-er-al*). Relating to the periphery. *P. iridectomy.* Excision of a small piece of iris from its peripheral edge. *P. nervous system.* Those parts of the nervous system lying outside the central nervous system. *P. neuritis.* Inflammation of terminal nerves. *P. resistance.* The resistance in the walls of the arterioles, which is a major factor in the control of blood pressure.

periphery (*per-if'-er-e*). The outer surface or circumference.

perisalpingitis (*per-e-sal-pin-ji'-tis*). Inflammation of the peritoneal covering of a uterine tube.

perisplenitis (*per-e-splen-i'-tis*). Inflammation of the peritoneum over the spleen.

peristalsis (*per-e-stal'-sis*). A wave-like contraction, preceded by a wave of dilatation, which travels along the walls of a tubular organ, tending to press its contents onwards. It occurs in the muscle coat of the alimentary canal. *Reversed p.* A wave of contraction in the alimentary canal which passes *towards* the mouth. *Visible p.* A wave of contraction in the alimentary canal that is visible on the surface of the abdomen. It can be seen in premature infants and in those who have pyloric stenosis.

peritomy (*per-it'-om-e*). Excision of a portion of the conjunctiva at the edge of the cornea, for the cure of pannus.

peritoneal (*per-e-to-ne'-al*). Referring to the peritoneum. *P. cavity.* The cavity between the parietal and the visceral peritoneum. *P. dialysis.* A method of removing waste products from the blood by passing a cannula into the peritoneal cavity, running in a dialysing fluid, and after an interval, draining it off.

peritoneoscope (*per-e-to'-ne-o-skope*). An endoscopic instrument for viewing the peritoneal cavity through an incision in the abdominal wall. A laparoscope.

peritoneoscopy (*per-e-to-ne-os'-kop-e*). Visual examination of the peritoneum by means of a peritoneoscope.

peritoneum (*per-e-to-ne'-um*). The serous membrane lining the abdominal cavity and forming a covering for the abdominal organs. *Parietal p.* That which lines the abdominal cavity. *Visceral p.* The inner layer which closely covers the abdominal organs, and includes the mesenteries.

peritonitis (*per-e-to-ni'-tis*). Inflammation of the peritoneum due to infection. This may occur from: (1) perforation of a viscus, e.g. the stomach; (2) infection of an organ, e.g. the appendix; (3) intestinal obstruction, as in strangulated hernia; (4) injury, such as a stab wound; (5) blood-borne infection, e.g. by pneumococci or other streptococci. *Pelvic p.* That confined to the pelvic peritoneum. *Septic p.* That due to a pyogenic organism. *Tuberculous p.* A chronic form due to the tubercle bacillus affecting the mesenteric glands.

peritonsillar (*per-e-ton'-sil-ar*). Around the tonsil. *P. abscess.* Quinsy.

perlèche (*pair-lesh'*). A superficial fissuring at the angles of the mouth often due to vitamin B deficiency.

permeability (*per-me-ab-il'-it-e*). The degree to which a fluid can pass from one structure through a wall or membrane to another.

pernicious (*per-nish'-us*). Highly destructive; fatal. *P. anaemia.* An anaemia due to lack of absorption of vitamin B_{12} for the formation of red blood cells.

perniosis (*per-ne-o'-sis*). A condition resulting from persistent exposure to cold which produces vascular spasm in the superficial arterioles of the hands and feet, causing thrombosis and necrosis. Perniosis includes chilblains and Raynaud's disease.

peromelia (*per-o-me'-le-ah*). A congenital malformation of a limb which resembles an amputation though bud-like remnants of the peripheral segments may exist.

peroneal (*per-o-ne'-al*). Relating to the fibula.

peroneus (*per-o-ne'-us*). One of the muscles of the leg arising from the fibula.

peroral (*per-or'-al*). By the mouth.

per os (*per os*). By the mouth (*Latin*).

perphenazine (*per-fen'-az-een*). An antiemetic and tranquillizing drug similar to chlorpromazine. Used in the treatment of nausea and vomiting, and of schizophrenia and other psychoses.

perseveration (*per-sev-er-a'-shun*). The constant recurrence of an idea or the tendency to keep repeating the same words or actions.

personality (*per-son-al'-it-e*). The sum total of heredity and inborn tendencies, with influences from environment and education, which goes to form the mental make-up of a person and influence his attitude to life. *Cycloid p.* An unstable person who has periods of great activity and elation followed by periods of depression. *Double* or *dual p.* A patient suffering from such a degree of dissociation that he leads two lives, one personality not knowing what the other is doing. *Hysterical p.* An emotionally unstable person whose behaviour is designed to attract attention. Such people are very open to suggestion, are self-centred and long for sympathy. *Schizoid p.* An introverted person who is shy and retiring. A poor mixer in society, given to day dreaming.

perspiration (*per-spir-a'-shun*). Sweat or the act of sweating. *Insensible p.* Water evaporation from the moist surfaces of the body, such as the respiratory tract and skin, that is not due to the activity of the sweat glands. It occurs at a constant rate of about 500 ml a day. When treating dehydration this loss must be taken into account. *Sensible p.* Sweat which is visible as droplets on the skin. Part of the mechanism for regulation of body temperature.

Perthes' disease (*G.C. Perthes, German surgeon, 1869–1927*). Osteochondritis of the head of the femur. Pseudo-coxalgia (Legg–Calvé–Perthes disease).

pertussis (*per-tus'-is*). Whooping-cough.

perversion (*per-ver'-shun*). Morbid diversion from a normal course. *Sexual p.* Abnormal sexual desires and behaviour. A deviation.

pes (*paze*). The foot, or any foot-like structure. *P. cavus.* A foot with an abnormally high arch. Claw-foot. *P. malleus valgus.* Hammer-toe. *P. planus.* Flat-foot.

pessary (*pes'-ar-e*). (1) A plastic or metal ring-shaped instrument which is inserted in the vagina to support a prolapsed uterus. (2) A medicated suppository inserted into the vagina for antiseptic or contraceptive purposes.

pesticide (*pes'-tis-ide*). A chemical agent that destroys pests.

pestilence (*pes'-til-ens*). Any deadly epidemic disease; a term commonly applied to plague.

pestis (*pes'-tis*). Plague.

petechia (*pe-te'-ke-ah*). *pl.* petechiae. A small spot due to an effusion of blood under the skin, as in purpura.

pethidine (*peth'-id-een*). A powerful analgesic drug much used in obstetrics and in pre- and post-operative medication.

petit mal (*pet'-e mal*). A mild form of epilepsy common in children and characterized by a sudden and brief loss of consciousness.

Petri dish (*R.J. Petri, German bacteriologist, 1852–1922*). A shallow glass or plastic dish with a lid, in which bacteria are grown on a culture medium.

pétrissage (*pa-tris-ahzh'*). A kneading action used in massage.

petroleum (*pet-ro'-le-um*). An oily liquid found in the earth of various parts of the world. *P. jelly.* Soft paraffin. Used as an ointment base.

petrositis (*pet-ro-si'-tis*). Inflammation of the petrous portion of the temporal bone usually spread from a middle-ear infection.

petrous (*pet'-rus*). Resembling a stone. *P. bone.* That part of the two temporal bones that forms the base of the skull and contains the middle and inner ear.

Peyer's glands or patches (*Johann Conrad Peyer, Swiss anatomist, 1653–1712*). Small lymph nodules situated in the mucous membrane of the lower part of the small intestine.

pH. A measure of the hydrogen ion concentration, and so the acidity or alkalinity of a solution. Expressed numerically 1 to 14; 7 is neutral, below this is acid and above alkaline. *See* Hydrogen ion concentration.

phaco-anaphylactic uveitis (*fak-o-an-ah-fil-ak'-tik u-ve-i'-tis*). Inflammation of the uveal tract occurring as a result of an allergy to lens protein following rupture of the lens capsule or after an extracapsular extraction.

phaco-emulsification (*fak-o-e-mul-sif-ik-a'-shun*). A method of cataract extraction whereby the lens is shattered by an electronic probe and the debris washed out through a very small incision.

phacoma (*fak-o'-mah*). A congenital tumour of the lens of the eye.

phaeochromocytoma (*fe-o-kro-mo-si-to'-mah*). A tumour of the adrenal medulla which gives rise to paroxysmal hypertension.

phage (*faje*). Bacteriophage. A virus which lives on bacteria but is confined to a particular strain. *P.-typing.* The identification of certain bacterial strains by determining the presence of strain-specific phages. Used in detecting the causative organisms of epidemics, especially food poisoning.

phagocyte (*fag'-o-site*). A blood cell that has the power of ingesting bacteria, protozoa and foreign bodies in the blood.

phagocytosis (*fag-o-si-to'-sis*). The engulfing and destruction of micro-organisms and foreign bodies by phagocytes in the blood.

phalanges (*fal-an'-jez*). *sing.* phalanx. The bones of the fingers or toes.

phalangitis (*fal-an-ji'-tis*). Inflammation of a finger or toe.

phalloplasty (*fal'-o-plas-te*). A plastic operation on the penis to repair deformity or after injury.

phallus (*fal'-us*). The penis.

phantasy (*fan'-tas-e*). A mental activity in which imagination weaves thoughts and feelings which bear little relation to reality.

phantom (*fan'-tom*). (1) An apparition. (2) A model of the whole or a part of the body. *P. limb*. A feeling that an arm or leg that has been amputated still exists. *P. tumour*. A tumour-like swelling of the abdomen caused by contraction of the muscles or by localized gas.

pharmaceutical (*far-mah-su'-tikl*). Relating to drugs.

pharmacist (*far'-mah-sist*). A dispensing chemist, qualified and authorized to dispense and sell medicines.

pharmacogenetics (*far-mah-ko-jen-et'-iks*). The study of genetically determined variations in drug metabolism and the response of the individual.

pharmacognosy (*far-mah-kog'-no-se*). The study of drugs of vegetable and animal origin, their preparation and their actions.

pharmacology (*far-mah-kol'-o-je*). The science of the nature and preparation of drugs and particularly of their effects on the body.

pharmacopoeia (*far-mah-ko-pe'-ah*). An authoritative publication which gives the standard formulae and preparations of drugs used in a given country. *British P.* That authorized for use in Great Britain.

pharmacy (*far'-mas-e*). (1) The art of preparing, compounding, and dispensing medicines. (2) The place where drugs are stored and dispensed.

pharyngeal (*far-in'-je-al*). Relating to the pharynx.

pharyngectomy (*far-in-jek'-tom-e*). Excision of a section of the pharynx.

pharyngitis (*far-in-ji'-tis*). Inflammation of the pharynx.

pharyngolaryngeal (*far-ing-go-lar-in-je'-al*). Referring to both the pharynx and larynx.

pharyngotympanic tube (*far-ing-go-tim-pan'-ik tube*). The tube which joins the middle ear to the pharynx. The eustachian tube.

pharynx (*far'-inks*). The muscular tube lined with mucous membrane situated at the back of the mouth. It leads into the oesophagus, and also communicates with the nose through the posterior nares, with the ears through the pharyngotympanic (eustachian) tubes, and with the larynx. *See* Laryngopharynx, Nasopharynx *and* Oropharynx.

phenazocine (*fen-az'-o-seen*). An analgesic drug used to relieve severe pain. It is a drug of addiction.

phenelzine (*fen-el'-zeen*). A monoamine oxidase inhibitor used in the treatment of depressive illness.

phenformin (*fen-for'-min*). An oral hypoglycaemic drug. A biguanide that aids the entry of glucose into the cells. Used in the treatment of diabetes mellitus.

phenindione (*fen-in-di'-one*). An anticoagulant drug used in the treatment of deep vein thrombosis.

pheniodol (*fen-i'-o-dol*). A radio-opaque contrast medium used in cholecystography.

phenobarbitone (*fe-no-bar'-bit-one*). A long-lasting barbiturate drug used to treat severe insomnia and also as an anticonvulsant drug in the treatment of epilepsy.

phenol (*fe'-nol*). Carbolic acid. A disinfectant derived from coal-tar.

phenomenon (*fen-om'-en-on*). *pl.* phenomena. An objective sign or symptom. A noteworthy occurrence.

phenothiazine (*fe-no-thi'-az-een*). One of a group of drugs used in the treatment of severe psychiatric disorders. The first to be used was chlorpromazine.

phenotype (*fen'-o-tipe*). The characteristics of an individual that are due both to his environment and to his genetic make-up.

phenoxybenzamine (*fen-oks-e-benz'-am-een*). A vasodilator drug used in the treatment of peripheral conditions such as Raynaud's disease.

phenoxymethylpenicillin (*fen-oks-e-meth-il-pen-is-il'-in*). A penicillinase-sensitive antibiotic similar in action to benzylpenicillin. Used mainly against streptococcal infections in children, it is taken orally. Penicillin V.

phentermine (*fen'-ter-meen*). An appetite-suppressant drug used in the treatment of obesity.

phentolamine (*fen-tol'-am-een*). A vasodilator, used to reduce the blood pressure in treating phaeochromocytoma.

phenylalanine (*fen-il-al'-an-een*). An essential amino acid that cannot be properly metabolized in persons suffering from phenylketonuria.

phenylbutazone (*fen-il-bu'-taz-one*). An analgesic antipyretic drug used in the treatment of gout and rheumatic disorders.

phenylketonuria (*fen-il-ke-ton-u'-re-ah*). The presence in the urine of phenylpyruvic acid due to the incomplete breakdown of phenylalanine. It is a hereditary abnormality leading to severe mental deficiency which if detected early can be treated by a diet that is low in phenylalanine.

phenylpyruvic acid (*fen-il-pi-ru'-vik as'-id*). An abnormal constituent of the urine present in phenylketonuria.

phenytoin (*fen-it-o'-in*). An anticonvulsant drug used in the treatment of major epileptic fits.

phial (*fi'-al*). A small glass container or bottle for drugs.

phimosis (*fi-mo'-sis*). Constriction of the prepuce so that it cannot be drawn back over the glans penis. The usual treatment is circumcision.

phlebectomy (*fleb-ek'-tom-e*). Excision of a vein or a portion of a vein.

phlebitis (*fleb-i'-tis*). Inflammation of a vein, usually in the leg, which tends to lead to the formation of a thrombus. The symptoms are: pain and swelling, and redness along the course of the vein, which is felt later as a hard, tender cord.

phlebography (*fleb-og'-raf-e*). (1) X-ray examination of a vein containing a contrast medium. (2) The graphic representation of the venous pulse.

phlebolith (*fleb'-o-lith*). A stone formed in a vein by calcification of a blood clot.

phlebothrombosis (*fleb-o-throm-bo'-sis*). Obstruction of a vein by a blood clot, without local inflammation. It is usually in the deep veins of the calf of the leg, causing tenderness and swelling. The clot may break away and cause an embolism.

Phlebotomus (*fleb-ot'-o-mus*). A genus of sandflies, the various species of which transmit leishmaniasis in its many forms, and also sandfly fever.

phlebotomy (*fleb-ot'-om-e*). The puncture of a vein for the withdrawal of blood. Venesection.

phlegm (*flem*). Mucus secreted by the lining of the air-passages.

phlegmasia (*fleg-ma'-ze-ah*). An inflammation. *P. alba dolens.* Acute oedema in a leg due to lymphatic blockage. 'White leg'. It occurs most frequently in women after child-birth.

phlegmatic (*fleg-mat'-ik*). Dull and apathetic.

phlycten (*flik'-ten*). (1) A small blister caused by a burn. (2) A small vesicle containing lymph occurring in the conjunctiva or cornea of the eye. Often associated with tuberculosis.

phlyctenule (*flik'-ten-ule*). A small vesicle on the conjunctiva or cornea.

phobia (*fo'-be-ah*). An irrational fear produced by a specific situation which the patient attempts to avoid.

phocomelia (*fo-ko-me'-le-ah*). A congenital deformity in which the long bones of the limbs are minimal or absent and the individual has hands or feet resembling the flippers of seals, or stump-like limbs of various lengths. The drug thalidomide, taken by the mother early in pregnancy, has produced this deformity.

pholcodine (*fol'-ko-deen*). A linctus for the suppression of a dry or painful cough.

phon (*fon*). A unit of loudness of sound.

phonation (*fo-na'-shun*). The art of uttering meaningful vocal sounds.

phonetic (*fo-net'-ik*). Representing sounds or pertaining to the voice. *P. spasm.* An affliction of singers and public speakers when they are unable to perform in public but can talk normally.

phonocardiogram (*fo-no-kar'-de-o-gram*). A record of the heart sounds made by a phonocardiograph.

phonocardiograph (*fo-no-kar'-de-o-graf*). An instrument that records graphically heart sounds and murmurs.

phonology (*fo-nol'-o-je*). The study of speech sounds, their production and the relationship between sounds as elements of language.

phosgene (*fos'-jeen*). A lung irritant war gas.

phosphatase (*fos'-fat-aze*). One of a group of enzymes involved in the metabolism of phosphate. *Alkaline p.* One formed by osteoblasts in the bone and by liver cells and excreted in the bile.

phosphate (*fos'-fate*). A salt or ester of phosphoric acid.

phosphaturia (*fos-fat-u'-re-ah*). Excess of phosphates in the urine.

phospholipid (*fos-fo-lip'-id*). A lipid of glycerol fats found in cells, especially those of the nervous system.

phosphonecrosis (*fos-fo-nek-ro'-sis*). Necrosis, usually of the jaw-bone, due to an excessive intake of phosphorus. An industrial disease.

phosphorus (*fos'-for-us*). *abbrev.* P. A non-metallic highly inflammable element. It is poisonous, causing fatty degeneration of organs, especially the liver.

phosphorylase (*fos-for'-il-aze*). An enzyme found in the liver and kidneys, which catalyses the breakdown of glycogen into glucose-1-phosphate.

photalgia (*fo-tal'-je-ah*). Pain in the eyes from exposure to too much light.

photocoagulation (*fo-to-ko-ag-ul-a'-shun*). The use of a powerful light source to induce inflammation of the retina and choroid to treat retinal detachment.

photon (*fo'-ton*). A 'packet' of energy, with no mass or electric charge. A 'particle' of light.

photophobia (*fo-to-fo'-be-ah*). Intolerance of light. It can occur in many eye conditions including conjunctivitis, corneal ulceration, iritis and keratitis.

photophthalmia (*pho-toff-thal'-me-ah*). Inflammation of the eye due to over-exposure to bright light, especially to ultra-violet light.

photopic (*fo-top'-ik*). Pertaining to bright light. *P. vision.* Vision in bright light when the cones of the retina provide the visual appreciation of colour and shape.

photopsia (*fo-top'-se-ah*). A sensation of flashes of light occurring sometimes in the early stages of retinal detachment.

photosensitivity (*fo-to-sen-sit-iv'-it-e*). An abnormal degree of sensitivity of the skin to sunlight.

photosynthesis (*fo-to-sin'-thes-is*). A chemical combination caused by the action of light; particularly the production by green-leaved plants of carbohydrates out of carbon dioxide and water.

phrenemphraxis (*fren-em-frak'-sis*). An operation in which a phrenic nerve is crushed to paralyse one half of the diaphragm.

phrenic (*fren'-ik*). (1) Relating to the mind. (2) Pertaining to the diaphragm. *P. avulsion.* The surgical extraction of a part of the phrenic nerve. *P. nerve.* One of a pair of nerves controlling the muscles of the diaphragm.

phrenicectomy (*fren-e-sek'-tom-e*). The excision of a part of the phrenic nerve.

phrenicotomy (*fren-e-kot'-om-e*). Division of a phrenic nerve.

phthalylsulphathiazole (*thal-il-sul-fah-thi'-az-ole*). An insoluble sulphonamide, poorly absorbed in the intestine and so used to kill intestinal bacteria prior to surgery.

Phthirus pubis (*thi'-rus pu'-bis*). The crab-louse.

phthisis (*thi'-sis*). Pulmonary tuberculosis. *P. bulbi.* A shrinking of the eyeball following inflammation or injury.

phylum (*fi'-lum*). *pl.* phyla. A primary classificatory division of animal and plant life, which is itself subdivided into classes.

physical (*fiz'-ik-al*). In medicine, relating to the body as opposed to the mental processes. *P. medicine.* The treatment and rehabilitation of patients with physical disabilities. It includes physiotherapy and manipulation. *P. signs.* Those observed by inspection, percussion, etc.

physician (*fiz-ish'-an*). One who practises medicine as opposed to surgery.

physics (*fiz'-iks*). The study of the laws and phenomena of nature.

physiological (*fiz-e-o-loj'-ik-al*).

Relating to physiology. Normal, as opposed to pathological. *P. jaundice. See* Jaundice. *P. solutions.* Those of the same salt composition and same osmotic pressure as blood plasma.

physiology (*fiz-e-ol'-o-je*). The science of the functioning of living organisms.

physiotherapy (*fiz-e-o-ther'-ap-e*). Treatment and rehabilitation by natural forces, e.g. heat, light, electricity, massage, manipulation and remedial exercises.

physique (*fiz-eek'*). The structure of the body.

physostigmine (*fi-so-stig'-meen*). Eserine. An alkaloid from the calabar bean. It is an antidote to curare; it constricts the pupils and is used with pilocarpine in the treatment of glaucoma.

phytomenadione (*fi-to-men-ah-di'-one*). An intravenous preparation of vitamin K, effective in treating haemorrhage occurring during anticoagulant therapy.

phytotoxin (*fi-to-toks'-in*). A poisonous substance derived from a plant.

pia mater (*pi'-ah ma'-ter*). The innermost membrane enveloping the brain and spinal cord consisting of a network of small blood vessels connected by areolar tissue. This dips down into all the folds of the nerve substance.

pica (*pi'-kah*). An unnatural craving for strange foods and for things not fit to be eaten. It may occur in pregnancy, and sometimes in mental diseases.

Pick's disease (*A. Pick, Czechoslovakian physician, 1851–1924*). A form of presenile dementia with atrophy of the frontal and temporal lobes of the cerebrum.

Pickwickian syndrome (*pik-wik'-e-an sin'-drome*). (named after the fat boy 'Joe' in *Pickwick Papers*). A condition in which extreme obesity is associated with severe congestive cardiac failure. The victims are cyanosed and have polycythaemia and marked oedema.

Picornavirus (*pi-korn'-ah-virus*). A family of small RNA-containing viruses including echoviruses and rhinoviruses.

picric acid (*pik'-rik as'-id*). Trinitrophenol.

pigeon-breast (*pij'-un-brest*). A deformity in which the sternum is unduly prominent. Usually a result of rickets.

pigment (*pig'-ment*). Colouring matter. *Bile p.'s.* Bilirubin and biliverdin. *Blood p.* Haemoglobin. *Melanotic p.* Melanin.

pigmentation (*pig-ment-a'-shun*). The deposition in the tissues of an abnormal amount of pigment.

pile (*pile*). A haemorrhoid.

pill (*pil*). A rounded mass of one or more drugs sometimes coated with sugar. Taken orally.

pilocarpine (*pi-lo-kar'-peen*). An alkaloid prepared from jaborandi leaves. It is used to constrict the pupils in the treatment of glaucoma.

pilomotor (*pi-lo-mo'-tor*). Capable of moving the hair. *P. nerves.* Sympathetic nerves which control muscles in the skin connected with hair follicles. Stimulation causes the hair to be erected, and also the condition of 'gooseflesh' of the skin.

pilonidal (*pi-lo-ni'-dal*). Having a growth of hair. *P. cyst.* A congenital infolding of hair-bearing skin over the coccyx. It may become infected and lead to sinus formation.

pilosebaceous (*pi-lo-se-ba'-shus*). Applied to sebaceous glands that open into the hair follicles.

pilosis (*pi-lo'-sis*). An abnormal growth of hair.

pilule (*pil'-ule*). A small pill.

pimple (*pimpl*). A small papule or pustule.

pineal (*pin'-e-al*). Shaped like a pine-cone. *P. body*. A small cone-shaped structure attached by a stalk to the posterior wall of the third ventricle of the brain and composed of glandular substance.

pinguecula (*pin-gwek'-u-lah*). A degenerative condition in which nodules appear on the conjunctiva near the edge of the cornea. It is often seen in elderly people who have led an open-air life.

pink disease (*pink diz-eez'*). Acrodynia.

pink-eye (*pink'-i*). Acute contagious conjunctivitis.

pinna (*pin'-ah*). The projecting part of the external ear; the auricle.

pinocytosis (*pi-no-si-to'-sis*). A process similar to phagocytosis by which molecules of protein enter or are absorbed by cells.

pinta (*pin'-tah*). A non-venereal skin infection caused by the *Treponema carateum* which is similar to the causative agent of syphilis. It is prevalent in the West Indies and Central America.

pinworm (*pin'-werm*). A threadworm. *Enterobius vermiculatus*.

piperazine (*pi-per'-az-een*). An anthelmintic drug used in the treatment of threadworms

and roundworms.

pipette (*pip-et'*). A glass tube for measuring or conveying small quantities of liquid.

piriform (*pir'-e-form*). Pear-shaped. *P. fossa*. One of a pair of depressions lying on either side of the opening into the larynx.

pisiform (*pi'-se-form*). Shaped like a pea. *P. bone*. A small carpal bone.

pitchblende (*pitch'-blend*). Uranium oxide, a black mineral from which radium is obtained.

pituitary (*pit-u'-it-are-e*). An endocrine gland suspended from the base of the brain and protected by the sella turcica in the sphenoid bone. It consists of two lobes: (1) *anterior*, which secretes a number of different hormones including adrenocorticotrophic hormone (ACTH), gonadotrophin, thyroid stimulating hormone (TSH) and prolactin, (2) *posterior*, which secretes oxytocin and vasopressin.

pityriasis (*pit-e-ri'-as-is*). A skin disease characterized by fine scaly desquamation. *P. alba*. A condition common in children, when white scaly patches appear on the face. *P. capitis*. Dandruff. *P. rosea*. An inflammatory form, in which the affected areas are macular and ring-shaped.

placebo (*plas-e'-bo*). Any inactive substance resembling medicine given during controlled experiments or to satisfy a patient.

placenta (*plas-en'-tah*). The afterbirth. A vascular structure inside the pregnant uterus supplying the fetus with nourishment through the connecting umbilical cord. The placenta develops about the third month of pregnancy, and is expelled after the birth of the child. *Battledore p.* One in which the cord is attached to the margin and not the centre. *P. praevia.* One attached to the lower part of the uterine wall. It may cause severe antepartum haemorrhage.

placidity (*plas-id'-it-e*). A calm state, the opposite of rage, in which it takes a strong stimulus to evoke a response.

Placido's disc (*A. Placido, Portuguese ophthalmologist, 1882–1916*). A disc marked with black and white circles used in the diagnosis of corneal distortion.

plagiocephaly (*pla-je-o-kef'-al-e*). Asymmetry of the head resulting from the irregular closing of the sutures.

plague (*pla'-g*). An acute fever endemic in Asia and Africa. The causative organism is *Pasteurella pestis* transmitted by the bites of fleas that have derived the infection from diseased rats. *Bubonic p.* Type in which the lymph glands are infected and buboes form in the groins and armpits. Known in mediaeval times as 'The Black Death'. *Pneumonic p.* Type in which the infection attacks chiefly the lung tissues. A fatal form. *Septicaemic p.* A very severe and fatal form when the infection enters the blood stream.

plantar (*plan'-tar*). Relating to the sole of the foot. *P. arch.* The arch made by anastomosis of the plantar arteries. *P. flexion.* Bending of the toes downward and so arching the foot. *P. reflex.* Contraction of the toes on stroking the sole of the foot.

plaque (*plahk*). (1) A flat patch on the skin. (2) A deposit of

food and bacteria on the enamel of teeth which may produce tartar and caries.

plasma (*plaz'-mah*). The yellow fluid part of blood. *Reconstituted p.* Dried plasma when again made liquid by addition of distilled water. *P. proteins.* Those present in the blood plasma: albumin, globulin and fibrinogen.

plasmacytoma (*plas-mah-si-to'-mah*). A malignant tumour of plasma cells akin to multiple myeloma.

plasmapheresis (*plaz-mah-fe'-re-sis*). A method of removing a portion of the plasma from circulation. Venesection is performed, the blood is allowed to settle, the plasma is removed, and the blood is then returned to circulation.

plasmin (*plaz'-min*). A fibrinolysin found in blood plasma which can dissolve fibrin clots.

plasminogen (*plas-min'-o-jen*). The inactive precursor of plasmin.

Plasmodium (*plas-mo'-de-um*). A genus of protozoan parasites, some of which cause malaria in man, which is transmitted by the *Anopheles* mosquito. *P. falciparum.* The cause of malignant tertian malaria. *P. malariae.* The cause of quartan malaria. *P. ovale.* The cause of a mild and non-recurrent form of the disease. *P. vivax.* The cause of benign tertian malaria.

plaster (*plah'-ster*). A substance for application to the surface of the body. It is prepared in various forms. *Adhesive p.* One used for (a) drawing together the edges of wounds, (b) holding in position small dressings, (c) support, e.g. of a sprained ankle. *Bohler's p.* Plaster for Pott's fracture. A leg splint of plaster of Paris, in which is embedded an iron stirrup extending below the foot, which enables the patient to walk without putting weight on the joint. *Corn p.* One impregnated with salicylic acid. *Frog p.* A plaster of Paris splint used to maintain the position after correction of the deformity due to congenital dislocation of the hip. *P. of Paris.* Calcium sulphate or gypsum which sets hard when water is added to it and is used to form a plaster cast to immobilize a part and in dentistry to make a model of the teeth.

plastic (*plas'-tik*). (1) Constructive. Tissue-forming. (2) Capable of being moulded. Pliable. *P. lymph.* The exudate which in wounds and inflamed serous tissues is organized into fibrous tissue and promotes healing. *P. surgery.* The branch of surgery which deals with the repair and reconstruction of deformed or injured parts of the body, including their replacement, by tissue grafting or other means.

platelet (*plate'-let*). A disc-shaped structure present in the blood and concerned in the process of clotting. A thrombocyte.

platyhelminth (*plat-e-hel'-minth*). A flat-bodied worm. The flatworms include tapeworms and flukes.

pleocytosis (*ple-o-si-to'-sis*). An excessive number of cells, usually lymphocytes, in the cerebrospinal fluid.

pleomastia (*ple-o-mas'-te-ah*). The presence in a human being of more than two mammary glands. Polymastia.

pleomorphism (*ple-o-morf'-izm*). Occurring in more than one form. The existence of several distinct types of the same species.

pleoptics (*ple-op'-tiks*). An orthoptic method of improving the sight in cases of strabismus by stimulating the use of the macular part of the retina.

plessor (*ples'-or*). A small hammer used in percussion of the chest or for testing nerve reflexes. A plexor.

plethysmography (*pleth-is-mog'-raf-e*). The measurement of changes in the volume of a limb due to alterations in blood pressure, using an oncometer.

pleura (*plu'-rah*). The serous membrane lining the thorax and enveloping each lung. *Parietal p.* The layer which lines the chest wall. *Visceral p.* The inner layer which is in close contact with the lung.

pleurisy (*plu'-ris-e*). Inflammation of the pleura. *Diaphragmatic p.* Such inflammation when that part covering the diaphragm is affected most. *Dry (fibrinous) p.* Pleurisy in which the membrane is inflamed and roughened, but no fluid is formed. This causes a purposeless cough and a sharp, stabbing pain on inspiration. *P. with effusion (wet pleurisy).* Type that is characterized by inflammation and exudation of serous fluid into the pleural cavity. Pain is less, but cardiac and respiratory function may be impeded to such an extent that the fluid has to be aspirated. This may result from infection or irritation of the pleura. *Purulent p.* or *empyema.* The formation of pus in the pleural cavity. An operation for drainage is usually necessary.

pleurocele (*plu'-ro-seel*). Hernia of the lung or pleura.

pleurodynia (*plu-ro-din'-e-ah*). Pain in the intercostal muscles, probably rheumatic in origin.

pleurolysis (*plu-rol'-is-is*). Pneumolysis.

plexor (*pleks'-or*). A small hammer used in percussion of the chest and for testing nerve reflexes. A plessor.

plexus (*pleks'us*). A network of veins or nerves. *Auerbach's p.* The nerve ganglion situated between the longitudinal and circular muscle fibres of the intestine. They are motor nerves. *Brachial p.* The network of nerves of the neck and axilla. *Choroid p.* A capillary network situated in the ventricles of the brain which forms the cerebrospinal fluid. *Meissner's p.* The sensory nerve ganglion situated in the submucous layer of the intestinal wall. *Rectal p.* The network of veins which surrounds the rectum and forms a direct communication between the systemic and portal circulations. *Solar* or *coeliac p.* The network of nerves and ganglia at the back of the stomach, which supply the abdominal viscera.

plicate (*pli'-kate*). Folded or plaited.

plumbism (*plum'-bizm*). Lead poisoning.

Plummer–Vinson syndrome (*H.S. Plummer, American physician, 1874–1936; P.P. Vinson, American physician, 1890–1959*). Difficulty in swallowing associated with glossitis and iron deficiency anaemia.

pneumatocele (*nu-mat'-o-seel*). (1) A swelling containing a collection of gas. (2) Hernia of the lung.

pneumaturia (*nu-mat-u'-re-ah*). The passing of flatus with the urine owing to a vesico-intestinal fistula and air from the bowel entering the bladder.

pneumocephalus (*nu-mo-kef'-al-us*). The presence of air in the ventricles of the brain caused usually by an anterior fracture of the base of the skull.

pneumococcus (*nu-mo-kok'-us*). The causative agent of lobar and bronchopneumonia and of other bronchial diseases. A gram-positive, ovoid diplococcus, the *Streptococcus pneumoniae.*

pneumoconiosis (*nu-mo-kone-o'-sis*). An industrial disease of the lung due to inhalation of dust particles. *See* Anthracosis, Asbestosis *and* Silicosis.

Pneumocystis (*nu-mo-sis'-tis*). A genus of micro-organisms of uncertain status, but usually considered to be protozoans. *P. carinii.* The causative organism of interstitial plasma cell pneumonia, particularly in immunosuppressed patients or small children.

pneumodynamics (*nu-mo-di-nam'-iks*). The mechanics of respiration.

pneumo-encephalography (*nu-mo-en-kef-al-og'-raf-e*). *See* Encephalography.

pneumogastric (*nu-mo-gas'-trik*). Pertaining to lungs and stomach. *P. nerve.* The tenth cranial nerve to the lungs, stomach, etc. The vagus nerve.

pneumolysis (*nu-mol'-is-is*). The operation of detaching the pleura from the chest wall in order to collapse the lung when the two pleural layers are adherent. Pleurolysis.

pneumomycosis (*nu-mo-mi-ko'-sis*). Infection of the lung by microfungi. *See* Bronchomycosis.

pneumonectomy (*nu-mon-ek'-tom-e*). Partial or total removal of a lung, usually because of malignant disease.

pneumonia (*nu-mo'-ne-ah*). Inflammation of the lung. *Aspiration p.* An acute condition caused by the aspiration of infected material into the lungs. *Broncho-p.* A descending infection starting around the bronchi and bronchioles. *Hypostatic p.* A mild form which occurs in weak, bedridden patients. *Lobar p.* An acute infectious disease caused by a pneumococcus and affecting whole lobes of either or both lungs. *Virus p.* Inflammation of the lung occurring during some virus disease and secondary to it.

pneumonitis (*nu-mon-i'-tis*). An imprecise term denoting any inflammatory condition of the lung.

pneumoperitoneum (*nu-mo-per-it-o-ne'-um*). Air or gas in the peritoneal cavity. The condition sometimes occurs as a result of a perforating wound or abscess of the bowel or stomach wall. Air may be introduced into the upper part of the cavity to limit movement of the diaphragm, and was a treatment for pulmonary tuberculosis affecting the base of the lung.

pneumopyothorax (*nu-mo-pi-o-thor'-aks*). *See* Pyopneumothorax.

pneumoradiography (*nu-mo-ra-de-og'-raf-e*). X-ray ex-

amination of a cavity or part after air or a gas has been injected into it.

pneumotaxic (*nu-mo-taks'-ik*). Regulating the rate of respiration. *P. centre.* The centre in the pons that influences inspiratory effort during respiration.

pneumothorax (*nu-mo-thor'-aks*). Air in the pleural cavity, caused by perforation of the chest wall or of the lung pleura, in which case air enters via the bronchi. Both cause the lung to collapse. *Artificial p.* The introduction of air into the pleural space, formerly much used in the treatment of pulmonary tuberculosis. *Extrapleural p.* The parietal pleura is stripped from the chest wall to enable air to be placed outside the pleura when adhesions are present. *Spontaneous p.* A pneumothorax due to rupture of an over-dilated air-sac, as in emphysema, which causes the air passages to communicate with the pleura.

pock (*pok*). The pustule of smallpox or chickenpox.

podagra (*pod-ag'-rah*). Gout, particularly of the big toe.

podalic (*pod-al'-ik*). Relating to the feet. *P. version.* A method of changing the lie of a fetus so that its feet will present.

podarthritis (*pod-ar-thri'-tis*). Inflammation of any of the joints of the foot.

poikilocyte (*poi'-kil-o-site*). An irregularly shaped red blood cell.

poikilocythaemia (*poi-kil-o-si-the'-me-ah*). Poikilocytosis.

poikilocytosis (*poi-kil-o-si-to'-sis*). The presence of poikilocytes in the blood. Poikilocythaemia.

poikilothermic (*poi-kil-o-ther'-*

mik). Cold-blooded. With a body temperature which varies widely with the environment.

pointillage (*pwahn'-til-ahzh*). A method of massage using the tips of the fingers.

poison (*poi'-zon*). Any substance which, applied to the body externally or taken internally, can cause injury to any part or cause death. *Corrosive p.* One which corrodes or destroys tissues with which it comes in contact. *Irritant p.* One which causes irritation of the surfaces with which it comes in contact.

polio-encephalitis (*pol-e-o-en-kef-al-i'-tis*). Acute inflammation of the cortex of the brain.

poliomyelitis (*pol-e-o-mi-el-i'-tis*). Acute inflammation of the grey matter of the spinal cord. *Acute anterior p.* Infantile paralysis. An infectious disease usually caused by a poliovirus. It mainly attacks young adults and children, and the inflammation of the anterior horn cells of the spinal cord may result in paralysis and wasting of muscle groups. *Bulbar p.* A severe form in which the medulla and spinal cord are affected; the respiratory and swallowing reflexes are lost and the use of a respirator may be required.

poliovirus (*pol-e-o-vi'-rus*). A small RNA-containing virus which is the commonest cause of poliomyelitis.

politzerization (*pol-it-zer-i-za'-shun*). Insufflation of the middle ear and the pharyngo-tympanic tube by a Politzer bag.

Politzer's bag (*A. Politzer, Australian otologist, 1835–1920*). A rubber bag attached to a eustachian catheter, for forcing air into the pharyngo-tympanic tube to clear it.

pollinosis (*pol-in-o'-sis*). Hay fever. An allergy caused by various kinds of pollen. Pollenosis.

pollution (*pol-u'-shun*). The act of destroying the purity of or contaminating something.

polyarteritis (*pol-e-ar-ter-i'-tis*). Inflammatory changes in the walls of the small arteries.

polyarthralgia (*pol-e-ar-thral'-je-ah*). Pain in several joints.

polyarthritis (*pol-e-ar-thri'-tis*). Inflammation of several joints at the same time, as seen in rheumatoid arthritis.

polycoria (*pol-e-kor'-e-ah*). A congenital abnormality in which there are one or more holes in the iris in addition to the pupil.

polycystic (*pol-e-sist'-ik*). Composed of many cysts. *P. disease of kidneys.* A congenital disease. The kidneys are much enlarged with many cysts. There is a slowly developing renal failure, hypertension and haematuria.

polycythaemia (*pol-e-si-the'-me-ah*). An abnormal increase in the number of red cells in the blood. Erythrocythaemia. *P. vera.* A rare disease in which there is a greatly increased production of red blood cells and also of leucocytes and platelets. The skin becomes flushed, with cyanosis, thrombosis and splenomegaly.

polydactylism (*pol-e-dak'-til-izm*). The condition of having more than the normal number of fingers or toes.

polydipsia (*pol-e-dip'-se-ah*). Abnormal thirst. It may be a symptom of diabetes.

polymastia (*pol-e-mas'-te-ah*). The presence in a human being of more than two mammary glands. Pleomastia.

polymorphonuclear (*pol-e-morf-o-nu'-kle-ar*). (1) *adj.* Having nuclei of many different shapes. (2) *n.* A polymorphonuclear leucocyte.

polymorphous (*pol-e-morf'-us*). Occurring in several or many different forms.

polymyalgia rheumatica (*pol-e-mi-al'-je-ah ru-mat'-ik-ah*). Persistent aching pain in the muscles often involving the shoulder or the pelvic girdle.

polymyositis (*pol-e-mi-o-si'-tis*). A generalized inflammation of the muscles with weakness and joint stiffness, particularly around the hips and shoulders.

polymyxin (*pol-e-miks'-in*). An antibiotic drug used in the treatment of gram-negative bacteria, particularly *Pseudomonas.*

polyneuritis (*pol-e-nu-ri'-tis*). Inflammation of many nerves at the same time.

polyneuropathy (*pol-e-nu-rop'-ath-e*). A number of disease conditions of the nervous system.

polyopia (*pol-e-o'-pe-ah*). The perception of two or more images of the same object. Multiple vision.

polyp (*pol'-ip*). A pedunculated tumour of mucous membrane. A polypus.

polyposis (*pol-e-po'-sis*). The presence of many polyps in an organ. *Familial p.* An hereditary condition in which large numbers of polypi develop in the colon, which may become malignant.

polypus (*pol'-e-pus*). *pl.* polypi. A polyp. A small pedunculated tumour arising from any mucous surface and especially in the nose and nasal

sinuses.

polyserositis (*pol-e-ser-o-si'-tis*). Inflammation of the serous membranes with effusion of fluid.

polyuria (*pol-e-u'-re-ah*). An abnormally large output of urine due to either an excessive intake of liquid or to disease, often diabetes.

pompholyx (*pom'-fo-liks*). An eczematous condition in which vesicles appear on the hands and feet, particularly on the palms and soles. The condition is temporary but tends to recur.

pons (*ponz*). A bridge of tissue connecting two parts of an organ. *P. varolii.* The part of the brain which connects the cerebrum, cerebellum and medulla oblongata.

popliteal (*pop-lit-e'-al*). Relating to the posterior part of the knee joint.

popliteus (*pop-lit-e'-us*). The flat triangular muscle at the back of the knee joint.

pore (*por*). A minute circular opening on a surface. *Sweat p.* An opening of a sweat gland on the skin surface.

porphyria (*por-fi'-re-ah*). An abnormality in the metabolism of porphyrins, resulting in porphyrinuria. *Acquired p.* Porphyria resulting from misuse of alcohol or drugs. The liver is affected. *Congenital p.* Porphyria affecting the bone marrow. There is photosensitivity, reddening of the skin, blistering, neuritis, abdominal pain and psychiatric disturbances.

porphyrin (*por'-fir-in*). One of a number of pigments used in the production of the haem portion of haemoglobin.

porphyrinuria (*por-fir-in-u'-re-ah*). The presence of an excess of porphyrin in the urine.

porta (*por'-tah*). An opening in an organ through which pass the main vessels.

portacaval (*por-tah-ka'-val*). Pertaining to the portal vein and the inferior vena cava. *P. anastomosis.* The joining of the portal vein to the inferior vena cava so that much of the blood by-passes the liver. It is used in the treatment of portal hypertension.

position (*po-zish'-un*). Attitude or posture. *Dorsal p.* Lying flat on the back. *Genupectoral or knee—chest p.* Resting on the knees and chest with arms crossed above the head. *Lithotomy p.* Lying on the back with thighs raised and knees supported and held widely apart. *Prone p.* Face down. *Sims' p.* or *semi-prone p.* Lying on the left side with the right knee well flexed and the left arm drawn back over the edge of the bed. *Trendelenburg p.* Lying down on a tilted plane (usually an operating table at an angle of 45° to the floor), with the head lowermost and the legs hanging over the raised end of the table.

posology (*po-sol'-o-je*). The science of the dosage of drugs.

Possum (*pos'-um*). Patient-Operated Selector Mechanism. A machine that can be operated with a very slight degree of pressure, or suction, using the mouth, if no other muscle movement is possible. It may transmit messages from a lighted panel or be adapted for typing, telephoning, or working certain machinery.

post-concussional syndrome (*po-st-kon-kush'-un-al sin'-drome*). Constant headaches with mental fatigue, difficulty

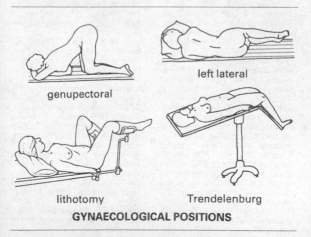

genupectoral

left lateral

lithotomy

Trendelenburg

GYNAECOLOGICAL POSITIONS

in concentration and insomnia that may persist after head injury.

posterior (*pos-te'-re-or*). Behind a part. Dorsal. *P. chamber*. That part of the aqueous chamber that lies behind the iris, but in front of the lens.

postero-anterior (*pos'-ter-o-an-teer'-e-or*). From the back to the front.

postganglionic (*po-st-gang-gle-on'-ik*). Situated posterior or distal to a ganglion. *P. fibre*. A nerve fibre posterior to a ganglion of the autonomic nervous system.

postgastrectomy syndrome (*po-st-gas-trek'-tom-e sin'-drome*). *See* Dumping.

posthitis (*pos-thi'-tis*). Inflammation of the prepuce.

posthumous (*post'-hu-mus*). Occurring after death. *P. birth*. One occurring after the death of the father, or by caesarean section after the death of the mother.

postmature (*po'-st-mat-ure*). Pertaining to a fetus before or a baby after birth when it has remained in the uterus longer than 280 days.

post mortem (*po-st mor'-tem*). After death. *P.-m. examination*. Autopsy.

postnatal (*po-st-na'-tal*). Occurring after birth.

postpartum (*po-st-par'-tum*). Occurring after labour.

postprandial (*po-st-pran'-de-al*). Occurring after a meal.

postural (*pos'-tu-ral*). Relating to a position or posture. *P. drainage*. Drainage of secretions from specific lobes or segments of the lung, aided by careful positioning of the patient.

potassium (*pot-as'-e-um*). *abbrev*. K. A metallic alkaline element which is a constituent of all plants and animals. Its salts are widely used in medicine. *P. chloride*. Salt used in the treatment of potassium deficiency. *P. citrate*. Salt used for alkalinizing the urine in mild cases of cystitis. *P. perchlorate*. Salt used in the treatment of thyrotoxicosis. *P. permanganate*. A dark purple, water-soluble compound used as a disinfectant and deodorant, as a gargle, and for cleaning wounds.

Pott's disease (*P. Pott, British surgeon, 1714–1788*). Tuberculosis of the spine.

Pott's fracture. A fracture-dislocation of the ankle, involving fracture of the lower end of the tibia, displacement of the talus and sometimes fracture of the medial malleolus.

pouch (*powch*). A pocket-like space or cavity. *P. of Douglas*. The lowest fold of the peritoneum between the uterus and rectum. *Morison's p*. A fold of peritoneum below the liver.

poultice (*pole'-tis*). A local application used to improve circulation and relieve pain as in the use of kaolin or linseed. A fomentation.

Poupart's ligament (*F. Poupart, French anatomist, 1616–1708*). The inguinal ligament. The tendinous lower border of the external oblique muscle of the abdominal wall, which passes from the anterior spine of the ilium to the os pubis.

powder (*pow'-der*). Fine dry particles. Usually a mixture of two or more drugs in this form.

pox (*poks*). Any disease characterized by an eruption on the skin.

poxvirus (*poks'-vi-rus*). A group of large DNA-containing viruses, two of which cause smallpox and cowpox.

practolol (*prak'-to-lol*). A drug used in the treatment of tachycardia and irregular heart rhythms. It is a beta-blocker and can only be given by injection.

precancerous (*pre-kan'-ser-us*). Applied to conditions or histological changes that may precede cancer.

precipitate (*pre-sip'-it-ate*). A deposit of solid matter which was previously in solution.

precipitin (*pre-sip'-it-in*). An antibody, present in the blood, which when mixed in solution with its antigen forms a precipitate.

precocious (*pre-ko'-shus*). Developed in advance of the norm either mentally or physically or both.

precognition (*pre-kog-nish'-un*). A direct perception of a future event which is beyond the reach of inference.

precordium (*pre-kord'-e-um*). The area lying over the heart.

predigestion (*pre-di-jest'-shun*). Partial digestion of food by artificial means before it is taken into the body.

predisposition (*pre-dis-po-zish'-un*). Susceptibility to a specific disease.

prednisolone (*pred-nis'-o-lone*). A synthetic corticosteroid used in the treatment of inflammatory and rheumatic conditions and of asthma and allergic skin diseases. Also used in the treatment of leukaemia.

prednisone (*pred'-ne-sone*). A synthetic drug with an action and usage similar to prednisolone.

pre-eclampsia (*pre-ek-lamp'-se-ah*). A condition occurring in late pregnancy. The symptoms include proteinuria, hypertension and oedema.

pregnancy (*preg'-nan-se*). Being with child; the condition from conception to the expulsion of the fetus. The normal period is 280 days or nine calendar months. *Ectopic* or *extra-uterine p.* Pregnancy occurring outside the uterus, in the uterine tube (*tubal p.*) or very rarely in the abdominal cavity. *P. tests.* Tests used to demonstrate whether conception has occurred. Usually a sample of the woman's urine is obtained to test for the presence of chorionic gonadotrophin. The urine is mixed with a test solution containing an antibody to this hormone. If positive the urine becomes a milky colour.

premature (*prem-at-ure'* or *prem'-at-ure*). Occurring before the anticipated time. *P. contraction.* A form of cardiac irregularity in which the ventricle contracts before its anticipated time. *See* Systole. *P. ejaculation.* Emission of semen before or at the beginning of sexual intercourse. *P. infant.* A child weighing 2500 g (5½ lb) or less at birth.

premedication (*pre-med-ik-a'-shun*). Drugs given preoperatively before the induction of general anaesthesia.

premenstrual (*pre-men'-stru-al*). Preceding menstruation. *P. endometrium.* The hypertrophied and vascular mucous lining of the uterus immediately before the menstrual flow starts. *P. tension.* Feelings of nervousness, depression and irritability experienced by some women in the days before their menstrual periods.

premolar (*pre-mo'-lar*). A bicuspid tooth in front of the molars on each side of the upper and lower jaws.

prenatal (*pre-na'-tal*). Before birth. Antenatal.

preoperative (*pre-op'-er-a-tiv*). Before operation. Usually referring to drugs, investigations, and treatment.

prepuce (*pre'-puse*). Foreskin. The loose fold of skin covering the glans penis.

presbycusis (*pres-be-ku'-sis*). Progressive bilateral deafness in old age.

presbyopia (*pres-be-o'-pe-ah*). Impairment of vision occurring in old age, due to loss of accommodating power of the lens. The near point of distinct vision is removed farther from the eye and reading glasses are required.

prescription (*pre-skrip'-shun*). A formula written by a physician, directing the pharmacist to prepare a remedy.

presenile (*pre-se'-nile*). Prematurely aged in mind and body. *See* Dementia.

presentation (*prez-ent-a'-shun*). In obstetrics, that portion of the fetus which

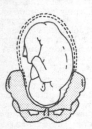
vertex

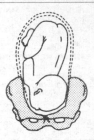
brow

face

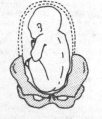
breech

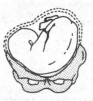
shoulder

PRESENTATIONS

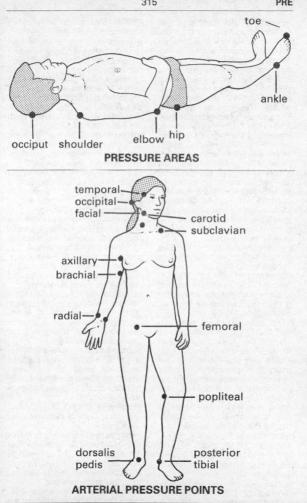

PRESSURE AREAS

ARTERIAL PRESSURE POINTS

appears in the centre of the neck of the uterus.

pressor (*pres'-or*). A substance that can cause a rise in the blood pressure.

pressure (*presh'-er*). Stress or strain. The force exerted by one object upon another. *P. areas.* Areas of the body where the tissues may be compressed between the bed and the underlying bone, especially the sacrum, greater trochanters and heels; the tissues become ischaemic. *P. point.* The point at which an artery can be compressed against a bone in order to stop bleeding. *P. sore.* A decubitus ulcer. A bedsore. Ulceration of the skin due to pressure, which causes interference with the blood supply to the area.

presystole (*pre-sist'-o-le*). The period in the cardiac cycle just before systole.

priapism (*pri'-ap-izm*). Persistent erection of the penis, usually without sexual desire. It may be caused by local or spinal cord injury.

Price precipitation reaction (*I.N.O. Price, British physician*). PPR. A serological test for syphilis.

prickle cell (*prik'-l sel*). A cell from the inner layer of the epidermis possessing delicate rod-shaped processes, by which it is connected to other cells. *P.c. layer.* The layer of the epidermis immediately above the basal-cell layer.

prickly heat (*prik'-le heet*). Miliaria. Heat rash. A skin eruption characterized by minute red spots with central vesicles.

primaquine (*prim'-ah-kween*). A drug used in the treatment of benign tertian malaria after initial treatment with other antimalarial drugs.

primidone (*prim'-e-done*). An anticonvulsant drug used in the treatment of major epilepsy.

primigravida (*pri-me-grav'-id-ah*). A woman who is pregnant for the first time.

primipara (*pri-mip'-ar-ah*). A woman who has given birth to her first child.

primordium (*pri-mor'-de-um*). The earliest discernible sign during embryonic development of an organ or part.

probe (*probe*). A slender metal rod for exploration of a wound or cavity. *Lacrimal p.* One for use in the tear ducts.

probenecid (*pro-ben'-es-id*). A drug which increases the excretion of uric acid and is used between attacks of gout to prevent their occurrence.

procainamide (*pro-kane'-am-ide*). A cardiac depressant drug used in the treatment of abnormal heart rhythms.

procaine (*pro'-kane*). A local anaesthetic used by infiltration. *P. penicillin.* A long-acting antibiotic drug, chiefly used in the treatment of venereal diseases.

procarbazine (*pro-kar'-baz-een*). A monoamine oxidase inhibitor used in the treatment of some malignant conditions such as lymphadenoma.

process (*pro'-ses*). In anatomy, a prominence or outgrowth of any part.

prochlorperazine (*pro-klor-per'-az-een*). A tranquillizing drug used in the treatment of schizophrenia and other psychoses and also of vertigo, nausea and vomiting.

procidentia (*pro-sid-en'-she-ah*). Complete prolapse of an organ, particularly the uterus so that the cervix extrudes through the vagina.

proctalgia (*prok-tal'-je-ah*). Pain in the rectum and anus. Proctodynia.

proctatresia (*prok-tat-re'-ze-ah*). Imperforate anus.

proctectomy (*prok-tek'-tom-e*). Surgical removal of the rectum.

proctitis (*prok-ti'-tis*). Inflammation of the rectum.

proctocele (*prok'-to-seel*). Prolapse of a part of the rectum into the vagina. Rectocele.

proctoclysis (*prok-tok'-lis-is*). Irrigation of the rectum.

proctocolectomy (*prok-to-kol-ek'-tom-e*). Surgical removal of the rectum and colon.

proctodynia (*prok-to-din'-e-ah*). Pain in the rectum and anus. Proctalgia.

proctorrhaphy (*prok-tor'-af-e*). Suture of a wound in the rectum or anus.

proctoscope (*prok'-to-skope*). An instrument for examination of the rectum. *Tuttle's p.* A speculum illuminated by an electric bulb, combined with an arrangement by which the rectum can be dilated with air.

proctosigmoiditis (*prok-to-sig-moid-i'-tis*). Inflammation of the rectum and sigmoid colon.

proctotomy (*prok-tot'-om-e*). Incision of the rectum or anus to relieve stricture.

procyclidine (*pro-si'-klid-een*). A drug used in the treatment of parkinsonism as it reduces muscle tremor and rigidity.

prodromal (*pro-dro'-mal*). Relating to a prodrome. *P. rash.* One which appears before the true rash, e.g. in measles.

prodrome (*pro'-drome*). A symptom which appears before the true diagnostic signs of a disease.

progeria (*pro-je'-re-ah*). Premature senility, the signs of which appear in childhood.

progesterone (*pro-jes'-ter-one*). A hormone of the corpus luteum, which plays an important part in the regulation of the menstrual cycle and in pregnancy.

progestogen (*pro-jes'-to-jen*). One of a group of steroid hormones having an action similar to that of progesterone.

proglottis (*pro-glot'-is*). A mature segment of a tapeworm.

prognathism (*prog'-nath-izm*). Enlargement and protrusion of one or both jaws.

prognosis (*prog-no'-sis*). A forecast of the course and duration of a disease.

proguanil (*pro-gwan'-il*). A widely used drug which is taken daily to prevent malarial infection.

projection (*pro-jek'-shun*). In psychology, an unconscious process by which painful thoughts or impulses are made acceptable by transferring them on to another person or object in the environment.

prolactin (*pro-lak'-tin*). A milk-producing hormone of the anterior lobe of the pituitary body, which stimulates the mammary gland. Now termed luteotrophin as it also stimulates the continued secretion of the corpus luteum.

prolapse (*pro'-laps*). The downward displacement of an organ or part of one. *P. of the cord.* Expulsion of the umbilical cord before the fetus presents. *P. of an intervertebral disc.* PID. Displacement of part of an intervertebral disc; 'slipped disc'. *P. of the iris.* Protrusion of a part of

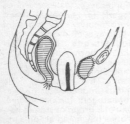 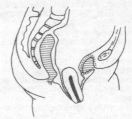

early stage   procidentia

PROLAPSE OF THE UTERUS

the iris through a wound in the cornea. *P. of the rectum.* Protrusion of the mucous membrane, through the anal canal to the exterior. *P. of the uterus.* Descent of the cervix or of the whole uterus into the vagina owing to a weakening of its supporting ligaments.

proliferation (*pro-lif-er-a'-shun*). Rapid multiplication of cells, as may occur in a malignant growth and during wound healing.

proline (*pro-leen*). One of the 22 amino acids formed by the digestion of dietary protein.

promazine (*pro'-maz-een*). A tranquillizing drug used to treat confusion and anxiety in elderly patients.

promethazine (*pro-meth'-az-een*). A powerful long-acting antihistamine drug used in conditions of hypersensitivity, e.g. hay fever, contact dermatitis, drug rashes, etc.

prominence (*prom'-in-ens*). In anatomy, a projection, usually on a bone.

pronation (*pro-na'-shun*). Turning the palm of the hand downward.

prone (*prone*). Lying face downward.

propantheline (*pro-pan'-thel-een*). An antispasmodic drug that blocks the impulses from the vagus nerve to the stomach and is used in the treatment of peptic ulcer and spastic colon.

prophylactic (*pro-fil-ak'-tik*). (1) *adj.* Relating to prophylaxis. (2) *n.* A drug used to prevent a disease developing.

prophylaxis (*pro-fil-ak'-sis*). Measures taken to prevent a disease.

propranolol (*pro-pran'-o-lol*). A beta-blocking drug used in the treatment of cardiac arrhythmias, angina, thyrotoxicosis and also of anxiety states.

proprietary name (*pro-pri'-e-tar-e name*). The name assigned to a drug by the firm which made it. A drug may have several different proprietary names.

proprioceptor (*pro-pre-o-sep'-tor*). One of the sensory end-organs that provide information about movements and position of the body. They occur chiefly in the muscles, tendons, joint capsules and labyrinth.

proptosis (*prop-to'-sis*). Forward displacement of the eyeball. Exophthalmus.

prostaglandin (*pros-tah-gland'-in*). One of several hormone substances produced in many body tissues including the brain, lungs, uterus and semen. They are active in many ways, having cardiac, gastric and respiratory effects and causing uterine contractions. They are sometimes used for the induction of abortion. Chemically they are fatty acids.

prostate (*pros'-tate*). The gland surrounding the male urethra at its junction with the bladder, which produces during ejaculation a fluid which forms part of the semen. It often becomes enlarged after middle age and may require removal, if it causes obstruction to the outflow of urine.

prostatectomy (*pros-tat-ek'-tom-e*). Surgical removal of the whole or a part of the prostate gland. *Retropubic p.* Removal of the gland by incising the capsule of the prostate after making a suprapubic abdominal incision. *Transurethral p.* Resection of the gland through the urethra using a resectoscope. *Transvesical p.* Removal of the gland by incising the bladder following a low abdominal incision.

prostatitis (*pros-tat-i'-tis*). Inflammation of the prostate gland.

prostatocystitis (*pros-tat-o-sis-ti'-tis*). Inflammation of the prostate and urinary bladder.

prostatorrhoea (*pros-tat-or-e'-ah*). A thin urethral discharge from the prostate gland, occurring in prostatitis.

prosthesis (*pros-the'-sis*). The fitting of artificial parts to the body, such as artificial limbs, dentures and pace-makers.

prostration (*pros-tra'-shun*). A condition of extreme exhaustion.

protamine (*pro'-tam-een*). One of a number of proteins occurring only in fish sperm. *P. sulphate.* A drug used to neutralize circulating heparin should haemorrhage arise during anticoagulant therapy. *P. zinc insulin.* See Insulin.

protanopia (*pro-tan-o'-pe-ah*). Partial colour blindness for red hues.

protease (*pro'-te-aze*). A proteolytic enzyme in the digestive juices that causes the breakdown of protein.

protein (*pro'-teen*). One of a group of complex organic nitrogenous compounds formed from amino acids and occurring in every living cell of animal and vegetable tissue. *Bence Jones p.* An abnormal protein found in the urine of patients suffering from multiple myeloma. *First class p.* One that provides the essential amino acids. Sources are meat, poultry, fish, cheese, eggs, and milk. *Second class p.* One that comes from a vegetable source (e.g. peas, beans and whole cereal), which cannot supply all the body's needs. *P.-bound iodine.* The iodine in the plasma which is combined with protein. Measurement of this is made when assessing thyroid function. *P.-losing enteropathy.* A condition in which protein is lost from the lumen of the intestine. This causes hypoproteinaemia and oedema.

proteinuria (*pro-teen-u'-re-ah*). A condition in which plasma proteins are present in the urine, often due to increased permeability of the tubules of the kidneys.

proteolysis (*pro-te-ol'-is-is*). The processes by which proteins are reduced to an absorbable form by digestive enzymes in the stomach and intestines.

proteose (*pro'-te-oze*). One of the first products in the breakdown of proteins.

Proteus (*pro'-te-us*). A genus of gram-negative bacteria common in the intestines of man and animals and in decaying matter. They are frequently to be found in secondary infections of wounds and in the urinary tract.

prothrombin (*pro-throm'-bin*). A constituent of blood plasma, the precursor of thrombin, which is formed in the presence of calcium salts and thrombokinase when blood is shed.

proton (*pro'-ton*). A positively charged particle which forms part of the nucleus of the atom.

protoplasm (*pro'-to-plazm*). The essential chemical compound of which living cells are made.

prototype (*pro'-to-tipe*). The original form from which all other forms are derived.

Protozoa (*pro-to-zo'-ah*). The most primitive class of animal organisms, some of which are pathogenic, including *Entamoeba histolytica* (cause of amoebic dysentery) and *Plasmodium vivax* (cause of malaria). A protozoon consists of a single cell. *See* Metazoa.

protozoology (*pro-to-zo-ol'-o-*

je). The study of Protozoa.

protriptylene (*pro-trip'-ti-leen*). An antidepressant drug used in the treatment of extreme apathy and withdrawal.

protuberance (*pro-tu'-ber-ans*). In anatomy, a rounded projecting part.

provitamin (*pro-vit'-am-in*). A precursor of a vitamin. *P. 'A'.* Carotene. *P. 'D'.* Ergosterol.

proximal (*proks'-im-al*). In anatomy, nearest that point which is considered the centre of a system. The opposite to distal.

prurigo (*pru-ri'-go*). A chronic skin disease with an irritating papular eruption.

pruritus (*pru-ri'-tus*). Great irritation of the skin. It may affect the whole surface of the body, as in certain skin diseases and nervous disorders, or it may be limited in area, especially involving the anus and vulva.

prussic acid (*prus'-ik as'-id*). Hydrocyanic acid.

pseudarthrosis (*su-dar-thro'-sis*). A false joint formed when the two parts of a fractured bone have failed to knit together.

pseudo-angina (*su-do-an-ji'-nah*). False angina. Precordial pain occurring in anxious individuals without evidence of organic heart disease.

pseudocoxalgia (*su-do-koks-al'-je-ah*). Osteochondritis of the head of the femur. Perthes' disease.

pseudocrisis (*su-do-kri'-sis*). A false crisis which is sometimes accompanied by the symptoms of true crisis, but in which the temperature rises again almost at once, and there is continuation of the disease.

pseudocroup (*su-do-kroop'*).

False croup. Laryngismus stridulus.

pseudocyesis (*su-do-si-e'-sis*). A false pregnancy in which subjective signs may be present: amenorrhoea, enlarged abdomen and breast changes, but no fetus. A 'phantom' pregnancy.

pseudogynaecomastia (*su-do-gi-ne-ko-mas'-te-ah*). The deposition of adipose tissue in the male breast that may give the appearance of enlarged mammary glands.

pseudohermaphroditism (*su-do-her-maf'-ro-di-tizm*). A congenital abnormality in which the external genitalia are characteristic of the opposite sex and confusion may arise as to the true sex of the individual.

pseudo-isochromatic chart (*su-do-i-so-kro-mat'-ik chart*). A chart of coloured dots for testing colour-blindness. Ishihara colour chart.

Pseudomonas (*su-do-mo'-nas*). A genus of gram-negative motile bacilli commonly found in decaying organic matter. *P. pyocyanea (P. aeruginosa).* One found in pus from wounds ('blue pus') and also in urinary tract infections.

pseudomyopia (*su-du-mi-o'-pe-ah*). Spasm of the ciliary muscle causing the same focusing defect as in myopia.

pseudoparalysis (*su-do-par-al'-is-is*). Apparent inability to move. Pseudoplegia.

pseudoplegia (*su-do-ple'-je-ah*). Apparent loss of muscle power but not true paralysis. It may be hysterical in origin.

pseudopodium (*su-do-po'-de-um*). A temporary protrusion of a part of an amoeba which enables it to move and to ingest food.

psittacosis (*sit-ah-ko'-sis*). A virus disease of parrots and budgerigars communicable to man. The symptoms resemble paratyphoid fever with bronchopneumonia.

psoas (*so'-as*). A long muscle originating from the lumbar spine with insertion into the lesser trochanter of the femur. It flexes the hip joint. *P. abscess.* One that arises in the lumbar region and is due to spinal caries as a result of tuberculous infection.

psoriasis (*sor-i'-as-is*). A chronic skin disease characterized by reddish marginated patches with profuse silvery scaling on extensor surfaces like the knees and elbows, but which may be more widespread. It is non-infectious and the cause is unknown.

psyche (*si'-ke*). The mind, both conscious and unconscious.

psychiatrist (*si-ki'-at-rist*). A physician who has devoted himself to the study of mental disorders and their treatment.

psychiatry (*si-ki'-at-re*). The branch of medicine which deals with mental disorders and their treatment.

psychoanalysis (*si-ko-an-al'-is-is*). A prolonged and intensive method of psychotherapy developed by Freud in which the patient is encouraged to speak freely concerning anything on his mind. Repressed material may be brought into consciousness. This may be helpful in partially or completely solving emotional problems and thus helping patients with neurotic traits or symptoms.

psychoanalyst (*si-ko-an'-al-ist*). One who specializes in psychoanalysis. He may or may not be medically qualified.

psychodrama (*si-ko-drah'-mah*). A form of group psychotherapy in which the patient, with other group members, acts out past incidents in his life. This is followed by group discussion, and under guidance of the psychiatrist an effort is made to give the patient a greater awareness of his behaviour and to try to solve the problem or conflict presented.

psychodynamics (*si-ko-di-nam'-iks*). The understanding and interpretation of psychiatric symptoms or abnormal behaviour in terms of unconscious mental mechanisms.

psychogenic (*si-ko-jen'-ik*). Originating in the mind. *P. illness.* A disorder having a psychological origin as opposed to an organic basis.

psychogeriatrics (*si-ko-jer-e-at'-riks*). The study and treatment of the psychological and psychiatric problems of the aged.

psychologist (*si-kol'-o-jist*). One who studies normal and abnormal mental processes, development and behaviour.

psychology (*si-kol'-o-je*). The study of the mind and mental processes.

psychometrics (*si-ko-met'-riks*). The measurement of mental characteristics by means of a series of tests.

psychomotor (*si-ko-mo'-tor*). Related to the motor effects of mental activity. The term is applied to those mental disorders which affect muscular activity.

psychoneurosis (*si-ko-nu-ro'-sis*). A mental disorder characterized by an abnormal mental response to a normal

stimulus. The psychoneuroses include anxiety states, depression, hysteria and obsessive-compulsive neurosis.

psychopath (*si'-ko-path*). A person with a defect in his personality. His actions will vary; he may be asocial, withdrawn, inadequate, and unable to take responsibility for himself or others; he may be antisocial, a criminal psychopath; or he may have long-standing sexual perversions.

psychopathic disorder (*si-ko-path'-ik dis-or'-der*). Mental Health Act 1983: A persistent disorder or disability of the mind (whether or not including significant impairment of intelligence) which results in abnormally aggressive or seriously irresponsible conduct on the part of the patient.

psychopathology (*si-ko-path-ol'-o-je*). The study of the causes and processes of mental disorders.

psychopharmacology (*si-ko-far-mah-kol'-o-je*). The study of drugs which have an action on the mind and how such action is produced.

psychoprophylaxis (*si-ko-pro-fil-ak'-sis*). (1) A psychological technique used to prevent emotional disturbances. (2) A technique involving breathing control and exercises used to relieve pain during childbirth.

psychosexual (*si-ko-seks'-u-al*). Relating to the mental aspects of sex. *P. development.* The stages through which an individual passes from birth to full maturity, especially in regard to sexual urges, in the total development of the person.

psychosis (*si-ko'-sis*). A severe mental illness affecting the whole personality. *Manic-depressive p.* Mild or severe attacks of elation or depression or both alternating. *Organic p.* That which may be due to trauma, new growth or degenerative changes. *Senile p.* That occurring in the aged. *Toxic p.* That which may be due to alcohol or metallic poisoning.

psychosomatic (*si-ko-so-mat'-ik*). Relating to the mind and the body. *P. disorders.* Those illnesses in which emotional factors have a profound influence, including eczema, migraine, asthma and ulcerative colitis.

psychotherapy (*si-ko-ther'-ap-e*). The treatment of disease by psychological methods. This may be by suggestion, persuasion, hypnosis or by psychoanalytical methods.

psychotomimetic (*si-kot-o-mi-met'-ik*). A drug that produces symptoms similar to those of a psychosis with an abnormal mental state, mood changes, and delusions.

psychotropic (*si-ko-tro'-pik*). Pertaining to drugs that have an effect on the psyche. These include antidepressants, stimulants, sedatives and tranquillizers.

pterygium (*te-rij'-e-um*). A patch of thickened conjunctiva which may develop over part of the cornea. It is commonest in hot, dusty and windy countries.

pterylglutamic acid (*ter-il-glu-tam'-ik as'-id*). Folic acid.

ptomaine (*to'-mane*). Any of a large number of alkaloid compounds formed by the putrefaction of animal or vegetable tissue.

ptosis (*to'-sis*). (1) Dropping of the upper eyelid due to para-

lysis of the third cranial nerve. It may be congenital or acquired. (2) Prolapse of an organ; e.g. gastroptosis.

ptyalin (*ti'-al-in*). An enzyme (amylase) in saliva which metabolizes starches.

ptyalism (*ti'-al-izm*). An abnormally large secretion of saliva. Sialorrhoea.

ptyalography (*ti'-al-og'-raf-e*). X-ray examination of the salivary glands after the introduction of a radio-opaque medium into the salivary ducts. Sialography.

ptyalolith (*ti'-al-o-lith*). A salivary calculus. A sialith.

puberty (*pu'-ber-te*). The period during which secondary sexual characteristics develop and the reproductive organs become functional. Generally between the 12th and 17th year.

pubes (*pu'-beez*). Pubic hair or the area on which it grows.

pubiotomy (*pu-be-ot'-om-e*). Surgical division of a pubic bone during labour to increase the pelvic diameter.

pubic (*pu'-bik*). Pertaining to the pubis.

pubis (*pu'-bis*). The anterior part of a hip-bone. The left and right pubic bones meet at the front of the pelvis at the pubic symphysis.

pudendum (*pu-den'-dum*). *pl.* pudenda. The external genitalia, especially those of a woman.

puerperal (*pu-er'-per-al*). Pertaining to childbirth. *P. fever* or *sepsis.* Infection of the genital tract following childbirth.

puerperium (*pu-er-pe'-re-um*). A period of about six weeks following childbirth when the reproductive organs are returning to their normal state.

Pulex (*pu'-leks*). A genus of fleas. *P. irritans*. That parasitic on man. The type which infests rats may transmit plague to man.

pulmonary (*pul'-mon-ar-e*). Pertaining to or affecting the lungs. *P. hypertension*. An increase of blood pressure in the lungs usually following disease of the lung. *P. infarction*. That due to the occlusion of a branch of the pulmonary artery by a clot, which causes death of the tissue supplied by that vessel. *P. oedema*. An excess of fluid in the lungs. *P. stenosis*. A narrowing of the passage between the right ventricle of the heart and the pulmonary artery. The condition is frequently congenital. *P. tuberculosis*. See Tuberculosis. *P. valve*. The valve at the point where the pulmonary artery leaves the heart.

pulp (*pulp*). Any soft, juicy animal or vegetable tissue. *Digital p*. The soft pads at the ends of the fingers and toes. *Splenic p*. The reddish-brown tissue of the spleen. *P. cavity*. The centre of a tooth containing blood tissue and nerves.

pulsation (*pul-sa'-shun*). A beating or throbbing.

pulse (*puls*). The local rhythmic expansion of an artery, which can be felt with the finger, corresponding to each contraction of the left ventricle of the heart. It may be felt in any artery sufficiently near the surface of the body which passes over a bone, and the normal adult rate is about 72 per minute. In childhood it is more rapid, varying from 130 in infants to 80 in older children. *Alternating p*. Alternate strong and weak beats. Pulsus alternans. *High-tension p*.

Cordy pulse. The duration of the impulse in the artery is long, and the artery feels firm and like a cord between the beats. *Low-tension p*. One easily obliterated by pressure. *Paradoxical p*. Pulsus paradoxus. The pulse rate slows on inspiration and quickens on expiration. It may occur in constrictive pericarditis. *Running p*. Little distinction between the beats. It occurs in haemorrhage. *Thready p*. Thin and almost imperceptible pressure. *Venous p*. That felt in a vein—it is usually taken in the right jugular vein. *Water-hammer p*. Corrigan's pulse. A full volume, but rapidly collapsing pulse occurring in aortic regurgitation. *P. deficit*. A sign of atrial fibrillation—the pulse rate is slower than the apex beat.

punctate (*punk'-tate*). Dotted. *P. erythema*. A rash of very fine spots.

punctum (*punk'-tum*). *pl.* puncta. A point or small spot. *P. lacrimalis*. One of the two openings of the lacrimal ducts at the inner canthus of the eye.

puncture (*punk'-chur*). (1) The act of piercing with a sharp object. (2) The wound so produced. *Cisternal p*. The withdrawal of fluid from the cisterna magna. *Lumbar p*. The removal of cerebrospinal fluid by puncture between the third and fourth lumbar vertebrae. *Sternal p*. The withdrawal of bone marrow from the manubrium of the sternum. *Ventricular p*. The withdrawal of cerebrospinal fluid from a cerebral ventricle.

pupil (*pu'-pil*). The circular aperture in the centre of the iris, through which light passes into the eye. *Argyll Robertson p.* Absence of response to light but not to accommodation; characteristic of syphilis of the central nervous system. *Artificial p.* One made by cutting a piece out of the iris when the centre part of the cornea or the lens is opaque. *Fixed p.* One that fails to respond to light or convergence. *Multiple p.* Two or more openings in the iris. *Tonic p.* One that reacts slowly to light or to convergence or both.

pupillary (*pu'-pil-ar-e*). Referring to the pupil.

purgative (*pur'-gat-iv*). A laxative. An aperient drug. Purgatives may be: (1) irritants like cascara, senna, rhubarb and castor oil, (2) lubricants like liquid paraffin, (3) mechanical agents that increase bulk like bran and agar preparations.

purine (*pu'-reen*). A nitrogen-containing organic compound. Adenine and guanine are essential constituents of DNA. Metabolism of purines results in the formation of uric acid. *See* Pyrimidine.

Purkinje cells (*J.E. Purkinje, Bohemian physiologist, 1787 –1869*). A layer of cells with an extensive dendritic network that are connector neurones in the cerebellar cortex.

Purkinje fibres. Cardiac muscle fibres found in subendocardial tissue.

purpura (*per'-pu-rah*). A condition characterized by extravasation of blood in the skin and mucous membranes, causing purple spots and patches. It may be a *primary* disease, most probably an auto-immune process, or a *secondary* sign in other diseases where there is failure of

platelet production. (1) *P. haemorrhagica* or *thrombocytopenic p.* A severe form with profuse haemorrhage, especially from the mucous membranes, any of which may be involved. (2) *Non-thrombocytopenic p.*: (i) *Henoch's p.* occurs in children and is characterized by purpura within the intestinal canal and the passage of blood and mucus in the stools. There is no reduction in the number of blood platelets. (ii) *Schönlein's p.* occurs in young adults. Crops of purpuric spots occur and haemorrhages into joints, causing painful swellings.

purulent (*pu'-ru-lent*). Containing or resembling pus.

pus (*pus*). A thick, yellow semi-liquid substance consisting of dead leucocytes and bacteria, debris of cells, and tissue fluids. It results from inflammation caused by invading bacteria, mainly *Staphylococcus aureus* and *Streptococcus haemolyticus* which have destroyed the phagocytes and set up local suppuration. *Blue p.* That produced by infection with *Pseudomonas pyocyanea*.

pustule (*pus'-tule*). A small pimple or elevation of the skin containing pus. *Malignant p. See* Anthrax.

putrefaction (*pu-tre-fak'-shun*). Decomposition of animal or vegetable matter under the influence of micro-organisms, usually accompanied by an offensive odour due to gas formation.

pyaemia (*pi-e'-me-ah*). A condition resulting from the circulation of pyogenic micro-organisms from some focus of infection. Multiple abscesses occur, the development of which causes rigor and high fever. *Portal p.* Pylephlebitis.

pyarthrosis (*pi-ar-thro'-sis*). Suppuration in a joint.

pyelography (*pi-el-og'-raf-e*). X-ray examination of the kidney using a radio-opaque dye. *Intravenous p.* Insertion of the dye into a vein, so that it is excreted by the renal tubules within about 10 minutes. *Retrograde p.* Insertion of the dye into the pelvis of the kidney using a cystoscope and ureteric catheters.

pyelolithotomy (*pi-el-o-lith-ot'-om-e*). The surgical removal of a stone from the renal pelvis.

pyelonephritis (*pi-el-o-nef-ri'-tis*). Inflammation of the renal pelvis and renal substance characterized by fever, acute loin pain, and increased frequency of micturition with the presence of pus and albumin in the urine. Due to an ascending infection from the ureters and below (urinary stasis or urinary obstruction being important contributory factors) or from the blood stream. Recurrent acute attacks may lead to chronic infection and eventual renal failure.

pyknic (*pik'-nik*). A type of physique—a stocky rounded figure with a good chest and abdominal capacity and a tendency to put on fat—that is said to go with the cheerful extroverted type of personality. One of the Kretschmer types whereby potential psychopathic tendencies are related to physical characteristics.

pylephlebitis (*pi-le-fleb-i'-tis*). Inflammation of the portal vein which gives rise to severe symptoms of septic-

aemia or pyaemia.

pylethrombosis (*pi-le-thrombo'-sis*). Thrombosis of the portal vein.

pyloric (*pi-lor'-ik*). Relating to the pylorus. *P. stenosis.* Stricture of the pyloric orifice. It may be: (1) Hypertrophic, when there is thickening of normal tissue. This is congenital and occurs in infants from 4 to 7 weeks old, usually males and first babies. (2) Cicatricial, when there is ulceration or a malignant growth near the pylorus.

pyloromyotomy (*pi-lor-o-mi-ot'-om-e*). Ramstedt's operation. An incision of the pylorus performed to relieve congenital pyloric stenosis.

pyloroplasty (*pi-lor'-o-plas-te*). Plastic operation on the pylorus to enlarge the outlet. A longitudinal incision is made and it is re-sutured transversely.

pylorospasm (*pi-lor'-o-spazm*). Forceful muscle contraction of the pylorus that delays emptying of the stomach and causes vomiting.

pylorus (*pi-lor'-us*). The opening into the duodenum at the lower end of the stomach. It is surrounded by a circular muscle, the *pyloric sphincter*, which contracts to close the opening.

pyocolpos (*pi-o-kol'-pos*). An accumulation of pus in the vagina.

pyocyanic (*pi-o-si-an'-ik*). Relating to the blue pus produced by infection with *Pseudomonas pyocyanea.*

pyogenic (*pi-o-jen'-ik*). Producing pus.

pyometra (*pi-o-me'-trah*). The presence of pus in the uterus.

pyonephrosis (*pi-o-nef-ro'-sis*). Obstruction and infection of

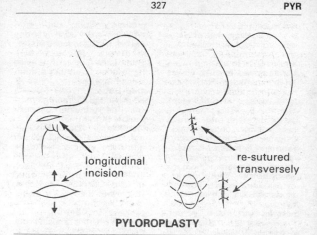

longitudinal
incision

re-sutured
transversely

PYLOROPLASTY

the pelvis of the kidney. The calyces and pelvis are dilated, and contain pus and usually calculi.

pyopericarditis (*pi-o-per-e-kard-i'-tis*). Suppurative infection of the pericardium.

pyopneumothorax (*pi-o-nu-mo-thor'-aks*). Pus and gas or air in the pleural cavity, usually associated with the partial or total collapse of the lung.

pyorrhoea (*pi-or-e'-ah*). A discharge of pus. *P. alveolaris.* Pus in the sockets of the teeth. Suppurative periodontitis.

pyosalpinx (*pi-o-sal'-pinks*). The presence of pus in a uterine tube.

pyosis (*pi-o'-sis*). Suppuration. The formation of pus.

pyothorax (*pi-o-thor'-aks*). The presence of pus in the pleural cavity. Empyema.

pyramidal (*pir-am'-id-al*). Of pyramid shape. *P. cells.* Cortical cells shaped like a pyramid from which originate nerve impulses to voluntary muscle. *P. tract.* The nerve fibres which transmit impulses from pyramidal cells through the cerebral cortex to the spinal cord.

pyrazinamide (*pi-raz-in'-am-ide*). A drug used in the treatment of tuberculosis, especially tuberculous meningitis.

pyretic (*pi-ret'-ik*). Pertaining to fever.

pyrexia (*pi-rek'-se-ah*). Fever; a rise of body temperature to any point between 37 and 40°C; above this is hyperpyrexis. Pyrexia can be (1) *continuous*, in which the temperature is high and does not vary more than 1°C in 24 hours, (2) *intermittent*, in which the temperature rises very high and falls below normal each day, or (3) *remittent*, in which the temperature varies more than 1°C but never reaches normal.

pyridostigmine (*pir-id-o-stig'-meen*). A drug that prevents destruction of acetylcholine at the neuromuscular junctions and is used in treating myasthenia gravis. It is less powerful than neostigmine but has a more prolonged action.

pyridoxine (*pir-id-oks'-een*). Vitamin B$_6$. This vitamin is concerned with protein metabolism and blood formation. It is found in many types of food and deficiency is rare.

pyrimidine (*pi-rim'-id-een*). A nitrogen-containing organic compound. Thymine and cytosine are essential constituents of DNA, and uracil and cytosine of RNA. *See* Purine.

pyrogen (*pi'-ro-jen*). A substance that can produce fever.

pyrogenic (*pi-ro-jen'-ik*). Producing fever.

pyromania (*pi-ro-ma'-ne-ah*). An irresistible desire to set things on fire.

pyrosis (*pi-ro'-sis*). Heartburn; a symptom of indigestion marked by a burning sensation in the stomach and oesophagus with eructation of acid fluid.

pyuria (*pi-u'-re-ah*). The presence of pus in the urine. It is visible as a whitish sediment; pus cells can be seen on microscopic examination.

Q

Q fever (*kew fe'-ver*). An acute infectious disease of cattle which is transmitted to man usually by infected milk. It is caused by a rickettsia, *Coxiella burneti*, and has symptoms resembling pneumonia.

quadrant (*kwod'-rant*). A quarter of a circle.

quadrantanopia (*kwod-rant-an-o'-pe-ah*). Loss of one quarter of the visual field.

quadratus (*kwod-ra'-tus*). Four-sided. The term is used to describe a number of four-sided muscles.

quadriceps (*kwod'-re-seps*). Four-headed. *Q. femoris muscle.* The principal extensor muscle of the thigh.

quadriplegia (*kwod-re-ple'-je-ah*). Paralysis in which all four limbs are affected. Tetraplegia.

quarantine (*kwor'-an-teen*). The period of isolation of an infectious or suspected case, to prevent the spread of disease. For contacts, this is the longest incubation period known for the specific disease.

quartan (*kwor'-tan*). Occurring at intervals of three days, i.e. on every fourth day. *Q. fever.* A malarial fever, caused by infection with *Plasmodium malariae*, recurring at 3-day intervals. Each attack corresponds with a fresh invasion of red corpuscles by the malarial parasites.

quartz (*kwortz*). Rock crystal. Ultra-violet rays can penetrate it. *Q. lamp.* A mercury-vapour lamp which produces ultra-violet rays.

Queckenstedt's test (*H.H.G. Queckenstedt, German physician, 1876–1918*). A test carried out during lumbar puncture by compression of the jugular veins. When normal there is a sharp rise in pressure, followed by a fall as the compression is released. Blockage of the spinal canal or thrombosis of the jugular vein will result in an absence of rise, or only a sluggish rise and fall.

'quickening' (*kwik'-en-ing*). The first perceptible fetal movement, felt by the mother usually between the fourth and fifth months of pregnancy.

quicklime (*kwik'-lime*). Calcium oxide.

quiescent (*kwi-es'-ent*). Inactive or at rest. Descriptive of a time when the symptoms of a disease are not evident.

quinalbarbitone (*kwin-al-bar'-bit-one*). An intermediate-acting barbiturate drug used in the treatment of severe insomnia.

quinestrol (*kwin-e'-strol*). A synthetic oestrogen used for the suppression of lactation after childbirth.

quinidine (*kwin'-id-een*). An alkaloid obtained from cinchona. It is used in the treatment of cardiac arrhythmias.

quinine (*kwin'-een*). An alkaloid obtained from cinchona. Formerly universally used in the prevention and treatment of malaria. Still used to treat malignant tertian malaria.

quininism (*kwin'-in-izm*). Cinchonism.

quinsy (*kwin'-ze*). A peritonsillar abscess. Acute inflammation of the tonsil and surrounding cellular tissue with suppuration. It is characterized by fever, abscess formation, and great pain and difficulty in swallowing. Antibiotic treatment may abort the attack but if suppuration occurs an incision of the abscess may be necessary.

quotidian (*kwo-tid'-e-an*). Recurring every day. *Q. fever.* A variety of malaria in which the fever recurs daily.

quotient (*kwo'-shent*). A number obtained by dividing one number by another. *Intelli-*gence q. IQ. The degree of intelligence estimated by dividing the mental age reckoned from standard tests by the age in years. *Respiratory q.* The ratio between the carbon dioxide expired and the oxygen inspired during a specified time.

R

R. Abbreviation for the *roentgen* unit.

Ra. Chemical symbol for *radium*.

rabid (*rab'-id*). Infected with rabies.

rabies (*ra'-beez*). Hydrophobia. An acute infectious disease of the central nervous system of animals, especially dogs, foxes, wolves and bats. The virus is found in the saliva of infected animals and is usually transmitted by a bite. Symptoms include fever, muscle spasms and intense excitement, followed by convulsions and paralysis, and death usually occurs within a few days.

racemose (*rase'-moze*). Grapelike. *R. gland.* A compound gland composed of a number of small sacs, e.g. the salivary gland.

rachitic (*rah-kit'-ik*). Pertaining to rickets.

radial (*ra'-de-al*). Relating to the radius. *R. artery.* The artery leading from the elbow to the wrist. *R. nerve.* A main nerve supplying the muscles of the upper arm and elbow, and some parts of the hand.

radiant (*ra'-de-ant*). Emitting rays. *R. heat bath.* Exposure of the whole or part of the body to infra-red rays generated by electricity.

radiation (*ra-de-a'-shun*). The emanation of energy in the form of electromagnetic waves, including gamma rays, X-rays, infra-red and ultra-violet rays, and visible light rays. Radiation may cause damage to living tissues. *R. pneumonitis.* Inflammatory changes in the alveoli and interstitial tissue due to radiation which may lead to fibrosis later. *R. sickness.* A toxic reaction of the body to radiation. Any or all of the following may be present: anorexia, nausea, vomiting and diarrhoea.

radical (*rad'-ik-al*). Dealing with the root or cause of a disease. *R. cure.* One which cures by complete removal of the cause.

radicle (*rad'-ikl*). In anatomy, a small root.

radioactive (*ra-de-o-ak'-tiv*). Having the power of radioactivity.

radioactivity (*ra-de-o-ak-tiv'-ite*). Disintegration of certain elements to ones of lower atomic weight, with the emission of alpha and beta particles and gamma rays. *Induced r.* That brought about by bombarding the nuclei of certain elements with neutrons.

radiobiology (*ra-de-o-bi-ol'-o-je*). The branch of medical science that studies the effect of radiation on live animal and human tissues.

radiocolloid (*ra-de-o-kol'-oid*). A radioactive isotope in the form of a large molecule solution which can be instilled into the body cavities to treat malignant ascites.

radiocurable (*ra-de-o-ku'-rabl*). Any disease which is curable by radiotherapy.

radiodermatitis (*ra-de-o-dermat-i'-tis*). A late skin complication of radiotherapy in which there is atrophy, scarring, pigmentation and telangiectases of the skin.

radiograph (*ra'-de-o-graf*). Skiagram. The picture obtained on a sensitive plate by X-rays passing through the body.

radiographer (*ra-de-og'-raf-er*). One who is trained to take X-ray pictures.

radiography (*ra-de-og'-raf-e*). The method of making X-ray photographic records. Some substances are less easily penetrated than others and therefore throw a shadow on the film or on a fluorescent screen. Bone and many diseased tissues are semiopaque. To assist diagnosis, drugs opaque to the rays may be introduced into the body.

radioisotope (*ra-de-o-i'-so-tope*). An isotope of an element that emits radioactivity. These isotopes may occur naturally or be produced artificially by bombardment with neutrons.

radiologist (*ra-de-ol'-o-jist*). A doctor who specializes in the science of radiology.

radiology (*ra-de-ol'-o-je*). The science of radiation. In medicine the term refers to its use in the diagnosis and treatment of disease.

radionuclide (*ra-de-o-nu'-klide*). A radioactive substance which is inherently unstable. It is used in both radiodiagnosis and in radiotherapy.

radio-opaque (*ra-de-o-o-pake'*). Capable of obstructing the passage of X-rays. *R. dye.* One used as a contrast medium in soft tissue radiography.

radioscopy (ra-de-os'-ko-pe). The examination of X-ray images on a fluorescent screen.

radiosensitive (ra-de-o-sen'-sit-iv). Pertaining to those structures that respond readily to radiotherapy.

radiotherapy (ra-de-o-ther'-ap-e). Treatment of disease by X-rays or radioactive isotopes.

radium (ra'-de-um). abbrev. Ra. A radioactive element obtained from pitchblende and other uranium ores, which gives off emanations of great radioactive power. Used in the treatment of some malignant diseases.

radius (ra'-de-us). The outer and smaller bone of the forearm.

râle (rahl). An abnormal rattling sound, heard on auscultation of the chest during respiration when there is fluid in the bronchi.

Ramstedt's operation (W.C. Ramstedt, German surgeon, b. 1867). Operation for congenital stricture of the pylorus in which the fibres of the sphincter muscle are divided but the mucous lining is left intact.

ramus (ra'-mus). pl. rami. (1) A branch, particularly of a nerve fibre or of a vein or artery. R. communicans. A branch connecting two nerves or two arteries. (2) A thin projection on a bone.

ranula (ran'-u-lah). A retention cyst usually under the tongue when blockage occurs in a submaxillary or sublingual duct, or in a mucous gland.

Ranvier's node (L.A. Ranvier, French pathologist, 1835–1922). See Node.

raphe (raf'-e). A seam or ridge

of tissue indicating the juncture of two parts.

rapport (rah-por'). In psychiatry, a satisfactory relationship between two persons, either the doctor and patient or nurse and patient, or the patient with any other person significant to him.

rarefaction (rair-e-fak'-shun). The process of becoming less dense.

rash (rash). A superficial eruption on the skin, frequently characteristic of some specific fever.

Rashkind catheter (W.J. Rashkind, American paediatric cardiologist, b. 1922). A balloon catheter used to increase the size of the atrial septal defect in children who have transposition of the great vessels.

raspatory (ras'-pat-or-e). An instrument used to scrape the periosteum from bone.

Rastelli's operation (G.C. Rastelli, American thoracic surgeon, b. 1933). Surgical procedure used in the treatment of transposition of the great vessels. The circulation of blood through the heart is diverted to effect adequate oxygenation.

Rathke's pouch (M.H. Rathke, German anatomist, 1793–1860). A diverticulum in the roof of the embryonic mouth which becomes part of the pituitary gland.

rationalization (rash-un-al-i-za'-shun). In psychiatry, the mental process by which an individual explains his behaviour, giving reasons that are advantageous to himself or are socially acceptable. It may be a conscious or an unconscious act.

Rauwolfia (raw-wol'-fe-ah). A genus of tropical trees and shrubs. The dried roots of one, *R. serpentina*, produces a number of alkaloids, including reserpine, which may be used in the treatment of hypertension.

ray (*ra*). A straight beam of electromagnetic radiation, including light and heat. Each ray has a precise wavelength. Light from the sun when split up has colours ranging from red, through orange, yellow, green, blue and indigo, to violet: this is the *visible spectrum*. Other kinds of rays exist beyond each end of the spectrum and these rays can be made apparent by photography or fluorescence. Those below the red rays (*infra-red*) include Hertzian or radio waves, while the invisible ones beyond the violet, the wavelengths of which are extremely short, include gamma rays, X-rays and ultraviolet rays.

Raynaud's phenomenon (*M. Raynaud, French physician, 1834–1881*). Reversible peripheral ischaemia, predominantly of the hands and feet. Attacks may be precipitated by cold or emotional stimuli. Pain, numbness and paraesthesia are common, accompanied by pallor and cyanosis. The extremities become red when re-warming. Analogous changes in blood flow have been observed in kidneys, heart and lungs. *See* scleroderma *and* sclerosis.

reaction (*re-ak'-shun*). Counteraction; a response to the application of a stimulus.

reactive (*re-ak'-tiv*). In psychiatry, used to describe a mental condition brought about by adverse external circumstances. *R. depression.*

One that arises in this way and is not endogenous.

reagent (*re-a'-jent*). A substance employed to produce a chemical reaction.

reamer (*re'-mer*). An instrument for enlarging root canals in dentistry.

recall (*re-kawl'*). To bring back to consciousness.

receptaculum (*re-sep-tak'-u-lum*). A vessel or receptacle. *R. chyli.* The pouch-like end of the thoracic duct.

receptor (*re-sep'-tor*). A sensory nerve ending that receives stimuli for transmission through the sensory nervous system.

recessive (*re-ses'-iv*). Tending to recede. The opposite to dominant. *R. gene.* A gene which will produce its characteristics only when present in a homozygous state—both parents need to possess the particular gene, and there is a 1 in 4 chance of a child inheriting it homozygously.

recipient (*re-sip'-e-ent*). (1) One who receives blood from another by transfusion. *Universal r.* A person who can receive blood from all groups of donors without harmful effect. *See* Blood grouping. (2) One who receives an organ or tissue from another by transplantation.

von Recklinghausen's disease (*F.D. von Recklinghausen, German pathologist, 1833–1910*). (1) *Neurofibromatosis.* A rare disease of skin pigmentation and multiple painless fibromata along the course of the peripheral nerves. (2) *Osteitis fibrosa cystica* or hyperparathyroidism of the bones in which the blood calcium is raised but there is decalcification of bone tissue.

recrudescence (re-kru-des'-ens). Renewed aggravation of symptoms following an interval of abatement.

rectal (rek'-tal). Relating to the rectum. *R. examination.* Inspection by insertion of a glove-covered finger or with the aid of a proctoscope.

rectocele (rek'-to-seel). Hernia or prolapse of the rectum usually caused by overstretching of the vaginal wall at childbirth. Proctocele.

rectoperineorrhaphy (rek-to-per-in-e-or'-af-e). The operation for repair of the perineum and rectal wall.

rectopexy (rek'-to-peks-e). The operation for fixation of a prolapsed rectum.

rectoscope (rek'-to-skope). See Proctoscope.

rectosigmoid (rek-to-sig'-moid). The junction of the pelvic colon to the rectum.

rectovaginal (rek-to-vaj-i'-nal). Concerning the rectum and vagina.

rectovesical (rek-to-ves'-ik-al). Concerning the rectum and bladder.

rectum (rek'-tum). The lower end of the large intestine from the sigmoid flexure to the anus.

rectus (rek'-tus). Straight. *R. abdomininis.* The straight muscle passing up the front of the abdomen from the pubis to the ribs. *R. femoris.* The straight muscle of the thigh; part of the quadriceps extensor. *R. muscle of the orbit.* One of the four straight muscles which move the eyeball.

recumbent (re-kum'-bent). Lying down in the dorsal position.

recuperation (re-ku-per-a'-shun). Convalescence.

recurrent (re-kur'-ent). (1) Liable to recur. *R. fever.* Relapsing fever. *R. haemorrhage.* See Haemorrhage. (2) In anatomy, turning back on itself to form a loop. *R. bandage.* A pattern used for stumps of limb, fingers, etc., when the bandage is made to turn back over itself in order to cover in the part.

reduction (re-duk'-shun). In surgery, the restoration of a displaced part to its normal position, e.g. a hernia, a dislocation or a fracture. *R. division.* A type of multiplication of sex cells in which the chromosomes separate into two duplicate strands, instead of splitting into two as they do in other cells. *R. en bloc (R. en masse).* An attempt to reduce a strangulated hernia, but in which the sac is pushed back intact, so that the bowel remains strangulated and the condition is not relieved.

re-education (re-ed-u-ka'-shun). The training of the physically or mentally handicapped person to enable him to regain completely, or in some degree, his former powers.

referred pain (re-furd' pane). That which occurs at a distance from the place of origin due to the sensory nerves entering the cord at the same level, e.g. the phrenic nerve supplying the diaphragm enters the cord in the cervical region, as do the nerves from the shoulder, and so an abscess on the diaphragm may cause pain in the shoulder. Synalgia.

reflex (re'-fleks). Reflected or thrown back. *R. action.* An involuntary action following immediately upon some stimu-

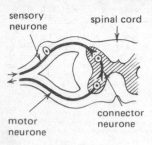

sensory neurone

spinal cord

motor neurone

connector neurone

REFLEX ARC

lus, e.g. the knee jerk, or the withdrawal of a limb from a pinprick. *R. arc.* The sensory and motor neurones together with the connector neurone which carry out a reflex action. *Accommodation r.* The alteration in the shape of the lens according to the distance of the image viewed. *Conditioned r.* That which is not natural, but is developed by association and frequent repetition until it appears natural. *Corneal r.* The automatic reaction of closing the eyelids following light pressure on the cornea. This is a test for unconsciousness which is absolute when there is no response. *Deep r.* A muscle reflex elicited by tapping the tendon or bone of attachment. *Light r.* Alteration of the size of the pupil in response to exposure to light. *Spinal r.* That which takes place through centres in the spinal cord. *Swallowing r.* Automatic reaction initiated by stimulation of the palate.

reflux (*re'-fluks*). A backward flow. Regurgitation.

refraction (*re-frak'-shun*). (1) The bending or deviation of rays of light, as they pass obliquely through one transparent medium and penetrate another of different density. (2) In ophthalmology, the testing of the eyes to ascertain the amount and variety of refractive error that may be present in each of them.

refractive (*re-frak'-tiv*). Relating to refraction. *R. error.* A defect that prevents light rays from converging on a single focus on the retina.

refractory (*re-frak'-tor-e*). Not yielding to, or resistant to, treatment. *R. period.* The period immediately after some activity during which a nerve or muscle is unable to react to a fresh impulse.

refrigeration (*re-frij-er-a'-shun*). The cooling of a part to reduce the metabolic requirements.

regeneration (*re-jen-er-a'-shun*). Renewal, as in new growth of tissue in its specific form after injury.

regimen (*rej'-im-en*). A prescribed course of treatment, especially diet and exercise.

region (*re'-jun*). A defined area of the body.

regression (*re-gresh'-un*). (1) A return to a previous state of health. (2) In psychiatry, a tendency to return to primitive or child-like modes of behaviour. This may be done as a means of solving a problem when under emotional stress.

regurgitation (*re-gur-jit-a'-shun*). Backward flow, e.g. of food from the stomach into the mouth. Fluids regurgitate through the nose in paralysis affecting the soft palate. *Aortic r.* Backward flow of blood into the left ventricle when the aortic valve is incompetent. *Mitral r.* Mitral incompetence. *See* Mitral.

rehabilitation (*re-hab-il-it-a'-shun*). Re-education, particularly of one who has been ill or injured, so that he may become capable of useful activity. *R. centre.* One which provides for organized employment within the capacity of the patient, and with especial regard to the psychical influence of the work.

Reiter's protein complement fixation (*H. Reiter, German bacteriologist, 1881–1969*). RPCF. A serological test used to aid the diagnosis of syphilis.

Reiter's syndrome. A non-specific urethritis, affecting males, in which there is also arthritis and conjunctivitis.

rejection (*re-jek'-shun*). In immunology, the formation of antibodies by the host against transplanted tissue with eventual destruction of the transplanted tissue.

relapse (*re-laps'*). The return of a disease, after an interval of convalescence.

relapsing fever (*re-laps'-ing fe'-ver*). One of a group of louse- or tick-borne tropical fevers. The fever lasts a few days, but relapses are common.

relaxant (*re-laks'-ant*). A drug or other agent that brings about muscle relaxation or relieves tension.

relaxin (*re-laks'-in*). A hormone that is produced by the corpus luteum of the ovary which softens the cervix and loosens the pelvic ligaments to aid the birth of the baby.

releasing factor (*re-le'-sing fak'-tor*). A substance produced in the hypothalamus which causes the anterior pituitary gland to release hormones.

remission (*re-mish'-un*). Subsidence of the symptoms of a disease for a time.

remittent (*re-mit'-ent*). Decreasing at intervals. *R. fever.* One in which a partial fall in the temperature occurs daily.

renal (*re'-nal*). Relating to the kidney. *R. asthma. See* Asthma. *R. calculus.* Stone in the kidney. *R. rickets,* or *infantilism.* A form of interstitial nephritis, sometimes occurring in children, associated with delayed growth and marked rickets. *R. threshold.* The level of the blood sugar, beyond which it is excreted in the urine—normally 0.18%. *R. tubule.* The thin tubular part of a nephron. A uriniferous tubule.

renin (*re'-nin*). A proteolytic enzyme released into the blood stream when the kidneys are ischaemic. It causes vasoconstriction and increases the blood pressure.

rennin (*ren'-in*). An enzyme present in gastric juice that curdles milk.

renography (*re-nog'-raf-e*). Radiography of the kidney. *Arterial r.* Insertion of a radio-opaque dye via the femoral artery or aorta to outline the blood supply in the kidney. This may reveal a non-vascular area indicating a tumour.

reorganization (*re-or-gan-i-za'-shun*). Healing by formation of new tissue identical to that which was injured or destroyed.

reovirus (*re-o-vi'-rus*). One of a group of small RNA-containing viruses. Sometimes found in children with respiratory or intestinal infections.

repellent (*re-pel'-ent*). A substance that keeps away insect pests.

replication (*rep-lik-a'-shun*). (1) The turning back of a tissue on itself. (2) The process by which DNA duplicates itself when the cell divides.

repolarization (*re-po-lar-i-za'-shun*). The re-forming of an electric charge at the neuromuscular junction after its dispersal by the passage of a nerve impulse.

repositor (*re-poz'-it-or*). An instrument for replacing a prolapsed organ. *Aveling r.* One for repositioning an inverted uterus. *Iris r.* One for replacing the iris following an intraocular operation.

repression (*re-presh'-un*). In psychoanalysis, the inability of an individual to recognize motives and feelings which are unacceptable to him. It is a defence mechanism by which painful experiences are forced out into, and kept in, the unconscious.

reproductive system (*re-pro-duk'-tiv sis'-tem*). All those parts of the male and female body associated with the production of children.

resection (*re-sek'-shun*). Surgical removal of a part. *Submucous r.* Removal of part of a deflected nasal septum, from beneath a flap of mucous membrane which is then replaced. *Transurethral r.* A method of removing portions of an enlarged prostate gland via the urethra.

resectoscope (*re-sek'-to-skope*). A telescopic instrument by which pieces of tissue can also be removed. Used for transurethral pros-

tatectomy.

reserpine (*res'-er-peen*). An alkaloid from *Rauwolfia*, a drug used to reduce the blood pressure in hypertension.

residual (*re-zid'-u-al*). Remaining. *R. air, R. volume.* The amount of air remaining in the lungs after breathing out fully. *R. urine.* See Urine.

resilience (*re-zil'-e-ens*). The ability to return to a normal shape after stretching or compression.

resistance (*re-zis'-tans*). The degree of opposition to a force. (1) In *electricity*, the opposition made by a non-conducting substance to the passage of a current. (2) In *psychology*, the opposition, stemming from the unconscious, to repressed ideas being brought to consciousness. *Cross r.* Resistance developed by micro-organisms to a certain antibiotic and to other antibiotics in the same group. *Peripheral r.* That offered to the passage of blood through small vessels and capillaries. *R. to infection.* The natural power of the body to withstand the toxins of disease. It can be maintained and increased by conserving the patient's strength by good diet, fresh air, rest, and freedom from mental worries. Artificially, it is increased by injection of vaccines and antitoxic sera.

resolution (*rez-o-lu'-shun*). (1) In medicine, the process of returning to normal. (2) The disappearance of inflammation without the formation of pus.

resonance (*rez'-on-ans*). In medicine, the reverberating sound obtained on percussion over a cavity or hollow organ, such as the lung.

resorcinol (*res-or'-sin-ol*). Resorcin. A phenol compound used in ointments and hair lotions in skin diseases.

resorption (*re-sorp'-shun*). The absorption of morbid deposits, such as the products of inflammation.

respiration (*res-pir-a'-shun*). The gaseous interchange between the tissue cells and the atmosphere. *Artificial r.* The production of respiratory movements by external effort. *External r.* Breathing, which comprises *inspiration*, when the external intercostal muscles and the diaphragm contract and air is drawn into the lungs, and *expiration*, when the air is breathed out. *Intermittent positive pressure respiration.* IPPR. Respiration produced by a ventilator. *Internal or tissue r.* The interchange of gases which occurs between tissues and blood through the walls of capillaries. *Laboured r.* That which is difficult and distressed. *Stertorous r.* Snoring. A noisy breathing. *See* Cheyne–Stokes respiration.

respirator (*res'-pir-a-tor*). A device to aid respiration. (1) *A face mask* for giving oxygen or a drug or for removing impurities or poison gases. (2) *Tank r.* The 'iron lung' into which the patient is put except for the head and respiration is brought about by intermittent negative pressure, drawing air into the lungs. (3) *Cuirass r.* An appliance strapped to the chest, leaving the limbs free. (4) *Intermittent positive pressure r.* A machine which blows air into the lungs via an intratracheal tube or tracheostomy. It may

be patient-triggered.

respiratory (*res-pir'-at-or-e*). Pertaining to respiration. *R. distress syndrome*. Dyspnoea occurring between soon after birth and the third day of life, Associated with prematurity it is characterized by severe retraction of the chest wall with expiratory grunting and cyanosis. Hyaline membrane disease.

resuscitation (*re-sus-it-a'-shun*). The bringing back to life of one who is apparently dead.

retardation (*re-tard-a'-shun*). A slowing down. *Mental r.* A state of arrested development of the mind that has existed from birth or from an early age. Subnormality. *Psychomotor r.* A slowing down of mental processes of speech and of bodily movement.

retching (*retch'-ing*). An involuntary spasmodic, but ineffectual effort to vomit.

retention (*re-ten'-shun*). Holding back. *R. cyst. See* Cyst. *R. defect.* A defect of memory. Inability to retain material in the mind so that it can be recalled when required. *R. of urine.* Inability to pass urine from the bladder, which may be due to obstruction or be of nervous origin.

reticular (*re-tik'-u-lar*). Resembling a network. *R. formation.* Areas in the brain stem from which nerve fibres extend to the cerebral cortex.

reticulocyte (*re-tik'-u-lo-site*). A red blood cell that is not fully mature—it retains strands of nuclear material.

reticulocytosis (*re-tik-u-lo-si-to'-sis*). The presence of an increased number of immature red cells in the blood, indicating overactivity of the bone marrow.

reticulo-endothelial system (*re-tik'-u-lo-en-do-the'-le-al sis'-tem*). A collection of endothelial cells in the liver, spleen, bone marrow and lymph glands that produce large mononuclear cells or macrophages. These are phagocytic; they destroy red blood cells and have the power of making some antibodies.

reticulosarcoma (*re-tik-u-lo-sar-ko'-mah*). A malignant disease of the blood in which the liver and spleen are involved. It is one of the reticuloses.

reticulosis (*re-tik-u-lo'-sis*). *pl.* reticuloses. Any of a group of rare malignant diseases of the reticulo-endothelial system. These include Hodgkin's disease, lymphosarcoma and reticulosarcoma.

reticulum (*re-tik'-u-lum*). A network, especially of blood vessels.

retina (*ret'-in-ah*). The innermost coat of the eyeball, formed of nerve cells and fibres, and from which the optic nerve leaves the eyeball and passes to the visual area of the cerebrum. The impression of the image is focused upon it.

retinal (*ret'-in-al*). Relating to the retina. *R. detachment.* Partial detachment of the retina from the underlying choroid layer, resulting in loss of vision. It may result from the presence of a tumour, from trauma or from high myopia.

retinitis (*ret-in-i'-tis*). Inflammation of the retina. *R. pigmentosa.* A hereditary pigment degeneration of the retina, commencing in childhood with night-blindness and leading to tunnel-vision and to loss of sight in middle age.

retinoblastoma (*ret-in-o-blas-to'-mah*). A malignant growth of nerve cells of the retina that have failed to develop normally. Occurring in infancy, it is congenital and may affect several members of one family.

retinopathy (*ret-in-op'-ath-e*). Degenerative changes occurring in the retinal blood vessels leading to loss of vision. *Diabetic r.* A complication occurring in diabetes. Retinal haemorrhages occur, resulting in permanent visual damage and retinal detachment may follow. *Hypertensive r.* Retinal change occurring as a result of high blood pressure.

retinoscope (*ret'-in-o-skope*). An electrically lit instrument for carrying out retinoscopy.

retinoscopy (*ret-in-os'-ko-pe*). The objective measurement of errors of refraction of the eye.

retractile (*re-trak'-tile*). Capable of being drawn back.

retraction (*re-trak'-shun*). A drawing back, as in the shortening of the muscle fibres of the uterus during labour to expel the fetus. *Clot r.* The contraction of a blood clot, which normally is completed in 24 hours. *R. ring.* A ridge sometimes felt above the pubes between the upper contracting part of the uterus and the lower dilatable part.

retractor (*re-trak'-tor*). A surgical instrument for drawing apart the edges of a wound to allow the deep structures to be more accessible.

retrobulbar (*ret-ro-bul'-bar*). Pertaining to the back of the eyeball. *R. neuritis.* Dimness of vision due to inflammation of the optic nerve. There is a central scotoma for colours. The condition normally lasts for a few weeks, but it may be an early symptom of multiple sclerosis.

retroflexion (*ret-ro-flek'-shun*). A bending back, particularly of the uterus when it is bent backward at an acute angle, the cervix being in its normal position. *See* Retroversion.

retrograde (*ret'-ro-grade*). Going backwards. *R. amnesia.* Forgetfulness of events occurring immediately before an illness or injury. *R. pyelography.* X-ray examination of the kidney by injecting an opaque substance into the renal pelvis through the urethra, using ureteric catheters.

retrogression (*ret-ro-gresh'-un*). A going backwards. Degeneration. A return to an earlier state.

retrolental fibroplasia (*ret-ro-len'-tal fi-bro-pla'-ze-ah*). A fibrous condition of the anterior vitreous body which develops when a premature infant is given too much oxygen. The condition now seldom occurs. Both eyes are affected and it may cause blindness.

retroperitoneal (*ret-ro-per-it-o-ne'-al*). Behind the peritoneum.

retropharyngeal (*ret-ro-far-in'-je-al*). Behind the pharynx. *R. abscess.* One between the pharynx and the spine. It may occur in caries of the cervical vertebrae, or in glandular affections.

retropubic (*ret-ro-pu'-bik*). Behind the pubic bone.

retrospection (*ret-ro-spek'-shun*). A morbid dwelling on memories.

retrosternal (*ret-ro-ster'-nal*). Behind the sternum.

retroversion (*ret-ro-ver'-shun*). A lifting backwards, particularly of the uterus when the whole organ is tilted backward. *See* Retroflexion.

Reverdin's graft (*J.L. Reverdin, Swiss surgeon, 1842–1929*). A form of skin graft in which pieces of skin are placed as islands over the area. *See* Thiersch's graft.

Reye's disease (*R.D.K. Reye, Australian pathologist*). An acute disease occurring in children in which there is fatty degeneration of the liver and other organs, accompanied by vomiting, convulsions and coma. Death usually follows within a few days. Encephalohepatitis.

rhabdomyoma (*rab-do-mi-o'-mah*). A tumour, usually benign, of striated muscle.

rhabdomyosarcoma (*rab-do-mi-o-sar-ko'-mah*). A rare malignant growth of striated muscle. It grows rapidly and metastasizes early.

rhagades (*rag'-ad-eez*). Cracks or fissures in the skin, especially those round the mouth.

rheostat (*re'-o-stat*). An instrument for regulating the force of resistance against an electric current.

Rhesus factor (*re'-sus fak'-tor*). Rh factor. The red blood cells of most humans carry a group of genetically determined antigens and are said to be Rhesus positive (Rh+). Those that do not are said to be Rhesus-negative (Rh−). This is of importance as a probable cause of anaemia and jaundice in the newly born when the infant is Rh+ and the mother Rh−. The result of this incompatibility is the formation of an antibody which causes excessive haemolysis in the child's blood. *See* Antirhesus serum.

rheum (*room*). Any watery catarrhal discharge.

rheumatic (*ru-mat'-ik*). Relating to rheumatism. *R. fever. See* Rheumatism. *R. nodules.* Specific lesions of acute rheumatism appearing as small fibrous swellings under the skin, especially over bony ridges, e.g. elbow, spine, occiput, etc. They are found chiefly in rheumatic fever and in rheumatoid arthritis.

rheumatism (*ru'-mat-izm*). (1) *Acute r.* or *rheumatic fever.* An acute fever associated with previous streptococcal infection and occurring most commonly in children. The onset is usually sudden with pain, swelling and stiffness in one or more joints. There is fever, sweating, and tachycardia, and carditis is present in most cases. Recurrences are likely and this disease is the commonest cause of mitral stenosis in later life as scar tissue results from the inflammation. In a subacute attack there may be no fever but fatigue, malaise and loss of weight. (2) The term may be loosely applied to any pain of unknown cause in the joints or muscles.

rheumatoid (*ru'-mat-oid*). Resembling rheumatism. *R. arthritis. See* Arthritis.

rheumatology (*ru-mat-ol'-o-je*). The branch of medicine dealing with disorders of the joints, muscles, tendons and ligaments.

rhinitis (*ri-ni'-tis*). Inflammation of the mucous membrane of the nose. *Acute catarrhal r.* The common cold. *Allergic r.* Hay fever. *Atrophic r.* Ozaena.

A degenerative condition of the nasal mucous membrane and inferior turbinate bones. *Chronic catarrhal r.* Inflammation of the membranes with a chronic excess of secretion.

rhinopathy (*ri-nop'-ath-e*). Any disease of the nose.

rhinoplasty (*ri'-no-plas-te*). A plastic operation on the nose; repairing a part or forming an entirely new nose.

rhinorrhoea (*ri-nor-e'-ah*). An abnormal discharge of mucus from the nose.

rhinoscope (*ri'-no-skope*). A nasal speculum with a mirror, used in posterior rhinoscopy.

rhinoscopy (*ri-nos'-kop-e*). Examination of the interior of the nose. *Anterior r.* Examination through the nostrils with the aid of a speculum. *Posterior r.* Examination through the nasopharynx by means of a rhinoscope.

rhinovirus (*ri-no-vi'-rus*). One of a genus of small RNA-containing viruses that cause respiratory diseases, including the common cold.

Rhipicephalus (*ri-pe-kef'-al-us*). A genus of ticks which can transmit the rickettsiae which cause typhus and relapsing fever.

rhizodontropy (*ri-zo-don'-tro-pe*). The fixing of an artificial crown on to a natural tooth root.

rhizoid (*ri'-zoid*). Like a root.

rhizotomy (*ri-zot'-om-e*). Division of a spinal nerve root for the relief of pain or of tic douloureux.

rhodopsin (*rod-op'-sin*). The visual purple of the retina, the formation of which is dependent upon vitamin A in the diet.

rhomboid (*rom'-boid*). Any one of two pairs of muscles in the upper back which control the shoulder-blades.

rhonchus (*rong'-kus*). A wheezing sound produced in the bronchial tubes which is caused by partial obstruction and can be heard on auscultation.

rhythm (*rithm*). A regular recurring action. *Cardiac r.* The smooth action of the heart when systole is followed by diastole. *R. method.* A contraceptive technique in which intercourse is limited to the 'safe period' (avoiding the 2–3 days immediately preceding and following ovulation).

rib (*rib*). Any one of the twelve pairs of long, flat curved bones of the thorax, each united by cartilage to the spinal vertebrae at the back. *Cervical r.* Elongation of the cervical processes towards the front of the chest. Pressure of this may cause impairment of nerve or vascular function. *See* Scalenus syndrome. *False r.* The last five pairs, the upper three of which are attached by cartilage to each other. *Floating r.* The last two pairs, connected only to the vertebrae. *True r.* The seven pairs attached directly to the sternum.

riboflavin (*ri-bo-fla'-veen*). A chemical factor in the vitamin B complex.

ribonuclease (*ri-bo-nu'-kle-aze*). An enzyme from the pancreas which is responsible for the breakdown of nucleic acid.

ribonucleic acid (*ri-bo-nu-kle'-ik as'-id*). RNA. A complex chemical found in the cytoplasm of animal cells and concerned with protein synthesis. Certain viruses contain RNA.

ribosome (*ri'-bo-some*). An

RNA and protein-containing particle which is the site of protein synthesis in the cell.

Richter's hernia (*A.G. Richter, German surgeon, 1742–1812*). One in which only a portion of the circumference of the intestine is contained within the hernial sac.

rickets (*rik'-ets*). A deficiency disease of young children from 6 months to 2 years of age. It is caused by a lack of vitamin D which results in a failure of calcium and phosphorus absorption from the diet. This leads to softening and irregular growth of the bones resulting in deformity, such as bowing of the long bones and enlargement of the epiphyses. The disease is preventable, and can be treated by giving adequate vitamin D and by exposure to sunlight or ultra-violet light.

Rickettsia (*rik-et'-se-ah*). A genus of micro-organisms which are parasitic in lice and similar insects. The bite of the host is thus the means of transmitting the organisms, some of which are disease-producing. *R. prowazeki.* A species that inhabits the digestive tract of lice and is the cause of epidemic typhus fever. *R. tsutsugamushi.* The cause of scrub typhus.

rifampicin (*rif-am'-pis-in*). An antibiotic drug used, often with other drugs such as isoniazid, in the treatment of tuberculosis.

rigor (*ri'-gor*). An attack of intense shivering occurring when the heat regulation is disturbed. The temperature rises rapidly and may either stay elevated or fall rapidly as profuse sweating occurs. *R. mortis.* Stiffening of the body which occurs soon after death owing to coagulation of the muscle plasma. It begins in the muscles of the neck and jaw, then proceeds to those of the chest and upper extremities, finally reaching those of the lower limbs. The time of its appearance varies (1 to 24 hours after death) and its duration may be from a few minutes to several days.

rima (*ri'-mah*). A narrow fissure or crack. *R. glottidis.* The cleft between the vocal cords.

Ringer's solution (*S. Ringer, British physiologist, 1835–1910*). A physiological solution of saline to which small amounts of calcium and potassium salts have been added. It is injected intravenously for fluid replacement in dehydration.

ringworm (*ring'-werm*). Tinea. A contagious skin disease, characterized by circular patches, pinkish in colour, with a desquamating surface, and due to a parasitic fungus.

Rinne's test (*H.A. Rinne, German biologist, 1819–1868*). A test for deafness in which the degree of conductivity through bone is tested by holding a vibrating tuning fork alternately in front of the ear and over the mastoid bone.

risus (*ri'-sus*). Laughter. *R. sardonicus.* A peculiar grin caused by muscle spasm around the mouth, seen in tetanus and in strychnine poisoning.

RNA. Ribonucleic acid. *RNA viruses.* Viruses which contain ribonucleic acid as their genetic material.

ROA. Right occipito-anterior. Referring to a possible position of the fetus in the uterus.

Rocky Mountain spotted fever (*rok'-e mown'-tane spot'-ed fe'-ver*). A tick-borne infection caused by a *Rickettsia*, common in the USA. Causes a rose-red rash to appear, with fever, muscle pain and often an enlarged liver. The disease lasts about three weeks.

rod (*rod*). A straight thin structure. *Retinal r.* One of the two types of light-sensitive endorgans of the retina, which contain rhodopsin and are responsible for night vision.

roentgen (*runt'-jen*). abbrev. R. A unit of dosage for X and gamma radiation.

roentgenography (*runt-jen-og'-raf-e*). Radiography.

Rolando's fissure (*L. Rolando, Italian anatomist, 1773–1831*). The central sulcus of the cerebrum.

Romberg's sign (*M.H. Romberg, German physician, 1795–1853*). Inability to stand erect without swaying if the eyes are closed. A sign of tabes dorsalis.

ROP. Right occipitoposterior. Referring to a possible position of the fetus in the uterus.

Rorschach test (*H. Rorschach, Swiss psychiatrist, 1884–1922*). A mental test that consists of ten ink-blot designs, some in colours and some in black and white. The patient is asked to look at the cards and tell what he sees. This test measures some aspects of personality.

rosacea (*ro-za'-se-ah*). See Acne rosacea.

roseola (*ro-ze'-o-lah*). A rose-coloured rash. *R. infantum.* An acute disease of infancy in which a high temperature which has persisted for several days falls as soon as the rash appears.

rotator (*ro-ta'-tor*). A muscle which causes rotation of a part, particularly the dorsal muscles which rotate the vertebrae.

Rothera's test (*A.C.H. Rothera, Australian biochemist, 1880–1915*). A test for the presence of acetone in urine.

Roth's spots (*M. Roth, Swiss physician, 1839–1915*). Small white spots in the retina which may be surrounded by haemorrhages. Seen in bacterial endocarditis, collagen diseases, leukaemia and pernicious anaemia.

roughage (*ruf'-aje*). Coarse vegetable fibres and cellulose that give bulk to the diet and stimulate peristalsis.

rouleau (*ru'-lo*). A rounded formation found in blood which has been shed and caused by red cells piling on each other.

roundworm (*rownd'-werm*). A nematode.

Rovsing's sign (*N.T. Rovsing, Danish surgeon, 1868–1927*). A test for acute appendicitis in which pressure in the left iliac fossa causes pain in the right iliac fossa.

RPCF. See Reiter.

rubefacient (*ru-be-fa'-shent*). An agent causing redness of the skin.

rubella (*ru-bel'-ah*). German measles. A mild contagious virus infection of short duration in which there is slight pyrexia, enlarged cervical lymph glands and a rash. The greatest risk from this disease is to the offspring of mothers who contract it during the early weeks of pregnancy. The child may be born with cataract or deformities, be a deaf mute or have other congenital defects.

ruga (*ru'-gah*). A ridge or crease, especially of the mucosa of the stomach.

rumination (*ru-min-a'-shun*). Recurring thoughts. *Obsessional r.* Thoughts which persistently recur against the patient's will and from which he cannot rid himself.

rupture (*rup'-chur*). (1) Tearing or bursting of a part, as in rupture of an aneurysm; of the membranes during labour; or of a tubal pregnancy. (2) A term commonly applied to hernia.

Russell traction (*R.H. Russell, Australian surgeon*). A form of extension by use of skin traction and sling supports without the use of a splint. *See* Traction.

S

Sabin vaccine (*A.B. Sabin, American biologist, b. 1906*). A live oral attenuated poliovirus vaccine active against poliomyelitis.

sac (*sak*). A pouch-like structure. *Air s.* An alveolus. The pouch-like dilatation terminating the bronchioles. *Conjunctival s.* The space between the conjunctiva covering the eyeball, and that lining the eyelid. *Hernial s.* The pouch of peritoneum containing the loop of intestine. *Lacrimal s.* The dilatation at the top of the lacrimal duct.

saccharide (*sak'-ar-ide*). One of a series of carbohydrates, including the sugars.

saccharin (*sak'-ar-in*). Gluside. A crystalline substance used as a substitute for sugar.

Saccharomyces (*sak-ar-o-mi'-seez*). A genus of fungi, of which yeast is an example.

sacculated (*sak'-u-la-ted*). Divided into small sacs.

saccule (*sak'-ule*). A small sac, particularly the smaller of the two sacs within the membranous labyrinth of the ear.

sacral (*sa'-kral*). Relating to the sacrum.

sacroiliac (*sa-kro-il'-e-ak*). Relating to the sacrum and the ilium.

sacrum (*sa'-krum*). A triangular bone composed of five united vertebrae, situated between the lowest lumbar vertebra and the coccyx. It forms the back of the pelvis.

sadism (*sa'-dizm*). A form of sexual perversion in which the individual takes pleasure in inflicting mental and physical pain on others.

sagittal (*saj'-it-al*). Arrow-shaped. *S. suture.* The junction of the parietal bones.

sal (*sal*). Salt. (*Latin*). *S. ammoniac.* Ammonium chloride. It is used as a diuretic and to produce acidosis. Also used as an expectorant. *S. volatile.* Aromatic ammonium carbonate. Diluted with water it may be given in cases of syncope.

salbutamol (*sal-bu'-tam-ol*). A sympathomimetic drug used in the treatment of bronchospasm.

salicylate (*sal-is'-il-ate*). A salt of salicylic acid. *Methyl s.* The active ingredient in ointments and lotions for joint pains and sprains. *Sodium s.* The specific drug used for rheumatic fever. It reduces the pyrexia and relieves the pain but does not prevent cardiac complications. Where there is intolerance aspirin or calcium aspirin may be substituted.

salicylic acid (*sal-is-il'-ik as'-id*). A drug used externally to destroy bacteria and fungi, to treat skin diseases such as psoriasis and eczema and, in concentrated form, to remove warts and corns.

saline (*sa'-line*). A solution of sodium chloride and water. *Hypertonic s.* A stronger than normal strength. *Hypotonic s.* A weaker than normal strength. *Normal* or *physiological s.* An 0.9% solution which is isotonic with blood.

saliva (*sal-i'-vah*). The secretion of the salivary glands which is poured into the mouth when food is taken. It moistens and dissolves certain substances, and partially digests carbohydrates by the action of its enzyme, ptyalin (amylase).

salivary (*sal'-iv-ar-e*). Relating to saliva. *S. calculus.* A stony concretion in a salivary duct. *S. fistula.* An unnatural opening on the skin of the face leading into a salivary duct or gland. *S. glands.* The parotid, submaxillary and sublingual glands.

salivation (*sal-iv-a'-shun*). Ptyalism, an excessive flow of saliva.

Salk vaccine (*J.E. Salk, American virologist, b. 1914*). The first poliomyelitis vaccine. *See* Vaccine.

Salmonella (*sal-mon-el'-ah*). A genus of gram-negative, non-sporing, rod-like bacteria that are parasites of the intestinal tract of man and animals. *S. typhi* and *S. paratyphi* are exclusively human pathogens which cause typhoid and paratyphoid fevers. Other strains, e.g. *S. typhimurium*, can give rise to acute gastroenteritis (food poisoning).

salmonellosis (*sal-mon-el-o'-sis*). Infection with salmonellae, especially paratyphoid fever and food poisoning; caused by the ingestion of food containing the organisms or their products.

salpingectomy (*sal-pin-jek'-tom-e*). Excision of one or both of the uterine tubes.

salpingemphraxis (*sal-pin-jem-fraks'-is*). (1) Obstruction of an auditory tube. (2) Obstruction of a uterine tube.

salpingitis (*sal-pin-ji'-tis*). (1) Inflammation of the uterine tubes. *Acute s.* Most often a bilateral ascending infection due to a streptococcus or a gonococcus. *Chronic s.* A less acute form that may be blood borne and may be due to the tubercle bacillus. (2) Inflammation of the pharyngotympanic (eustachian) tubes.

salpingography (*sal-ping-gog'-raf-e*). X-ray examination of the uterine tubes after injection of a radio-opaque substance to determine their patency.

salpingo-oöphorectomy (*salping'-go-o-off-or-ek'-tom-e*). Removal of a uterine tube and its ovary.

salpingostomy (*sal-ping-gos'-tom-e*). The making of a surgical opening in a uterine tube near the uterus to restore patency.

salpinx (*sal'-pinks*). A tube—applied to the uterine or pharyngotympanic (eustachian) tubes.

salt (*sawlt*). (1) Sodium chloride, common salt, used in solution as a cleansing lotion, a stimulating bath, or for infusion into the blood, etc. (2) Any compound of an acid with an alkali or base. (3) A saline purgative such as Epsom salts. *Smelling s.'s.* Aromatic ammonium carbon-ate. A restorative in fainting. *S. depletion.* A loss of salt from the body due to sweating or persistent diarrhoea or vomiting. Common in hot climates when it may be prevented by the taking of salt tablets.

salve (*salv*). An ointment.

sanatorium (*san-at-or'-e-um*). A building used for restoring to health, usually used for the treatment of long-term illness like tuberculosis.

sandfly (*sand'-fli*). A very small fly of the genus *Phlebotomus*, common in tropical climates and the vector of most types of leishmaniasis. *S. fever.* A fever transmitted by the bites of sandflies, and common in Mediterranean countries. Similar to *dengue* and sometimes known as *three-day fever.*

sanguineous (*san-gwin'-e-us*). Pertaining to or containing blood.

sanies (*sa'-ne-eez*). A fetid discharge from a wound consisting of serum, pus and blood.

sanitary (*san'-it-ar-e*). Relating to or promoting health.

saphena (*saf-e'-nah*). One of two superficial veins that carry blood from the foot upwards.

saphenous (*saf-e'-nus*). Relating to the saphena.

sapo (*sa'-po*). Soap (*Latin*).

saponaceous (*sap-on-a'-she-us*). Soapy; having the nature of soap.

saponification (*sap-on-if-ik-a'-shun*). The making of soap by combining a fat and an alkali.

sapphism (*saf'-izm*). Female homosexuality. Lesbianism.

sapraemia (*sap-re'-me-ah*). A form of toxaemia. The toxins are produced by saprophytes and circulate in the blood.

saprophyte (*sap'-ro-fite*). An organism bred in and living on putrefying animal or plant matter.

sarcoid (*sar'-koid*). (1) A fleshy tumour. (2) Sarcoidosis.

sarcoidosis (*sar-koid-o'-sis*). A rare disease in some ways similar to tuberculosis. It chiefly affects the skin, the lymphatic glands, the liver and the lungs.

sarcolemma (*sar-ko-lem'-ah*). A delicate membrane enveloping each striated or cardiac muscle fibre.

sarcoma (*sar-ko'-mah*). A malignant tumour developed from connective tissue cells, and their stroma. *Chondro-s.* One arising in cartilage. *Fibros.* One containing much fibrous tissue; this may arise in the fibrous sheath of a muscle. *Melanotic s.* A highly malignant type, pigmented with melanin. *Round-celled s.* A highly malignant growth, composed of a primitive type of cell.

sarcomatosis (*sar-ko-mat-o'-sis*). Multiple sarcomatous growths in various parts of the body.

Sarcoptes (*sar-kop'-teez*). A genus of mites. *S. scabiei.* The cause of scabies.

sardonic (*sar-don'-ik*). Pertaining to the grinning expression sometimes displayed in tetanus. *See* Risus sardonicus.

sartorius (*sar-tor'-e-us*). A long muscle of the thigh, which flexes both the thigh and the lower leg.

saturated (*sat'-u-ra-ted*). Pertaining to a solution containing the largest amount of a solid which can be dissolved in it without forming a precipitate.

satyriasis (*sat-ir-i'-as-is*). Abnormally excessive sexual appetite in men.

Sayre's jacket (*L.A. Sayre, American surgeon, 1820–1900*). A jacket made of plaster of Paris used to support the back in cases of spinal disease.

Sb. Chemical symbol for *antimony* (stibium).

scab (*skab*). The crust on a superficial wound consisting of dried blood, pus, etc.

scabies (*ska'-beez*). 'The itch'. A contagious skin disease caused by the itch mite (*Sarcoptes scabiei*), the female of which burrows beneath the skin and deposits eggs at intervals. It is intensely irritating, and the rash is aggravated by scratching. The sites affected are chiefly between the fingers and toes, the axillae, and groins.

scald (*skawld*). A burn caused by hot liquid or vapour.

scale (*skale*). (1) *n.* A scheme or instrument by which something can be measured. A pair of scales is a balance for measuring weight. (2) *n.* Compact layers of dead epithelial tissue shed from the skin. (3) *v.* To scrape deposits of tartar from the teeth.

scalenus (*ska-le'-nus*). One of four muscles which move the neck to either side and raise the first and second ribs during inspiration. *S. syndrome.* Symptoms of pain and tenderness in the shoulder, with sensory loss and wasting of the medial aspect of the arm. It may be caused by pressure on the brachial plexus, by spasm of the scalenus anterior muscle or by a cervical rib.

scaler (*ska'-ler*). An instrument for removing deposits of tartar from the teeth.

scalp (*skalp*). The hairy skin which covers the cranium.

scalpel (*skal'-pel*). A small pointed surgical knife with a convex edge to the blade.

scan (*skan*). A two-dimensional representation of deep tissues produced by a scanner, a machine using gamma radiation. Used instead of X-rays. Radio-opaque contrast media are not required.

scanner (*skan'-er*). An instrument used for scanning, e.g. a scintiscanner.

scanning (*skan'-ing*). (1) Visual examination of an area. (2) A speech disorder that may be present in cerebellar disease. The syllables are inappropriately separated from each other and are evenly stressed with rhythmically occurring pauses between them.

scaphocephaly (*skaf-o-kef'-ale*). Abnormal boat-shape of the head due to premature closure of the sagittal suture of the skull. Mental subnormality is usually found.

scaphoid (*skaf'-oid* or *ska'-foid*). Boat-shaped. *S. bone.* A boat-shaped bone of the wrist which articulates with the radius and with the trapezium and the trapezoid bones.

scapula (*skap'-u-lah*). The large flat triangular bone forming the shoulder-blade.

scar (*skar*). The mark left after a wound has healed with the formation of connective tissue.

scarification (*skar-if-ik-a'-shun*). The making of small cuts or punctures of the skin to allow a vaccine to enter the body.

scarlet fever (*skar'-let fe'-ver*). Scarlatina. An acute infectious disease which of latter years has much decreased in severity. It is caused by a haemolytic streptococcus. There is sore throat, high fever and a punctate rash. Now it is readily treated by antibiotics and the complications of nephritis and middle ear infection are less common.

scatter (*skat'-er*). In radiology, the deviation of radioactive rays caused by passing through a medium such as human tissue.

Scheuermann's disease (*H.W. Scheuermann, Danish surgeon, 1877–1960*). Osteochondritis of the spine affecting the rings of cartilage and bone around the margin of the superior and inferior surfaces of the vertebral bodies.

Schick test (*B. Schick, Austrian paediatrician, 1877–1967*). A skin test of susceptibility to diphtheria. A small amount of diphtheria toxin is injected intradermally.

Schilling test (*R.F. Schilling, American haematologist, b. 1919*). A test used to confirm the diagnosis of pernicious anaemia by estimating the absorption of ingested radioactive vitamin B_{12}.

Schirmer's test (*O.W. Schirmer, German ophthalmologist, b. 1864*). A method of determining the quantity of lacrimal secretion by using standard-sized pieces of filter paper to collect the liquid produced in 5 minutes.

Schistosoma (*shis-to-so'-mah*). A genus of minute blood flukes, some of which are parasitic in man. *S. haematobium*. A species which infests the urinary bladder; widely found in Africa and the Middle East, especially in Egypt. *S. japonicum* and *S. mansoni*. Species which infest the large intestine. They are found respectively in China, Japan and the Philippines, and in Africa, the West Indies and tropical America.

schistosomiasis (*shis-to-so-mi'-as-is*). A parasitic infection of the intestinal or urinary tract by *Schistosoma*. The parasite enters the skin from contaminated water, and causes diarrhoea, haematuria, and anaemia. The secondary hosts are freshwater snails. Bilharziasis.

schizoid (*skits'-oid*). Resembling schizophrenia. *S. personality*. One that is marked by introspection, self-consciousness, solitariness and a failure in affection towards others. Some schizophrenics have this personality, but only a few who are schizoid become schizophrenic.

Schizomycetes (*skits-o-mi-se'-teez*). A class of minute vegetable organisms that reproduce themselves by fission; bacteria and fungi are of this type.

schizophrenia (*skits-o-fre'-ne-ah*). A psychosis of unknown cause but showing hereditary links. Characteristically the patient feels himself to be influenced in a strange way by external forces and suffers delusions and hallucinations; his thought processes are disordered. *Paranoid s.* Predominance of delusions of a persecutory nature. *Simple s.* A progressive deterioration of the patient's efficiency with increasing social withdrawal. *See* Hebephrenia *and* Catatonia.

schizosis (*skits-o'-sis*). A mental state with a marked tendency to avoid contact with the outside world, and to shun social responsibilities.

Schlatter's disease (*C. Schlatter, Swiss surgeon, 1864–1934*). Osteochondrosis of the tibial tuberosity.

Schlemm's canal (*F. Schlemm, German anatomist, 1795–1858*). A venous channel at the junction of the cornea and sclera for the draining of aqueous humour.

Schönlein–Henoch purpura or **syndrome** (*J.L. Schönlein, German physician, 1793–1864; E.H. Henoch, German paediatrician, 1820–1910*). *See* Purpura.

Schultz–Charlton test (*W. Schultz, German physician, 1878–1947; W. Charlton, German physician, b. 1889*). A test in which an intradermal injection of scarlet fever antitoxin is made into an area of rash. Blanching will occur at the injection site if the patient has scarlet fever.

Schwartze's operation (*H.H.R. Schwartze, German otologist, 1837–1910*). Opening of the mastoid cells, without involvement of the middle ear, in order to drain a mastoid abscess.

sciatic (*si-at'-ik*). Relating to the largest nerve in the leg, which runs down the back of the thigh.

sciatica (*si-at'-ik-ah*). Pain down the back of the leg in the area supplied by the sciatic nerve. It is usually caused by pressure on the nerve roots by a protrusion of an intervertebral disc.

scintigraphy (*sin-tig'-raf-e*). The recording of the distribution of radioactivity in an organ following injection of a small dose of a radioactive substance that is specifically taken up by that organ.

scintillography (*sin-til-og'-raf-e*). The method of examination by means of gamma-rays on a fluorescent screen.

scirrhous (*skir'-us*). Hard; indurated; resembling a scirrhus.

scirrhus (*skir'-us*). A hard carcinoma containing much connective tissue.

sclera (*skle'-rah*). The fibrous coat of the eyeball—the white of the eye, which covers the posterior part and in front becomes the cornea.

scleritis (*skler-i'-tis*). Inflammation of the sclera.

scleroderma (*skler-o-der'-mah*). A disease marked by progressive hardening of the skin in patches or diffusely, with rigidity of the underlying tissues. It is often a chronic condition. *See* Raynaud's phenomenon.

scleroma (*skler-o'-mah*). A patch of hardened tissue.

sclerosis (*skler-o'-sis*). The hardening of any part from an overgrowth of fibrous and connective tissue, often due to chronic inflammation. *Amyotrophic lateral s.* Rapid degeneration of the pyramidal (motor nerves) tract and anterior horn cells in the spinal cord. Characterized by weakness and spasm of limb muscles with wasting of the muscle, difficulty with talking and swallowing. *Arterio-s.* The changes occurring in walls of arteries which cause hardening and loss of elasticity. *Athero-s.* The deposition of fatty plaques and hardening and fibrosis of the artery lining. *Disseminated s. See* Multiple s. *Mönckeberg's s.* Extensive degeneration with atrophy and calcareous deposits in the middle muscle coat of arteries, especially of the small ones. *Multiple s.* Scattered (disseminated) patches of degeneration in the nerve sheaths in the brain and spinal cord. Characterized by relapses and remissions. Symptoms include disturbances of speech, vision and micturition and muscular weakness of a limb or limbs. *Systemic s. (scleroderma)* A generalized multisystem disease characterized by dense fibrosis of involved organs and a widespread vascular disorder. *See* Raynaud's phenomenon.

sclerotherapy (*skler-o-ther'-ap-e*). Treatment of varicose veins and haemorrhoids by the injection of sclerosing solutions to produce fibrosis.

sclerotic (*skler-ot'-ik*). (1) Hard; indurated; affected by sclerosis. (2) Pertaining to the sclera of the eye. *S. coat.* The tough membrane forming the outer covering of the eyeball, excepting in front of the iris, where it becomes the clear horny cornea.

sclerotomy (*skler-ot'-om-e*). Incision of the sclerotic coat, usually for the removal of a foreign body or for the relief of glaucoma.

scolex (*sko'-leks*). The head of a tapeworm. It is provided with hooks and suckers with which to hold on to the wall of the intestine.

scoliosis (*skol-e-o'-sis*). Lateral curvature of the spine. *See* Lordosis *and* Kyphosis.

scopolamine (*sko-pol'-am-een*). Hyoscine.

scorbutic (*skor-bu'-tik*). Affected with or related to scurvy.

scotoma (*sko-to'-mah*). A blind

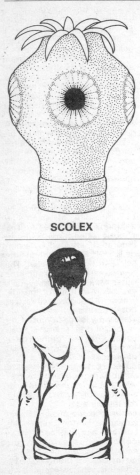

SCOLEX

SCOLIOSIS

area in the field of vision, due to some lesion of the retina. It is also found in glaucoma and in detachment of the retina.

screening (*skre'-ning*). (1) Fluoroscopy. (2) The carrying out of a test on a large number of people to determine the proportion of them that have a particular disease.

scrotum (*skro'-tum*). The pouch of skin and soft tissues containing the testicles.

scrub typhus (*skrub ti'-fus*). Tsutsugamushi disease.

scrumpox (*skrum'-poks*). Contagious impetigo.

scurf (*skerf*). Dandruff.

scurvy (*sker'-ve*). Avitaminosis C. A deficiency disease due to incorrect diet, i.e. one lacking in raw fruits and vegetables and therefore in vitamin C. It rapidly improves with adequate diet. *Infantile s.* A type that may occur in artificially fed infants as milk is a poor source of vitamin C. To prevent it such children should be given orange, tomato or rose hip juice daily.

scybalum (*sib'-al-um*). *pl.* scybala. A mass of abnormally hard faecal matter in the intestine.

sebaceous (*se-ba'-shus*). Fatty, or pertaining to the sebum. *S. glands* are found in the skin, communicating with the hair follicles and secreting sebum. *S. cyst. See* Cyst.

seborrhoea (*se-bor-e'-ah*). A disease of the sebaceous glands, marked by an excessive secretion of sebum which collects on the skin in oily scales.

sebum (*se'-bum*). The fatty secretion of the sebaceous glands.

secondary (*sek'-on-dar-e*). Second in order of time or

importance. *S. deposits. See* Metastases.

secretagogue *(se-kre'-tag-og).* Any agent that stimulates the secretion of a gland.

secrete *(se-kreet').* To separate and alter the constituents of the blood and body fluids and produce a substance that emerges as a secretion.

secretin *(se-kre'-tin).* The hormone originating in the duodenum which, in the presence of bile salts, is absorbed into the blood stream and stimulates the secretion of pancreatic juice.

secretion *(se-kre'-shun).* (1) The process whereby various substances are separated. (2) The substance which is secreted from the blood by glands. Secretions are (a) used for special purposes in the body, e.g. the digestive juices and the hormones, or (b) excreted, e.g. urine and sweat.

section *(sek'-shun).* (1) In surgery, the act of cutting. (2) A portion which has been cut through. *Frozen s.* A thin slice that has been cut from frozen tissue for examination under a microscope.

sedation *(sed-a'-shun).* The allaying of irritability or the relief of pain or mental distress, particularly by drugs.

sedative *(sed'-at-iv).* A drug which lessens excitement and relieves tension. Tranquillizers are primarily used, as are hypnotic drugs such as the barbiturates.

sedentary *(sed'-en-tar-e).* Pertaining to sitting; physically inactive.

sedimentation *(sed-im-en-ta'-shun).* The deposit of solid particles at the bottom of a liquid. *Erythrocyte s. rate.*

ESR. *See* Erythrocyte.

segment *(seg'-ment).* A small piece separated from any part by an actual or imaginary line.

segregation *(seg-re-ga'-shun).* The separation of a number of people from others, e.g. infectious patients.

sella turcica *(sel-ah ter'-sik-ah).* A depression in the sphenoid body which protects the pituitary gland.

semen *(se'-men).* The secretion of the testicles containing spermatozoa, which is ejaculated from the penis during sexual intercourse. Seminal fluid.

semicircular *(sem-e-ser'-ku-lar).* Formed in a half-circle. *S. canals.* Part of the labyrinth of the internal ear, consisting of three canals in the form of arches which contain fluid, and by their nerve supply are connected with the cerebellum. Impressions of change of position of the body are registered in these canals by oscillation of the fluid, and are conveyed by the nerves to the cerebellum.

semicomatose *(sem-e-ko'-mat-oze).* In a condition of unconsciousness from which the patient can be roused.

semilunar *(sem-e-lu'-nar).* Shaped like a half-moon. *S. cartilages.* Two crescent-shaped cartilages in the knee-joint. *S. valve. See* Valve.

seminal *(sem'-in-al).* Relating to the semen.

seminoma *(se-min-o'-mah).* A malignant tumour of the testis, which is highly radiosensitive.

semipermeable *(sem-e-per'-me-abl).* Of a membrane, permitting the passage of some molecules and hindering that of others.

semiprone (*sem-e-prone'*). Partly prone. Applied to a position in which the patient is lying face down but the knees are turned to one side.

senescence (*sen-es'-ens*). The process of growing old.

Sengstaken's tube (*R.W. Sengstaken, American neurosurgeon, b. 1923*). A compression tube used in the treatment of bleeding oesophageal varices.

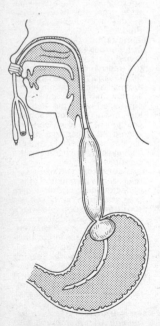

SENGSTAKEN'S TUBE

senile (*se'-nile*). Related to the involutional changes associated with old age. *S. dementia.* Deterioration of mental activity in the elderly associated with an impaired blood supply to the brain.

senility (*sen-il'-it-e*). A state of mental and physical deterioration resulting from old age.

senna (*sen'-ah*). A laxative derived from the cassia plant, given in the form of an infusion of the pods in water. Proprietary standardized preparations are available as tablets or granules.

sensation (*sen-sa'-shun*). A feeling resulting from impulses sent to the brain by the sensory nerves.

sense (*sens*). The faculty by which conditions and properties of things are perceived, e.g. hunger or pain. *Special s.* Any one of the faculties of sight, hearing, touch, smell, taste, and muscle sense, through which the consciousness receives impressions from the environment. *S. organ.* One which receives a sensory stimulus, for instance the eyes and ears.

sensible (*sen'-sibl*). (1) Capable of being perceived. *S. perspiration.* That obvious on the skin as moisture. (2) Sensitive.

sensitive (*sen'-sit-iv*). Capable of reacting to a stimulus.

sensitization (*sen-sit-i-za'-shun*). (1) The process of rendering susceptible. (2) An increase in the body's response to a certain stimulus, as in the development of an allergy. *Protein s.* The condition occurring in an individual when a foreign protein is absorbed into the body, e.g.

shellfish causing urticaria when eaten. *See* Desensitization.

sensory (*sen'-sor-e*). Relating to sensation. *S. cortex.* That part of the cerebral cortex to which information is relayed by the sensory nerves. *S. nerve.* An afferent nerve conveying impressions from the peripheral nerve endings to the brain or spinal cord.

sentiment (*sen'-tim-ent*). An emotion directed towards some object or person. Sentiments are acquired and profoundly influence a person's actions.

sepsis (*sep'-sis*). An infection of the body by pus-forming bacteria. *Focal s.* A local focus of infection which produces general symptoms. *Oral s.* Infection of the mouth which causes general ill-health by absorption of toxins. *Puerperal s.* Infection of the uterus occurring after labour.

septal (*sep'-tal*). Relating to a septum. *S. defect.* A congenital defect when there is an opening in the septum between the two atria or two ventricles of the heart.

septic (*sep'-tik*). Relating to or caused by sepsis. *S. tank.* A tank receiving sewage which is liquefied and purified by anaerobic organisms.

septicaemia (*sep-tis-e'-me-ah*). The presence in the blood of large numbers of bacteria and their toxins. The symptoms are: a rapid rise of temperature, which is later intermittent, rigors, sweating, and all the signs of acute fever.

septum (*sep'-tum*). A division or partition. *Atrial s., atrioventricular s., ventricular s.* The partitions dividing the various cavities of the heart. *Nasal s.*

The structure made of bone and cartilage which separates the nasal cavities.

sequela (*se-kwe'-lah*). *pl.* sequelae. A morbid condition following a disease and resulting from it.

sequestrectomy (*se-kwestrek'-tom-e*). The removal of a sequestrum.

sequestrum (*se-kwes'-trum*). *pl.* sequestra. A piece of dead bone. Inflammation in bone leads to pressure and thrombosis of blood vessels resulting in necrosis of the affected part, which separates from the living structure.

serological (*se-ro-loj'-ik-al*). Relating to serum. *S. tests.* Those that are dependent on the formation of antibodies in the blood as a response to specific organisms or proteins.

serology (*se-rol'-o-je*). The scientific study of blood sera, their actions and reactions. A branch of medicine particularly concerned with diagnosis and immunity.

serosa (*se-ro'-sah*). A serous membrane. It consists of two layers—the *visceral,* in close contact with the organ, and the *parietal,* lining the cavity. The serum exudes, and lubricates between the layers, giving a smooth movement without friction.

serotonin (*se-ro-to'-nin*). An amine present in blood platelets, the intestine and the central nervous system, which acts as a vasoconstrictor. It is derived from the amino acid tryptophan and is inactivated by monoamine oxidase.

serous (*se'-rus*). Related to serum. *S. effusion.* An effusion of serous exudate. *S. in-*

flammation. Inflammation of a serous membrane. Serositis. *S. membrane.* A serosa.

serpiginous (*ser-pij'-in-us*). Creeping from one place to another. Applied to skin lesions such as those of ringworm.

serrated (*ser-a'-ted*). With a saw-like edge.

serum (*se'-rum*). The clear, fluid residue of blood, from which the corpuscles and fibrin have been removed. *S. hepatitis.* Jaundice caused by hepatitis B virus, usually following a blood transfusion or an injection with contaminated material. *S. sickness.* An allergic reaction usually 8 to 10 days after a serum injection. It may be manifest by an irritating urticaria, pyrexia and painful joints. It readily responds to adrenaline and antihistaminic drugs. *See* Anaphylaxis. *S. therapy.* The treatment of an infectious disease by injection of a serum containing antibodies to the micro-organism causing the disease. The antiserum if taken prophylactically will produce temporary passive immunity.

sesamoid (*ses'-am-oid*). Resembling a sesame seed. *S. bone.* A nodule of bone developed in a tendon, e.g. the patella and the pisiform bone.

sessile (*ses'-ile*). Attached by a base. *S. tumour.* A tumour without a stalk or peduncle.

sex (*seks*). (1) *n.* Either of the two divisions of organic organisms described respectively as male and female. *S. chromosome.* A chromosome that determines sex. Women have two X chromosomes and men have one X chromosome and one Y chromo-some. *S. hormone.* A steroid hormone produced by the ovaries or the testes and controlling sexual development. *S.-limited.* Pertaining to a characteristic found in only one sex. *S.-linked.* Pertaining to a characteristic that is transmitted by genes that are located on the sex chromosomes, e.g. haemophilia. (2) *v.* To discover the sex of an organism.

SGOT. Serum glutamic oxalacetic transaminase, an enzyme excreted by damaged heart muscle. A raised serum level occurs in myocardial infarction.

SGPT. Serum glutamic pyruvic transaminase, an enzyme excreted by the parenchymal cells of the liver. There is a raised blood level in infectious hepatitis.

Sheehan's syndrome (*H.L. Sheehan, British pathologist, b. 1900*). Hypopituitarism caused by thrombosis of the pituitary blood supply. It occurs in association with post-partum haemorrhage.

Shigella (*shig-el'-ah*). A genus of gram-negative rod-like bacteria. Some species cause bacillary dysentery. *S. flexneri* and *S. shiga* are common in Asia, *S. dysenteriae* in the USA, and *S. sonnei* in Western Europe.

shin (*shin*). The bony front of the leg below the knee. The tibia.

shingles (*shing'-glz*). Herpes zoster.

Shirodkar's suture (*Shirodkar, Indian obstetrician*). A 'purse-string' suture that is placed round an incompetent cervix during pregnancy to prevent abortion. It is removed at the thirty-eighth week.

shock (*shok*). A condition in which there is a sudden fall in blood pressure. This, untreated, will lead to lack of oxygen in the tissues and greater permeability of the capillary walls, so increasing the degree of shock, by greater loss of fluid. The patient has a cold moist skin, a feeble pulse, a low blood pressure and is distressed and restless. *Allergic* or *Anaphylactic s.* Shock produced by the injection of a protein to which the patient is sensitive. *Cardiac s.* Shock resulting from heart failure, often following a coronary thrombosis. *Hypovolaemic s.* Shock resulting from a reduction in the volume of blood in circulation, following haemorrhage or severe burns. *Neurogenic s.* Shock due to nervous or emotional factors. *Primary s.* Shock occurring immediately after the causative trauma or event. *Shell s.* A psychoneurotic condition caused by the stresses of warfare. *Surgical* or *postoperative s.* A severe state of shock following operation or injuries such as those suffered in road accidents.

short-sightedness (*short-si'-ted-nes*). Myopia.

shoulder (*shold'-er*). The junction of the clavicle and the scapula where the arm joins the body.

show (*sho*). The blood-stained discharge which occurs at the onset of labour.

shunt (*shunt*). A diversion, particularly of blood, due to a congenital defect, disease or surgery.

SI units. The metric system of measurement forming the Système International d'Unités (International System of Units) and now generally accepted for all scientific and technical uses.

sialogogue (*si-al'-o-gog*). A drug increasing the flow of saliva.

sialography (*si-al-og'-raf-e*). X-ray examination of the salivary ducts following the insertion of a radio-opaque dye.

sialolith (*si-al'-o-lith*). A salivary calculus.

sialorrhoea (*si-al-o-re'-ah*). Ptyalism.

sibilant (*sib'-il-ant*). Whistling or hissing. Applied to a high-pitched sound heard on auscultation.

sibling (*sib'-ling*). One of a family of children having the same parents. Applied in psychology to one of two or more children of the same parent or substitute parent figure. *S. rivalry.* Jealousy, compounded of love and hate of one child for its sibling.

sickle-cell anaemia (*sikl'-sel an-e'-me-ah*). An inherited disease in which the red blood cells are crescent-shaped and very friable. Occurs almost exclusively in Negroes.

siderosis (*sid-er-o'-sis*). (1) Chronic inflammation of the lung due to inhalation of particles of iron. (2) Excess iron in the blood. (3) The deposit of iron in the tissues.

sigmoid (*sig'-moid*). Shaped like the Greek letter Σ. *S. colon* or *flexure.* That part of the colon in the left iliac fossa just above the rectum.

sigmoidoscope (*sig-moid'-o-skope*). An instrument by which the interior of the rectum and sigmoid colon can be seen.

sigmoidostomy (*sig-moid-os'-tom-e*). The making of an

artificial opening between the sigmoid colon and the skin.

sign (*sine*). An indication of the presence of disease that can be seen or elicited by a physician, but of which the patient may be unaware.

silicosis (*sil-ik-o'-sis*). Fibrosis of the lung due to the inhalation of silica dust particles. It occurs in miners, stone masons and quarry workers.

silver (*sil'-ver*). *abbrev.* Ag. A metallic element. *S. nitrate.* AgNO₃. A crystalline salt. In solid form it is used as a caustic for destroying warts and reducing excessive granulation tissue. In solution it is antiseptic and astringent.

Simmonds's disease (*M. Simmonds, German physician, 1855–1925*). A condition of anterior pituitary deficiency, causing arrest of growth and premature senility. It most commonly occurs in women after postpartum haemorrhage.

Sims's position (*J.M. Sims, American gynaecologist, 1813–1883*). A semi-prone position. *See* Position.

sinciput (*sin'-sip-ut*). The upper and frontal part of the skull.

sinew (*sin'-u*). A tendon.

sino-atrial (*si-no-a'-tre-al*). Situated between the sinus venosus and the atrium of the heart. *S. node.* The pacemaker of the heart. *See* Node.

sinography (*si-nog'-raf-e*). Radiographic examination of the extent of a sinus using a radio-opaque dye.

sinus (*si'-nus*). (1) A cavity in a bone. *Air s.* A cavity in a bone containing air. *Ethmoidal s.* Air spaces in the ethmoid bone. *Frontal s.* Air spaces in the frontal bone. *Sphenoidal*

s. Air spaces in the sphenoid bone. (2) A venous channel, especially within the cranium. *Cavernous s.* A venous sinus of the dura mater which lies along the body of the sphenoid bone. *Coronary s.* The vein which returns the blood from the heart muscle into the right atrium. *S. arrhythmia.* *See* Arrhythmia. *S. thrombosis.* Clotting of blood in a cranial venous channel. In the lateral sinus it is a complication of mastoiditis. (3) An unhealed passage leading from an abscess or internal lesion to the surface.

sinusitis (*si-nu-si'-tis*). Inflammation of the lining of a sinus, especially applied to the bony cavities of the face.

sinusoid (*si'-nu-soid*). Like a sinus. Used to describe the irregular channels by which blood vessels anastomose in certain organs, such as the liver and suprarenal glands.

siphonage (*si'-fon-aje*). A method of drawing a liquid from one vessel into another. Used in gastric lavage.

Sjögren's disease (*H.S.C. Sjögren, Swedish ophthalmologist, b. 1899*). A deficiency in lacrimation usually found in women in middle age. Keratoconjunctivitis, rhinitis or laryngitis may occur.

skatole (*skat'-ole*). A product of protein decomposition in the intestine which is present in faeces.

skeleton (*skel'-et-on*). The bony framework of the body, supporting and protecting the organs and soft tissues.

Skene's gland (*A.J.C. Skene, American gynaecologist, 1838–1900*). One of a pair of glands which open into the posterior urethral orifice in the female. These glands usually become infected in acute gonorrhoea.

skin (*skin*). The outer protective covering of the body. It consists of an outer layer, the *epidermis* or cuticle, and an inner layer, the *dermis* or corium, which is known as 'true skin'. The skin and nervous system are developed from the same primitive layer of cells in the embryo, and keep this deep-rooted relationship through life, as is often seen in disease. *S. grafting.* Transplantation of pieces of healthy skin to an area where loss of surface tissue has occurred.

skull (*skul*). The bony framework of the head, consisting of the cranium and facial bones.

sleeping sickness (*sle'-ping sik'-nes*). Trypanosomiasis. A tropical fever occurring in parts of Africa, caused by a protozoal parasite (*Trypanosoma*) which is conveyed by the tsetse fly.

sling (*sling*). A bandage for support of the upper limb.

slipped disc (*slipd disk*). A prolapsed intervertebral disc which causes pressure on the spinal nerves. It may be very painful.

slit lamp (*slit lamp*). A special light source so arranged with a microscope that examination of the interior of the eye can be carried out at the level of each layer.

slough (*sluf*). Dead tissue caused by injury or inflammation. It separates from the healthy tissue and is ultimately washed away by exuded serum, leaving a granulating surface.

smallpox (*smawl'-poks*). Variola.

smear (*smeer*). A specimen for microscopic examination that has been prepared by spreading a thin film of the material across a glass slide.

smegma (*smeg'-mah*). The secretion of sebaceous glands of the clitoris and prepuce.

Smith-Petersen nail (*M.N. Smith-Petersen, American surgeon, 1886–1953*). A metal nail used to fix the fragments of bone in intracapsular fracture of the head of the femur.

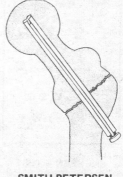

SMITH-PETERSEN NAIL

snake (*snake*). A limbless reptile. A serpent. The bites of many snakes are poisonous to man. *S. venom antitoxin.* Antivenin. A serum made from animals, usually horses, which have been immunized against the venom of a specific type of snake.

snare (*snair*). A wire loop used for removing pedunculated tumours (polyps).

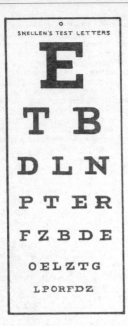

SNELLEN'S TEST LETTERS

Snellen's test letters (*H. Snellen, Dutch ophthalmologist, 1834–1908*). Square-shaped letters on a chart, used for sight testing.

snow (*sno*). Frozen water vapour. *S. blindness.* Photophobia due to the glare of snow. *Carbon dioxide s.* Solid CO_2 which is used as a refrigerant. 'Dry ice'.

snuffles (*snuf'-lz*). A chronic discharge from the nose occurring in children, usually those with congenital syphilis, due to infection of the nasal mucous membrane.

sociology (*so-se-ol'-o-je*). The scientific study of the development of man's social relationships and organization, i.e. interpersonal and intergroup behaviour as distinct from the behaviour of an individual.

sodium (*so'-de-um*). *abbrev.* Na. A metallic alkaline element widely distributed in nature, and forming an important constituent of animal tissue. *S. aminosalicylate.* An antituberculous drug used in conjunction with streptomycin and isoniazid. *S. bicarbonate.* An antacid widely used to treat digestive disorders, especially flatulence. Repeated use can cause alkalosis. *S. chloride.* Common salt. Its presence in the diet is necessary to health. Sometimes used in solution by injection to increase the quantity of electrolytes in the body. *S. citrate.* Compound used to prevent clotting of blood during blood transfusions. *S. cromoglycate.* A drug used as an inhalant in the treatment of asthma. *S. fluoride.* A salt used in the fluoridation of water and also locally on the teeth to prevent the formation of caries. *S. hydroxide.* Caustic soda. A powerful corrosive drug used to destroy warts. It can cause severe chemical burns. *S. hypochlorite.* A compound with germicidal properties used in solution to disinfect utensils. In diluted form (Dakin's solution) it is used for wound irrigation and as a local antibacterial. *S. phosphate.* A purgative. *S. salicylate.* An antipyretic drug used in the treatment of rheumatic fever. *S. sulphate.* A purgative. *S. valproate.* A drug used in the treatment of epilepsy.

solar plexus (*so'-lar pleks'-us*). Coeliac plexus. A network of sympathetic nerve ganglia in the abdomen; the nerve supply to abdominal organs below the diaphragm.

solarium (*sol-ar'-e-um*). (1) A room designed to admit as much sunlight as possible. (2) A room in which artificial sunlight treatment is given.

solution (*so-lu'-shun*). A liquid in which one or more substances have been dissolved.

solvent (*sol'-vent*). A liquid which dissolves or has power to dissolve.

soma (*so'-mah*). (1) The body as distinct from the mind. (2) The body tissue as distinct from the germ cells.

somatic (*so-mat'-ik*). (1) Relating to the body as opposed to the mind. (2) Relating to the body wall as distinct from the viscera.

somite (*so'-mite*). One of the paired blocks of mesoderm present in the early embryo from which the body tissues are developed.

somnambulism (*som-nam'-bu-lizm*). Walking and carrying out other complex activities during a state of sleep. It is a state of dissociation and may occur in hysteria, in epilepsy and in a hypnotic state.

Sonne dysentery (*C.O. Sonne, Danish bacteriologist, 1882–1948*). A mild form of bacillary dysentery which is common in Britain. The symptoms are diarrhoea, vomiting and abdominal pain. The causative agent is *Shigella sonnei.*

sonometer (*so-nom'-e-ter*). An instrument for measuring the acuity of heating or the frequency and pitch of sound waves.

sopor (*so'-por*). Profound sleep.

soporific (*sop-or-if'-ik*). A drug that causes sleep.

sorbefacient (*sor-be-fa'-shent*). An agent that promotes absorption.

sorbitol (*sor'-bit-ol*). A sweetening agent which is converted into sugar in the body though it is slowly absorbed from the intestine. It is used in some diabetic foods and in intravenous feeding.

sordes (*sor'-dez*). Brown crusts which form on the teeth and lips of unconscious patients, or those suffering from acute or prolonged fevers.

sore (*sor*). A general term for any ulcer or open skin lesion. *Cold s.* Herpes simplex. *Hard s.* A syphilitic chancre. *Pressure s.* A sore caused by pressure from the bed (decubitus ulcer) or a splint. *Soft s.* A chancroid ulcer. *S. throat.* Inflammation of the larynx or pharynx, including tonsillitis.

souffle (*soo'-fl*). A blowing sound heard on auscultation.

sound (*sownd*). In surgery, an instrument shaped like a probe for exploring cavities and detecting the presence of foreign bodies. Also, an instrument used for the dilatation of a canal.

Spanish fly (*span'-ish fli*). A species of beetle from which cantharidin, a blistering agent, is derived.

spasm (*spazm*). A sudden involuntary muscle contraction. *Carpopedal s.* Spasm of the hands and feet. A sign of tetany. *Clonic s.* Alternate muscle rigidity and relaxation. *Habit s.* A tic. *Nictitating s.* Spasmodic twitching of the eyelid. *Tetanic s.* Violent muscle spasms, including opisthotonos. *Tonic s.* A sustained muscle rigidity.

spasmodic (*spaz-mod'-ik*). (1) Related to a spasm. (2) Occurring and recurring, as in spasms.

spasmolytic (*spaz-mo-lit'-ik*). A drug which reduces spasm.

spastic (*spas'-tik*). (1) Caused by spasm; convulsive. *S. colon.* Irritable bowel syndrome. *S. paralysis.* Paralysis associated with lesions of the upper motor neurone as in cerebral vascular accidents and characterized by increased muscle tone and rigidity. (2) One affected by spasticity, often applied to persons suffering from congenital paralysis due to some cerebral lesion or impairment.

spasticity (*spas-tis'-it-e*). Marked rigidity of muscle.

spatial (*spa'-shal*). Pertaining to space.

spatula (*spat'-u-lah*). (1) A flexible blunt blade used for spreading ointment. (2) A rigid blade-shaped instrument for depressing the tongue in throat examination, etc.

spatulate (*spat'-u-late*). Flattened like a spatula.

species (*spe'-sheez*). A subdivision of a genus.

specific (*spes-if'-ik*). (1) *adj.* Relating to a species. (2) *n.* A remedy which has a distinct curative influence on a particular disease, e.g. quinine in malaria. (3) *adj.* Related to a unit mass of a substance. *S. gravity.* The density of fluid compared with that of an equal volume of water.

specimen (*spes'-im-en*). A sample or part taken to show the nature of the whole, e.g. for chemical testing or microscopic survey.

spectacles (*spek'-taklz*). A frame containing lenses worn in front of the eyes to correct errors of vision or to protect from glare.

spectrometer (*spek-trom'-e-ter*). An instrument for measuring the strength and wavelengths of visible or invisible electromagnetic radiations.

spectroscope (*spek'-tro-skope*). An instrument used for analysing the spectra of light and other radiations.

spectrum (*spek'-trum*). *pl.* spectra. (1) The range of colours produced when white light is split up into its component parts. (2) The full range of wavelengths of electromagnetic radiation.

speech (*speech*). The act of communicating by sounds by means of a linguistic code. *Clipped s.* Speech in which the words are cut short. *Deaf s.* The characteristic utterance of people with severe hearing loss. *Explosive s.* Loud sudden utterances, a sign of mental disorder. *Incoherent s.* Disconnected utterances made when the sequence of thought is disturbed, as in delirium. *Oesophageal s.* Speech produced following laryngectomy by swallowing air and using it to vibrate within the oesophagus against the closed cricopharyngeal sphincter. *Scanning s.* Speech in which the syllables are inappropriately separated from each other and are evenly stressed. Characteristic of cerebellar damage. *Staccato* *s.* Speech in which each syllable is separately pronounced. Characteristic of multiple sclerosis.

Spencer Wells forceps (*Sir T. Spencer Wells, British surgeon, 1818–1897*). Artery forceps. *See* Forceps.

sperm (*sperm*). (1) A spermatozoon. (2) The semen.

spermatocele (*sper'-mat-o-seel*). A cystic swelling in the epididymis, containing semen.

spermatorrhoea (*sper-mat-or-e'-ah*). An involuntary discharge of semen, without orgasm.

spermatozoon (*sper-mat-o-zo'-on*). *pl.* Spermatozoa. A mature male germ cell consisting of a flat-shaped head, a short middle part and a long tail. There are 300–500 million sperms in a normal ejaculate.

spermicide (*sper'-mis-ide*). Any agent which will destroy spermatozoa.

sphenoid (*sfe'-noid*). Wedge-shaped. *S. bone.* The central part of the base of the skull.

spherocytosis (*sfer-o-si-to'-sis*). The presence in the blood of erythrocytes which are more nearly spherical than biconcave. Characteristic of acholuric jaundice, it may also be hereditary.

sphincter (*sfingk'-ter*). A ring-shaped muscle, contraction of which closes a natural orifice.

sphincterectomy (*sfingk-ter-ek'-tom-e*). (1) The excision of a sphincter. (2) In ophthalmology, an operation to free the sphincter of the iris when it has become attached to the back of the cornea.

sphincterotomy (*sfingk-ter-ot'-om-e*). The incision of a sphincter to relieve constriction.

sphygmic (*sfig'-mik*). Relating to the pulse.

sphygmocardiograph (*sfig-mo-kard'-e-o-graf*). An instrument that records both the pulse waves and heartbeat.

sphygmograph (*sfig'-mo-graf*). An instrument which registers graphically the force and character of the arterial pulse.

sphygmomanometer (*sfig-mo-man-om'-e-ter*). An instrument for measuring the arterial blood pressure.

spica (*spi'-kah*). A bandage applied to a joint in a series of 'figures of eight'.

spicule (*spik'-ule*). A splinter-like fragment of bone.

Spigelius's lobe (*A. van Spieghel (Spigelius), Flemish anatomist, 1578–1625*). The small lobe on the under surface of the liver.

spigot (*spig'-ot*). A small plastic peg to close the opening of a tube.

spina (*spi'-nah*). (1) The vertebral column. The spine. *S. bifida.* A congenital defect of non-union of one or more vertebral arches, allowing protrusion of the meninges and possibly their contents. *See* Meningocele *and* Meningomyelocele. (2) Any sharp bony projection.

spinal (*spi'-nal*). Relating to the spine. *S. anaesthesia. See* Anaesthesia. *S. canal.* The hollow in the spine formed by the neural arches of the vertebrae. It contains the spinal cord, meninges, and cerebrospinal fluid. *S. caries.* Disease of the vertebrae, usually tuberculous. *See* Pott's disease. *S. column.* The backbone. The vertebral column. *S. cord. See* Cord. *S. curvature.* Abnormal curving of the spine. If associated with caries, it is known as Pott's disease. (*See* Kyphosis, Lordosis *and* Scoliosis.) *S. jacket.* A support for the spine, made of plaster of Paris, or other material, and used to give rest after injury to or operation on the spine. *S. nerves.* The 31 pairs of nerves which leave the spinal cord at regular intervals throughout its length. They pass out in pairs one on either side between each of the vertebrae, and are distributed to the periphery. *S. puncture.* Lumbar or cisternal puncture.

spine (*spine*). (1) The backbone or vertebral column, consisting of 33 vertebrae, separated by fibrocartilaginous discs, and enclosing the spinal cord. (2) A sharp process of bone.

spinnbarkeit (*spin'-bar-kite*). A thread of mucus secreted by the cervix uteri. Used to determine ovulation as this usually coincides with when the mucus can be drawn out on a glass slide to its maximum length.

spiral (*spi'-ral*). Winding, as the method of applying a roller bandage. *S. fracture.* One that is usually due to a rotational strain.

Spirillum (*spi-ril'-um*). A genus of spiral-shaped bacteria. *S. minus.* A species carried by rats and causing one type of rat-bite fever.

spirit (*spir'-it*). An alcoholic solution of a volatile substance.

spirochaete (*spi'-ro-keet*). One of a group of micro-organisms in the form of a spiral, some of which are found in impure fresh or salt water. The group includes the species *Treponema*, *Borrelia* and *Leptospira*.

spirograph (*spi'-ro-graf*). An instrument for registering respiratory movements.

spirometer (*spi-rom'-e-ter*). An instrument for measuring the air capacity of the lungs.

spironolactone (*spi-ron-o-lak'-tone*). A diuretic drug used when there is excess secretion of aldosterone. It promotes the excretion of sodium and water but the retention of potassium. Used in the treatment of oedema caused by cirrhosis of the liver and of chronic heart failure.

Spitz–Holter valve (*Spitz, American engineer; J.W. Holter, American engineer*). A device used in the treatment of hydrocephalus to drain the cerebrospinal fluid from the ventricles into the superior vena cava or the right atrium.

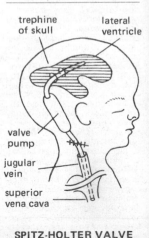

SPITZ-HOLTER VALVE

splanchnic (*splangk'-nik*). Pertaining to the viscera. *S. nerves*. Sympathetic nerves to the viscera.

spleen (*spleen*). A large, very vascular gland-like but ductless organ, coloured a reddish purple and situated in the left hypochondrium under the border of the stomach. It manufactures lymphocytes and breaks down red blood corpuscles.

splenectomy (*splen-ek'-tom-e*). Excision of the spleen.

spleneolus (*splen-e-o'-lus*). An accessory spleen.

splenitis (*splen-i'-tis*). Inflammation of the spleen.

splenomegaly (*splen-o-meg'-al-e*). Enlargement of the spleen.

splenorenal (*splen-o-re'-nal*). Relating to the spleen and the kidney. *S. anastomosis*. An operation carried out to treat portal hypertension. The spleen is excised and the splenic vein is inserted into the renal vein.

splint (*splint*). An appliance used to support or immobilize a part while healing takes place or to correct or prevent deformity.

spondylitis (*spon-dil-i'-tis*). Inflammation of the vertebrae. *Ankylosing s.* A rheumatic disease chiefly of young males in which there is abnormal ossification with pain and rigidity of the intervertebral, hip and sacroiliac joints.

spondylolisthesis (*spon-dil-o-lis-the'-sis*). A sliding forwards or displacement of one vertebra over another, usually the fifth lumbar over the sacrum, causing symptoms such as low back pain due to pressure on the nerve roots.

spondylosis (*spon-dil-o'-sis*). Ankylosis of the vertebral joints usually caused by a degenerative disease of the intervertebral discs, such as osteo-arthritis.

sponging (*spun'-jing*). A method of reducing a high temperature by encouraging evaporation from the skin. The temperatures suggested for the sponge water are approximate, but suitable ones are: *cold s.* 20°C, *tepid s.* 30°C, *hot s.* 40°C.

spongioblastoma (*spun-je-o-blas-to'-mah*). A rapidly growing brain tumour that is highly malignant. A glioma.

spontaneous (*spon-ta'-ne-us*). Occurring without apparent cause. Applied to certain types of fracture and to recovery from a disease without any specific treatment.

sporadic (*spor-ad'-ik*). Pertaining to isolated cases of a disease which occurs in various and scattered places (compare endemic and epidemic).

spore (*spor*). (1) A reproductive stage of some of the lowest forms of vegetable life, e.g. moulds. (2) A protective state which some bacteria are able to assume in adverse conditions, such as lack of moisture, food, or heat. In this form the organism can remain alive, but inert, for years.

spotted fever (*spot'-ed fe'-ver*). A name given both to cerebrospinal fever and to rickettsial Rocky Mountain fever on account of the purpuric rash which may be present in either disease.

sprain (*sprane*). Wrenching of a joint, producing laceration of the capsule or stretching of the ligaments, with consequent swelling, which is due to effusion of fluid into the affected part.

Sprengel's deformity (*O.G.K. Sprengel, German surgeon, 1852–1915*). A congenital condition in which one shoulderblade is higher than the other, causing some limitation of abduction power.

sprue (*sproo*). A disease of malabsorption in the intestine, which may be tropical or non-tropical in form. There is steatorrhoea, diarrhoea, glossitis, and anaemia.

spud (*spud*). A flat, blunt blade used for removing foreign bodies from the eye.

spur (*sper*). A projecting piece of bone.

sputum (*spu'-tum*). Material expelled from the air passages through the mouth. It consists chiefly of mucus and saliva, but in diseased conditions of the air passages it may be purulent, bloodstained and frothy and contain many bacteria. It must always be regarded as highly infectious. *Rusty s.* That in which altered blood permeates the mucus. Characteristic of acute lobar pneumonia.

squamous (*skwa'-mus*). Scaly. *S. bone.* The thin part of the temporal bone which articulates with the parietal and frontal bones. *S. epithelium.* Epithelium composed of flat and scale-like cells.

squint (*skwint*). See Strabismus.

Sr. Chemical symbol for *strontium.*

stadium (*sta'-de-um*). The stage of a disease. *S. decrementi.* The period of decline in severity. Defervescence. *S. incrementi.* The stage of advance when symptoms are developing. *S. in-* *cubationis* or *invasionis.* The incubation period.

staging (*sta'-jing*). The classification of malignant diseases according to the extent of tumour infiltration, the involvement of lymph nodes and the presence or absence of metastases.

stain (*stane*). In medicine, a dye used to colour tissues and other material for microscopical examination.

stammering (*stam'-er-ing*). Stuttering. A speech disorder in which the utterance is broken by hesitation and repetition or prolongation of words and syllables.

stapedectomy (*sta-pe-dek'-tom-e*). Removal of the stapes and insertion of a vein graft or other device to re-establish conduction of sound waves in otosclerosis.

stapediolysis (*sta-pe-de-ol'-is-is*). An operation in which the footpiece of the stapes is mobilized to aid conduction in deafness from otosclerosis.

stapes (*sta'-peez*). The stirrup-shaped bone of the middle ear.

staphylectomy (*staf-il-ek'-tom-e*). Surgical removal of the uvula. Uvulectomy.

Staphylococcus (*staf-il-o-kok'-us*). A genus of gram-positive non-mobile bacteria which, under the microscope, appear grouped together in small masses like bunches of grapes. They are normally present on the skin and mucous membranes. *S. pyogenes* (or *S. aureus*) is a common cause of boils, carbuncles and abscesses.

staphyloma (*staf-il-o'-mah*). A protrusion of the cornea or the sclerotic coat of the eyeball as the result of inflammation or wound.

staphylorrhaphy (*staf-il-or'-af-e*). An operation to suture a cleft soft palate and uvula.

starch (*starch*). A carbohydrate occurring in many vegetable tissues.

starvation (*star-va'-shun*). A prolonged lack of food, and the condition arising from it.

stasis (*sta'-sis*). The stagnation or stoppage of the flow of a fluid. *Intestinal s.* Sluggish movement of faeces through the bowel, due to partial obstruction or to impairment of the action of the intestinal muscles. *Venous s.* Congestion of blood in the veins.

static (*stat'-ik*). Stationary; at rest. *S. electricity.* The build-up of an electrical charge in a non-conductor, which may cause a spark, and an explosion of oxygen or an explosive anaesthetic gas if such are present.

status (*sta'-tus*). Condition. *S. asthmaticus.* A severe and prolonged attack of asthma. *S. epilepticus.* A condition in which there is a rapid succession of epileptic fits. *S. lymphaticus.* A condition in which all lymphatic tissues are hypertrophied, especially the thymus gland.

staxis (*staks'-is*). Haemorrhage.

steapsin (*ste-ap'-sin*). *See* Lipase.

steatoma (*ste-at-o'-mah*). (1) A sebaceous cyst. (2) A lipoma; a fatty tumour.

steatopygia (*ste-at-o-pij'-e-ah*). Excessive deposit of fat in the buttocks.

steatorrhoea (*ste-at-or-e'-ah*). The presence of an excess of fat in the stools due to malabsorption of fat by the intestines.

steatosis (*ste-at-o'-sis*). Fatty degeneration.

Stein–Leventhal syndrome (*I.F. Stein, American gynaecologist, b. 1887; M.L. Leventhal, American gynaecologist, 1901–1971*). Condition affecting females in which obesity, hirsutism and sterility are associated with polycystic ovaries and menstrual irregularities.

Steinmann's pin (*F. Steinmann, Swiss surgeon, 1872–1932*). A fine metal rod passed through bone, by which extension is applied to overcome muscle contraction in certain fractures. *See* Kirschner's wire.

stellate (*stel'-ate*). Star-shaped. *S. fracture.* A radiating fracture of the patella. *S. ganglion.* The inferior cervical ganglion. A star-shaped collection of nerve cells at the base of the neck.

Stellwag's sign (*C. Stellwag von Carion, Austrian ophthalmologist, 1823–1904*). A 'widening' of the eyes with infrequent blinking, as may occur in exophthalmos.

stenocardia (*sten-o-kar'-de-ah*). Angina pectoris.

stenosis (*sten-o'-sis*). Abnormal narrowing or contraction of a channel or opening. *Aortic s.* Narrowing of the opening of the aortic valve due to scar tissue formation as the result of inflammation. *Mitral s.* Narrowing of the orifice of the mitral valve, usually following rheumatic fever. *Pulmonary s.* A congenital narrowing of the opening from the right ventricle of the heart into the pulmonary artery. *Pyloric s.* Narrowing of the pyloric orifice of the stomach due to scar tissue, new growth, or congenital hypertrophy.

Stensen's duct (*H. Stensen, Danish physician, 1638–1686*). The duct of the parotid gland, opening into the mouth opposite the second upper molar.

stercobilin (*ster-ko-bi'-lin*). A brown-orange pigment derived from bile and present in faeces.

stercolith (*ster'-ko-lith*). A hard mass of faeces in the bowel. A faecalith.

stercoraceous (*ster-kor-a'-shus*). Faecal, or containing faeces. *S. vomit.* Vomit containing faeces. Caused by an overflow of faeces into the stomach due to intestinal obstruction.

stereognosis (*steer-e-og-no'-sis*). The ability to visualize the shape of an object by touch alone.

stereoscopy (*steer-e-os'-ko-pe*). In radiography, the making of a pair of radiographs for viewing with binocular vision.

stereotypy(*steer-e-o-ti'-pe*).Repetitive actions carried out or maintained for long periods in a monotonous fashion.

sterile (*ster'-ile*). (1) Barren; incapable of producing young. (2) Aseptic; free from micro-organisms.

sterility (*ster-il'-it-e*). (1) The inability of a woman to become pregnant, or of a man to produce potent spermatozoa. (2) The state of being free from micro-organisms.

sterilization (*ster-il-i-za'-shun*). (1) Rendering incapable of reproduction by any means, e.g. bilateral severing of the uterine tubes in the female, or bilateral severing of the vas deferens in the male. (2)

Rendering dressings, instruments, etc., aseptic by destroying or removing all microbial life.

sterilizer (*ster'-il-i-zer*). An apparatus in which objects can be sterilized. *See* Autoclave.

sternal (*ster'-nal*). Relating to the sternum.

sternocleidomastoid (*ster-no-kli-do-mas'-toid*). A muscle group stretching from the mastoid process to the sternum and clavicle.

sternotomy (*ster-not'-om-e*). The operation in which the sternum is cut through to enable the heart to be reached.

sternum (*ster'-num*). The breast-bone; the flat narrow bone in the centre of the anterior wall of the thorax.

sternutator (*ster'-nu-ta-tor*). A substance which causes wheezing.

steroid (*ster'-oid*). One of a group of hormones chemically related to cholesterol. They include oestrogen and androgen, progesterone and the corticosteroids. They may be naturally occurring or they may be synthesized.

sterol (*ster'-ol*). One of a group of steroid alcohols which includes cholesterol and ergosterol.

stertorous (*ster'-tor-us*). Snore-like; applied to a snoring sound produced in breathing during sleep or in coma.

stethometer (*steth-om'-e-ter*). An instrument for measuring the expansion of the chest.

stethoscope (*steth'-o-skope*). The instrument used in mediate auscultation for listening to internal sounds from the heart and lung. It consists of a hollow tube, one end of which is placed over the part to be examined and the other at the ear of the examiner. *Binaural s.* One with two flexible tubes, one for each ear of the examiner.

Stevens–Johnson syndrome (*A.M. Stevens, American paediatrician, 1884–1945; F.C. Johnson, American paediatrician, 1894–1934*). A form of erythema multiforme in which ulcers occur on the conjunctiva, sometimes leading to corneal ulceration, and on the anogenital mucosa and round the mouth, accompanied by fever.

sthenia (*sthe´-ne-ah*). A condition of abnormally great strength and activity.

sthenic (*sthen´-ik*). Strong, active. *S. fever.* One marked by high temperature, rapid strong pulse and sometimes delirium.

stibophen (*stib´-o-fen*). A sodium salt of antimony given intramuscularly in the treatment of schistosomiasis.

stigma (*stig´-mah*). *pl.* stigmata. (1) A small spot or mark on the skin. (2) Any mark characteristic of a condition or defect, or of a disease. It refers to visible signs rather than symptoms.

stilboestrol (*stil-be´-strol*). A synthetic oestrogen preparation used in the treatment of cancer of the prostate and also of post-menopausal breast cancer.

stillbirth (*stil´-berth*). As defined by the Central Midwives Board: a fetus, born after the twenty-eighth week of pregnancy, which, after complete expulsion, has not breathed or shown any sign of life.

Still's disease (*Sir G.F. Still, British paediatrician, 1868–1941*). A form of rheumatoid arthritis in children sometimes associated with enlargement of the lymph glands.

stimulant (*stim´-u-lant*). An agent which causes increased energy or functional activity of any organ.

stimulus (*stim´-u-lus*). Any agent that produces a functional reaction from a cell tissue or other structure.

stirrup bone (*stir´-up bone*). *See* Stapes.

stitch (*stitch*). (1) A sudden sharp pain usually due to spasm of the diaphragm. (2) A suture. *S. abscess.* Pus formation where a stitch has been inserted.

Stokes–Adams syndrome (*Sir W. Stokes, Irish surgeon, 1804–1878; R. Adams, Irish physician, 1791–1875*). Attacks of syncope or fainting due to cerebral anaemia in some cases of complete heart block. The heart stops temporarily but breathing continues. It is treated by using an artificial pace-maker.

stoma (*sto´-mah*). (1) A mouth or mouthlike opening. (2) An artificial opening in the skin surface leading into one of the tubes forming the alimentary canal. *See* Colostomy *and* Ileostomy.

stomach (*stum´-ak*). The dilated portion of the alimentary canal between the oesophagus and the duodenum, just below the diaphragm. *Bilocular* or *hourglass s.* One divided into two parts by a constriction. *Leather bottle s.* Induration and thickening of the gastric wall, usually the result of malignant disease. *S. pump.* One that removes the contents of the stomach by suction. *S.*

tube. A flexible tube used for washing out the stomach, or for the administration of liquid food.

stomachic (*stum-ak'-ik*). (1) *adj.* Pertaining to the stomach. (2) *n.* A gastric tonic. A drug which stimulates and improves gastric function.

stomatitis (*sto-mat-i'-tis*). Inflammation of the mouth, either simple or with ulceration caused by a vitamin deficiency or by a bacterial or fungal infection. *Angular s.* Cracking at the corners of the mouth, usually due to riboflavine deficiency. *Aphthous s.* That characterized by small, white, painful ulcers on the mucous membrane. *Ulcerative s.* Painful shallow ulcers on the tongue, cheeks and lips. A severe type which may produce serious constitutional effects.

stomatology (*sto-mat-ol'-o-je*). The study of diseases of the mouth.

stomatonoma (*sto-mat-o-no'-mah*). Gangrene of the mouth.

stone (*stone*). A calculus.

stool (*stool*). A motion or discharge from the bowels. *Fatty s.* That which contains undigested fat. *Hunger s.* Stool passed by underfed infants: frequent, small and green. *Rice-water s.* The watery stool, containing small white flakes, seen in cholera. *Tarry s.* A black tarry stool due to the presence of blood from a peptic ulcer.

stop-needle (*stop-ne'-dl*). A surgical needle with an enlargement on the shank to prevent deep penetration, e.g. a sternal marrow puncture needle.

strabismus (*strab-iz'-mus*). Squint. Heterotropia. A deviation of the eye from its normal direction. It is called *convergent* when the eye turns in toward the nose, and *divergent* when it turns outward. *Concomitant s.* A squint in which the angle of deviation stays constant.

strabotomy (*strab-ot'-om-e*). The division of ocular muscles in the treatment of strabismus.

strain (*strane*). (1) *n.* Over-use or stretching of a part, e.g. a muscle or tendon. (2) *n.* A group of micro-organisms within a species. (3) *v.* To pass a liquid through a filter.

stramonium (*stra-mo'-ne-um*). A vegetable drug containing the alkaloid hyoscyamine, which in its action resembles belladonna.

strangulated (*strang'-gu-la-ted*). Compressed or constricted so that the circulation of the blood is arrested. *S. hernia. See Hernia.*

strangulation (*strang-gu-la'-shun*). (1) Choking caused by compression of the air passages. (2) Arrested circulation to a part, which will result in gangrene.

strangury (*strang'-gu-re*). A frequent desire to micturate, but in which only a few drops or urine are passed with difficulty and pain. It results from local inflammatory conditions and muscle spasm.

stratified (*strat'-e-fide*). Arranged in layers. *S. tissue.* A covering tissue in which the cells are arranged in layers. The germinating cells are the lowest, and as surface cells are shed there is continual replacement.

stratum (*strah'-tum*). *pl.* strata. A layer; applied to structures such as the skin and mucous membranes. *S. corneum.* The outer, horny layer of the epidermis.

Streptococcus (*strep-to-kok'-us*). A genus of gram-positive spherical bacteria occurring in chain-like formation. Many of them are haemolytic and these strains are divided into Lancefield groups, of which group A is the most important in medicine. *S. faecalis.* A group D strain which is found in the intestines. *S. pneumoniae.* The pneumococcus which is a cause of pneumonia. *S. pyogenes.* A group A strain which is responsible for most streptococcal infections. It may be the cause of acute tonsillitis, cellulitis, otitis media, scarlet fever, septicaemia, and puerperal fever. Its toxins cause haemolysis of red blood cells. *S. viridans.* A group A strain similar to *S. pyogenes.* It causes subacute bacterial endocarditis.

streptodornase (*strep-to-dorn'-aze*). An enzyme produced by some haemolytic streptococci. It is capable of liquefying pus. Often used in combination with streptokinase in the management of deep wounds.

streptokinase (*strep-to-ki'-naze*). An enzyme derived from a streptococcal culture and used to liquefy clotted blood and pus.

Streptomyces (*strep-to-mi'-seez*). A genus of soil bacteria from which a large number of antibiotics are derived.

streptomycin (*strep-to-mi'-sin*). An antibiotic drug derived from *Streptomyces griseus* used particularly in the treatment of tuberculosis, and then usually given in conjunction with calcium or sodium aminosalicylate or isoniazid.

stress (*stres*). Any factor, mental or physical, the pressure of which can adversely affect the functioning of the body. *S. disorders.* Those resulting from an individual's inability to withstand stress. *S. incontinence.* Incontinence, usually of urine, when the intra-abdominal pressure is raised such as in coughing, sneezing or laughing. Usually occurs in elderly women with lax abdominal muscles.

stria (*stri'-ah*). *pl.* striae. A line or stripe. *Striae gravidarum.* The lines which appear on the abdomen of pregnant women. They are red in first pregnancy, but white subsequently and are due to stretching and rupture of the elastic fibres.

striated (*stri-a'-ted*). Striped. *S. muscle.* Voluntary muscle. See Muscle.

stricture (*strik'-chur*). A narrowing or local contraction of a canal. It may be caused by muscle spasm, new growth, or scar tissue formation following inflammation.

stridor (*stri'-dor*). A harsh, vibrating, shrill sound, produced during respiration when there is partial obstruction of the larynx or trachea.

stridulous (*strid'-u-lus*). Relating to stridor. See Laryngismus.

stroke (*stroke*). A popular term to describe the sudden onset of symptoms, especially those of cerebral origin. *Apoplectic s.* Cerebral haemorrhage. *Heat s.* A hyperpyrexia accompanied by cerebral symptoms. It may occur in someone newly arrived in a very hot climate.

stroma (*stro'-mah*). The connective tissue forming the foundation and framework of an organ which supports the functioning cells.

Strongyloides (*stron-jil-oid'-eez*). A genus of nematode worms, one of which, *S. stercoralis*, is common in tropical countries and causes diarrhoea and intestinal ulcers.

strontium (*stron'-she-um*). *abbrev.* Sr. A metallic element. *S. 90*. A radioactive isotope used in radiotherapy in the treatment of skin and eye malignancies.

strychnine (*strik'-neen*). A highly poisonous alkaloid made from the seeds of *Strychnos nox-vomica*. At one time it was widely used in small amounts in 'tonics'.

stupor (*stu'-por*). A state of semi-unconsciousness occurring in the course of many varieties of mental illness, where the patient does not move or speak, and makes no response to stimuli.

stuporous (*stu'-por-us*). In a semi-conscious state.

Sturge–Weber syndrome (*W.A. Sturge, British physician, 1850–1919; Sir H.D. Weber, British physician, 1824–1918*). A congenital abnormality in which there is a port wine stain on the face with an angioma of the meninges on the same side. Glaucoma may ensue and there is often brain damage and mental subnormality.

stuttering (*stut'-er-ing*). *See* Stammering.

stye (*sti*). *See* Hordeolum.

stylet (*sti'-let*). A wire or rod for keeping clear the lumen of catheters, cannulae and hollow needles.

styloid (*sti'-loid*). Like a pen. *S.*

process. A long pointed spine, particularly one projecting from the temporal bone. Also processes on the ulna and radius.

styptic (*stip'-tik*). An astringent which, applied locally, arrests haemorrhage, e.g. alum and tannic acid.

subacute (*sub'-ak-ute*). Moderately acute. Applied to a disease that progresses moderately rapidly, but does not become acute.

subarachnoid (*sub-ar-ak'-noid*). Below the arachnoid. *S. space.* Between the arachnoid and pia mater of the brain and spinal cord, and containing cerebrospinal fluid.

subclavian (*sub-kla'-ve-an*). Beneath the clavicle. *S. artery*. The main vessel of supply to the neck and arms.

subclinical (*sub-klin'-ik-al*). Pertaining to an infection in which the signs and symptoms are so mild that a diagnosis is not made.

subconscious (*sub-kon'-shus*). (1) *adj.* Not conscious yet able to be recalled to consciousness. (2) *n.* In psychoanalysis, the part of the mind which retains memories which cannot without much effort be recalled to mind.

subcutaneous (*sub-ku-ta'-ne-us*). Beneath the skin. *S. injection.* One given hypodermically.

subdural (*sub-du'-ral*). Below the dura mater. *S. haematoma.* A blood clot between the arachnoid and dura mater. It may be acute or arise slowly from a minor injury, particularly in elderly people.

subinvolution (*sub-in-vo-lu'-shun*). Incomplete contraction of the uterus after labour.

subjective (*sub-jek'-tiv*). Related to the individual. *S. symptoms.* Those of which the patient is aware by sensory stimulation, but which cannot easily be seen by others. *Cf.* Objective.

sublimate (*sub'-lim-ate*). A substance obtained by sublimation.

sublimation (*sub-lim-a'-shun*). (1) The vaporization of a solid and its condensation into a solid deposit. (2) In psychoanalysis, a redirecting of energy at an unconscious level. The transference into socially acceptable channels of tendencies that cannot be expressed. An important aspect of maturity.

subliminal (*sub-lim'-in-al*). Below the threshold of perception.

sublingual (*sub-ling'-gwal*). Beneath the tongue. *S. glands.* Two small salivary glands in the floor of the mouth.

subluxation (*sub-luks-a'-shun*). Partial dislocation of a joint.

submaxillary (*sub-maks-il'-ar-e*). Beneath the lower jaw. *S. glands.* Two salivary glands situated under the lower jaw.

submucous (*sub-mu'-kus*). Beneath mucous membrane. *S. resection.* An operation to correct a deflected nasal septum.

subnormality (*sub-nor-mal'-it-e*). A term used in the Mental Health Act 1959, but which has been superseded by mental handicap and mental impairment. *See* Mental.

subphrenic (*sub-fren'-ik*). Beneath the diaphragm. *S. abscess.* One which develops below the diaphragm, usually after peritonitis or from postoperative infection.

substitution (*sub-stit-u'-shun*).

The act of putting one thing in place of another. In psychology, this may be the nurse or foster mother in the place of the child's own mother. In psychotherapy, the nurse or therapist may be substituted for someone in the patient's background.

substrate (*sub'-strate*). A substance on which an enzyme acts.

subtertian (*sub-ter'-shan*). Pertaining to a form of malaria in which there is continuous fever, caused by infection by *Plasmodium falciparum.*

subtotal (*sub-to'-tal*). Incomplete.

succinylsulphathiazole (*suk-sin-il-sul-fah-thi'-az-ole*). A sulphonamide preparation used for intestinal infections. It is not absorbed from the alimentary tract.

succus (*suk'-us*). A juice. *S. entericus.* A digestive fluid secreted by intestinal glands. *S. gastricus.* Gastric juice.

succussion (*suk-ush'-un*). A method of determining when free fluid is present in a cavity in the body. A sound of splashing is heard when the patient moves or is deliberately moved.

sucrose (*su'-krose*). A disaccharide obtained from cane or beet sugar.

suction (*suk'-shun*). (1) The process of sucking. (2) The removal of gas or fluid from a cavity or other container by means of reduced pressure. *Post-tussive s.* A sucking noise heard in the lungs just after a cough.

sudamen (*su-da'-men*). *pl.* sudamina. A small white vesicle formed in the sweat glands after prolonged sweating and sometimes occurring in febrile conditions.

sudor (*su'-dor*). Sweat. Perspiration.

sudorific (*su-dor-if'-ik*). Diaphoretic; an agent causing sweating.

suffocation (*suf-o-ka'-shun*). Asphyxiation. A cessation of breathing caused by occlusion of the air passages, leading to unconsciousness and ultimately to death.

suffusion (*suf-u'-zhun*). A sudden flushing of the skin, as in blushing.

sugar (*shoo'-gar*). A group of sweet carbohydrates classified chemically as monosaccharides or disaccharides. The following are included: *Beet s.* Obtained from sugar beet. *Cane s.* Obtained from sugar cane. *Fructose.* Fruit sugar. *Grape s.* Dextrose. Glucose. *Milk s.* Lactose. *Muscle s.* Inositol; a sugar-like compound found in animal tissue, particularly in muscle, and also in many plant tissues.

suggestibility (*suj-es-tib-il'-it-e*). A condition in which there is an abnormal susceptibility to suggestion.

suggestion (*suj-est'-shun*). A tool of psychotherapy in which an idea is presented to a patient and accepted by him. *Post-hypnotic s.* One implanted in a patient under hypnosis, which lasts after his return to normal condition.

suicide (*su'-is-ide*). The act of killing oneself.

sulcus (*sul'-kus*). *pl.* sulci. A furrow or fissure; applied especially to those of the brain.

sulphacetamide (*sul-fah-set'-am-ide*). A soluble sulphonamide used as eye-drops to treat corneal and conjunctival infections.

sulphadiazine (*sul-fah-di'-az-een*). A slow-acting sulphonamide drug which is relatively non-toxic. Used in the treatment of meningococcal meningitis.

sulphadimidine (*sul-fah-di'-mid-een*). A sulphonamide of which a high blood level can be obtained but toxic effects are rare. Used in the treatment of urinary tract infections.

sulphaemoglobin (*sulf-he-mo-glo'-bin*). The substance produced in the blood by an excess of sulphur, which gives rise to sulphaemoglobinaemia. Sulphmethaemoglobin.

sulphaemoglobinaemia (*sulf-he-mo-glo-bin-e'-me-ah*). A condition of cyanosis that used to arise during the administration of the earlier sulphonamides. Sulphmethaemoglobinaemia.

sulphafurazole (*sul-fah-fur'-az-ole*). A soluble, rapidly excreted sulphonamide useful in treating urinary tract infections.

sulphaguanidine (*sul-fah-gwan'-id-een*). A mild sulphonamide used in the treatment of bacillary dysentery.

sulphamethizole (*sul-fah-meth'-e-zole*). A sulphonamide used in urinary infection as it is rapidly excreted in an active form.

sulphanilamide (*sul-fan-il'-am-ide*). The first of the sulphonamide drugs, less potent than many that have been later developed.

sulphasalazine (*sul-fah-sal'-az-een*). A sulphonamide used in the treatment of ulcerative colitis.

sulphate (*sul'-fate*). A salt of sulphuric acid.

sulphathiazole (*sul-fah-thi'-az-ole*). A very active but now seldom used preparation; liable to give rise to rashes and drug fever; very rapidly excreted from the body.

sulphmethaemoglobin (*sulfmet-he-mo-glo'-bin*). See Sulphaemoglobin.

sulphonamide (*sul-fon'-amide*). The generic term for all aminobenzene-sulphonamide preparations including the bactericidal sulpha drugs.

sulphone (*sul'-fone*). One of a group of drugs which with prolonged use have been successful in treating leprosy. Dapsone is the most widely used.

sulphonylurea (*sul-fon-il-u'-re-ah*). One of a group of drugs used in the treatment of diabetes mellitus.

sulphuric acid (*sul-fu'-rik as'-id*). H_2SO_4. Oil of vitriol. A heavy colourless liquid and corrosive poison, which burns any organic substance with which it comes into contact.

sulthiame (*sul-thi'-ame*). An anticonvulsant drug used in the treatment of epilepsy.

sunburn (*sun'-bern*). A dermatitis due to exposure to the sun's rays, causing burning and redness.

sunstroke (*sun'-stroke*). Overwhelming prostration caused by exposure to excessive heat from the sun. See Heat stroke.

superciliary (*su-per-sil'-e-ar-e*). Relating to the eyebrow.

supercilium (*su-per-sil'-e-um*). The eyebrow.

superego (*su-per-e'-go*). That part of the personality that is concerned with moral standards and ideals that are derived unconsciously from the parents, teachers and environment, and influence the person's whole mental make-up, acting as a control on impulses of the ego.

superfecundation (*su-per-fekun-da'-shun*). The fertilization of two or more ova, produced during the same menstrual cycle, by spermatozoa from separate coital acts.

superfetation (*su-per-fe-ta'-shun*). The fertilization of a second ovum when pregnancy has already started, producing two fetuses of different maturity.

superficial (*su-per-fish'-al*). On or near the surface. Often applied to those blood vessels near the skin.

superior (*su-pe'-re-or*). Above; the upper of two parts.

supination (*su-pi-na'-shun*). (1) The act of lying on one's back. (2) The turning of the palm of the hand upwards. (See Pronation.)

supine (*su'-pine*). Lying on the back, with the face upward.

suppository (*sup-oz'-it-or-e*). A medicated solid substance, prepared for insertion into the rectum or vagina, which will dissolve at body temperature.

suppression (*sup-resh'-un*). (1) Complete cessation of a secretion. *S. of urine.* No secretion of urine by the kidneys. (2) In psychology, *conscious* inhibition as distinct from *repression*, which is *unconscious.*

suppuration (*sup-u-ra'-shun*). The formation of pus.

supracondylar (*su-prah-kondi'-lar*). Above the condyles. *S. fracture.* One above the lower end of the humerus or femur.

supra-orbital (*su-prah-or'-bital*). Above the orbit of the eye.

suprapubic (*su-prah-pu'-bik*). Above the pubic bones. *S.*

cystotomy. Surgical incision of the urinary bladder just above the pubic bones.

suprarenal (*su-prah-re'-nal*). Above the kidney. *S. gland.* Adrenal gland. One of a pair of triangular endocrine glands situated on the upper surface of the kidneys. *See* Adrenal.

surgeon (*ser'-jun*). A medical practitioner who specializes in surgery.

surgery (*ser'-jer-e*). The branch of medicine that treats disease by operative measures.

surgical (*ser'-jik-al*). Pertaining to surgery. *S. neck.* The narrower part of the humerus, just below the tuberosities.

surrogate (*sur'-o-gate*). A real or imaginary substitute for a person or object in someone's life.

susceptibility (*sus-ep-tib-il'-it-e*). Lack of resistance to infection. The opposite to immunity.

suspensory (*sus-pen'-sor-e*). Supporting a part. *S. bandage.* One applied to support a part of the body, particularly the scrotum or the lower jaw. *S. ligament.* A ligament that supports or suspends an organ, e.g. that of the lens of the eye.

suture (*su'-chur*). (1) A stitch or series of stitches used to close a wound. *Atraumatic s.* A suture fused to the needle, to obtain a single thickness through each puncture of the needle. *Continuous s.* A form of oversewing with one length of suture. *Everting s.* A type of mattress stitch that turns the edges outwards to give a closer approximation. *Fascial s.* A strip of fascia taken from the patient and used to form a suture. *Interrupted s.* A series of separate

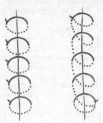

interrupted   continuous

mattress

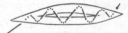

subcuticular

SUTURES

sutures. *Mattress s.* One in which each suture is taken twice through the wound, giving a loop one side and a knot the other. *Purse-string s.* A circular continuous suture round a small wound or appendix stump. *Subcuticular s.* A continuous suture placed just below the skin. *Tension s.* or *relaxation s.* One taking a large bite and relieving the tension on the true stitch line. (2) The jagged line of junction of the bones of the cranium. *Coronal s.* The junction between the frontal and parietal bones. *Lambdoidal s.* The junction between the parietal and occipital bones. *Sagittal s.* The junction between the two occipital bones.

suxamethonium (*suks-ah-meth-o'-ne-um*). A short-acting muscle-relaxant drug that may be used to get good muscle relaxation during surgery performed under general anaesthesia and during electroconvulsive therapy.

swab (*swob*). (1) A small piece of wool or gauze. (2) In pathology, a dressed stick used in taking bacteriological specimens.

swallowing (*swol'-o-ing*). The act of deglutition, in which food is passed from the mouth to the oesophagus.

sweat (*swet*). Perspiration. A clear watery fluid secreted by the sweat-glands. *S.-glands.* Coiled tubular glands situated in the dermis with long ducts to the skin surface.

sweetbread (*sweet'-bred*). The pancreas or thymus of a food animal.

sycosis (*si-ko'-sis*). A bacterial inflammation of the hair follicles, especially those of the beard and moustache. It is characterized by pustules which form into scabs. *S. barbae.* That affecting the beard. Barber's itch.

Sydenham's chorea (*T. Sydenham, British physician, 1624–1689*). A disease, chiefly affecting children, in which there is inability to control movement. It is often associated with rheumatic fever.

symbiosis (*sim-bi-o'-sis*). In parasitology, an intimate association between two different organisms for the mutual benefit of both.

symblepharon (*sim-blef'-ar-on*). Adhesion of an eyelid to the eyeball. This occurs as a result of acid burns, injury or ulceration, or following pemphigus or trachoma.

symbol (*sim'-bol*). (1) A letter or mark used by convention to denote a substance or process. (2) An object or activity representing and substituting for something else.

symbolism (*sim'-bol-izm*). In psychology, an abnormal mental condition in which events or objects are interpreted as symbols of the patient's own thoughts. In psychiatry, the re-entry into consciousness of repressed material in an acceptable form. A child's play may be symbolic, as may a painting by an emotionally disturbed patient.

Syme's amputation (*J. Syme, British surgeon, 1799–1870*). Amputation of the foot at the ankle-joint.

sympathectomy (*sim-path-ek'-tom-e*). Division of autonomic nerve fibres which control specific involuntary muscles. An operation performed for many conditions, among them Raynaud's disease.

sympathetic (*sim-path-et'-ik*). (1) Exhibiting sympathy. *S. ophthalmia.* Inflammation leading to loss of sight in the opposite eye following a perforating injury in the ciliary region. (2) Relating to the autonomic nervous system. *S. nervous system.* One of the two divisions of the autonomic nervous system. It supplies involuntary muscle and glands; it stimulates the ductless glands and the circulatory and respiratory systems, but inhibits the digestive system.

sympatholytic (*sim-path-o-lit'-ik*). Pertaining to drugs which oppose the action of the sympathetic nervous system.

sympathomimetic (*sim-path-o-mim-et'-ik*). Pertaining to drugs which produce effects similar to those caused by a stimulation of the sympathetic nervous system.

symphysiectomy (*sim-fiz-e-ek'-tom-e*). Surgical removal of a part of the symphysis pubis to facilitate a subsequent delivery.

symphysiotomy (*sim-fiz-e-ot'-om-e*). Surgical division of the symphysis pubis to enlarge the pelvic diameter and aid delivery.

symphysis (*sim'-fis-is*). A cartilaginous joint along the line of union of two bones. *S. pubis.* The cartilaginous junction of the two pubic bones.

symptom (*simp'-tum*). Any evidence as to the nature and location of a disease. It is *subjective*, i.e. noted by the patient; *signs* are noted by the observer and are therefore *objective*. Thus the phrase 'signs and symptoms'. *Withdrawal s.* That arising when a drug or alcohol is withheld from an individual who is addicted.

symptomatology (*simp-to-mat-ol'-o-je*). (1) The study of the symptoms of disease. (2) The symptoms of a particular disease, taken together.

synalgia (*sin-al'-je-ah*). Pain felt in one part of the body but caused by inflammation of or injury to another part. Referred pain.

synapse (*sin'-aps*). The termination of an axon with the dendrites of another nerve cell. Chemical transmitters pass the impulse across the space.

synarthrosis (*sin-ar-thro'-sis*). A fibrous joint, in which the bones are fixed immovably together with no intervening synovial membrane, e.g. cranial sutures.

synchrondrosis (*sin-kon-dro'-sis*). A cartilaginous joint between two bones.

synchysis (*sin'-kis-is*). Liquefaction of the vitreous humour of the eye.

syncope (*sin'-ko-pe*). A simple faint or temporary loss of consciousness due to cerebral ischaemia, often caused by dilatation of the peripheral blood vessels and a sudden fall in blood pressure.

syncytium (*sin-sit'-e-um*). A mass of protoplasm containing a number of nuclei.

syndactylism (*sin-dak'-til-izm*). Possessing webbed fingers or toes. A condition in which two or more fingers or toes are joined together.

syndrome (*sin'-drome*). A group of signs or symptoms typical of a distinctive disease, which frequently occur together and form a distinctive clinical picture.

synechia (*sin-e'-ke-ah*). Adhesion of the iris to the cornea in front (*anterior s.*) or the capsule of the lens behind (*posterior s.*).

synergist (*sin'-er-jist*). (1) A muscle which works in conjunction with another muscle. (2) A drug which works in combination with another drug, the two drugs having a greater effect when taken together than when taken separately.

synergy (*sin'-er-je*). The harmonious action of two agents or muscles working together.

synovectomy (*si-no-vek'-tom-e*). Excision of a diseased synovial membrane to restore joint movement.

synovia (*si-no'-ve-ah*). The fluid which surrounds a joint and is secreted by the synovial membrane. It is a thick, colourless, lubricating substance.

synovial membrane (*si-no'-ve-al mem'-brane*). A serous membrane lining the articular capsule of a movable joint, and terminating at the edge of the articular cartilage.

synovitis (*si-no-vi'-tis*). Inflammation of a synovial membrane, usually with an effusion of fluid within the joint. Arthritis occurs and ankylosis may follow prolonged inflammation.

synthesis (*sin'-thes-is*). The building up of a more complex structure from simple components. This may apply to drugs or to plant or animal tissues.

synthetic (*sin-thet'-ik*). Artificial; made by synthesis.

syphilid (*sif'-il-id*). A skin rash occurring during the secondary stage of syphilis. It is highly contagious and may be erythematous, vesicular or pustular.

syphilis (*sif'-il-is*). A contagious venereal disease caused by *Treponema pallidum*. *Acquired s.* That commonly transmitted by sexual intercourse; there is an early infectious stage, followed by a latent period of many years before the non-infectious late stage when serious disorders of the nervous and vascular systems arise. *Congenital s.* That transmitted by the mother to the fetus; it is preventable if the mother receives a full course of penicillin during her pregnancy.

syringe (*sir-inj'*). An instrument for injecting fluids or for aspirating or irrigating body cavities. It consists of a hollow tube with a tight-fitting piston. A hollow needle or a thin tube can be fitted to the end.

syringobulbia (*sir-ing-go-bul'-be-ah*). The formation of cavities in the medulla oblongata.

syringomyelia (*sir-ing-go-mi-e'-le-ah*). The formation of cavities filled with fluid inside the spinal cord. Impairment of muscle function and sensation result at the level of and below the lesion. Painless injury may be the first symptom. It is a progressive disease.

syringomyelitis (*sir-ing-go-mi-el-i'-tis*). Inflammation of the spinal cord, as the result of which cavities are formed in it.

syringomyelocele (*sir-ing-go-mi'-el-o-seel*). A type of spina bifida in which the protruded sac of fluid communicates with the central canal of the spinal cord.

syrup (*sir'-up*). An aqueous solution of refined sugar to which drugs may be added.

system (*sis'-tem*). In anatomy, a combination of organs in the performance of a common function, e.g. the organs of digestion = the digestive system.

systemic (*sis-tem'-ik*). Pertaining to or affecting the body as a whole. *S. circulation.* Circulation of the blood throughout the whole body, other than the pulmonary circulation. *See* sclerosis.

systole (*sis'-to-le*). The period of contraction of the heart. (*See* Diastole.) *Atrial s.* The contraction of the heart by which the blood is pumped from the atria into the ventricles. *Extra-s.* A premature contraction of the atrium or ventricle, without alteration of the fundamental rhythm of the pace-maker. *Ventricular s.* The contraction of the heart by which the blood is pumped into the aorta and pulmonary artery.

systolic (*sis-tol'-ik*). Relating to a systole. *S. murmur.* An abnormal sound produced during systole, in heart affections. *S. pressure.* The highest pressure of the blood reached during systole.

T

T cell (*te sel*). A lymphocyte which is derived from the thymus and is responsible for cell-mediated immunity.

TAB. Typhoid-paratyphoid A and B vaccine. A sterile suspension of the salmonellae causing these diseases. Used as a preventive it provides an active immunity.

tabes (*ta'-beez*). A wasting away. *T. dorsalis.* Locomotor ataxia. A slowly progressive disease of the nervous system affecting the posterior nerve roots and spinal cord. It is a late manifestation of syphilis.

tablet (*tab'-let*). A solid dosage form consisting of compressed powder.

taboparesis (*ta-bo-par-e'-sis*). The presence of the symptoms of both tabes dorsalis and general paralysis of the insane in a patient suffering from late syphilis.

tachycardia (*tak-e-kar'-de-ah*). Abnormally rapid action of the heart and consequent increase in pulse rate. (*See* Bradycardia.) *Paroxysmal t.*

Spasmodic increase in cardiac contractions of sudden onset lasting a variable time from a few seconds to hours. Sometimes a sign of ailing heart muscle, but in young people especially it may be of nervous origin.

tachylalia (*tak-e-la'-le-ah*). Extreme rapidity of speech.

tachyphrasia (*tak-e-fra'-ze-ah*). Extreme volubility of speech. It may be a sign of mental disorder.

tachyphrenia (*tak-e-fre'-ne-ah*). Hyperactivity of the mental processes.

tachypnoea (*tak-e-pne'-ah*). Rapid, shallow respirations; a reflex response to stimulation of the vagus nerve endings in the pulmonary vessels.

tactile (*tak'-tile*). Relating to the sense of touch.

Taenia (*te'-ne-ah*). A genus of tapeworms. *T. saginata.* The beef tapeworm. The commonest type of tapeworm found in the human intestine. *T. solium.* The pork tapeworm. Can also be parasitic in man, causing cysticercosis. *See* Tapeworm.

taeniafuge (*te'-ne-ah-fuje*). A drug which expels tapeworms.

taeniasis (*te-ni'-as-is*). An infestation with tapeworms.

TAF. Toxoid-antitoxin floccules. A vaccine used for diphtheria immunization. *See* Toxoid.

talc, talcum (*talk, tal'-kum*). French chalk. A preparation of magnesium silicate, used as a dusting powder.

talipes (*tal'-ip-eez*). Club-foot. A deformity caused by a congenital or acquired contraction of the muscles or tendons of the foot. *T. calcaneous.* The heel alone touches the

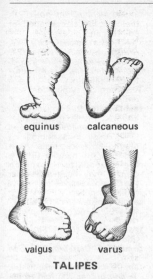

equinus | calcaneous

valgus | varus

TALIPES

ground on standing. *T. equinus.* The toes touch the ground but not the heel. *T. valgus.* The inner edge of the foot only is in contact with the ground. *T. varus.* The person walks on the outer edge of the foot.

talus (*ta'-lus*). The astragalus or ankle-bone.

tampon (*tam'-pon*). A plug of absorbent material inserted in the vagina, the nose or other orifice to restrain haemorrhage or absorb secretion.

tamponade (*tam'-pon-ade*). The surgical use of tampons. *Cardiac t.* Impairment of heart action by haemorrhage or effusion into the pericardium; may be due to a stab wound or follow surgery.

tannin (*tan'-in*). Tannic acid. A yellowish powder prepared from vegetable substances, e.g. from tea. A powerful astringent and haemostatic, which on contact with any mucous membrane causes contraction and diminishes secretions.

tantalum (*tan'-tal-um*). *abbrev. Ta.* Metallic element used for prostheses and wire sutures.

tantrum (*tan'-trum*). An outburst of ill temper. *Temper t.* A behaviour disorder of childhood. A display of bad temper in which the child performs uncontrolled actions in a state of emotional stress.

tapeworm (*tape'-werm*). Any of a group of cestode flatworms, including the *Taenia* genus, which are parasitic in the intestines of man and many animals. The adult consists of a round head with suckers or hooklets for attachment (scolex). From this numerous segments (proglottides) arise, each of which produces ova capable of independent existence for a considerable length of time. Treatment is by drugs to expel the parasite, and cure is not complete until the head is discharged or destroyed.

tapotement (*tap-ote-mon'*). A tapping movement used in massage.

tapping (*tap'-ing*). *See* Paracentesis.

tar (*tar*). A dark brown or black viscid fluid, derived from the bark of various species of pine. Used externally in certain skin diseases. *Coal-t.* That obtained from coal or petroleum. The source of phenol, cresol, xylene, benzene, etc.

tarsal (*tar'-sal*). Relating to a tarsus. *T. bones.* The seven small bones of the ankle and instep. *T. cyst.* Meibomian cyst. Chalazion. *T. glands.* Meibomian glands of the eyelids. *T. plates.* Small cartilages in the upper and lower eyelids.

tarsalgia (*tar-sal'-je-ah*). Pain in the foot, usually associated with flattening of the arch.

tarsoplasty (*tar'-so-plas-te*). Plastic surgery of the eyelid.

tarsorrhaphy (*tar-sor'-af-e*). Stitching of the eyelids together to protect the cornea or to allow healing of an abrasion.

tarsus (*tar'-sus*). (1) The seven small bones of the ankle and instep. (2) The firm fibrous tissue which forms the framework of the eyelids.

tartar (*tar'-tar*). (1) Potassium bitartrate (*cream of t.*). (2) A hard incrustation deposited on the teeth and on dentures. *T. emetic.* Antimony potassium tartrate. A salt used in the treatment of schistosomiasis and leishmaniasis.

taste (*ta'-st*). The sense by which it is possible to identify what is eaten and drunk. Taste receptors (buds) lie on the tongue and give the sensations of sweet, sour, salt and bitter.

Taussig's operation (*Helen B. Taussig, American paediatrician, b. 1898*). Block dissection of the pelvic lymphatic glands to prevent spread of carcinoma of the uterus.

Tawara's node (*S. Tawara, Japanese pathologist, b. 1873*). The atrioventricular node. *See* Node.

taxis (*taks'-is*). Manipulation by hand to restore any part to its normal position. It can be used to reduce a hernia or a dislocation.

taxonomy (*taks-on'-om-e*). In biology, the classification of animals and plants.

Tay–Sachs disease (*W. Tay, British physician, 1843–1927; B. Sachs, American neurologist, 1858–1944*). *See* Amaurotic familial idiocy.

Tc. Chemical symbol for *technetium.*

technetium (*tek-ne'-she-um*). *abbrev.* Tc. A metallic element. *Radioactive t.* Isotope (^{99}Tc) used in a number of diagnostic tracer tests. As it has a short half-life (6 h), a high dose for scanning organs may be given whilst the patient receives only a low radiation dose.

technique (*tek-neek'*). The details of a method or procedure.

teething (*tee'-thing*). *See* Dentition.

tegument (*teg'-u-ment*). The skin.

tela (*te'-lah*). A web-like tissue. *T. choroidea.* The fold of pia mater containing a network of blood vessels found in the ventricles of the brain from which the cerebrospinal fluid originates.

telangiectasis (*tel-an-je-ek'-tas-is*). A group of dilated capillary blood vessels, web-like or radiating in form.

telangioma (*tel-an-je-o'-mah*). A tumour of the blood capillaries.

teleceptor (*tel-e-sep'-tor*). A telereceptor.

telepathy (*tel-ep'-ath-e*). The transmission of thought without any normal means of communication between two persons.

telereceptor (*tel-e-re-sep'-tor*). A sensory nerve ending which can respond to distant stimuli. Those of the eyes, ears and nose are examples. Teleceptor.

teletherapy (tel-e-ther'-ap-e). Treatment of malignant disease by radiation where the source is at a distance from the tumour. *External beam therapy. See* Brachytherapy.

telophase (tel'-o-faze). The last stage in the division of cells when the chromosomes have been reconstituted in the nuclei at either end of the cell and the cell cytoplasm divides to form two new cells.

temperature (tem'-per-at-cher). The degree of heat of a substance or body as measured by a thermometer. *Normal t.* of the human body is 37°C (98.6°F) with a slight decrease in the early morning, and a slight increase at night. It indicates the balance between heat production and heat loss. A thermometer inserted under the tongue or into the rectum will register slightly higher than one placed in the axilla or groin. *Subnormal t.* is below the normal. A sign of shock. *See* Pyrexis *and* Fever.

template (tem'-plate). A mould or pattern. In radiotherapy, a map of the area of the patient requiring treatment and of those areas to be protected from radiation.

temple (tem'-pl). The region on either side of the head above the zygomatic arch.

temporal (tem'-por-al). Pertaining to the side of the head. *T. bone.* One of a pair of bones on either side of the skull and containing the organ of hearing. *T. arteritis.* Giant cell arteritis. A chronic inflammatory condition of the carotid arterial system, occurring usually in elderly people.

There is persistent headache and partial or total blindness may result. *T. lobe.* The part of the cerebrum below the lateral sulcus.

temporomandibular (tem-por-o-man-dib'u-lar). Relating to the temporal bone and the mandible. *T. joint.* The hinge of the lower jaw.

tenacious (ten-a'-shus). Thick and viscid, as applied to sputum or other body fluids.

tenaculum (ten-ak'-u-lum). A hook-shaped surgical instrument used to pick up and hold pieces of tissue.

tendinitis (ten-din-i'-tis). Inflammation of a tendon and its attachments.

tendinous (ten'-din-us). Having the nature of a tendon.

tendon (ten'-don). A band of fibrous tissue, forming the termination of a muscle and attaching it to a bone. *Achilles t.* That inserted into the calcaneum. *T. grafting.* An operation which repairs a defect in one tendon by a graft from another. *T. insertion.* The point of attachment of a muscle to a bone which it moves. *T. reflex.* The muscular contraction produced on percussing a tendon.

tenesmus (ten-ez'-mus). A painful ineffectual straining to empty the bowel or bladder.

tennis elbow (ten'-is el'-bo). A painful disorder which affects the extensor muscles of the forearm at their attachment to the external epicondyle.

tenonitis (ten-on-i'-tis). Inflammation of Tenon's capsule. Proptosis of the eyeball occurs, often accompanied by pain and pyrexia.

Tenon's capsule (J.R. Tenon, French surgeon, 1724–1816). The fibrous tissue in which the eyeball is situated.

tenoplasty (*ten'-o-plas-te*). Plastic surgery on a tendon.

tenorrhaphy (*ten-or'-af-e*). The suturing together of the ends of a divided tendon.

tenosynovitis (*ten-o-si-no-vi'-tis*). Inflammation of a tendon sheath.

tenotomy (*ten-ot'-om-e*). The surgical division of a tendon, to correct a deformity caused by its shortening. In ophthalmology, performed to correct a squint.

tension (*ten'-shun*). The act of stretching or the state of being stretched. *Arterial t.* The pressure of blood on the vessel wall during cardiac contraction. *Intra-ocular t.* The pressure of the contents of the eye on its walls, measured by a tonometer. *Intravenous t.* The pressure of blood within the veins. *Premenstrual t.* Symptoms of abdominal distension, headache, emotional lability and depression occurring a few days before the onset of menstruation. *See* Cyclical syndrome. *Surface t.* Tension or resistance which acts to preserve the integrity of a surface, particularly the surface of a liquid.

tensor (*ten'-sor*). A muscle which stretches a part.

tent (*tent*). (1) A small cone-shaped plug, often of compressed seaweed, which swells considerably on the absorption of moisture. It may be used to dilate the cervix. *See* Laminaria. (2) A cover, usually of canvas or plastic, placed over a bed into which a gas or vapour can be infiltrated.

tentorium (*ten-tor'-e-um*). The dividing wall of dura mater between the cerebrum and the cerebellum.

teratogenesis (*ter-at-o-jen'-es-is*). The process leading to the development of a monster or a child with gross congenital abnormalities.

teratoma (*ter-at-o'-mah*). A solid tumour containing tissues similar to those of a dermoid cyst. Found most often in the ovaries and testes, many of these tumours are malignant.

teres (*teer'-eez*). Long and round (*Latin*). Applied to such muscles, particularly those of the shoulder, running from the scapula to the humerus.

terminal (*ter'-min-al*). Placed at or forming the extremity. *T-infection.* An infection occurring shortly before or hastening death.

terminology (*ter-min-ol'-o-je*). The vocabulary of scientific and technical subjects.

tertian (*ter'-shan*). Recurring every 48 hours. *See* Malaria.

tertiary (*ter'-she-ar-e*). Third. *T. syphilis.* The non-infectious stage of neurosyphilis.

test (*test*). (1) A trial. *T. meal.* A procedure used to test the digestive powers of the gastric juice. *Fractional t. meal.* One designed to estimate the activity of the gastric glands in producing hydrochloric acid. Alcohol, histamine or pentagastrin may be used and successive specimens taken to estimate the acid content. *T. type.* A card of letters of varying size for testing the acuity of sight. (2) Analysis of the composition of a substance by the use of chemical reagents.

testicle (*tes'-tikl*). A testis. One of the two glands in the scrotum which produce spermatozoa. *Undescended t.* Condition in which the organ remains in the pelvis or inguinal canal.

testis (*tes'-tis*). *pl.* Testes. A testicle.

testosterone (*tes-tos'-ter-one*). The hormone produced by the testes which stimulates the development of sex characteristics. Now made synthetically. It is used medicinally in cases of failure of sex function and as a palliative treatment in some cases of advanced metastatic breast cancer in females.

tetanus (*tet'-an-us*). An acute disease of the nervous system caused by the contamination of wounds by the spores of a soil bacterium, *Clostridium tetani*. Muscle stiffness around the site of the wound occurs followed by rigidity of face and neck muscles; hence *'lockjaw'*. All muscles are then affected and opisthotonos may occur. *T. vaccine* or *toxoid* will give an active immunity. *T. antitoxin*. A serum that gives a short-term passive immunity and may be used with penicillin for immediate treatment of a case of tetanus.

tetany (*tet'-an-e*). An increased excitability of the nerves due to a lack of available calcium, accompanied by painful muscle spasm of the hands and feet (*carpopedal spasm*). The cause may be hypoparathyroidism or alkalosis owing to excessive vomiting or hyperventilation.

tetrachloroethylene (*tet-rah-klor-o-eth'-il-een*). An anthelmintic drug widely used to treat hookworm disease.

tetracycline (*tet-rah-si'-kleen*). An antibiotic drug belonging to the group known as the **tetracyclines** which are used

to treat infections caused by brucella, chlamydia, mycoplasma and rickettsia.

tetradactylous (*tet-rah-dak'-til-us*). Having four digits on each hand or foot.

tetralogy (*tet-ral'-o-je*). A series of four. *T. of Fallot. See* Fallot's tetralogy.

tetraplegia (*tet-rah-ple'-je-ah*). Quadriplegia. Paralysis of all four limbs.

thalamotomy (*thal-am-ot'-om-e*). Surgical destruction of the nucleus in the thalamus to relieve symptoms of severe anxiety. The area needs to be carefully localized first.

thalamus (*thal'-am-us*). A mass of nerve cells at the base of the cerebrum. Most sensory impulses from the body pass to this area and are transmitted to the cortex.

thalassaemia (*thal-as-e'-me-ah*). A group of disorders mostly found in the Mediterranean region and the Far East, caused by the inheritance of abnormal haemoglobin. *T. major.* Cooley's anaemia, the severest form of thalassaemia with death usually occurring before adolescence. *T. minor.* A mild form of the disease with few symptoms. Those suffering from it can pass the disease on to their children.

thalassotherapy (*thal-as-o-ther'-ap-e*). Treatment involving sea bathing or a sea voyage.

Thalidomide (*thal-id'-o-mide*). A proprietary drug formerly used as a sedative but now withdrawn because many pregnant women took it during the first trimester of pregnancy and gave birth to children with abnormalities of the limbs.

theca (*the'-kah*). A sheath, such as the covering of a tendon. *T. folliculi.* The covering of a graafian follicle. *T. vertebralis.* The membranes enclosing the spinal cord. The dura mater.

theine (*the'-een*). The alkaloid found in tea. A form of caffeine.

theism (*the'-izm*). Chronic poisoning resulting from excessive tea drinking. Theinism.

thenar (*the'-nar*). (1) The palm of the hand. (2) The fleshy part at the base of the thumb.

theobromine (*the-o-bro'-meen*). An alkaloid derived from the cocoa bean. Used as a heart stimulant and as a mild diuretic.

theophylline (*the-off-il'-een*). An alkaloid derived from tea-leaves, and with action similar to that of theobromine. Used mainly in the treatment of bronchospasm.

therapeutics (*ther-ap-u'-tiks*). The science and art of healing and the treatment of disease.

therapy (*ther'-ap-e*). The treatment of disease. *Group t.* A form of psychotherapy. *See* Group. *Occupational t.* Treatment by providing interesting and congenial work within the limitations of the patient in mental diseases and in order to re-educate and coordinate muscles in physical defect. *See* Rehabilitation. *Role t.* A method of psychiatric treatment in which the patient casts the nurse or psychotherapist into the role of someone who has had a great influence on his past. The nurse, under guidance of the psychiatrist, assists by behaving in the manner of the object of the patient's emotion.

therm (*therm*). A unit of heat equal to 100,000 British Thermal Units. *See* Unit.

thermal (*ther'-mal*). Relating to heat.

thermocautery (*ther-mo-kaw'-ter-e*). The deliberate destruction of tissue by means of heat. *See* Cautery.

thermogenesis (*ther-mo-jen'-es-is*). The production of heat.

thermography (*ther-mog'-raf-e*). A method of measuring the amount of heat produced by different areas of the body, using infra-red photography. Employed in early detection of breast cancer, it depends on the greater blood supply of a cancerous growth compared to that of the surrounding tissue.

thermolysis (*ther-mol'-is-is*). The loss of body heat by radiation, by excretion and by the evaporation of sweat.

thermometer (*ther-mom'-e-ter*). An instrument for measuring temperature. *Clinical t.* One used to measure the body temperature. *Electronic t.* A clinical thermometer which works electrically. It contains electronic devices whose characteristics change with temperature. The reading is recorded within seconds and displayed visually. Usually an audible tone tells the user when the temperature has reached its maximum reading.

thermoreceptor (*ther-mo-re-sep'-tor*). A nerve ending that responds to heat and cold.

thermostat (*ther'-mo-stat*). An apparatus which automatically regulates the temperature and maintains it at a specified level.

thermotaxis (*ther-mo-taks'-is*). The normal regulation of body temperature by maintaining the balance between heat production and heat loss.

thermotherapy (*ther-mo-ther'-ap-e*). The treatment of disease by application of heat.

thiamine (*thi'-am-een*). Vitamin B₁, or aneurine. An essential vitamin involved in carbohydrate metabolism. A deficiency causes beri beri. The source is liver and unrefined cereals.

Thiersch's skin graft (*l. Thiersch, German surgeon, 1822–1895*). The transplantation of areas of partial thickness skin. A pinch graft. *See* Graft.

thigh (*thi*). The part of the leg between the pelvis and the knee.

thioguanine (*thi-o-gwan'-een*). An antimetabolite used in the treatment of acute leukaemia.

thiopentone (*thi-o-pen'-tone*). A basal narcotic of the barbiturate group given intravenously as a short-acting anaesthetic and in preoperative preparation.

thiopropazate (*thi-o-pro'-pazate*), A tranquillizer used in the treatment of schizophrenia and psychoneuroses.

thiotepa (*thi-o-te'-pah*). An intravenous cytotoxic drug used in the treatment of cancer, particularly of the bladder or ovary.

thiouracil (*thi-o-u'-ras-il*). A drug used in the treatment of thyrotoxicosis. A derivative, propylthiouracil, which is more active and less toxic, is now more often used.

thirst (*therst*). An uncomfortable sensation of dryness of the mouth and throat with a desire for oral fluids. *Abnormal t.* Polydipsia.

Thomas's splint (*H.O. Thomas, British orthopaedic surgeon, 1834–1891*). A splint consist-

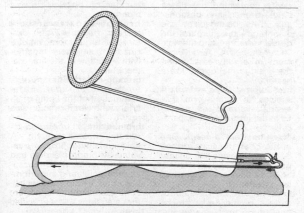

THOMAS'S SPLINT

ing of an oval iron ring which fits over the lower limb. Attached to the ring are two round iron rods which are bent into a W-shape at the lower end. It is used to support the limb and move the weight from the knee-joint to the pelvis.

thoracic (thor-as'-ik). Relating to the thorax. *T. duct.* The large lymphatic vessel situated in the thorax along the spine. It opens into the left subclavian vein.

thoracocentesis (thor-ak-o-sen-te'-sis). Puncture of the wall of the thorax to allow aspiration of the pleural fluid.

thoracoscopy (thor-ak-os'-kop-e). Examination of the pleural cavity by means of an endoscopic instrument.

thoracotomy (thor-ak-ot'-ome). A surgical incision into the thorax.

thorax (thor'-aks). The chest; a cavity containing the heart, lungs, bronchi and oesophagus. It is bounded by the diaphragm, the sternum, the dorsal vertebrae, and the ribs. *Barrel-shaped t.* A development in emphysema, when the chest is malformed like a barrel.

threadworm (thred'-werm). A species of roundworm, *Enterobius vermicularis*, parasitic in the large intestine, particularly of children.

threonine (thre'-o-neen). One of the 22 amino acids formed by the digestion of dietary protein.

thrill (thril). A tremor discerned by palpation.

throat (throte). (1) The anterior surface of the neck. (2) The pharynx. *Sore t.* Pharyngitis. *Clergyman's sore t.* Laryngitis.

thrombectomy (throm-bek'-tom-e). Surgical excision of a clot from a vein or an artery.

thrombin (throm'-bin). An enzyme which converts fibrinogen to fibrin during the later stages of blood clotting.

thrombo-angeitis (throm-bo-an-je-i'-tis). Inflammation of blood vessels with clot formation. *T. obliterans.* Inflammation of the arteries, usually of the legs of young males, causing intermittent claudication and gangrene. Buerger's disease.

thrombocyte (throm'-bo-site). A blood platelet. Disc-shaped, essential for the clotting of shed blood.

thrombocytopenia (throm-bo-si-to-pe'-ne-ah). A reduction in the number of platelets in the blood. Spontaneous bleeding may occur.

thrombocytosis (throm-bo-si-to'-sis). An increase in the number of platelets in the blood.

thrombo-endarterectomy (throm'-bo-end-art-er-ek'-tom-e). Surgical removal of a clot from an artery together with a portion of the lining of the artery.

thrombo-endarteritis (throm'-bo-end-art-er-i'-tis). Inflammation of the lining of an artery with clot formation as a result.

thrombokinase (throm-bo-ki'-naze). Thromboplastin. A lipid-containing protein activated by blood platelets and injured tissues, which is capable of activating prothrombin to form thrombin which, combined with fibrinogen, forms a clot.

thrombolysis (throm-bol'-is-is). The disintegration or dissolving of a clot.

thrombophlebitis (*throm-bo-fleb-i'-tis*). The formation of a clot, associated with inflammation of the lining of a vein.

thromboplastin (*throm-bo-plas'-tin*). See Thrombokinase.

thrombosis (*throm-bo'-sis*). The formation of a thrombus. *Cavernous sinus t.* Thrombosis of the cavernous sinus, usually the result of infection of the face, when the veins in the sinus are affected via ophthalmic vessels. *Cerebral t.* The occlusion of a cerebral artery—the most common cause of cerebral infarction (a 'stroke'). *Coronary t.* The occlusion of a coronary vessel, by which the heart muscle is deprived of blood, causing myocardial ischaemia, and leading often to myocardial infarction (a 'heart attack'). *Lateral sinus t.* A complication of mastoiditis when infection of the lateral sinus of the dura mater occurs and there is clot formation.

thrombus (*throm'-bus*). A stationary blood clot caused by coagulation of the blood in the heart or in an artery or a vein.

thrush (*thrush*). An infection of the mucous membrane of the mouth by a fungus, *Candida albicans*. It occurs in infants and also in older persons suffering from a debilitating disease.

thymectomy (*thi-mek'-tom-e*). Surgical removal of the thymus. A treatment for myasthenia gravis.

thymine (*thi'-meen*). One of the pyrimidine bases found in DNA.

thymokesis (*thi-mo-ke'-sis*). Persistence of the thymus gland in an adult.

thymol (*thi'-mol*). An aromatic antiseptic used in solution as a mouth wash.

thymoma (*thi-mo'-mah*). A tumour that originates in thymus tissue and is found to be present in a number of patients suffering from myasthenia gravis.

thymus (*thi'-mus*). A gland-like structure situated in the upper thorax and neck. Present in early life, it reaches its maximum size at 10 to 12 years and then slowly regresses. Its only known function is the formation of lymphocytes.

thyrocricotomy (*thi-ro-kri-kot'-om-e*). An opening made between the thyroid and cricoid cartilages.

thyroglobulin (*thi-ro-glob'-u-lin*). The protein in thyroxine, the endocrine secretion of the thyroid.

thyroglossal (*thi-ro-glos'-al*). Relating to the thyroid and the tongue. *T. cyst. See* Cyst.

thyroid (*thi'-roid*). (1) Shaped like a shield. (2) Pertaining to the thyroid gland. *T. cartilage.* The largest cartilage of the larynx. It forms the 'Adam's apple' in the front of the throat. *T. gland.* A large gland consisting of two lobes, situated in front and on either side of the trachea. It secretes the hormones thyroxine and tri-iodothyronine which are concerned in regulating the metabolic rate. *T.-stimulating hormone.* TSH. Thyrotrophin. A hormone produced by the anterior pituitary gland which controls the activity of the thyroid gland. *Intrathoracic* or *retrosternal t.* Position of the gland low in the neck and wholly or in part behind the sternum.

thyroidectomy (*thi-roid-ek'-tom-e*). Partial or complete removal of the thyroid gland.

thyroparathyroidectomy (*thi'-ro-par-ah-thi-roid-ek'-tom-e*). Surgical removal of the thyroid and parathyroid glands.

thyrotomy (*thi-rot'-om-e*). Surgical incision of the thyroid cartilage or of the gland.

thyrotoxicosis (*thi-ro-toks-ik-o'-sis*). Hyperthyroidism. The symptoms arising when there is overactivity of the thyroid gland. The metabolism is speeded up and there is enlargement of the gland and exophthalmos.

thyrotrophin (*thi-ro-trof'-in*). *See* Thyroid-stimulating hormone.

thyroxine (*thi-roks'-een*). One of the two hormones secreted by the thyroid gland. It is used in the treatment of hypothyroidism.

tibia (*tib'-e-ah*). The shin-bone. The larger of the two bones of the leg, extending from knee to ankle.

tic (*tik*). A spasmodic twitching of certain muscles, usually of the face, neck or shoulder. *T. douloureux.* Paroxysmal trigeminal neuralgia.

ticarcillin (*tik'-ar-sil-in*). A semisynthetic penicillin which is active against both gram-negative and gram-positive bacteria.

tick (*tik*). A blood-sucking parasite which may transmit the organisms of disease.

tincture (*tink'-chur*). An alcoholic solution of an animal or vegetable drug.

tinea (*tin'-e-ah*). A group of skin infections caused by a variety of fungi and named after the area of the body affected, thus: *T. barbae*—the beard; *T. capitis*—the head; *T. circinata* or *T. corporis*—the body; *T. cruris*—the groin; and *T. pedis*—the feet. *See* Ringworm.

tinnitus (*tin'-it-us*). A ringing, buzzing or roaring sound in the ears.

tintometer (*tin-tom'-e-ter*). An instrument by which changes in colour of a fluid can be measured.

tissue (*tis'-u*). A mass of cells or fibres forming one of the structures of which the body is composed. *Adipose t.* Fatty tissue. *Areolar t.* Connective tissue of bundles of white fibres, elastic fibres and connective tissue cells. *Cancellous t.* The honeycomb arrangement of bone cells beneath the compact layer, especially at the ends of long bones, and in the centre of such bones as the clavicle, sternum, ribs, cranium and vertebrae. It contains red bone marrow. *Compact t.* The close arrangement of bone cells which forms the outer layer of all bones and is especially thick in the shafts. *Connective t.* A general term for all those tissues of the body which support and connect the various organs and other structures. *Elastic t.* Connective tissue chiefly composed of yellow elastic fibres. *Fibrous t.* Connective tissue composed of bundles of white fibres. *Homologous t.* One similar in structure to another. *Parenchymatous t.* The essential functioning cells of an organ, as distinct from its supporting tissues. *T. fluid.* The extracellular fluid, formed by capillary filtration, which surrounds all body cells. *T. typing.* The matching of tissue types for the purpose of grafting tissue from one person to another.

titration (*ti-tra'-shun*). A method of estimating the weight of a solute in solution by dropping a measured amount of a reagent into a measured quantity of solution until the expected colour change or reaction occurs.

tobramycin (*to-brah-mi'-sin*). An antibiotic drug used chiefly in the treatment of *Pseudomonas* infection.

tocography (*to-kog'-raf-e*). The measurement of alterations in the intra-uterine pressure during labour.

tocopherol (*to-kof'-er-ol*). Vitamin E, present in wheat germ, green leaves and milk.

tolazamide (*tol-az'-am-ide*). An oral hypoglycaemic drug used in the treatment of diabetes mellitus.

tolazoline (*tol-az'-ol-een*). A vasodilator drug of the peripheral blood vessels, used in the treatment of peripheral vascular disease.

tolbutamide (*tol-bu'-tam-ide*). An oral drug that appears to stimulate the release of insulin from the pancreas. Used in the treatment of diabetes mellitus and of diabetes insipidus of hypothalamic or pituitary origin.

tolerance (*tol'-er-ans*). The capacity for assimilating unusually large amounts of a drug or food without apparent harmful effects.

tomography (*to-mog'-raf-e*). Body section radiography in which X-rays or ultrasound waves are used to produce an image of a layer of tissue at any depth.

tone (*tone*). (1) The normal degree of tension, e.g. in a muscle. (2) A particular quality of

sound.

tongue (*tung*). A muscular organ attached to the floor of the mouth and concerned in taste, mastication, swallowing and speech. It is covered by a mucous membrane from which project numerous papillae.

tonic (*ton'-ik*). (1) *n.* A term popularly applied to any drug supposed to brace or tone up the body or any particular part or organ. (2) *adj.* Possessing tone in a state of contraction, e.g. muscles. *T. spasm.* A prolonged contraction of one or several muscles. *See* Clonic.

tonicity (*to-nis'-it-e*). (1) The normal state of muscular tension. (2) The effective osmotic pressure of a fluid.

tonography (*to-nog'-raf-e*). The measurement made by an electric tonometer recording the intra-ocular pressure and so indirectly the drainage of aqueous humour from the eye.

tonometer (*to-nom'-e-ter*). An instrument for measuring intra-ocular pressure.

tonsil (*ton'-sil*). A mass of lymphoid tissue, particularly one of two small almond-shaped bodies, situated one on each side between the pillars of the fauces. It is covered by mucous membrane, and its surface is pitted with follicles. *Pharyngeal t.* The lymphadenoid tissue of the pharynx between the pharyngotympanic tubes. Adenoids.

tonsillectomy (*ton-sil-ek'-tom-e*). Excision of one or both tonsils.

tonsillitis (*ton-sil-i'-tis*). Inflammation of the tonsils. *Follicular t.* Inflammation affecting chiefly the follicles, and causing purulent patches on

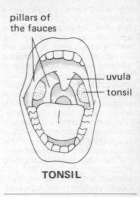

pillars of
the fauces

uvula

tonsil

TONSIL

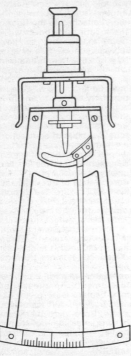

TONOMETER

the tonsils, formed by pus exuded from the follicles.

tonsillotome (*ton-sil'-o-tome*). An instrument for excising tonsils.

tonsillotomy (*ton-sil-ot'-om-e*). (1) Incision of a tonsil. (2) Excision of a part of a tonsil.

tonus (*to'-nus*). The normal state of partial contraction of the muscles.

tooth (*tooth*). *pl.* teeth. A structure in the mouth designed for the mastication of food. Each is composed of a crown, neck and root with one or more fangs. The main bulk is of dentine enclosing a central pulp; the crown is covered with a hard white substance called enamel. *See* Dentition. *Canine t.* One of the so-called 'dog-teeth'. There are four, one on each side of the upper and lower jaws. *Deciduous (milk) t.* One of the first set, later replaced by the permanent dentition. *Eye-t.* A canine tooth in the upper jaw. *Impacted t.* One which is unable to erupt owing to its position in the jaw. *Wisdom-t.* One of the last molars to appear, at either end of each jaw. It is often missing or fails to erupt.

tophus (*to'-fus*). A small, hard, chalky deposit in the skin and cartilage occurring in gout, and sometimes appearing on the auricle of the ear. It is composed of sodium biurate.

topical (*top'-ik-al*). Relating to a particular spot; local. *T. lotion.* One for local or external application.

topography (*to-pog'-raf-e*). The study of the surface of the body in relation to the underlying structures.

torpor (*tor'-por*). A sluggish condition, in which response to stimuli is absent or very slow.

torque (*tork*). A rotatory force.

torsion (*tor'-shun*). Twisting: (1) of an artery to arrest haemorrhage; (2) of the pedicle of a cyst which produces venous congestion in the cyst and consequent gangrene—a possible complication of ovarian cyst.

torso (*tor'-so*). The body, excluding the head and the limbs. The trunk.

torticollis (*tor-te-kol'-is*). Wryneck, a contraction of one or more of the cervical muscles on one side only, resulting in an abnormal position of the head. *Congenital t.* That due to injury to the sternocleidomastoid muscle at birth. It becomes a fibrous cord. *Spasmodic t.* Intermittent twisting of the neck due to spasmodic contraction of the sternomastoid muscle.

tourniquet (*toor'-ne-ka*). A constrictive band applied to a limb to arrest arterial haemorrhage. No longer used in First Aid since its use may cause permanent damage to muscles or nerve supply.

toxaemia (*toks-e'-me-ah*). Poisoning of the blood by the absorption of bacterial toxins. *T. of pregnancy.* A condition affecting pregnant women and characterized by albuminuria, hypertension and oedema, with the possibility of pre-eclampsia and eclampsia developing.

toxic (*toks'-ik*). (1) Poisonous, relating to a poison. (2) Caused by a toxin.

toxicity (*toks-is'-it-e*). The degree of virulence of a poison.

toxicology (*toks-ik-ol'-o-je*). The science dealing with poisons.

toxicosis (*toks-ik-o'-sis*). The state of poisoning by toxins.

toxin (*toks'-in*). Any poisonous compound, usually referring to that produced by bacteria.

Toxocara (*toks-o-ka'-rah*). A genus of nematode worms, parasitic in the intestines of dogs and cats, which may also infest man, especially children. The spleen, liver and lungs are most often affected, but the parasite may also infest the retina, causing inflammation and granulation.

toxocariasis (*toks-o-ka-ri'-as-is*). Infestation by *Toxocara*.

toxoid (*toks'-oid*). A toxin which has been deprived of some of its harmful properties but is still capable of producing immunity and may be used in a vaccine. *Diphtheria t.* Toxin which has been treated with formaldehyde. Used for immunization against diphtheria. *See* TAF *and* APT.

Toxoplasma (*toks-o-plaz'-mah*). A genus of protozoa which infests birds and animals and may be transmitted from them to man.

toxoplasmosis (*toks-o-plaz-mo'-sis*). A condition of enlarged glands and fever caused by a protozoon, the *Toxoplasma.* May cause hydrocephalus and other disorders, including severe retardation in infants born of infected mothers.

trabecula (*trab-ek'-u-lah*). A dividing band or septum, extending from the capsule of an organ into its interior and holding the functioning cells in position.

trabeculectomy (*trab-ek-u-lek'-tom-e*). An operation to relieve glaucoma. The conjunctiva and sclera are opened and a piece of iris, with some of the trabecular meshwork, is removed to allow drainage.

trabeculotomy (*trab-ek-u-lot'-om-e*). An operation for glaucoma. An incision is made into the trabecular network.

tracer (*tra'-ser*). A substance that can be used to gain information about metabolic processes. For example, radioactive isotopes may be used to investigate disease of the thyroid gland.

trachea (*trak-e'-ah*). The windpipe: a cartilaginous tube lined with ciliated mucous membrane, extending from the lower part of the larynx to the commencement of the bronchi.

tracheitis (*trak-e-i'-tis*). Inflammation of the trachea causing pain in the chest, with coughing.

trachelorrhaphy (*trak-el-or'-af-e*). An operation for suturing lacerations of the cervix of the uterus.

tracheobronchitis (*trak-e-o-brong-ki'-tis*). Acute infection of the trachea and bronchi due to viruses or bacteria.

tracheostomy (*trak-e-os'-tom-e*). An operation to make an opening into the trachea through the neck. *T. tubes.* Those used to maintain an airway following this operation either permanently or until the normal use of the air-

passages is regained.

tracheotomy (*trak-e-ot'-om-e*). Surgical incision of the trachea. *Inferior* or *low t.* That in which the opening is made below the thyroid isthmus. *Superior* or *high t.* That in which the opening is made above the thyroid isthmus.

trachoma (*trak-o'-mah*). A contagious conjunctivitis marked by granulations on the membrane and contractions of the lids to scar tissue formation. Blindness often ensues. The causative organism is a species of *Chlamydia* and the disease is prevalent in tropical countries.

tract (*trakt*). In anatomy, a structure along which something can pass, for instance the *alimentary t.*, the *biliary t.* and the many different tracts consisting of nerve fibres.

traction (*trak'-shun*). The act of pulling or drawing. *Hamilton−Russell t.* A form of traction of the leg in which there is an upward pull over a beam and the cord is continuous with a series of pulleys attached to the limb by skin traction horizontally. *Head t.* Traction exerted on the head in the treatment of cervical injury. *Skeletal t.* A method of keeping the fractured ends of bone in position by traction on the bone. A metal pin or wire is passed through the distal fragment or adjacent bone to overcome muscle contraction. *Skin t. See* Extension.

tragus (*tra'-gus*). *pl.* tragi. (1) The small prominence of cartilage at the external meatus of the ear. (2) One of the hairs at the external auditory meatus.

trait (*trate*). An inherited or developed physical or mental

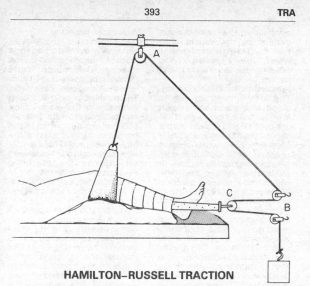

HAMILTON–RUSSELL TRACTION

characteristic.

trance (*trahns*). A condition of semi-consciousness of hysterical, cataleptic or hypnotic origin. It is not due to organic disease.

tranquillizer (*tran'-kwil-i-zer*). A drug which allays anxiety, relieves tension and has a calming effect on the patient.

transaminase (*trans-am'-in-aze*). One of a group of enzymes which catalyse the transfer of an amine group from one amino acid into another, together with a new keto acid. Transaminases include *glutamic-oxalacetic t.* (GO-T) and *glutamic-pyruvic t.* (GP-T).

transducer (*trans-du'-ser*). One of the data sources or electrodes attached to the patient

to enable recordings to be made. One physical quantity is translated to another, e.g. temperature to an electrical signal. *See* Monitoring.

transduction (*trans-duk'-shun*). The transfer of DNA from one micro-organism to another by a bacteriophage.

transection (*trans-ek'-shun*). (1) A cross-section of a tissue. (2) Section across the long axis of a part, e.g. *t. of the stomach*, which is performed in partial gastrectomy.

transfer RNA (*trans'-fer ar-en-a*). tRNA. Molecules of ribonucleic acid which are important in the formation of protein in that they attach the amino acids in the correct order at the ribosome.

transference (*trans-fer'-ens*). In

psychiatry, the unconscious transfer by the patient onto the psychiatrist of feelings which are appropriate to other people significant to the patient.

transfusion (*trans-fu'-zhun*). The introduction of whole blood or a blood component into a vein, performed in cases of severe loss of blood, shock, septicaemia, etc. It is used to supply actual volume of blood, or to introduce constituents as clotting factors, or antibodies, which are deficient in the patient. *Direct t.* The transfer of blood directly from a donor to a recipient. *Exchange, exsanguination* or *replacement t.* The removal of most or all of the recipient's blood and its replacement with fresh blood. Often used with infants suffering from erythroblastosis or acute leukaemia. *See* Rhesus factor. *Intra-arterial t.* The passing of blood into an artery under positive pressure in cases where large quantities are required rapidly, as in cardiovascular surgery.

transillumination (*trans-il-u-min-a'-shun*). The illumination of a translucent body structure by a strong light as an aid to diagnosis, particularly of tumours of the retina and of abnormalities in the ethmoidal and frontal sinuses.

translocation (*trans-lo-ka'-shun*). In morphology the transfer of a segment of a chromosome to a different site on the same chromosome or to a different chromosome. It can be a cause of congenital abnormality.

translucent (*trans-lu'-sent*). Allowing light rays to pass

through indistinctly.

transmigration (*trans-mi-gra'-shun*). A movement from one place to another, as in the passage of blood cells through the walls of the capillaries. Diapedesis. *External t.* The passage of an ovum from its ovary to the uterine tube on the opposite side. *Internal t.* The movement of an ovum from one uterine tube to the other through the uterus.

transplacental (*trans-plas-ent'-al*). Across the placenta. Movement may be from mother to fetus or vice versa. *T. infection* may affect the unborn child.

transplantation (*trans-plant-a'-shun*). The removal of a section of tissue (a graft) from one part to another, or to another body. *Organ t.* The transfer of a complete organ, e.g. a kidney from a donor, to replace a diseased organ. *Tendon t.* The transfer of a strip of tendon from a healthy muscle to a paralysed one. *T. of the ureters.* A necessary accompaniment to excision of the bladder. The ureters are usually implanted in the colon or loop of ileum.

transposition (*trans-po-zish'-un*). (1) Displacement of any of the viscera to the opposite side of the body. (2) The operation which partially removes a piece of tissue from one part of the body to another, the complete severance being delayed until it has become established in its new position. *T. of the great vessels.* A congenital abnormality of the heart in which the positions of the pulmonary artery and aorta are reversed.

transsexualism (*tran-seks'-u-al-izm*). A sexual aberration.

The person is convinced that his or her sex is the opposite to his or her physical state.

transudate (*trans'-u-date*). Any fluid which passes through a membrane.

transurethral (*trans-u-re'-thral*). Passing via the urethra.

transverse (*trans'-verse*). Cross-wise. *T. presentation.* Position of the fetus, whereby it lies across the pelvis, which position must be corrected before normal birth can take place.

transvestitism (*trans-vest'-it-izm*). A sexual aberration in which the patient dresses as a member of the opposite sex.

tranylcypromine (*tran-il-si'-pro-meen*). A monoamine oxidase inhibitor used in psychiatry for the treatment of depression.

trapezium (*trap-e'-ze-um*). A bone of the wrist in the distal row of the carpus.

trapezius (*trap-e'-ze-us*). One of two large muscles situated between the shoulders and at the back of the neck. It controls some of the movements of the scapula and draws the head backward and to the side.

trauma (*traw'-mah*). A wound or injury. *Psychic t.* An emotional disturbance which can lead to neurosis.

traumatic (*traw-mat'-ik*). Caused by injury. *T. fever.* That following an operation or injury when no bacterial infection is present.

treatment (*treet'-ment*). The mode of dealing with a patient or disease. *Active t.* That in which specific medical or surgical treatment is undertaken. *Conservative t.* That which aims at preserving and restoring injured parts by

natural means, e.g. rest, fluid replacement, etc., as opposed to radical or surgical methods. *Empirical t.* Treatment based on observation of symptoms and not on science. *Expectant t.* That in which symptoms only are treated, leaving nature to cure the disease. *Palliative t.* That which relieves distressing symptoms but does not cure the disease. *Prophylactic t.* That which aims at the prevention of disease.

Trematoda (*trem-at-o'-dah*). A class of fluke worms, some of which are parasitic in man. Many of them have freshwater snails as secondary hosts.

tremor (*trem'-or*). An involuntary, muscular quivering which may be due to fatigue, emotion or disease. Tremor, first of one hand, and later affecting the other limbs, is the first symptom of parkinsonism. *Intention t.* One which occurs on attempting a movement, as in disseminated sclerosis.

Trendelenburg's position (*F. Trendelenburg, German surgeon, 1844–1924*). See Position.

Trendelenburg's sign. An aid in diagnosis of congenital dislocation of the hip. The patient stands on the affected leg and flexes the other knee and hip. If there is dislocation the pelvis is lower on the side of the flexed leg, which is the reverse of normal.

trephine (*tre-fine'*). An instrument for cutting out a circular piece of bone, usually from the skull. *Corneal t.* One used to cut out a piece of cornea in keratoplasty.

Treponema (*trep-o-ne'-mah*).

A genus of spirochaetes. Anaerobic bacteria, they are motile, spiral and parasitic in man and animals. *T. careatum.* The causative agent of pinta. *T. pallidum.* The causative agent of syphilis. *T.p. immobilization test.* A serological test for syphilis. *T. pertenue.* The causative agent of yaws (framboesia).

triamcinolone (*tri-am-sin'-o-lone*). A glucocorticoid steroid which does not cause salt and water retention.

triamterine (*tri-am'-ter-een*). A diuretic that acts by antagonizing aldosterone and does not cause potassium loss. Used in the treatment of oedema.

triceps (*tri'-seps*). Having three heads. *T. muscle.* That situated on the back of the upper arm, which extends the forearm.

trichiasis (*trik-i'-as-is*). Friction and irritation of the cornea due to the eyelashes growing inwards.

trichinosis (*trik-in-o'-sis*). A disease caused by eating underdone pork containing a parasite, *Trichinella spiralis.* This becomes deposited in muscle, and causes stiffness and painful swelling. There may also be nausea, diarrhoea and fever. Trichiniasis.

trichloroethylene (*tri-klor-o-eth'-il-een*). A weak inhalation anaesthetic. Used in midwifery, for painful dressings and in general anaesthesia in combination with other anaesthetics.

trichology (*trik-ol'-o-je*). The study of hair.

Trichomonas (*trik-o-mo'-nas*). A genus of flagellate protozoa that are parasitic to man. *T. hominis* infests the bowel and may cause dysentery. *T. tenax* infests the mouth and may be present in cases of pyorrhoea. *T. vaginalis* is commonly present in the vagina and may cause leucorrhoea and vaginitis.

trichomoniasis (*trik-o-mon-i'-as-is*). Infestation with a parasite of the genus *Trichomonas.*

Trichophyton (*trik-o-fi'-ton*). A genus of fungi which affects the skin, nails and hair.

trichophytosis (*trik-o-fi-to'-sis*). Infection of the skin, nails or hair with one of the genus *Trichophyton. See* Tinea.

trichorrhexis (*trik-o-reks'-is*). Brittleness of the hair, which splits and breaks off easily.

trichosis (*trik-o'-sis*). Any abnormal growth of hair.

trichuriasis (*trik-u-ri'-as-is*). Infestation by the whipworm.

Trichuris (*trik-u'-ris*). A genus of nematode worms which may infest the colon and cause diarrhoea. A whipworm.

tricuspid (*tri-kus'-pid*). Having three flaps or cusps. *T. valve.* That at the opening between the right atrium and the right ventricle of the heart.

trifluoperazine (*tri-flu-o-per'-az-een*). A potent tranquillizing drug that is used in the treatment of schizophrenia and of psychoneuroses.

trifocal (*tri-fo'-kal*). Pertaining to a spectacle lens which has three foci, one for distant, one for intermediate and one for near vision.

trigeminal (*tri-jem'-in-al*). Divided into three. *T. nerve.* The fifth pair of cranial nerves, each of which is divided into three main branches and supplies one side of the face. *T. neuralgia.* Pain in the face which is confined to branches of the trigeminal nerve. Tic douloureux.

trigeminy (*tri-jem'-in-e*). The type of pulse in which there are three beats and then a missed beat. A regular irregularity. Pulsus trigeminus.

trigger finger (*trig'-er fing'-ger*). A stenosing of the tendon sheath at the metacarpophalangeal joint, allowing flexion of the finger but not extension without assistance, when it 'clicks' into position.

triglyceride (*tri-glis'-er-ide*). An ester of glycerol and three fatty acids.

trigone (*tri'-gone*). A triangular area. *T. of the bladder.* The triangular space on the floor of the bladder, between the ureteric openings and the urethral orifice.

tri-iodothyronine (*tri-i-o-do-thi'-ro-neen*). A hormone produced by the thyroid gland together with thyroxine.

trimeprazine (*tri-mep'-raz-een*). A sedative drug used for preoperative medication, in the treatment of pruritus and to sedate children.

trimester (*tri-mes'-ter*). A period of three months. *First t. of pregnancy.* The first three months, during which rapid development is taking place.

trimipramine (*tri-mip'-ram-een*). An antidepressant drug used particularly when anxiety and insomnia accompany depression.

triplopia (*tri-plo'-pe-ah*). A condition in which three images of an object are seen at the same time.

trismus (*triz'-mus*). Lock-jaw. A tonic spasm of the muscles of the jaw.

trisomy (*tri'-so-me*). The presence of an extra chromosome in each cell in addition to the normal paired set of 46. The cause of several chromosome disorders including Down's syndrome (mongolism) and Klinefelter's syndrome.

tritium (*trit'-e-um*). An isotope of hydrogen (H_3) that emits beta rays and is used as a tracer in studies of metabolism.

trocar (*tro'-kar*). A pointed instrument used with a canula for performing paracentesis.

trochanter (*tro-kan'-ter*). Either of two bony prominences, below the neck of the femur. *Greater t.* That on the outer side forming the bony prominence of the hip. *Lesser t.* That on the inner side at the neck of the femur.

troche (*tro'-ke*). A medicated lozenge used to treat infections of the mouth or throat or of the alimentary tract.

trochlea (*trok'-le-ah*). Any pulley-shaped structure, but particularly the fibrocartilage near the inner angular process of the frontal bone through which passes the tendon of the superior oblique muscle of the eye.

trochlear (*trok'-le-ar*). Relating to a trochlea. Pulley-shaped. *T. nerve.* The 4th cranial nerve.

trophic (*trof'-ik*). Relating to nutrition. *T. nerves.* Those which control the nutrition of a part. *T. ulcer.* One arising from a failure in the nutrition of a part.

trophoblast (*trof'-o-blast*). The layer of cells surrounding the blastocyst at the time of and responsible for implantation.

trophoblastoma (*trof'-o-blast-o'-mah*). Choriocarcinoma.

trophoneurosis (*trof-o-nu-ro'-*

sis). Malnutrition of a part, due to disturbance of the trophic nerves.

tropia (*tro'-pe-ah*). A manifest squint. One that is present when both eyes are open.

tropical (*trop'-ik-al*). Relating to the areas north and south of the equator termed the tropics. *T. medicine*. That concerned with diseases that are more prevalent in hot climates.

Trousseau's sign (*A. Trousseau, French physician, 1801–1867*). Sign indicating increased excitability of nerves caused by a lowered plasma calcium level. It is demonstrated by compressing the upper arm. This stimulates the underlying nerves and causes carpospasm.

truancy (*tru'-an-se*). Absence of a child from school without leave. A disorder of conduct which may result from emotional insecurity or a feeling of unfairness.

truncus (*trunk'-us*). A trunk. The main part of the body, or of a part of it, from which other parts spring. *T. arteriosus*. The arterial trunk connected to the fetal heart which develops into the aortic and pulmonary arteries. *Persistent t.a.* A rare congenital deformity in which this persists, causing a mixing of the systemic and pulmonary circulations.

truss (*trus*). An apparatus in the form of a belt with a pressure pad, for retaining a hernia in place after reduction.

Trypanosoma (*trip-an-o-so'-mah*). A genus of protozoan parasites which pass some of their life cycle in the blood of vertebrates, including man. *T. gambiense* and *T. rhodensiense* are transmitted

by the bite of the tsetse fly, and are the cause of sleeping sickness.

trypanosomiasis (*trip-an-o-so-mi'-as-is*). A disease caused by infestation with *Trypanosoma*. Sleeping sickness.

trypsin (*trip'-sin*). A digestive enzyme converting protein into amino acids.

trypsinogen (*trip-sin'-o-jen*). The precursor of trypsin. It is secreted in the pancreatic juice, and activated by the enterokinase of the intestinal juices into trypsin.

tryptophan (*trip'-to-fan*). One of the essential amino acids.

tsetse fly (*tset'-se fli*). A fly of the genus *Glossina* which transmits the parasite *Trypanosoma* to man, causing trypanosomiasis.

tsutsugamushi disease (*tsutsu-gah-mu'-shi diz-eez'*). Scrub typhus that occurs in Japan and is transmitted by the bite of a mite.

tubal (*tu'-bal*). Relating to a tube. *T. pregnancy*. Extrauterine pregnancy where the embryo develops in the uterine tube. Ectopic pregnancy.

tubectomy (*tu-bek'-tom-e*). Excision of a portion of a uterine tube.

tuber (*tu'-ber*). A protuberance. *T. cinereum*. A protruding part of the hypothalamus connected by the infundibulum to the pituitary gland.

tubercle (*tu'-ber-kl*). (1) A small nodule or a rounded prominence on a bone. (2) The specific lesion—a small nodule—produced by the tubercle bacillus.

tubercular (*tu-ber'-ku-lar*). Pertaining to tubercles.

tuberculid (*tu-ber'-ku-lid*). A papular eruption occurring on the skin of tuberculous patients.

tuberculin (tu-ber'-ku-lin). The filtrate from a fluid medium in which Mycobacterium tuberculosis has been grown and which contains its toxins. *Old t.* is prepared from the human bacillus. It is used in skin tests in diagnosing tuberculosis. *See* Mantoux test.

tuberculosis (tu-ber-ku-lo'-sis). An infectious disease produced by the tubercle bacillus, Myocobacterium tuberculosis, discovered by Koch in 1882. *Bovine t.* A form found in cattle and spread by infected milk. *Miliary t.* A severe form with small tuberculous lesions spread throughout the body with severe toxaemia. *Open t.* Any type of tuberculosis in which the organisms are being excreted from the body. *Pulmonary t.* That affecting the lungs; also termed phthisis. *T. of the spine.* Pott's disease.

tuberculous (tu-ber'-ku-lus). Infected with or relating to tuberculosis.

tuberosity (tu-ber-os'-it-e). A flat protuberance on a bone. *T. of the radius.* A prominence on the shaft of the radius into which the tendon of the biceps muscle is inserted. *T. of the tibia.* A raised and roughened surface on the tibia.

tuberous (tu'-ber-us). Covered with tubers. *T. sclerosis.* Epiloia.

tubocurarine (tu-bo-ku-rar'-ine). A preparation of curare used to secure skeletal muscle relaxation.

tubular (tu'-bu-lar). Relating to or resembling a tube.

tubule (tu'-bule). A small tube. *Renal* or *uriniferous t.* The essential secreting tube of the kidney.

tularaemia (tu-lar-e'-me-ah). An acute infectious fever caused by a bacterium, Pasteurella tularense. The disease originates in squirrels, rabbits and other rodents and may be transmitted by bloodsucking ticks or flies. The lymph glands are involved and they may suppurate.

tulle gras (tule grah'). A preparation of gauze impregnated with petroleum jelly. Other drugs may be added. Most useful on a granulating surface to stop a dressing adhering.

tumefaction (tu-me-fak'-shun). A swelling or the process of becoming swollen. Tumescence.

tumescence (tu-mes'-ens). The condition of being swollen. A swelling.

tumour (tu'-mer). An abnormal swelling. The term is usually applied to a morbid growth of tissue which may be benign or malignant. A neoplasm. *Benign* or *innocent t.* One that does not infiltrate or cause metastases, and is unlikely to recur if removed. *Malignant t.* One which invades and destroys tissue and can spread to neighbouring tissues, and to more distant sites via the blood and the lymphatic systems. *Phantom t.* An abdominal swelling, usually of gas, which may imitate a tumour.

tunica (tu'-nik-ah). A coat, a covering, or the lining of a vessel. *T. adventitia, t. media, t. intima.* The outer, middle and inner coats of an artery, respectively. *T. vaginalis.* The membrane covering the front and sides of the testis.

tuning fork (tu'-ning fork). A metal instrument used for testing hearing by means of the sounds produced by its vibration. *See* Rinne's *and* Weber's tests.

tunnel (*tun'-el*). In anatomy, a canal through a structure. *Carpal t.* The osteofibrous channel in the wrist between the carpal bones and tissue covering the flexor tendons. *C.t. syndrome.* Pain and tingling in the hand and fingers caused by compression of the median nerve in the carpal tunnel. *T. vision.* Vision that is restricted to the central field. Occurs in chronic glaucoma and in retinitis pigmentosa.

turbinate (*ter'-bin-ate*). Scroll-shaped. *T. bone.* One of the three thin long plates that form the walls of the nasal cavity.

turbinectomy (*ter-bin-ek'-tom-e*). Excision of a turbinate bone.

turgescence (*ter-jes'-ens*). Swelling due to congestion of blood or other fluid.

turgid (*ter'-jid*). Swollen and congested.

turgor (*ter'-gor*). The state of being swollen or distended.

Turner's syndrome (*H.H. Turner, American physician, 1892–1970*). A congenital condition in women in which there is absence of one X chromosome. The women are usually mentally retarded, are without ovaries and have infantile sex characteristics and webbing of the neck.

tussis (*tus'-is*). A cough.

twilight state (*twi'-lite state*). A period of dissociation in which a patient may perform acts of which he is not conscious later on. Though rare, such a state may follow an epileptic fit. *Hysterical t.s.* Mild clouding of conscious-ness giving rise to irrelevant speech or clumsy actions.

twin (*twin*). One of a pair of individuals who have developed in the uterus together. *Binovular (dizygotic) t.* Each twin has developed from a separate ovum. Fraternal twins. *Uniovular (monozygotic) t.* Both twins have developed from the same cell. Identical twins.

tylosis (*ti-lo'-sis*). The formation of a hard patch of skin. A callosity.

tympanectomy (*tim-pan-ek'-tom-e*). Excision of the tympanic membrane.

tympanic (*tim-pan'-ik*). Relating to the tympanum. *T. membrane.* The ear-drum.

tympanites (*tim-pan-i'-teez*). Distension of the abdomen by accumulation of gas in the intestine or the peritoneal cavity.

tympanitis (*tim-pan-i'-tis*). Inflammation of the middle ear. Otitis media.

tympanoplasty (*tim-pan-o-plas'-te*). An operation to reconstruct the ear-drum and restore conductivity to the middle ear. Myringoplasty.

tympanosclerosis (*tim-pan-o-skler-o'-sis*). Fibrosis and the formation of calcified deposits in the middle ear that lead to deafness.

tympanum (*tim'-pan-um*). (1) The middle ear. (2) The ear-drum or tympanic membrane.

typhlitis (*tif-li'-tis*). Inflammation of the caecum.

typhlon (*tif'-lon*). The caecum.

typhoid fever (*ti'-foid fe'-ver*). Enteric fever. An acute infectious disease caused by *Salmonella typhi*, which is transmitted by food, milk or water that has been contaminated by patients or by carriers.

There is high fever, a red rash, delirium and sometimes intestinal haemorrhage. Recovery usually begins during the fourth week of the disease.

typhus (*ti'-fus*). Any one of a group of fevers caused by rickettsiae. There is high fever, a widespread red rash and severe headache. Typhus is likely to occur where there is overcrowding, lack of personal cleanliness, and bad hygienic conditions, as the infection is spread by bites of infected lice or by rat fleas. *Scrub t.* A form spread by mites and widespread in the Far East. Tsutsugamushi disease.

tyramine (*ti'-ram-een*). An enzyme present in cheese, game, broad bean pods, yeast extracts, wine and strong beer, which has a similar effect in the body to that of adrenaline. Foodstuffs containing tyramine should be avoided by patients taking monoamine oxidase inhibitors.

tyrosine (*ti'-ro-seen*). An essential amino acid, which is the product of phenylalanine metabolism. In some diseases, especially of the liver, it is present as a deposit in the urine. It is a precursor of catecholamines, melanin and thyroid hormones.

tyrosinosis (*ti-ro-sin-o'-sis*). A congenital condition in which there is an error of metabolism and phenylalanine cannot be reduced to tyrosine. Hepatic failure may occur.

U

U. Chemical symbol for *uranium*.

ulcer (*ul'-ser*). An erosion or loss of continuity of the skin or of a mucous membrane, often accompanied by suppuration. *Decubitus u.* A pressure sore caused by lying immobile for long periods of time. *Duodenal u.* A peptic ulcer in the duodenum. *Gastric u.* One in the lining of the stomach. *Gravitational u.* A varicose ulcer of the leg which is difficult to heal because of its dependent position and the poor venous return. *Gummatous u.* One arising in late non-infective syphilis; it is slow to heal. *Indolent u.* One which is painless and heals slowly. *Peptic u.* One that occurs on the mucous membrane of either the stomach or duodenum. *Perforating u.* One that erodes through the thickness of the wall of an organ. *Rodent u.* A slow-growing epithelioma of the face which may cause much local destruction and ulceration, but does not give rise to metastases. Basal cell carcinoma. *Trophic u.* One due to a failure of nutrition of a part. *Varicose u.* Gravitational ulcer.

ulcerative (*ul'-ser-a-tiv*). Characterized by ulceration (the formation of ulcers). *U. colitis.* Inflammation and ulceration of the colon and rectum of unknown cause.

ulna (*ul'-nah*). The bone on the inner side of the forearm from elbow to wrist.

ulnar (*ul'-nar*). Relating to the ulna.

ultramicroscope (*ul-trah-mi'-kro-skope*). An instrument for examining minute particles suspended in water or gas and intensely lit from behind.

ultrasonic (*ul-trah-son'-ik*). Relating to sound waves having a frequency range beyond the upper limit perceived by the human ear. These waves are widely used instead of X-rays, particularly in the examination of structures not opaque to X-rays, and in obstetrics to replace X-ray pelvimetry.

ultrasonics (*ul-trah-son'-iks*). The study of ultrasound.

ultrasonography (*ul-trah-son-og'-raf-e*). The use of ultrasound to produce soft tissue scans.

ultrasound (*ul'-trah-sownd*). Ultrasonic waves used to examine the interior organs of the body. These waves can also be used in the treatment of soft tissue pain, and to break up renal calculi or the crystalline lens when cataract is present.

ultra-violet rays (*ul'-trah-vi'-o-let raze*). Short wavelength electromagnetic rays. They are present in sunlight and cause tanning and sunburn. *U.-v. light* is used to promote vitamin D formation and for the treatment of certain skin conditions.

umbilical (*um-bil'-ik-al*). Relating to the umbilicus.

umbilicated (*um-bil'-ik-a-ted*). Having a depression like that of the navel, as on a smallpox vesicle.

umbilicus (*um-bil'-ik-us*). The navel; the circular depressed scar in the centre of the abdomen where the umbilical cord of the fetus was attached.

unciform (*un'-se-form*). Hook-shaped. *U. bone.* A hook-shaped bone in the carpus. The hamate bone.

uncinate (*un'-sin-ate*). Hooked or barbed. *U. process.* A hooked part of the ethmoid bone.

unconscious (*un-kon'-shus*). Receiving no sensory impulses. Insensible. *U. mind.* In psychology, that part of the mind containing the urges, feelings and experiences of which the individual is unaware and which he cannot normally recall although they influence his actions.

unconsciousness (*un-kon'-shus-nes*). The state of being unconscious. This may vary in depth from (1) *deep u.,* when no response can be obtained, through (2) lesser degrees of unconsciousness, when the patient can be roused by painful stimuli, to (3) when the patient can be roused by speech or non-painful stimuli.

undecenoic acid (*un-de-sen-o'-ik as'-id*). An antifungal agent used in the treatment of such infections as athlete's foot. May be used in powder, ointment, lotion or spray form.

undifferentiated (*un-dif-er-en'-she-a-ted*). In pathology, used to denote primitive or unrecognizable cells.

undine (*un'-dine*). A glass flask with long spout formerly used for irrigation of the eye. Now largely replaced by the use of continuous flow irrigation solutions.

undulant (*un'-du-lant*). Rising and falling like a wave. *U. fever.* Brucellosis. A recurrent fever with enlargement of spleen, swelling of joints, neuralgic pains, and profuse sweating. Repeated attacks cause weakness and anaemia. The cause is *Brucella abortus,* transmitted in cow's milk, or *Brucella melitensis,* from goat's milk (*Malta fever*).

ungual (*ung'-gwal*). Relating to the finger- or toe-nails.

unguentum (*ung-gwen'-tum*).

An ointment.

unguis (*ung'-gwis*). A finger- or toe-nail.

unicellular (*u-ne-sel'-u-lah*). Consisting of one cell.

unilateral (*u-ne-lat'-er-al*). On one side only.

union (*u'-ne-on*). (1) A joining together. (2) The repair of tissue after separation by incision or fracture. *See* Callus *and* Healing.

uni-ovular (*u-ne-o'-vu-lar*). From one ovum. *U. twins.* Identical twins, developed from one ovum.

unipara (*u-nip'-ar-ah*). A woman who has had only one child.

unit (*u'-nit*). (1) A single thing. *Intensive care u.* A hospital department reserved for those with severe medical or surgical disorders. (2) A standard of measurement. *International insulin u.* A measurement of the pure crystalline insulin arrived at by biological assay. *SI unit.* One of the various units of measurement making up the Système International d'Unités (International System of Units).

urachal (*u-ra'-kal*). Referring to the urachus. *U. cyst.* A congenital abnormality when a small cyst persists along the course of the urachus. *U. fistula.* One that forms when the urachus fails to close. Urine may leak from the umbilicus.

urachus (*u'-ra-kus*). A tubular canal existing in the fetus, connecting the bladder with the umbilicus. In the adult it persists in the form of a solid fibrous cord.

uracil (*u'-ras-il*). One of the nucleic bases found in RNA.

uraemia (*u-re'-me-ah*). A condition of high blood urea, muscle weakness and increasing drowsiness caused by renal failure. *Extrarenal u.* High blood urea when the cause is outside the kidney, such as circulatory failure due to shock or haemorrhage.

uraniscorrhaphy (*u-ran-is-kor'-af-e*). Suture of a cleft palate. Staphylorrhaphy.

uranium (*u-ra'-ne-um*). abbrev. U. A radioactive metallic element.

urataemia (*u-rat-e'-me-ah*). An accumulation of urates in the blood.

urate (*u'-rate*). A salt of uric acid. *Sodium u.* A compound generally found in concentration around joints in cases of gout.

uraturia (*u-rat-u'-re-ah*). An excess of urates in the urine. Lithuria.

urea (*u-re'-ah*). Carbamide. A white crystalline substance which is an end-product of protein metabolism and the chief nitrogenous constituent of urine. It is a diuretic. The normal daily output is about 33 g. *Blood u.* That which is present in the blood. Normal is 20 to 40 mg per 100 ml.

urecchysis (*u-rek'-is-is*). The extravasation of urine into cellular tissue, e.g. in rupture of the bladder as a complication of fractured pelvis.

uresis (*u-re'-sis*). Urination.

ureter (*u-re'-ter*). One of the two long narrow tubes which convey the urine from the kidney to the bladder.

ureterectomy (*u-re-ter-ek'-tom-e*). The surgical removal of a ureter.

ureteric (*u-re-ter'-ik*). Relating to the ureter. *U. catheter.* A fine catheter for insertion via the ureter into the pelvis of the kidney, either for drainage or for retrograde pyelography. *U. transplantation.* Operation in which the ureters are divided from the bladder and implanted in the colon or loop of ileum. Congenital defects or malignant growth may make this necessary.

ureteritis (*u-re-ter-i´-tis*). Inflammation of the ureter.

ureterocele (*u-re´-ter-o-seel*). A cystic enlargement of the wall of the ureter at its entry into the bladder.

ureterocolostomy (*u-re-ter-o-kol-os´-tom-e*). Anastomosis of a ureter to the colon.

uretero-enterostomy (*u-re-ter-o-en-ter-os´-tom-e*). Surgical implantation of a ureter into the intestine.

ureterolith (*u-re´-ter-o-lith*). A calculus in a ureter.

ureterolithotomy (*u-re-ter-o-lith-ot´-om-e*). Removal of a calculus from the ureter.

ureteronephrectomy (*u-re-ter-o-nef-rek´-tom-e*). Surgical removal of a kidney and its ureter.

ureterosigmoidostomy (*u-re-ter-o-sig-moid-os´-tom-e*). Surgical implantation of the ureters into the sigmoid colon.

ureterostomy (*u-re-ter-os´-tom-e*). The surgical creation of a permanent opening through which the ureter discharges urine.

ureterovaginal (*u-re-ter-o-vaj-i´-nal*). Relating to the ureter and vagina. *U. fistula.* An opening into the ureter by which urine escapes via the vagina. It may be congenital, due to erosion as in carcinoma of the cervix, or to an error in operative technique.

urethra (*u-re´-thrah*). The canal through which the urine is discharged from the bladder. In a man it measures 20 to 23 cm (8 to 9 in.) in length; in a woman 4 cm (1.5 in.).

urethral (*u-re´-thral*). Relating to the urethra.

urethritis (*u-re-thri´-tis*). Inflammation of the urethra. *Non-specific u.* Inflammation caused by a venereal infection other than a gonococcus or another specific microorganism. *Simple* or *specific u.* Inflammation caused by a specific micro-organism, usually gonorrhoeal (*gonococcal u.*).

urethrocele (*u-re´-thro-seel*). A prolapse of the female urethral wall which may result from damage to the pelvic floor during childbirth.

urethrography (*u-re-throg´-raf-e*). X-ray examination of the urethra. A radio-opaque dye is inserted by catheter.

urethroplasty (*u-re´-thro-plas-te*). A surgical repair of the urethra.

urethroscope (*u-re´-thro-skope*). An instrument for examining the interior of the urethra.

urethrostenosis (*u-re-thro-sten-o´-sis*). Stricture of the urethra.

urethrostomy (*u-re-thros´-tom-e*). The creation of a permanent opening of the male urethra in the perineum.

urethrotomy (*u-re-throt´-om-e*). Incision of the urethra, to remedy stricture.

uric acid (*u´-rik as´-id*). Lithic acid, the end-product of nucleic acid metabolism, a normal constituent of urine. Its accumulation in the blood produces uricacidaemia. Renal calculi are frequently formed of it.

uricacidaemia (*u-rik-as-id-e´-me-ah*). The presence of an excess of uric acid in the blood.

uricosuric (*u-rik-o-su'-rik*). A drug that promotes the excretion of uric acid in the urine.

uridrosis (*u-rid-ro'-sis*). The presence of urinary constituents, such as urea and uric acid, in the perspiration. They may become deposited as crystals upon the skin. A symptom of uraemia.

urinalysis (*u-rin-al'-is-is*). The bacteriological or chemical examination of the urine.

urinary (*u'-rin-ar-e*). Relating to urine. *U. tract.* The system which leads urine from the kidneys to the exterior, including the ureters, the bladder and the urethra.

urination (*u-rin-a'-shun*). Micturition. The act of passing urine.

urine (*u'-rin*). The fluid secreted by the kidneys and excreted through the bladder and urethra. It is 96% water and 4% solid constituents, the most important being urea and uric acid. *Residual u.* That which remains in the bladder after micturition, as in cases of cystocele or enlargement of the prostate gland.

uriniferous (*u-rin-if'-er-us*). Capable of conveying urine. *U. tubule.* A renal tubule. *See* Tubule.

urinometer (*u-rin-om'-e-ter*). A glass instrument consisting of a graduated stem weighted with a mercury bulb, used for measuring the specific gravity of urine.

urobilin (*u-ro-bi'-lin*). The main pigment of urine, derived from urobilinogen.

urobilinogen (*u-ro-bi-lin'-o-jen*). A pigment derived from bilirubin which on oxidation forms urobilin.

urochrome (*u'-ro-krome*). The

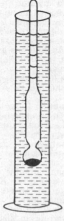

URINOMETER

yellow pigment which colours urine.

urogenital (*u-ro-jen'-it-al*). Relating to the urinary and genital organs. Urinogenital.

urography (*u-rog'-raf-e*). X-ray examination of any part of the urinary tract.

urokinase (*u-ro-kin'-aze*). An enzyme in urine which is secreted by the kidneys and causes fibrinolysis. In certain diseases it may cause bleeding from the kidneys.

urolith (*u'-ro-lith*). A calculus in the urinary tract.

urology (*u-rol'-o-je*). The study of diseases of the urinary tract.

uropathy (*u-rop'-ath-e*). Any disease condition affecting the urinary tract.

urticaria (*er-tik-air'-e-ah*). Nettle-rash or hives. An acute or chronic skin condition characterized by the recurrent appearance of an eruption of weals, causing great irritation. The condition is probably due to hypersensitiveness to certain foods. *See* Allergy.

uterine (*u'-ter-ine*). Relating to the uterus.

uterocele (*u'-ter-o-seel*). A hernia of the uterus. A hysterocele.

uterogestation (*u-ter-o-jes-ta'-shun*). Th development of a fetus within the uterus. A normal pregnancy.

uterography (*u-ter-og'-raf-e*). X-ray examination of the uterus.

uterosalpingography (*u-ter-o-sal-ping-gog'-raf-e*). X-ray examination of the uterus and the uterine tubes.

uterovesical (*u-ter-o-ves'-ik-al*). Referring to the uterus and bladder. *U. pouch.* The fold of peritoneum between the two organs.

uterus (*u'-ter-us*). The womb: a triangular, hollow, muscle organ situated in the pelvic cavity between the bladder and the rectum. Its function is the nourishment and protection of the fetus during pregnancy and its expulsion at term. *Bicornuate u.* One having two horns. A congenital malformation. *Gravid u.* The pregnant uterus. *U. didelphys.* A double uterus owing to the failure of union of the two Müllerian ducts from which it is formed.

utricle (*u'-trik-l*). The delicate membranous sac in the bony vestibule of the ear.

uvea (*u'-ve-ah*). Uveal tract. The pigmented layer of the eye, consisting of the iris, ciliary body and choroid.

uveitis (*u-ve-i'-tis*). Inflammation of the uveal tract.

uvula (*u'-vu-lah*). The small fleshy appendage which is the free edge of the soft palate,

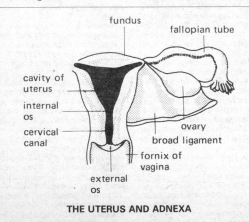

fundus

fallopian tube

cavity of uterus

internal os

cervical canal

ovary

broad ligament

fornix of vagina

external os

THE UTERUS AND ADNEXA

hanging from the roof of the mouth.

uvulectomy (*u-vu-lek'-tom-e*). The surgical excision of the uvula.

uvulitis (*u-vu-li'-tis*). Inflammation of the uvula.

uvulotomy (*u-vu-lot'-om-e*). The operation of cutting off a part or the whole of the uvula.

V

V. Abbreviation for the SI unit, the *volt*.

vaccination (*vak-sin-a'-shun*). The injection of a vaccine in order to produce artificial active immunity to a specific disease.

vaccine (*vak'-seen*). A suspension of killed or attenuated organisms in normal saline designed to protect the body against a specific disease by stimulating the formation of antibodies. *Attenuated v.* One prepared from living organisms which through long cultivation have lost their virulence. *Bacille Calmette Guérin v.* An attenuated bovine bacillus *v.* giving immunity from tuberculosis. *Triple v.* One that protects against diphtheria, tetanus and whooping cough. *Sabin v.* An attenuated poliovirus v. that can be administered by mouth, in a syrup or on sugar. *Salk v.* One prepared from an inactivated strain of poliomyelitis virus. *TAB v.* A sterile solution of the organisms that cause typhoid and paratyphoid A and B. Paratyphoid C may now be included. *V. lymph.* A preparation from healthy calves inoculated with smallpox, formerly used to prevent smallpox.

vaccinia (*vak-sin'-e-ah*). Cowpox. A virus infection of cows, which may be transmitted to man by contact with the lesions. A local pustular eruption is produced.

vaccinotherapy (*vak-sin-other'-ap-e*). Treatment by means of vaccines.

vacuole (*vak'-u-ole*). A cavity within the cytoplasm of a cell.

vacuum (*vak'-u-um*). A space from which air or gas has been extracted. *V. extractor.* An instrument to assist delivery of the fetus. A suction cup is attached to the head and a vacuum created slowly. Traction is applied during uterine contractions.

vagal (*va'-gal*). Relating to the vagus nerve.

vagina (*vaj-i'-nah*). The canal, lined with mucous membrane, which leads from the cervix of the uterus to the vulva.

vaginismus (*vaj-in-iz'-mus*). A painful spasm of the muscles of the vagina, occurring usually when the vulva or vagina is touched. Sexual intercourse may prove impracticable.

vaginitis (*vaj-in-i'-tis*). Inflammation of the vagina. *Atrophic* or *postmenopausal v.* Inflammation caused by degenerative changes in the mucous lining of the vagina and insufficient oestrogen secretion. Adhesions may occur, partially closing the vagina. *Trichomonas v.* Infection caused by *T. vaginalis*, a protozoon which causes a thin, yellowish discharge, giving rise to local tenderness and pruritus.

vagotomy (*va-got'-om-e*). Surgical incision of the vagus nerve or any of its branches. A treatment for peptic ulcer.

vagus (*va'-gus*). The tenth cranial nerve, arising in the medulla and providing the parasympathetic nerve supply to the organs in the thorax and abdomen. *V. resection.* Vagotomy.

valgus (*val'-gus*). A displacement outwards, particularly of the feet. *Genu valgum.* Knock-knee, with the ankles set apart. *Hallux v.* Twisting of the big toe outwards towards the other toes. *Talipes v.* Club-foot with the inner edge only in contact with the ground, and the foot turned outwards.

valine (*val'-een*). One of the 22 amino acids formed by the digestion of dietary protein.

Valsalva's manoeuvre (*A.M. Valsalva, Italian anatomist, 1666–1723*). Technique for increasing the intrathoracic pressure by closing the mouth and nostrils and blowing out the cheeks, thereby forcing air back into the nasopharynx. Used during the insertion of a catheter into the right atrium (a 'central venous line') and during the changing of tubing on such a line, to prevent the occurrence of an air embolism.

valve (*valv*). (1) A means of regulating the flow of liquid or gas through a pipe. (2) A fold of membrane in a passage or tube, so placed as to permit passage of fluid in one direction only. They are important structures in the heart, in veins and in lymph vessels. *Atrioventricular v's.* The bicuspid and tricuspid valves of the heart. *Houston's v's.* Folds of mucous membrane in the rectum. *Ileocaecal v.* Membranous folds at the junction of the ileum and caecum. *Pulmonary v.* A valve where the pulmonary artery emerges from the right ventricle. *Pyloric v.* A fold of mucous membrane at the junction of the stomach and duodenum. *Semilunar v.* Either of two valves at the junction of the pulmonary artery and aorta respectively, with the heart. *V. replacement.* A cardiac operation to replace a diseased aortic or mitral valve.

valvotomy (*val-vot'-om-e*). Valvulotomy. A surgical operation to open up a fibrosed valve, e.g. mitral valvotomy to relieve mitral stenosis.

valvula (*val'-vu-lah*). *pl.* valvulae. A small valve. *Valvulae conniventes.* Transverse folds of mucous membrane in the lining of the small intestine.

valvulitis (*val-vu-li'-tis*). Inflammation of a valve, particularly of the heart.

van den Bergh's test (*A.A.H. van den Bergh, Dutch physician, 1869–1943*). A chemical test of bilirubin in serum to aid the diagnosis of jaundice.

vaporizer (*va'-por-i-zer*). An apparatus for producing a very fine spray of a liquid.

varicectomy (*var-is-ek'-tom-e*). Phlebectomy. Surgical excision of a varicose vein.

varicella (*var-is-el'-ah*). Chickenpox. An infectious disease of childhood having an incubation period of 12–20 days. There is slight fever and an eruption of transparent vesicles on the chest on the first day of disease, which comes out in successive crops all over the body. The vesicles soon dry up, sometimes leaving shallow pits in the skin. Complications are rare.

varicocele (*var'-ik-o-seel*). A dilatation of the veins of the spermatic cord.

varicocelectomy (*var-ik-o-se-lek'-tom-e*). Operation for removal of dilated veins from the scrotum.

varicose (*var'-ik-oze*). Swollen or dilated. *V. veins.* A dilated and twisted condition of the veins (usually those of the leg), due to structural changes in the walls or valves of the vessels. *V. ulcer.* Gravitational ulcer. *See* Ulcer.

varicotomy (*var-ik-ot'-om-e*). Surgical incision of a varicose vein.

variola (*var-e-o'-lah*). Smallpox. A highly contagious and frequently fatal disease formerly occurring worldwide. Public Health measures have now totally eradicated the disease.

varix (*var'-iks*). *pl.* varices. An enlarged or varicose vein.

varus (*va'-rus*). A displacement inwards. *Genu varum.* Bowleg, with the ankles close together. *Hallux v.* Twisting of the big toe inwards, away from the other toes. *Talipes v.* Club-foot with the outer edge only in contact with the ground and the foot turned inwards.

vas (*vas*). *pl.* vasa. A vessel or duct. *V. deferens.* One of a pair of excretory ducts conveying the semen from the epididymis to the urethra. *V. efferens.* One of the many small tubes that convey semen from the testis to the epididymis. *Vasa vasorum.* The minute nutrient vessels that supply the walls of the arteries and veins.

vascular (*vas'-ku-lar*). Relating to, or consisting largely of blood vessels. *V. system.* The cardiovascular system.

vascularization (*vas-ku-lar-i-za'-shun*). The development of new blood vessels within a tissue.

vasculitis (*vas-ku-li'-tis*). Angiitis. Inflammation of a blood vessel. *Allergic v.* A severe allergic response to drugs or to cold. Arising in small arteries or veins, with fibrosis and thrombi formation.

vasectomy (*vas-ek'-tom-e*). Excision of a part of the vas deferens. If performed bilaterally sterility results. Now employed as a method of contraception.

vasoconstrictor (*va-zo-kon-strik'-tor*). A nerve or a drug that causes contraction of a blood vessel wall, and therefore a decrease in the blood flow and a rise in the blood pressure.

vasodilator (*va-zo-di-la'-tor*). A drug or motor nerve that causes an increase in the lumen of blood vessels, and therefore an increase in the blood flow and a fall in the blood pressure.

vasomotor (*va-zo-mo'-tor*). Controlling the muscles of blood vessels, both dilator and constrictor. *V. centre.* Nerve cells in the medulla oblongata controlling the vasomotor nerves. *V. nerves.* Sympathetic nerves regulating the tension of the blood vessels.

vasopressin (*va-zo-pres'-in*). Antidiuretic hormone (ADH). A hormone from the posterior lobe of the pituitary gland which causes constriction of plain muscle fibres and reabsorption of water in the renal tubules. It is used to relieve symptoms in diabetes insipidus.

vasovagal (va-zo-va'-gal). Vascular and vagal. *V. attack.* Fainting or syncope from psychogenic causes such as fear or witnessing an unpleasant sight. There is postural hypotension.

vasovesiculitis (va-zo-ves-ik-u-li'-tis). Inflammation of the vas deferens and seminal vesicles.

Vater's ampulla (*A. Vater, German anatomist, 1684–1751*). Dilatation at the point where the common bile duct enters the duodenum.

vectis (vek'-tis). A curved instrument used to hasten delivery of the fetal head in parturition.

vector (vek'-tor). (1) An animal that carries organisms or parasites from one host to another, either of the same species or to one of another species. (2) A quantity with magnitude and direction. *Electrocardiographic v.* The area of the heart which is monitored during electrocardiographic investigation.

vectorcardiography (vek-tor-kar-de-og'-raf-e). Electrocardiographic investigation of the heart in which individual vectors are monitored.

vegan (ve'-gan). A vegetarian who excludes all animal protein from his diet.

vegetation (vej-e-ta'-shun). In pathology, a plant-like outgrowth. *Adenoid v.* Overgrowth of lymphoid tissue in the nasopharynx.

vehicle (ve'-ikl). In pharmacy, a substance or medium in which a drug is administered.

vein (vane). A vessel carrying blood from the capillaries back to the heart. It has thin walls and a lining endothel-

ium from which the venous valves are formed.

vena (ve'-nah). *pl.* venae. A vein. *V. cava.* Either of the two large veins which return the venous blood to the right atrium of the heart.

venepuncture (ve-ne-punk'-cher). The insertion of a needle into a vein, usually to obtain a blood specimen.

venereal (ven-eer'-e-al). Pertaining to or caused by sexual intercourse. *V. diseases.* Those transmitted by sexual intercourse. The most important are syphilis, gonorrhoea, and soft chancre.

venereology (ven-eer-e-ol'-o-je). The study and treatment of venereal diseases.

venesection (ve-ne-sek'-shun). Phlebotomy. Surgical bloodletting by opening a vein or introducing a wide-bore needle. Commonly performed on blood donors and occasionally to relieve venous congestion.

venoclysis (ve-nok'-lis-is). The introduction of fluids directly into veins.

venogram (ve'-no-gram). (1) A graphic recording of the pulse in a vein. (2) An X-ray taken during venography.

venography (ve-nog'-raf-e). X-ray examination of a vein after the insertion of a dye to trace its pathway.

venom (ven'-om). A poison secreted by an insect, snake or other animal for injection into an enemy or its prey. *V. antiserum.* An antitoxin containing antibodies against the bites of poisonous snakes.

venomotor (ve-no-mo'-tor). Enlarging or reducing the calibre of a vein. *V. tone.* Muscle tone in the walls of the veins which can produce changes in the capacity of the circulation without affecting their resistance to blood flow.

venous (*ve'-nus*). Pertaining to the veins. *V. sinus.* One of 14 channels, similar to veins, by which blood leaves the cerebral circulation.

ventilation (*ven-til-a'-shun*). (1) The passage of air through the respiratory tract into and out of the lungs. (2) The process of removing vitiated air (the products of respiration, combustion, or putrefaction), and replacing it with fresh air. *Artificial v.* The supply of fresh air by propulsion and extraction methods, as is used for large buildings, mines, underground railways, etc. *Natural v.* The supply of fresh air by natural diffusion of air controlled by windows, doors, and ventilating devices.

ventilator (*ven'-til-a-tor*). In medicine, a machine which inflates the lungs by positive pressure through an endotracheal or tracheostomy tube, in a rhythmic manner. A respirator.

ventral (*ven'-tral*). Pertaining to a hollow structure or belly.

ventricle (*ven'-trikl*). A small pouch or cavity; applied especially to the lower chambers of the heart, and to the four cavities of the brain.

ventricular (*ven-trik'-u-lah*). Pertaining to a ventricle. *V. folds.* The outer folds of mucous membrane forming the false vocal cords. *V. septal defect.* VSD. Congenital abnormality in which there is communication between the two ventricles of the heart due to maldevelopment of the intraventricular septum.

ventriculitis (*ven-trik-u-li'-tis*).

Inflammation of the ventricles in the brain.

ventriculography (*ven-trik-u-log'-raf-e*). (1) X-ray examination of the ventricles of the heart using a radio-opaque contrast medium. (2) X-ray examination of the ventricles of the brain following the injection of air or a contrast medium through a burr hole. Used to help locate a cerebral tumour.

ventriculoscope (*ven-trik'-u-lo-skope*). An instrument for viewing the inside of the ventricles of the brain.

ventrofixation (*ven-tro-fiks-a'-shun*). Stitching a retroverted uterus or other abdominal organ to the abdominal wall.

ventrosuspension (*ven-tro-sus-pen'-shun*). An abdominal operation performed to remedy a displacement of the uterus.

venule (*ven'-ule*). A minute vein that collects blood from the capillaries.

verapamil (*ver-ap'-am-il*). A coronary dilator used in the treatment of supraventricular tachycardia and of angina pectoris.

verbigeration (*ver-bij-er-a'-shun*). The monotonous repetition of phrases. A disturbance of behaviour that may be present in schizophrenia.

vermicide (*ver'-me-side*). An agent which destroys intestinal worms; an anthelmintic.

vermiform (*ver'-me-form*). Worm-shaped. *V. appendix.* The worm-shaped structure attached to the caecum.

vermifuge (*ver'-me-fuje*). An agent which expels intestinal worms; an anthelmintic.

verminous (*ver'-min-us*). Infested with worms or other animal parasites, such as lice.

vermix (*ver'-miks*). The vermiform appendix.

vernix (*ver'-niks*). Varnish. *V.
caseosa.* The fatty covering
on the skin of the fetus during
the last months of pregnancy.
It consists of cells and
sebaceous material.

verruca (*ver-u'-kah*). A wart. A
localized hypertrophy of the
prickle cell layer of the
epidermis and thickening of
the horny layer. A virus is the
causative organism. *V. acumi-
nata.* A venereal wart that
appears on the external genitalia and may be associated
with gonorrhoea.

version (*ver'-shun*). The turning of a part; applied particularly to the turning of a fetus
in order to facilitate delivery.
External v. Manipulation of
the uterus through the abdominal wall in order to change
the position of the child. *Internal v.* Rotation of the fetus by
means of manipulation with
one hand in the vagina. *Podalic v.* Turning of the fetus so
that the head is uppermost
and the feet presenting. *Spontaneous v.* One that occurs
naturally without the application of force.

vertebra (*ver'-te-brah*). *pl.* vertebrae. One of the 33 irregular
bones forming the spinal column. They are divided into: 7
cervical, 12 *dorsal*, 5 *lumbar*, 5
sacral (sacrum), and 4 *coccygeal* (coccyx) vertebrae.

vertebral (*ver'-te-bral*). Pertaining to a vertebra. *V. column.*
The spine or backbone.

vertebrate (*ver'-te-brate*). Possessing a vertebral column.

vertebrobasilar (*ver-te-bro-
bas'-il-ar*). Pertaining to the
vertebral and the basilar arteries. *V. disease.* A condition
affecting the flow of blood

through the vertebral and
basilar arteries which causes
recurrent attacks of blindness,
diplopia, vertigo, dysarthria
and hemiparesis.

vertex (*ver'-teks*). The crown of
the head. *V. presentation.*
Position of the fetus such that
the crown of the head appears
in the vagina first.

vertigo (*ver'-tig-o*). A feeling of
rotation or of going round, in
either oneself or one's surroundings, particularly
associated with disease of the
cerebellum and the vestibular
nerve of the ear. It may occur
in diplopia or Ménière's syndrome.

vesica (*ves-i'-kah*). A bladder;
usually referring to the urinary bladder.

vesical (*ves'-ik-al*). Relating to
the urinary bladder.

vesicant (*ves'-ik-ant*). A blistering agent.

vesicle (*ves'-ikl*). (1) In anatomy, a small bladder usually
containing fluid. *Seminal v.*
One of a pair of sacs which
arise from the vas deferens
near the bladder and contain
semen. (2) A very small blister
usually containing serum.

vesico-ureteric (*ves-ik-o-u-re-
ter'-ik*). Relating to the urinary
bladder and the ureters. *V.
reflux.* The passing of urine
backwards up the ureter during micturition. A cause of
pyelonephritis in children.

vesicovaginal (*ves-ik-o-vaj-i'-
nal*). Relating to the bladder
and vagina. *See* Fistula.

vesicular (*ves-ik'-u-lar*). Relating to or containing vesicles.
V. breathing. The soft murmur of normal respiration, as
heard on auscultation. *V.
mole.* Hydatidiform mole.

vesiculitis (*ves-ik-u-li'-tis*). Inflammation of a vesicle, parti-

cularly the seminal vesicles.

vesiculopapular (*ves-ik-u-lo-pap'-u-lar*). Describing an eruption of both vesicles and papules.

vesiculopustular (*ves-ik-u-lo-pus'-tu-lar*). Describing an eruption of both vesicles and pustules.

vessel (*ves'-el*). A tube or canal for conveying fluid, usually blood or lymph.

vestibular (*ves-tib'-u-lar*). Relating to a vestibule. *V. glands.* Those in the vestibule of the vagina, including Bartholin's glands. *V. nerve.* A branch of the auditory nerve supplying the semicircular canals and concerned with balance and equilibrium.

vestibule (*ves'-tib-ule*). In anatomy, a space at the entrance to a canal. *V. of the ear.* The cavity at the entrance to the cochlea. *V. of the vagina.* The space between the labia minora at the entrance to the vagina.

vestibulocochlear (*ves-tib-u-lo-kok'-le-ah*). Pertaining to the vestibule of the ear and the cochlea. *V. nerve.* The eighth cranial nerve. Also known as the auditory nerve.

vestigial (*ves-tij'-e-al*). Rudimentary. Referring to the remains of an anatomical structure, which being of no further use has atrophied.

viable (*vi'-ab-l*). Capable of independent life. Applied to the fetus after 28 weeks of intra-uterine life.

Vibrio (*vib'-re-o*). A genus of gram-negative bacteria, curved and motile by means of flagellae. *Vibrio cholerae*, or *V. comma*, is that which causes cholera.

vicarious (*vi-ka'-re-us*). Substituted for another; used when one organ functions instead of another.

villus (*vil'-us*). *pl.* villi. A small finger-like process projecting from a surface. *Chorionic v. See* Chorionic. *Intestinal v.* Those of the mucous membrane of the small intestine, each of which contains a blood capillary and a lacteal.

vinblastine (*vin-blas'-teen*). A cytotoxic drug used in the treatment of lymphomas and of malignant teratomata.

Vincent's angina (*J.H. Vincent, French physician, 1862–1950*). *See* Angina.

vincristine (*vin-kris'-teen*). A cytotoxic drug used in the treatment of acute lympho-blastic leukaemia.

vinyl (*vi'-nil*). A plastic material now used extensively for medical equipment. *V. ether.* A short-acting inhalation anaesthetic drug used mainly for inducing anaesthesia and for minor surgery.

viraemia (*vi-re'-me-ah*). The presence of viruses in the blood.

viral (*vi'-ral*). Pertaining to a virus.

virilism (*vir'-il-izm*). Masculine traits exhibited by a female owing to the production of excessive amounts of androgenic hormone either in the adrenal cortex or from an ovarian tumour. *See* Arrheno-blastoma.

virology (*vi-rol'-o-je*). The scientific study of viruses, their growth and the diseases caused by them.

virulence (*vir'-u-lens*). The power of a micro-organism to produce toxins or poisons. In infection this depends on (1) the number and power of the invading organisms, and (2) the resistance of the patient.

virulent (*vir'-u-lent*). Dangerously poisonous.

virus (*vi'-rus*). One of a large number of minute microorganisms. They are smaller than bacteria and can be seen only with the aid of an electron microscope. They cause many diseases including influenza, chickenpox, mumps, measles, poliomyelitis and the common cold.

viscera (*vis'-er-ah*). *See* Viscus.

visceroptosis (*vis-er-op-to'-sis*). A general tendency to prolapse of the abdominal organs.

viscid (*vis'-id*). Sticky and glutinous.

viscosity (*vis-kos'-it-e*). Resistance to flowing. A sticky and glutinous quality.

viscus (*vis'-kus*). *pl.* viscera. Any of the organs contained in the body cavities, especially in the abdomen.

vision (*vish'-un*). The faculty of seeing. Sight.

visual (*viz'-u-al*). Relating to sight. *V. acuity.* Sharpness of vision. It is assessed by reading test types. *V. cells.* The rods and cones of the retina. *V. field.* The area within which objects can be seen when looking straight ahead. *V. purple.* The pigment in the outer layers of the retina. Rhodopsin.

vita glass (*vi'-tah glahs*). Quartz glass which is capable of transmitting ultra-violet rays of light.

vital (*vi'-tal*). Relating to life. *V. capacity.* The amount of air which can be expelled from the lungs after a full inspiration. *V. statistics.* The records kept of births and deaths among the population, including the causes of death, and the factors which seem to influence their rise and fall.

vitallium (*vi-tal'-e-um*). A metal alloy used in dentistry and for prostheses in bone surgery.

vitamin (*vit'-am-in*). Any of a group of accessory food factors which are contained in foodstuffs and are essential to life, growth, and reproduction.

vitellin (*vi-tel'-in*). The chief protein of egg yolk.

vitellus (*vi-tel'-us*). The yolk of an egg.

vitiligo (*vit-il-i'-go*). A skin disease marked by an absence of pigment, producing white patches on the face and body. Leucoderma.

vitrectomy (*vit-rek'-tom-e*). Surgical extraction of the vitreous humour and its replacement by a physiological solution in the treatment of vitreous haemorrhage following diabetic retinopathy.

vitreous (*vit'-re-us*). Glassy. *V. humour.* The transparent jelly-like substance filling the posterior of the eye, from lens to retina.

viviparous (*viv-ip'-ar-us*). Able to produce living young developed in the maternal body and not in the form of eggs.

vivisection (*viv-e-sek'-shun*). The use of living animals for experimental purposes. The procedures are carefully controlled by law and the animals are usually anaesthetized if surgery is being used.

VMA. Vanilmandelic acid. A metabolite of catecholamines which is excreted in small amounts in the urine. Excessive amounts of VMA in the urine may indicate that the patient has an adrenal medullary tumour.

vocal (*vo'-kal*). Pertaining to the voice or the organs which produce the voice. *V. cords.* The two folds of tissue in the larynx, formed of fibrous tissue covered with squamous epithelium. *V. resonance.* The normal sounds of speech heard through the chest wall by means of a stethoscope.

volatile (*vol'-at-ile*). Having a tendency to evaporate readily.

volition (*vo-lish'-un*). The conscious adoption by the individual of a line of action.

volitional (*vo-lish'-un-al*). Being impelled by will-power.

Volkmann's ischaemic contracture (*R. von Volkmann, German surgeon, 1830–1889*). Atrophy and fibrosis occurring in the muscles owing to an impaired blood supply. Usually applied to the upper limb when the brachial artery is compressed by a fracture of the lower end of the humerus.

volsella (*vol-sel'-ah*). A forceps the blades of which are tipped with claw-like hooks. Vulsella.

volt (*volt*). *abbrev.* V. The SI unit of electromotive force.

voltmeter (*volt'-me-ter*). An instrument for measuring an electromotive force.

volume (*vol'-ume*). The space occupied by a substance. *Minute v.* The total volume of air breathed in or out in 1 minute. *Packed cell v.* That occupied by the blood cells after centrifuging—about 45% of the blood sample. *Residual v.* The amount of air left in the lungs after breathing out fully.

voluntary (*vol'-un-tar-e*). Under the control of the will. *See* Involuntary.

volvulus (*vol'-vu-lus*). Twisting of a part of the intestine, causing obstruction. Most common in the sigmoid colon.

vomer (*vo'-mer*). A thin plate of bone forming the posterior septum of the nose.

vomit (*vom'-it*). (1) *n.* Matter ejected from the stomach through the mouth. (2) *v.* To eject material in this way. *Bilious v.* Vomit mixed with bile. The vomit is stained yellow or green. *Coffee-ground v.* Ejected matter that contains small quantities of altered blood, which has this appearance. *Faecal* or *stercoraceous v.* Vomit mixed with faeces. Occurs in intestinal obstruction when the contents of the upper intestine regurgitate back into the stomach. It is dark brown with an unpleasant odour.

vomiting (*vom'-it-ing*). A reflex act of expulsion of the stomach contents via the oesophagus and mouth. It may be preceded by nausea and excess salivation if the cause is local irritation in the stomach. *Cyclical v.* Recurrent attacks of vomiting often occurring in children and associated with acidosis. *Projectile v.* The forcible ejection of the gastric contents, usually without warning. Present in hypertrophic pyloric stenosis, and in cerebral diseases. *V. of pregnancy.* Vomiting occurring in the early months of pregnancy. Morning sickness.

vulnerability (*vul-ner-ab-il'-it-e*). Weakness. Susceptibility to injury or infection.

vulsella (*vul-sel'-ah*). Volsella.

vulva (*vul'-vah*). The external female genital organs.

vulvectomy (*vul-vek'-tom-e*). Excision of the vulva.

vulvitis (*vul-vi'-tis*). Inflammation of the vulva.

vulvovaginitis (*vul-vo-vaj-in-i'-tis*). Inflammation of the vulva and vagina.

W

W. Abbreviation for the SI unit, the *watt*.

wafer (*wa'-fer*). A thin double layer of flour paste sometimes used to enclose a dose of medicinal powder. A cachet.

Waldeyer's ring (*H.W.G. von Waldeyer-Hartz, German anatomist, 1836–1921*). The circle of lymphoid tissue in the pharynx formed by the lingual, faucial, and pharyngeal tonsils.

Wangensteen tube (*O.H. Wangensteen, American surgeon, b. 1898*). A gastrointestinal aspiration tube with a tip that is opaque to X-rays.

warfarin (*wor'-far-in*). An oral anticoagulant drug that depresses the prothrombin level. Used mainly in the treatment of coronary and venous thrombosis.

wart (*wort*). An elevation of the skin, which is often of a brownish colour, caused by hypertrophy of papillae in the dermis, usually due to a virus infection. *Plantar w's.* Large warts occurring on the soles of the feet and causing much discomfort. *See* Verruca *and* Condyloma.

Wassermann reaction (*A.P. von Wassermann, German bacteriologist, 1866–1925*). A method of testing the blood serum of a patient to aid in the diagnosis of syphilis.

water (*waw'-ter*). A clear, colourless, tasteless liquid composed of hydrogen and oxygen (H_2O). *W. balance.* Fluid balance. That between the fluid taken in by all routes (oral, intravenous and rectal) and the fluid lost by all routes (urine, vomit or drainage from

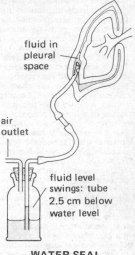

fluid in pleural space

air outlet

fluid level swings: tube 2.5 cm below water level

WATER-SEAL DRAINAGE

any body cavity). *W.-borne.* Descriptive of certain diseases that are spread by contaminated water. *W-brash.* The eructation of dilute acid from the stomach to the pharynx, giving a burning sensation. Pyrosis. Heartburn. *W.-seal drainage.* A closed method of drainage from the pleural space allowing the escape of fluid and air but preventing air entering as the drainage tube discharges under water.

Waterhouse–Friderichsen syndrome (*R. Waterhouse, British physician, 1873–1958; C. Friderichsen, Danish physician, b. 1886*). Peripheral vascular collapse which occurs in meningococcal septicaemia. It is the result of adrenal haemorrhage and is usually seen in children.

Waterston's operation (*D. Waterston, British paediatric surgeon, b. 1910*). A palliative operation of anastomosis of the right pulmonary artery to the ascending aorta. Used in the treatment of tricuspid atresia in the young child.

Watson–Crick hypothesis (*J.D. Watson, American geneticist, b. 1928; F. Crick, British biochemist, b. 1916*). Hypothesis proposed by Watson and Crick, who were awarded the Nobel Prize in 1962, to describe the structure of the DNA molecule as a double helix.

watt (*wot*). *abbrev*. W. The SI unit of power, equal to 1 joule per second.

wave (*wave*). A uniform advancing undulation. *Electromagnetic w's*. The entire range of waves, including light waves, in the ether. They all move with the speed of light but are differentiated by wide variations in wavelength.

wavelength (*wave'-length*). The measurement from the crest of one wave to the crest of the next one. Applied to the electromagnetic spectrum, the longest are radio waves and the shortest are X-rays and gamma rays.

wax (*waks*). In pharmacy, *beeswax*, used for making ointments. *Ear-w. See* Cerumen. *Bone w*. An aseptic form used for stopping bleeding from bone, especially whilst performing operations on the skull.

waxy flexibility (*wak'-se flek-*

sib-il'-it-e). A cataleptic state in which a patient's limbs are held indefinitely in any position in which they have been placed. *See* Catatonia.

weal (*weel*). A raised stripe on the skin, as is caused by the lash of a whip. Typical of urticaria.

weaning (*ween'-ing*). The change from breast or bottle to normal feeding. It should be effected gradually from about the fourth month.

webbing (*web'-ing*). The state of being connected by a membrane or a fold of skin. *W. of hands or feet*. Congenital abnormality in which the digits are not separated from each other. Syndactyly. *W. of neck*. Folds of skin in the neck, giving it a webbed appearance. Occurs in certain congenital conditions, e.g. Turner's syndrome.

Weber's test (*F.E. Weber-Liel, German otologist, 1832–1891*). A test for hearing. A vibrating tuning fork is held in the centre of the forehead. Sound is normally heard equally in both ears. If the sound is heard louder in one ear it may be indicative of conductive deafness in that ear.

Weil's disease (*A. Weil, German physician, 1848–1916*). Spirochaetal jaundice. The organism, *Leptospira icterohaemorrhagiae*, is harboured and excreted by rats and enters through a bite or skin abrasion, or infected food or water.

Weil–Felix reaction (*E. Weil, Austrian physician, 1880–1922; A Felix, Czech bacteriologist, 1887–1956*). An agglutination test of blood serum used in the diagnosis of typhus.

Welch's bacillus (*W.H. Welch, American pathologist, 1850–1934*). *Clostridium welchii*, the organism most usually found in gas gangrene. *See* Clostridium.

wen (*wen*). A small sebaceous cyst. A steatoma.

Wenckebach's phenomenon (*K.F. Wenckebach, Dutch physician, 1864–1940*). Abnormal heart rhythm in which the P–R interval gradually increases until a beat is missed.

Werdnig–Hoffmann disease (*G. Werdnig, Austrian neurologist, b. 1862; J.E. Hoffmann, German neurologist, 1857–1919*). Disease characterized by progressive spinal muscular atrophy affecting the shoulder, neck, pelvis and eventually the respiratory muscles of infants.

Werner's syndrome (*C.W.O. Werner, German physician*). A hereditary condition characterized by cataracts, osteoporosis, stunted growth and premature greying of the hair.

Wernicke's encephalopathy (*K. Wernicke, German neurologist, 1848–1905*). A neurological condition due to vitamin B$_1$ deficiency. Untreated it progresses from mental confusion and double vision to lethargy and coma. It is most commonly seen in chronic alcoholism.

Wertheim's operation (*E. Wertheim, Austrian gynaecologist, 1864–1920*). See Hysterectomy.

Wharton's duct (*T. Wharton, British physician, 1614–1673*). The duct of the submandibular gland.

Wharton's jelly. The connective tissue of the umbilical cord.

wheeze (*hweez*). To breathe with difficulty, producing a hoarse whistling sound.

whiplash injury (*hwip'-lash in'-jur-e*). Injury to the spinal cord, nerve roots, ligaments or vertebrae in the cervical region due to a sudden jerking back of the head and neck. Common in road traffic accidents where there is sudden acceleration or deceleration of the vehicle.

Whipple's operation (*A.O. Whipple, American surgeon, 1881–1963*). Radical pancreoduodenectomy performed for

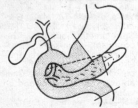
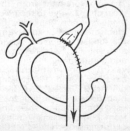

WHIPPLE'S OPERATION

carcinoma of the head of the pancreas. Most of the pancreas, the pylorus, duodenum and the common bile duct are excised. Gastrojejunostomy is performed with anastomosis of the tail of the pancreas and gall-bladder to the jejunum.

whipworm (*hwip'-werm*). *See* Trichuris.

white leg (*hwite leg*). Milk leg. *See* Phlegmasia.

Whitfield's ointment (*A. Whitfield, British dermatologist, 1868–1947*). Compound ointment of benzoic acid used in the treatment of fungal diseases.

whitlow (*hwit'-lo*). A felon. A suppurating inflammation of a finger near the nail. *Subperiosteal w.* One in which the infection involves the bone covering. *Superficial w.* A pustule between the true skin and cuticle. *See* Paronychia.

whooping cough (*hoop'-ing kof*). Pertussis. An acute infectious disease usually occurring in children, characterized by acute respiratory catarrh, with paroxysms of coughing. These terminate with a long-drawn noisy inspiration giving the typical *whoop.*

Widal reaction (*G.F.I. Widal, French physician, 1862–1929*). A blood agglutination test for typhoid fever. Sufficient antibodies are usually present from the second week to confirm diagnosis.

von Willebrand's disease (*E.A. von Willebrand, Finnish physician*). A form of non-thrombocytopenic purpura in which there is a deficiency in blood clotting.

Wilms' tumour (*M. Wilms, German surgeon, 1867–1918*). A highly malignant tumour of the kidney occurring in young children. A nephroblastoma.

Wilson's disease (*S.A.K. Wilson, British neurologist, 1878–1937*). Hepatolenticular degeneration. A congenital abnormality in the metabolism of copper leading to neurological degeneration. A brown ring appears at the outer edge of the cornea.

windpipe (*wind'-pipe*). The trachea.

wiring (*wi'-ring*). The fixing together of a broken or split bone by the use of a wire. Commonly used for the jaw, the patella and the sternum.

wisdom teeth (*wiz'-dom teeth*). The back molar teeth, the appearance of which is often delayed until maturity.

wish fulfilment (*wish ful-fil'-ment*). A desire, not always acknowledged consciously by the person, which is fulfilled through dreams or by daydreaming.

witch hazel (*wich ha'-zl*). Hamamelis.

withdrawal (*with-draw'-al*). In psychology, a defence mechanism in which an individual turns into himself and away from the world. *W. bleeding.* Bleeding that occurs from the uterus following the cessation of giving oestrogens for therapeutic reasons. *W. symptoms.* Symptoms which occur when drugs or alcohol are withdrawn from those who are dependent upon them. These may include nausea, tremor and hallucinations.

Wolff–Parkinson–White syndrome (*L. Wolff, American cardiologist, b. 1898; Sir J. Parkinson, British physician, 1885–1976; P.D. White, American cardiologist, 1886–1973*). Abnormal heart rhythm caused by an accessory bundle between the atria and ventricles. A congenital disorder.

wolffian body (K.F. Wolff, German anatomist, 1733–1794). One of two small organs in the embryo, representing the primitive kidneys. A mesonephros.

womb (woom). The uterus.

Wood's light (R.W. Wood, American physicist, 1868–1953). Ultra-violet light transmitted through a filter glass containing nickel oxide. It produces fluorescence of infected hairs when placed over a scalp affected with ringworm.

woolsorter's disease (wool'-sor-terz diz-eez'). Pulmonary anthrax.

word blindness (werd bli'-ndnes). See Dyslexia.

word salad (werd sal'-ad). Rapid speech in which the words are strung together without meaning.

worm (werm). Any one of a number of groups of long soft-bodied invertebrates, some of which are parasitic to man.

wound (woond). A cut or break in continuity of any tissue, caused by injury or operation. It is classified according to its nature, as follows: Abrased w. The skin is scraped off, but there is no deeper injury. Aseptic w. A non-infected one. Contused w. With bruising of the surrounding tissue. Incised w. Usually the result of operation, and produced by a knife or similar instrument. The edges of the wound can remain in apposition, and it should heal by first intention. Lacerated w. One with torn edges and tissues, usually the result of accident or injury. It

is often septic and heals by second intention. Open w. A gaping wound on the body surface. Penetrating w. Often made by gunshot, shrapnel, etc. There may be an inlet and outlet hole and vital organs are often penetrated by the missile. Punctured w. Made by a pointed or spiked instrument. Septic w. Any type into which infection has been introduced, causing suppurative inflammation. It heals by second intention. See Healing.

wrist (rist). The joint of the carpus and bones of the forearm. W. drop. Loss of power in the muscles of the hand. It may be due to nerve or tendon injury, but can result from lack of sufficient support by splint or sling.

writer's cramp (ri'-terz kramp). A colloquial term for painful spasm of the hand and forearm, caused by excessive writing and poor posture.

wry-neck (ri'-nek). See Torticollis.

Wuchereria (vook-er-eer'-e-ah). A genus of nematode worms which are the principal vectors of filariasis. W. bancrofti is the most common species in tropical and subtropical areas.

X

xanthelasma (zan-thel-az'-mah). A disease marked by the formation of flat or slightly raised yellow patches on the eyelids. Most frequently seen in the middle-aged and elderly.

xanthine (zan'-theen). A compound found in plant and animal tissues, the forerunner of uric acid in nucleoprotein metabolism.

xanthochromia (*zan-tho-kro'-me-ah*). (1) The presence of yellow patches on the skin. (2) The yellow colouring of cerebrospinal fluid seen in patients who have had a subarachnoid haemorrhage.

xanthoma (*zan-tho'-mah*). *pl.* xanthomata. The presence in the skin of flat areas of yellowish pigmentation due to deposits of lipoids. There are several varieties. *X. palpebrarum.* Xanthelasma.

xanthopsia (*zan-thop'-se-ah*). A disturbance of vision in which all objects appear yellow.

xanthosis (*zan-tho'-sis*). A yellow skin pigmentation, seen in some cases of diabetes and poliomyelitis.

X-chromosome (*eks-kro'-mo-some*). The female sex chromosome, being present in all female gametes and only half the male gametes. When union takes place two X-c's result in a female child (*XX*) but one of each results in a male child (*XY*). *See* Y-chromosome.

Xe. Chemical symbol for *xenon.*

xenograft (*zen'-o-graft*). A tissue graft between animals of different species. A heterograft.

xenon (*zen'-on*). *abbrev.* Xe. An inert gaseous element. *Radioactive x.* [133]Xe. In solution it is used in regional blood flow clearance tests. Also used in gaseous form in lung ventilation studies.

xenophobia (*zen-o-fo'-be-ah*). An unreasoning dislike of strangers and foreigners.

Xenopsylla (*zen-op-sil'-ah*). A genus of fleas, some of which are vectors of plague. *X. cheopis.* The rat flea, which transmits bubonic plague.

xeroderma (*zer-o-der'-mah*). An hereditary condition in which there is excessive dryness of the skin. A mild form of ichthyosis. *X. pigmentosum.* A rare hereditary and often fatal disease in which there is extreme sensitivity of the skin and eyes to light. It begins in childhood and rapidly progresses. The formation of malignant neoplasms is common.

xerography (*zer-og'-raf-e*). Radiography using selenium-coated metal plates. This is a rapid method and it provides a clear image of the soft tissue structures. It is used primarily in X-ray examination of the female breast.

xerophthalmia (*zer-off-thal'-me-ah*). A condition in which the cornea and conjunctiva become horny and necrosed owing to a deficiency of vitamin A. Xeroma.

xerosis (*zer-o'-sis*). A condition in which the conjunctiva appears dry and lustreless. Small white patches of horny epithelium appear on the cornea (*Bitôt's spots*).

xerostomia (*zer-o-sto'-me-ah*). Dryness of the mouth due to a failure of the salivary glands.

xiphoid (*zif'-oid*). Sword-shaped. *X. cartilage* or *x. process.* The lowest part of the sternum.

X-rays (*eks-raze*). Röntgen rays. Electromagnetic waves of short length which are capable of penetrating many substances and of producing chemical changes and reactions in living matter. They are used both to aid diagnosis and to treat disease.

xylene (*zi'-lene*). Xylol. Dimethylbenzene. A clear inflammable liquid resembling benzene. Used as a solvent for rubber and in microscopy.

xylose (*zi'-lose*). A pentose sugar found in connective tissue and sometimes in urine, which is not metabolized in the body.

XYY syndrome (*eks-wi-wi sin'-drome*). An extremely rare condition in males in which there is an extra Y chromosome, making a total of 47 in each body cell. Often the affected individuals are very tall and liable to exhibit aggressive and antisocial behavioural patterns.

tion of alcoholic solutions such as beer and wines.

yellow fever (*yel'-o fe'-ver*). An acute infectious disease of the tropics caused by a virus and transmitted by a mosquito (*Aëdes aegypti*). The virus attacks the liver and kidney and the symptoms include rigor, headache, pain in the back and limbs, high fever and black vomit. Haemorrhage from the intestinal mucous membrane may occur. There is a high mortality rate.

yttrium (*it'-re-um*). *abbrev.* Y. An element used as radioactive yttrium (^{90}Y) in the treatment of malignant effusions.

Y

Y. Chemical symbol for *yttrium.*

yawning (*yawn'-ing*). An involuntary act in which the mouth is opened wide and air is drawn in and exhaled. It may accompany tiredness or boredom.

yaws (*yawz*). Framboesia. A skin infection common in tropical countries caused by *Treponema pertenue.* It is not a venereal disease but it is associated with dirt and poverty.

Y-chromosome (*wi-kro'-mo-some*). The male sex chromosome, being present in half the male gametes and none of the female. It carries few major genes. *See* X-chromosome.

yeast (*ye'-st*). Any of the fungi of the genus *Saccharomyces.* They produce fermentation in malt, and in sweetened fruit juices, resulting in the forma-

Z

zein (*ze'-in*). Maize protein.

zero (*ze'-ro*). Nought. Nothing. The point on any scale from which measurements start.

Ziehl–Neelsen's method (*F. Ziehl, German bacteriologist, 1857–1926; F.K.A. Neelsen, 1854–1894*). A method of staining tubercle bacilli for microscopic study.

zinc (*zink*). *abbrev.* Zn. A bluish-white metallic element. *Z. ointment.* An emollient dressing.

Zn. Chemical symbol for *zinc.*

Zollinger–Ellison syndrome (*R.M. Zollinger, American physician, b. 1903; E.H. Ellison, American physician, 1918–1970*). A rare condition in which a pancreatic tumour causes excessive outpouring of gastric juice. Peptic ulcers may occur.

zona (*zo'-nah*). (1) A zone. *Z. pellucida.* The membrane surrounding the ovum. (2)

Herpes zoster. Shingles. *Z. facialis.* Herpes of the face.

zonula (*zo'-nu-lah*). A zonule. In anatomy, a small usually circular area. *Ciliary z.* The area surrounded by the suspensory ligaments of the eye.

zonular (*zo'-nu-lar*). Pertaining to a zonule. *Z. fibres.* The suspensory ligaments that suspend the lens behind the iris.

zonulolysis (*zo-nu-lol'-is-is*). Dissolving of the zonular fibres by zonulysin to aid cataract extraction.

zonulysin (*zo-nu-li'-sin*). A proteolytic enzyme that may be used in eye surgery to dissolve the suspensory ligament.

zoology (*zo-ol'-o-je*). The science of animals.

zoonosis (*zo-o-no'-sis*). A disease of animals that is transmissible to man, e.g. anthrax, cat-scratch fever, etc.

zoster (*zos'-ter*). *See* Herpes.

Z-plasty (*zed'-plas-te*). A plastic operation for removing and repairing deformity resulting from a contraction scar.

zygoma (*zi-go'-mah*). The arch formed by the union of the temporal with the malar bone in front of the ear.

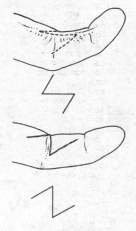

Z-PLASTY

zygote (*zi'-got*). A single fertilized cell formed from the union of a male and a female gamete.

zymosis (*zi-mo'-sis*). (1) Fermentation. (2) The development of an infectious disease.

REFERENCE SECTION

1
PREFIXES AND SUFFIXES

a-, an-	not, without	cheir-, chir-	hand
ab-	away from	chlor-	green
acr-	extremity, peak	chol-	bile
ad-	towards	chondr-	cartilage
aden-	gland	chrom-	colour
adip-	fat	-cide	killing
-aemia	blood	cine-, kine-	motion
aer-	air	-cle	small
-aesthesia	sensation	co-, col-,	together, with
-algia	pain	com- con-,	
amyl-	starch	colp-	vagina
ana-	up	contra-	against, counter
andr-	male	cortic-	bark, rind
angi-	(blood) vessel	cost-	rib
ante-	before, in front	cox-	hip
anti-	against	crani-	skull
apo-	away, from	cryo-	cold
arthr-	joint	crypt-	hidden, concealed
-asis	state of	cyan-	blue
aut-	self	cyst-	bladder
bi-, bis-	two	cyt-	cell
bil-	bile	-cyte	cell
bio-	life	dacry-	tear
blast-	bud	dactyl-	finger
blephar-	eyelid	de-	down, from
brachi-	arm	dec-	ten
brachy-	short	demi-	half
brady-	slow	dent-	tooth
bronch-	windpipe	derm-	skin
calc-	chalk	-desis	binding
carcin-	cancer	dextr-	right
card-	heart	di-, diplo-	two, double
carp-	wrist	dia-	through
cata-, kata-	down, negative	dis-	apart, away from
cav-	hollow	dors-	back
-cele	swelling	dys-	difficult, abnormal
cent-	hundred	ect-	outside
-centesis	piercing	-ectasis	stretching
cephal-	head	-ectomy	cutting out
cerebr-	brain	em-, en-,	in, inside, within
cervic-	neck	end-, ent-	
cheil-, chil-	lip	enter-	intestine

epi-	upon, over	medi-	middle
erythr-	red	megal-	large
eu-	good, normal	-megaly	enlargement
ex-, exo-	out of	melan-	black
extra-	outside	meso-	middle
faci-	face	meta-	after
-facient	making	metr-	uterus
flav-	yellow	micr-	small
galact-	milk	milli-	thousand
gastr-	stomach	mono-	single
-genic	producing	-morph	form
ger-	old age	muco-	mucus
gloss-	tongue	multi-	many
glyc-	sweet	myc-	fungus
gnath-	jaw	myel-	marrow
-gram	tracing	myo-	muscle
-graph	tracing	narc-	numb
gynae-	female	naso-	nose
haem-	blood	necr-	corpse
hemi-	half	neo-	new
hepat-	liver	nephr-	kidney
hex-	six	neur-	nerve
hist-	tissue, web	ocul-	eye
hom-	same, like	odont-	tooth
hydr-	water	-odynia	pain
hyper-	above	-oid	like
hypno-	sleep	oligo-	few
hypo-	below	-ology	study
hyster-	womb	-oma	tumour
-ia, -iasis	state, condition	onc-	mass
idi-	peculiar, distinct	onych-	nail
infra-	below	oö-	egg
inter-	between	ophthalm-	eye
intra-	within	-opsy	looking
intro-	inwards	or-	mouth
iso-	equal	orchid-	testis
-itis	inflammation of	orth-	straight
kary-	nut, nucleus	os-	mouth
kerat-	horn, cornea	os-, oste-	bone
-kinesis,	motion	-osis	pathological state
-kinetic		-ostomy	opening
lact-	milk	ot-	ear
laryng-	windpipe	-otomy	cutting
later-	side	ovi-	egg
leuc-, leuk-	white	pachy-	thick
-lith	stone	paed-	child
-lysis	destruction	pan-	all
macr-	large	para-	beside, beyond
mal-	bad, abnormal	path-	suffering, disease
-malacia	softening	-pathy	disease
mamm-	breast	-penia	lack
mast-	breast	pent-	five

per-	through	sclero-	hard
peri-	around	-scope	viewing instrument
-pexy	fixing	-scopy	looking
-phagia	swallowing	semi-	half
pharmac-	drug	sept-	seven
-phasia	speech	-sonic	sound
phleb-	vein	sphygm-	pulse
-phobia	irrational fear	splen-	spleen
phon-	sound	spondy-	vertebra
photo-	light	steat-	fat
phren-	diaphragm, mind	sub-	below
-phylaxis	prevention, protection	super-, supra-	above
physi-	form, nature	syn-	with
-plegia	paralysis	tachy-	quick
pneum-	lung	tars-	eyelid, instep
pod-	foot	-taxia, -taxis	arrangement, order
-poiesis	formation	tetra-	four
poly-	many	therm-	heat
post-	after	thorac-	chest
prae-, pre-, pro-	before, in front	thromb-	clot
proct-	anus	-tome	cutting instrument
pseud-	false	toxic-	poison
psych-	mind	trans-	through, across
pyo-	pus, matter	tri-	three
pyr-	fire, fever	trich-	hair
quadr-	four	troph-	nourishment
quint-	five	-tropy	turning
radi-	ray	tympano-	middle ear
re-	back, again	ultra-	beyond
ren-	kidney	uni-	one
retro-	backwards	uri-	urine
rhin-	nose	-uria	urine
-rrhoea	discharge	vas-	vessel
-rrhaphy	repair	xanth-	yellow
rub-	red	xero-	dry
salping-	(uterine) tube	zoo-	animal
sarc-	flesh		

FIRST AID AND BANDAGING

FIRST AID

Nurses are not usually very knowledgeable about first aid, owing mainly to the fact that they rarely have to use the skills involved. In an emergency, however, valuable time can be saved, and further injury to the victim prevented, if the nurse or helper can quickly assess the situation and has a good knowledge of priorities and the most efficient treatment.

Medical assistance should be obtained as soon as possible and the helper should remember that only the minimum of treatment can be administered at the scene of an accident.

Unconsciousness

Unconsciousness may be due to many different causes, such as asphyxia, trauma, shock or poisoning, but in all cases the first two conditions to be treated are cessation of breathing and cessation of heartbeat. The helper should note if there is continuing danger from fire, fumes, electric current or traffic and eliminate the source or remove the patient from it.

Next make sure the airway is clear by loosening constrictive clothing and clearing the mouth with the fingers; tilt the head backwards and draw the jaw forward. If breathing is established, place the patient in the semi-prone position (Fig. 1) and continue

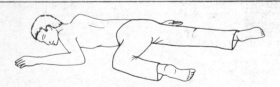

Fig. 1. The semi-prone position. The head is tilted slightly forward and no cushion is used.

to observe him closely. Should breathing not resume immediately, expired air artificial respiration must be started without delay. Full details are given and illustrated on pp. 439 and 440.

After artificial respiration has been started by breathing into the patient's lungs three times, the pulse must be felt (Fig. 2) in order to establish whether the heart is beating and, if it is not, external

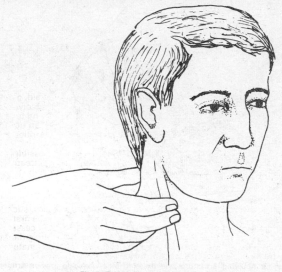

Fig. 2. Taking the carotid pulse.

cardiac massage must be begun. Full details of this are given on pp. 441–443.

Once the heart is beating and respiration has been established other measures can be taken.

Haemorrhage

External bleeding

When the bleeding is visible, examine the wound to see whether any cause, such as projecting metal or glass, can be seen. When there is danger that either may still be present in the wound, the area should be lightly covered with a clean cloth or first aid dressing (Fig. 3) while pressure, for not longer than 15 minutes, is applied to the artery proximal to the injury. In the event of a stab wound, take whatever measures may be necessary to resuscitate the patient, but do not remove the knife, as profuse bleeding may occur. Should a fracture be present or suspected, the same treatment is applied, followed by fracture treatment as described on pp. 443 and 444.

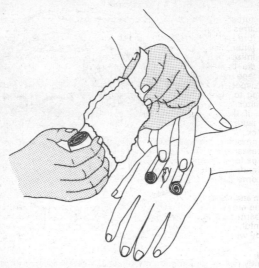

Fig. 3. Applying an improvised dressing to a wound to prevent further damage from an embedded fragment.

In other cases of bleeding from a wound apply a firm pad and bandage over the wound and apply direct pressure with the fingers for 5 to 15 minutes. With a large wound area press the sides of the wound firmly but gently together. If a limb is involved elevate the part. If the bleeding has been severe or shock is present treat as described below.

Internal bleeding

The signs of haemorrhage are an increasing pulse rate, pallor and deep sighing respirations. The patient will be restless and anxious and may complain of thirst, a feeling of faintness and blurred vision. This patient is in a state of shock due to depletion of circulating blood and the helper must treat this and at the same time send for a doctor.

Whilst waiting for medical aid, reassure and calm the patient. Lay him flat with the head low. Cover him, but do not apply heat and give nothing by mouth. Record the pulse and respiration every 15 minutes.

Fractures

Fractures may be either closed, simple fractures or compound fractures in which there is communication between the site of the fracture and the air through either the skin or a mucous surface. In the latter case the risk of infection entering the wound must be minimized and in treating any fractures the first aid worker must handle the injured part with great care in order that further damage may not be done.

Suspected fractures should be treated as fractures without trying to elicit signs of fracture such as unnatural mobility and crepitus. Cover any wound with as clean a dressing as is available and if there is much bleeding apply pressure to the arterial pressure point proximal to the wound. Give the treatment for shock.

Immobilize the fracture by moving the injured part as little as is necessary. Untrained workers are advised to use the body and slings for immobilizing the part.

Bandages should be checked every 15 minutes as they may become too tight owing to swelling of the injured tissues.

Arm and shoulder

If the elbow can be flexed without increasing the pain, place the forearm across the chest and apply a sling. Should flexion be too painful, use a broad bandage or scarf and tie the arm against the body with the palm facing inwards.

Leg

Gently pull the uninjured limb to rest against the injured one and place pads or a padded splint between the legs. With scarves or bandages tie the feet and knees together or the legs above and below the site of fracture, putting no pressure on the fracture. If it is necessary to move the injured limb, apply and maintain gentle traction until the two limbs have been tied together.

Pelvis

A broad folded cloth may be placed around the pelvis to give support or just keep the patient flat. As the bladder or urethra may be damaged ask the patient to try not to pass urine.

Spine

When there is a suspected injury to the spine do not move the patient until there is a stretcher available and a sufficient number of helpers. The whole body must be lifted or turned in unison with two of the team exerting slight traction on the head and feet. Place pads on the stretcher for the neck, lumbar curve, and ankles, and transport the patient in the dorsal position.

Skull

Lay the patient down and record the pulse every 15 minutes. Observe the condition of the eyes and pupils and note whether there is any bleeding or fluid discharge from the ears or nose. If the patient is unconscious, treat as described on p. 438. Facial injuries may necessitate the Holger–Nielsen method of artificial respiration (p. 439 and 441).

Patients suffering from fractures should be removed to hospital as quickly and gently as possible. Rough handling will greatly increase the degree of shock.

Road Accidents

Only remove the injured person (whether in a vehicle or on the roadway) if he is in danger, e.g. from fire or oncoming traffic. Unnecessary movement may worsen the injuries.

Send for help and whilst waiting, carry out the following as required in descending order:

- Treat asphyxia (p. 438)
- Treat cardiac arrest (pp. 441–443).
- Arrest haemorrhage (pp. 431–432).
- Keep the patient calm
- Immobilize fractures (p. 433)
- Cleanse and cover wounds

Poisoning

Take a quick note of the surroundings to establish the cause of the poisoning if possible and send for medical aid, stating the drug if known. If the patient is unconscious, notice whether he is breathing and whether his pulse can be felt. Should these signs be absent, follow the instructions on pp. 438–443. If respiration and circulation are present or restored but the patient is unconscious, no attempt must be made to make him vomit and no stomach washout should be carried out until medical aid is present.

Corrosive poisoning
The lips may be stained grey or yellowish and the patient may have a burning pain in the mouth and throat, denoting that a corrosive has been taken. Do not make the patient vomit, but give demulcent drinks such as milk or egg white to soothe and dilute the poison. If an acid has been taken it can be neutralized by magnesium oxide or other mild alkali, and an alkaline poison by giving diluted vinegar (100 ml to 0.5 litre of water).

Non-corrosive poisoning
When the poison taken is non-corrosive and the patient is conscious try to establish the substance taken—do not give an emetic or try to make the patient vomit. Seek the assistance of the emergency services and transfer the patient to hospital immediately.

Aspirin
Should the cause be aspirin or iron tablets an emetic may be given as a first aid measure before transport to hospital.

Barbiturates
Barbiturates and tranquillizers are commonly consumed poisons and the danger of overdosage is greatly increased if taken at the same time as alcohol. Drowsiness may cause accidental over-dosage if the container is by the bedside.

Inhalation of poisonous gas
Where possible turn off the gas and remove the patient to the fresh air or an open window. Loosen tight clothing and begin artificial respiration and cardiac massage if required (pp. 438 –443).

Hospital care
Patients suffering from poisoning need the facilities available in hospital for their treatment and there should be no delay in transporting them there, guarding against shock and respiratory failure in transit.

Poisons Information Centres
National Poisons Information Centres have been set up from which a doctor may obtain advice in a case where he is in doubt about the correct treatment for a particular drug. There are five national and three regional centres altogether and their addresses are as follows:

National centres

London
Poisons Reference Service
New Cross Hospital
Avonley Road
London SE14 5ER
Tel. 01-407 7600

Edinburgh
Scottish Poisons Information
 Bureau
The Royal Infirmary
Lauriston Place
Edinburgh EH3 9YW
Tel. 031-229 2477

Belfast
Poisons Information Centre
Casualty Department
Royal Victoria Hospital
Grosvenor Road
Belfast BT12 6BA
Tel. 0232-40503

Cardiff
Poisons Information Centre
c/o Medical Records Depart-
 ment
Cardiff Royal Infirmary
Cardiff
South Glamorgan
Tel. 0222-569200

Dublin
Poisons Information Centre
Jarvis Street Hospital
Dublin
Tel. Dublin 745588

Regional centres
Birmingham
West Midlands Regional
 Poisons Unit
Dudley Road Hospital
Dudley Road
Birmingham B18 7QH
Tel. 021-554 3801

Newcastle
Newcastle A.H.A. (Teaching)
Central Sector
Royal Victoria Infirmary
Queen Victoria Road
Newcastle-upon-Tyne   NE14
1LT
Tel. 0632 325131

Leeds
The Leeds Poisons Information
 Centre
Leeds General Infirmary
Great George Street
Leeds LS1 3EX
Tel. 0532 430715 *or* 0532 43299

Burns

Extinguish burning clothing by smothering the flames with a rug
or coat. Reassure and calm the patient and relatives while im-
mersing the burnt part in cold water if feasible. Do not remove
adherent burnt clothing but cover the area with a freshly laun-
dered cotton article. Treat the patient for shock and transfer him to
hospital as quickly as possible.

Chemical burns
To remove the chemical, wash the burnt area by flooding the part
thoroughly with gallons of water to which a neutralizing agent
may be added. Use slowly running water, ensuring that it drains
away freely and safely. Remove contaminated clothing if possible
at the same time. Treat an acid burn with a solution of sodium
bicarbonate and a corrosive alkali burn with weak vinegar or
lemon juice. Speed in treatment is essential: if obtaining the
correct antidote would entail loss of time, the use of plain water is
to be preferred; this particularly applies to splash injuries to the
eye.

Scalds
Remove clothing if possible as this will retain the heat from the
hot liquid. Run cold water over the scalded area in order to
minimize the severity of the injury.

BANDAGING

Bandages are being used less but they still have a place in
nursing. At the present time a wide choice of bandages is on the
market and in deciding which bandage to use the nurse should
consider the purpose for which it is to be applied, the comfort of
the patient and the cost of the bandage. The following are some
examples:

Roller Bandages

White openwove
The traditional bandage, which is used when a light bandage is
required, and is normally discarded after use.

Domette

Domette is a mixture of cotton and wool. It is a strong bandage and may be used to apply pressure following an operation on the knee. A pressure bandage in this case consists of alternate layers of wool and bandage. It is a useful material for making up into many-tailed and T bandages, for making a collar and cuff sling, and for dressing a Thomas's or Braun's splint.

Crêpe

This is an elasticated cotton bandage which has the advantage of conforming to body contours and giving a measure of support. It is useful as a head bandage following mastoidectomy or enuclea-tion of the eye. It may also be used as a chest bandage following mastectomy or for the legs when a degree of pressure is required to aid venous return or to prevent oedema.

Elastic web

This bandage is often referred to as a blue- or red-line bandage from the coloured line appearing throughout its length. It is a strongly supporting bandage and is used on the lower limb for the treatment of varicose ulcers.

Rayon elastic

This has more elasticity than the plain crêpe and is advocated for application to amputation stumps to aid healing with the forma-tion of a good firm stump by preventing oedema.

Conforming bandage

This is a very light bandage of fine cotton mesh and is particularly useful when a dressing requires supporting with the minimum of material and the avoidance of even slight pressure or the use of adhesive. This applies to the extremities when the blood supply to the area is much reduced.

Tubular Bandages

Tubular gauze

Light-weight bandages knitted in a tubular form that can be applied to any part of the body. In many cases a special applicator is required. The bandages can be applied with varying degrees of tension and they are cool and comfortable to wear. Tubular gauze is particularly recommended for finger and head dressings and where extensive covering is required in the treatment of skin disease.

Elastic net

This is a tubular mesh bandage of cotton and elastic fibres and stretches widely without being constrictive. It is a more expensive bandage but this is offset by the comfort to the patient in securing a dressing in an area that is awkward to bandage by the older methods. It can be applied to most areas of the body.

3
RESUSCITATION

In all conditions of unconsciousness, from whatever cause, the first consideration is maintenance of the airway. In hospital the commonest form of unconsciousness, apart from sleep, is that induced at operation, and every student is instructed at an early stage of training in the care of these patients. The necessary equipment should always be at hand. This should include a mouth gag, an angled spatula, sponge-holding forceps and swabs and a tongue clip. Equipment for oxygen administration, for suction and for artificial respiration should also be available.

For the sake of safety, unconscious patients are best transported and placed in bed in the lateral or semi-prone position. This enables the tongue to fall forward, preventing blockage of the larynx, and allows the secretions to collect in the lower cheek or run out of the mouth. If this position is not possible, owing to the patient's condition, the angle of the jaw should be drawn forward and supported. The patient must be breathing quietly and adequately and no cyanosis should be present.

ARTIFICIAL RESPIRATION

Obstructed airway
Should the breathing appear laboured, the nostrils dilated or the soft tissues of the neck and upper thorax be sucked inwards, obstruction of the airway must be suspected. The jaw and tongue should be drawn forward, but if this does not relieve the obstruction, a gag must be inserted, the tongue drawn forward and the back of the throat cleared using swabs and sponge-holding forceps. This emergency is unlikely to arise with good positioning of the patient, but it may occur owing to inhalation of food or foreign bodies. If immediate steps are not taken to dislodge the obstruction, either by sweeping the finger across the back of the throat or, as in the case of a child, holding the head down and giving a few taps on the back of the chest, asphyxia may easily result.

Cessation of breathing
If breathing has ceased, artificial respiration must be started at once to supply oxygen to the blood and the blood must reach the brain within 3 minutes or irreparable damage will be done.

Expired-Air Artificial Respiration

Mouth-to-nose respiration (Fig. 4)

(1) Sweep the finger round the back of the patient's mouth to remove any obstructing matter.

(2) Grasp the patient's head with one hand and extend his neck by pressing his head backwards and at the same time lifting his jaw upwards and forwards with the other hand. Close his mouth with the thumb.

(3) Take a deep breath, place the mouth over the patient's nostrils and exhale forcibly into his lungs. Chest expansion should be observed.

(4) Withdraw the mouth and take another deep breath while the patient exhales. Repeat the cycle 10 to 12 times a minute. The first six breaths should be given as rapidly as possible.

(5) In a child both his mouth and nose may be covered by the lips and the breaths should be gentler.

Mouth-to-mouth respiration

This method may be preferred, in which case the patient's nostrils should be closed by pressing with the finger and thumb and the breath exhaled into his mouth. Apart from this the procedure is the same as for mouth-to-nose respiration.

An *artificial mouthpiece and airway*, if available, may be used. Draw the patient's jaw forward, open his mouth and insert the airway, directing it first towards the roof of the mouth and then rotating it downwards behind the tongue.

The stomach may become blown up with air, especially if the head is not properly extended. If this occurs, apply pressure over the upper part of the abdomen.

Holger–Nielsen Method of Artificial Respiration

This method (Fig. 5) may be suitably used when it is impossible to use the expired-air method of artificial respiration because the face is badly damaged.

(1) With the patient prone, flex his arms and rest his forehead on his hands, so as to keep the nose and mouth free.

(2) Kneel at the head, placing one knee near the head and the other foot by the elbow.

(3) Place the hands over the shoulder-blades, with the thumbs touching on the midline and the fingers spread out, the arms being kept straight (Fig. 5A).

(4) Bend forward with arms straight, applying light pressure, while counting 'one, two, three' (Fig. 5B). This is expiration.

(5) Release pressure gradually and slide the hands to just above the elbows of the patient. Count 'four'.

(6) Raise the arms and shoulders by bending backwards until you feel resistance and tension, without lifting the chest off the ground, while counting 'five, six, seven' (Fig. 5C). This is inspiration.

(7) Lay the arms down and replace your hands on the patient's back while counting 'eight'.

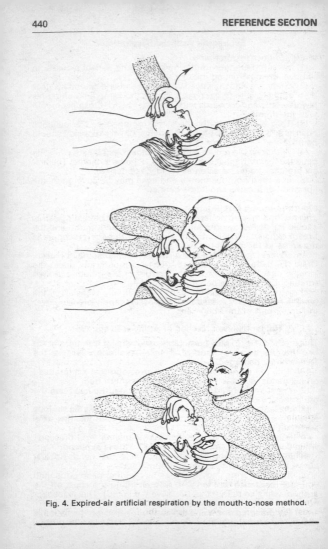

Fig. 4. Expired-air artificial respiration by the mouth-to-nose method.

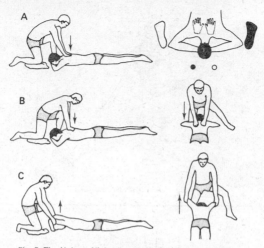

Fig. 5. The Holger–Nielsen method of artificial respiration.

(8) Repeat (3) to (7) with a rhythmic movement at the rate of 9 times a minute.

(9) When breathing is re-established, carry out arm raising and lowering (6 and 7 above) alone, 12 times a minute. Arm-raising—one, two, three (inspiration). Arm-lowering—four, five, six (expiration).

Manual Resuscitators

There are several simple devices that can be manually operated to maintain respiration by blowing air into the lungs. The most commonly available is the Ambu resuscitator bag (Fig. 6).

Where artificial respiration has to be maintained for a prolonged period, such methods are inadequate and a power-driven mechanical respirator is required.

EXTERNAL CARDIAC MASSAGE

Once the lungs have been inflated several times, the operator must feel for the patient's pulse in the carotid artery, or on the radial or femoral pressure point. Should no pulse be present

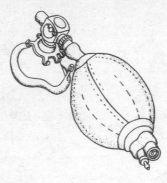

Fig. 6. Ambu resuscitator bag.

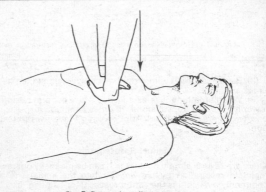

Fig. 7. External cardiac massage.

cardiac arrest has occurred and another helper must start external cardiac massage. If no assistant is present the operator must carry out artificial respiration and cardiac massage alternately.

(1) Place the patient on a firm surface, e.g. the floor, a trolley, or a board placed on a bed.

(2) Place the heel of one hand on the lower third of the patient's sternum and superimpose the other hand upon it.

(3) Depress the sternum rhythmically 3 to 4 cm towards the spine and repeat 50 or 60 times per minute until the patient's circulation becomes re-established.

(4) If a second person is not available to carry out mouth-to-mouth resuscitation the operator should ventilate the patient's lungs every six pressure strokes.

This procedure entails the risk of fracturing the ribs, a factor which makes practice difficult, and should not be carried out unless necessary. However, models are available and the operator can check the success of his efforts, as blood pressure readings can be taken and the lungs can be seen to inflate.

4

RESPIRATION AND ADMINISTRATION OF OXYGEN

RESPIRATION

Oxygen supply to the tissues depends on:
- adequate respiratory effort
- healthy alveolar tissue
- sufficient circulating red blood cells
- calibre of the blood vessels

Lack of any of these will result in oxygen deficiency.

Impairment in function of any of the links in the oxygen transport chain may necessitate administration of oxygen. The choice of method will vary with the cause of the oxygen insufficiency.

The air passages are never entirely free from air. At the end of expiration they hold about 150 ml of air which, on inspiration, will be the first to enter the alveoli, followed, in quiet respiration, by 250 ml of fresh air. However, part of the inhaled air never enters the depths of the lungs but remains in the area known as the anatomical dead space where no gas exchange can take place (i.e. the trachea and main bronchi down as far as the bronchioles) (Fig. 8). The volume retained at the end of inspiration is about 150 ml

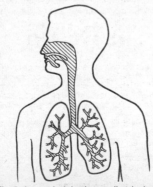

Fig. 8. Anatomical dead space (hatched area).

but varies with the depth of breathing. It is referred to as the effective dead space and on expiration it is the first air to be expelled, followed by 200 ml from the alveoli. This still leaves 150 ml in the respiratory passages, the so-called alveolar gas or alveolar air. Coming from the alveoli it has a high carbon dioxide content (5.5% as compared with 0.04% in atmospheric air) and a low oxygen content (14% as compared with 20% in atmospheric air).

ADMINISTRATION OF OXYGEN

There are two groups of patients requiring oxygen therapy— those who need it in controlled amounts and those who need it in high concentration.

Controlled oxygen therapy

Used for patients with a degree of respiratory failure, mainly those with chronic bronchitis. Such patients may need a low arterial oxygen level as a stimulus for them to maintain respiration. Too large an amount of inspired oxygen will raise the blood level and abolish this stimulus, stopping respiration and causing carbon dioxide retention, with resultant coma. These patients should be given only 24 to 28% oxygen, which will raise the blood level without stopping respiration (*see* Ventimask).

High percentage oxygen therapy

Used for patients who have a low arterial oxygen level not due to respiratory failure, such as those with heart failure or low blood pressure and postoperative patients. Oxygen (30 to 60%) is required, but provided it is high enough the percentage does not need to be carefully controlled.

Methods of Administration

Masks (see Fig. 9)
Ventimask. The Ventimask is a plastic disposable mask which gives a consistent alveolar concentration of oxygen and there is no rebreathing. The thin stream of oxygen draws in a good volume of air, which helps to flush out the dead space air. It is the best type of face mask for use where there is serious impairment of lung ventilation.

There are three models, giving a controlled intake of 24% or 28% at 4 litres of oxygen per minute, or 35% oxygen at a flow rate of 8 litres per minute.

Hudson mask. A soft plastic disposable mask which moulds gently to the patient's face and prevents oxygen leaking into the corner of the eyes. The oxygen concentration can be determined by controlling the oxygen flow rate, e.g. 2 litres per minute = 23% average oxygen concentration.

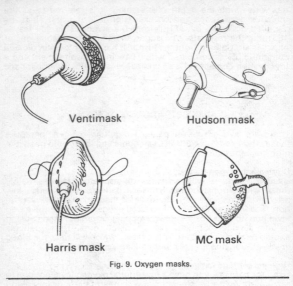

Ventimask   Hudson mask

Harris mask   MC mask

Fig. 9. Oxygen masks.

Harris mask. The Harris mask is a stiff transparent plastic disposable mask with good air entry holes. It does not cause rebreathing
or increase the dead space air. Where a controlled intake is not
necessary it is a cheaper model than the Ventimask.

MC and Edinburgh masks. These are transparent semi-rigid
plastic masks, comfortable to wear and very useful if no controlled oxygen percentage is required as the concentration does vary
with the lung ventilation. There is some rebreathing but less than
with soft plastic masks.

Nasal catheters
Nasal catheters used with a humidifier have the advantage that
there is no rebreathing and oxygen administration can be continued during meals. The percentage of oxygen received is considerably higher if the patient breathes through the nose than
through the mouth. The catheters need to be cleaned and lubri-
cated regularly.

Tracheostomy or endotracheal tubes
Oxygen may, if required, be given to a patient who has undergone

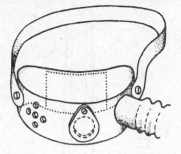

Fig. 10. A soft plastic tracheostomy mask (Hudson). The mask should be fitted snugly, though not tightly, over the tracheostomy. The strap is made long for easy fitting and so that the mask can be dropped down when suction is required. The tubing adaptor can be swivelled to any position desired.

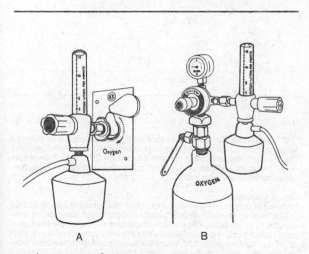

Fig. 11. An oxygen humidifer—A: attached to the wall supply; B: attached to an oxygen cylinder.

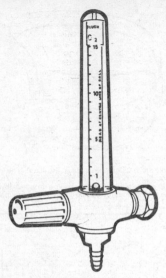

Fig. 12. Oxygen flowmeter.

tracheostomy by means of a mask which fits over the tube (Fig. 10).

If oxygen is administered in this way, humidification of the gas is required to prevent the mucous membrane from drying. This can be done by attaching a humidifier (Fig. 11) to the flowmeter (Fig. 12) on the oxygen cylinder or to a wall supply. The humidifier can also be used as a nebulizer to administer drugs.

Oxygen tents

In modern oxygen tents every effort has been made to control the oxygen concentration, the carbon dioxide content, the humidity and the temperature. The control of oxygen concentration is not easy as the patient treated in a tent is the very person who requires repeated physiotherapy and nursing attention which necessitates opening the tent. With improved tracheostomy and endotracheal care the tents are used less often than formerly, but are still useful for young children or adults who cannot tolerate a face mask or nasal catheters.

Mechanical respirators
The intermittent positive-pressure machine. Use of this machine, by which air is blown into the lungs, is at present the most favoured method for maintaining artificial respiration. A tracheostomy is frequently performed first and a cuffed tracheostomy tube inserted. This has the advantage of protecting the bronchi from the entry of secretions and makes removal of normal secretions by suction much easier. The air can be humidified and the oxygen content varied according to the needs of the individual patient. The nurse can then attend to all the patient's other bodily requirements quite easily and there is no restriction of movement of the limbs.

This type of artificial respiration is used for a great variety of conditions where the patient cannot adequately maintain normal breathing or where the nerve supply to the pharyngeal muscles is impaired and the protective mechanisms of the larynx are lost.

Nursing Observations

During oxygen administration the nurse should observe the rate and depth of respiration, the rate and strength of the pulse and the colour of the skin. A patient who becomes pink, who is difficult to rouse and whose respiration has become shallow and infrequent is likely to be suffering from a serious degree of carbon dioxide retention.

The apparatus used should be checked frequently to ensure that it is working correctly. Precautions must be taken against the risk of fire. Smoking must not therefore be allowed in the vicinity.

Hyperbaric Oxygen

This is oxygen under increased pressure and allows more oxygen to be carried in the blood. Normally the haemoglobin in the red blood cells is fully oxygenated on leaving the lungs and the amount of oxygen carried can only be increased by increasing the number of red blood cells. If the pressure of oxygen is increased then oxygen is dissolved in the plasma and so transported to the tissues. Raised atmospheric pressure increases the partial pressures of the individual gases that comprise it, in proportion to their percentage of the whole. These gases are chiefly oxygen and nitrogen. Hyperbaric oxygen may be administered in two ways:

(1) The patient is placed in an individual chamber or capsule with a transparent canopy in which the oxygen pressure will be raised. He can, however, remain in the chamber for only limited periods since nursing treatment cannot be carried out while he is enclosed. This type of chamber has been used with success for persons suffering from gas gangrene, frost-bite and carbon monoxide poisoning.

Radiotherapy may be carried out with the patient in a hyperbaric oxygen capsule. The increased oxygen supply to the tumour cells renders them more susceptible to radiation.

(2) The patient is placed in a large air-tight chamber constructed to hold an operating team or a group of patients and in which the air pressure can be raised to 2, 3 or 4 atm. The medical and nursing staff will work while breathing air but the patient will receive oxygen by a face mask. With the exception of radiotherapy, treatment for all these conditions can be given in this type of chamber and it can also be used for operating on congenital heart lesions.

If more than 2 atm of pressure are used there is serious risk on decompression of the release of nitrogen bubbles in the blood giving rise to decompression sickness. This is characterized by abdominal pain, cramp, vomiting, and pain in the joints. It may, however, be avoided by slow decompression, as used for deep-sea divers.

The fire risk is high and every possible precaution must be taken against a spark discharge. All towels and clothing must be fire-resistant and the monitoring equipment must be placed outside the chamber with only the leads to the patient inside the chamber. All equipment necessary must be tested to ensure that it is suitable for use at high pressures.

GAS CYLINDERS

Gases for inhalation, either by patients requiring assisted ventilation or by those undergoing anaesthesia, are usually delivered by pipeline to the wards and operating theatres.

In older hospitals they may be supplied in cylinders, which are colour-coded to denote the gas they contain and great care must be taken to ensure that the correct gas is administered.

Oxygen is supplied in cylinders painted black with white shoulders.
Air is supplied in cylinders painted grey with black and white shoulders.
Nitrous oxide is supplied in cylinders painted blue.
Carbon dioxide is supplied in cylinders painted grey.
Cyclopropane is supplied in cylinders painted orange.

METHODS OF STERILIZATION

Method	Action	Uses
Autoclaving	Dry steam under pressure at 135°C, destroying organisms and spores.	All linen and cotton articles, including garments and dressings. Polypropylene jugs, bowls and kidney dishes.
Hot-air oven	Dry heat at 160°C for 1 hour.	Delicate instruments, syringes.
Boiling	Total immersion in boiling water for 2 minutes, destroys *non-spore-forming* pathogenic bacteria.	Metal tracheostomy tubes, glass hypodermic or insulin syringes.
Gamma radiation	Exposure to radioactive cobalt; used as a commercial method of radiation.	Mainly disposable items: syringes, catheters, Ryle's tubes, tracheostomy tubes.
Formalin	Solid formalin is placed in a formalin cabinet and heat causes the rapid formation of formalin gas which will destroy bacteria and spores providing it comes into contact with all surfaces.	Mainly in operating theatres for sterilizing electrical equipment and the outside of glass ampoules (providing the contents are not for intravenous or intrathecal use); may also be used for decontamination of mattresses and bedding.
Chlorine and chlorine compounds	0.5–1.0% available chlorine in a hypochlorite solution is effective in killing bacteria and spores providing no organic matter is present.	Sterilizing clean glassware. Disinfection of baths, basins and toilet seats, etc.
	Milton 1:80.	
Sudol	Proprietary coal-tar derivative for crude disinfection. Used in 10% solution for 1 hour.	Sterilizing glassware, babies' feeding bottles, enteral feeding containers and tubes.
Glutaraldehyde	Potent antimicrobial agent against hepatitis viruses. Used in 2% solution for 1 hour.	Infected excreta, bed-pans and urinals of infected patients. Bed-pans and urinals of infected patients.
Ethylene oxide gas	Gas vapour used in conditions of humidity—rubber and similar substances absorb the gas, so the gas must be allowed to disperse before use.	Embolectomy catheters, cardiac pace-makers, criothermy electrodes and probes, heart valve prostheses. Large equipment, e.g. respirators, suction machines and incubators, should be allowed a cycle of 24 hours in an atmosphere of 10% ethylene oxide.

6
SI UNITS

The Système International d'Unités was introduced to British hospitals on 1 December 1975.

Basic Units

The SI system comprises seven basic units. The definitions of these are as follows:

Kilogram (kg)
The kilogram is based on the weight of a cylinder of platinum iridium which is kept in France at Sèvres, near Paris. The use of this was adopted in 1875.

Metre (m)
The international metre was adopted for use in 1962 and is based on the wavelength of an orange line in the krypton spectrum.

Second (s)
The unit is now based on the frequency of radiation of the caesium atom.

Ampere (A)
This unit is based on the attractive force produced when an electric current flows through two straight and parallel conductors which are 1 metre apart.

Kelvin (K)
The kelvin is defined in relation to degrees Celsius (centigrade): absolute zero $0 K = -273.15°C$. For practical purposes degrees Celsius will continue to be used. Body temperature 38°C is equal to 311°K.

Candela (cd)
A candela is 1/60th of the luminous intensity per square metre of platinum at 1773°C.

Mole (mol)
A mole is the amount of substance which contains the same number of elementary units as there are atoms to be found in 12 g of carbon 12. In practical terms a mole is the molecular weight of a substance expressed in grams. As this unit is of great importance in medicine, further explanation will be given later.

Derived Units

In addition to the seven basic units there are a number which have been obtained or derived from a combination of these. They are as follows:

Newton (N)

The newton is the force which will accelerate a mass of 1 kilogram by 1 metre a second per second.

Pascal (Pa)

The pascal is a unit of pressure which is derived by relating force to area, and results from the application of 1 newton per square metre. This should be the unit for the recording of blood pressure, but the old method of using mmHg still continues as the expense of changing every sphygmomanometer is at the moment prohibitive. Blood gas estimations will, however, be expressed in kilopascals (kPa).

Joule (J)

The joule is described as the potential energy which is released when 1 kg weight falls through 1 m by the force of gravity. The joule is the alternative unit to the calorie as the measure of nutritional energy. The Metrication Board have, however, decided to retain the calorie for the present, which means that two units are now being used because some hospitals had already effected the change by the time that this decision was taken.

As the joule is smaller than the calorie, dieticians (who have long been using the Calorie, or kilocalorie) are using the kilojoule which is one thousand times greater than the joule. While the change-over is being effected there will be a period during which there may be considerable confusion. In order to ameliorate this situation the conversion from calories to joules is given below:

$$1 \text{ calorie} = 4.184 \text{ joules}$$
$$1000 \text{ Calories} = 1 \text{ Calorie or kilocalorie}$$
$$1 \text{ Calorie} = 4184 \text{ joules or } 4.184 \text{ kilojoules}$$
$$1000 \text{ Calories} = 4184 \text{ kilojoules}$$

Litre (l)

The unit of volume is the cubic metre (m^3). This, however, is too large for use in biochemistry and so the cubic decimetre (1000 cubic centimetres) has been substituted. The universally accepted term for this is the litre, and it will continue to be used in medicine. Most nurses have been familiar with the litre for a considerable time since it has been common practice to measure the fluid intake and output of patients in this way. In common usage litre is best not abbreviated, to avoid confusion with the numeral 1.

Millimole (mmol)

Since the introduction of SI units, the majority of biochemical results have been expressed in millimoles per litre, and it is the unit which causes the greatest confusion.

It is useful at this point to return to the definition of the mole. A mole is the molecular weight of a substance expressed in grams. For example sodium chloride comprises one atom of sodium and one of chlorine. The weight of sodium is 23 and that of chlorine 35.5, and so molecular weight of sodium chloride is 23 + 35.5 = 58.5. A mole of sodium chloride is therefore 58.5 g.

The mole is a very large unit and is impractical for use in biochemistry. As a result, the unit that is most commonly used in medicine is the millimole, which is one thousand times smaller. It is used for substances, such as potassium chloride, which are added to intravenous infusions, as well as for the results of laboratory investigations. Concentrations are given in millimoles per litre (mmol/litre).

If the exact molecular weight of a substance is uncertain, the molar system cannot be used. This means that the concentration of a substance has still to be expressed in grams or milligrams per litre. One such substance is serum protein, which instead of being expressed in grams per 100 ml (g%) is now expressed in grams per litre. For example, a reading of serum protein at 7 g/100 ml will now be recorded as 70 g/litre. Haemoglobin, which is a complex molecule, will be expressed, as hitherto, in grams per 100 millilitres (g/100 ml).

Rules for Use of SI Units

In order to reduce the margin of error, the General Conference on Weights and Measures stipulated the way in which the symbols should be abbreviated and written down. It was decided that the abbreviations should not alter in the plural.

Therefore when describing weight:

One kilogram = 1 kg
Ten kilograms = 10 kg

It is *incorrect* to add an 's' to the symbol.

Multiples and submultiples

Multiples and submultiples are formed by using prefixes, e.g.

1 milligram = 1/1000th of 1 gram
1 kilogram = 1 gram × 1000

Time

Time is always expressed in seconds and is not converted into minutes and hours.

Decimal points

The decimal point is shown as a full stop on the line. A raised point now indicates a multiplication sign. In addition, in western Europe, it is acceptable to use a comma as a decimal point. Thus, two and a half might be written as 2.5 or 2,5 but not as 2·5, as this means two times five and equals ten.

When writing large numbers the figures should be grouped in threes with a space between the figure groups. Four figure units are usually written without space. This means that five million five hundred thousand should be written in the following way: 5 500 000. The number can be expressed more shortly as 5.5×10^6 or $5,5 \times 10^6$.

The tables below show the basic and derived units for the SI system with their abbreviations, and also the prefixes which are commonly used when denoting multiplication or division of units.

Units

Physical quantity	Name of unit	Symbol
Basic units		
Mass	kilogram	kg
Length	metre	m
Time	second	s
Electric current	ampere	A
Temperature	kelvin	K
Luminous intensity	candela	cd
Amount of substance	mole	mol
Derived units		
Force	newton	N
Pressure	pascal	Pa
Energy (work)	joule	J
Volume	litre	l

Prefixes

Prefix	Factor	Symbol
deci	10^{-1}	d
centi	10^{-2}	c
milli	10^{-3}	m
micro	10^{-6}	μ
nano	10^{-9}	n
pico	10^{-12}	p
femto	10^{-15}	f
atto	10^{-18}	a
deca	10^{1}	da
hecto	10^{2}	h
kilo	10^{3}	k
mega	10^{6}	M
giga	10^{9}	G

7
COMPARATIVE WEIGHTS, MEASURES AND TEMPERATURES

COMPARATIVE WEIGHTS AND MEASURES

Measures of Length

1 kilometre	=	1000 metres
1 metre	=	1000 millimetres
		100 centimetres
1 centimetre	=	10 millimetres
1 millimetre	=	1000 micrometres
1 mile	=	1.6 kilometres
1 yard	=	0.9 metre
1 foot	=	0.3 metre
1 inch	=	25.4 millimetres

Measures of Capacity

1 litre	=	1000 millilitres
1 gallon	=	4.5 litres
1 pint	=	0.57 litres
		568.37 millilitres
1 fluid ounce	=	28.42 millilitres

Measures of Weight

1 kilogram	=	1000 grams
1 gram	=	1000 milligrams
1 milligram	=	1000 micrograms
1 ton	=	1016 kilograms
1 pound	=	0.454 kilogram
		454 grams
1 ounce	=	28.35 grams

AVERAGE WEIGHTS AND HEIGHTS

Children from Birth to Eighteen Years

Boys		Age	Girls	
Weight (kg)	Height (cm)		Weight (kg)	Height (cm)
3.4	50.6	Birth	3.34	50.2
10.07	75.2	1 year	9.75	74.2
12.56	87.5	2 years	12.29	86.6
14.61	96.2	3 years	14.42	95.7
16.51	103.4	4 years	16.42	103.2
18.89	110.0	5 years	18.58	109.4
21.91	117.5	6 years	21.09	115.9
24.54	124.1	7 years	23.68	122.3
27.26	130.0	8 years	26.25	128.0
29.94	135.5	9 years	28.94	132.9
32.61	140.3	10 years	31.89	138.6
35.20	144.2	11 years	35.74	144.7
38.28	148.6	12 years	39.74	151.9
42.18	155.0	13 years	44.95	157.1
48.81	162.7	14 years	49.17	159.6
54.48	167.8	15 years	51.48	161.1
58.83	171.6	16 years	53.07	162.2
61.78	172.7	17 years	54.02	162.5
63.05	174.5	18 years	54.39	162.8

These figures only represent average heights and weights. Many children will therefore not conform to them. There are a number of factors which can cause a child to be considerably below or above average.

Adults Aged Thirty Years

Height (cm)	Weight (kg)		
	Small build	Medium build	Large build
Women			
152.5	48.5	53.9	60.7
157.5	51.2	56.6	63.9
162.5	53.9	59.8	67.5
167.5	57.1	63.4	71.6
172.5	60.2	67.0	75.7
178.0	63.4	70.2	78.9
Men			
167.5	58.4	64.8	72.9
172.5	61.6	68.4	77.0
177.5	65.7	72.9	82.0
183.0	70.7	78.4	87.9
188.0	75.7	83.8	94.2

COMPARATIVE TEMPERATURES

Celsius °C		Fahrenheit °F	Celsius °C		Fahrenheit °F
100	Boiling point	212	38.5		101.3
95		203	38		100.4
90		194	37.5		99.5
85		185	37		98.6
80		176	36.5		97.7
75		167	36		96.8
70		158	35.5		95.9
65		149	35		95
60		140	34		93.2
55		131	33		91.4
50		122	32		89.6
45		113	31		87.8
44		112.2	30		86
43		109.4	25		77
42		107.6	20		68
41		105.8	15		59
40		104	10		50
39.5		103.1	5		41
39		102.2	0	Freezing point	32

To convert readings of the Fahrenheit scale into Celsius degrees subtract 32, multiply by 5, and divide by 9, as follows:

$98 - 32 = 66 \times 5 = 330 \div 9 = 36.6$. Therefore $98°$ F $= 36.6°$C.

To convert readings of the Celsius scale into Fahrenheit degrees multiply by 9, divide by 5, and add 32, as follows:

$36.6 \times 9 = 330 \div 5 = 66 + 32 = 98$. Therefore $36.6°$C $= 98°$F.

The term 'Celsius' (from the name of the Swede who invented the scale in 1742) is now being internationally used instead of 'centigrade', which term is employed in some countries to denote fractions of an angle.

8
FLUIDS, ELECTROLYTES AND TRANSFUSION FLUIDS

FLUID

An average-sized man has some 45 litres of water in his body, and this water accounts for approximately 70% of his weight. The quantity present remains relatively constant and the balance between the quantities of water and of electrolytes present in the body fluids is controlled by a most delicate mechanism. To understand how this balance can be upset during disease or surgical procedures it is necessary to have some knowledge of the normal functioning of the salt and water balance in the body.

Fluid is normally lost by the body:

- in the urine
- through the skin in sweat and in sensible loss
- in expired air
- in the faeces.

The body normally obtains its fluid from:

- the fluids taken in liquid form
- the high fluid content of most foods eaten
- the metabolism of food and cell activity.

Much of the latter is a process of oxidation in which water is released.

This can be illustrated by an example:

1 molecule glucose + 6 molecules oxygen
= 6 molecules carbon dioxide + 6 molecules water + energy
$$C_6H_{12}O_6 + 6O_2 = 6CO_2 + 6H_2O + energy$$

In health the balance between fluid intake and fluid output depends mainly on the kidneys, which are able to excrete large amounts of dilute urine when the fluid intake is high and excrete only small quantities of concentrated urine when less fluid is available. The latter condition may be the result of a lessened fluid intake or of an increased fluid loss from the body.

The skin is primarily concerned with the regulation of body temperature—the amount of fluid evaporated from the skin depends on the body's need either to lose or to conserve heat. If the body is warm or the atmospheric temperature is high, much sweat will be excreted and evaporated in an attempt to cool the body. Under cool conditions the sweat glands will be less active in an endeavour to retain more heat within the body, although some loss occurs all the time.

The fluid in the body is present in three different compartments:

(1) The smallest quantity is the circulating fluid or blood plasma. This constitutes 3 litres.

(2) The fluid in the tissues or interstitial spaces constitutes 12 litres.

(1) and (2) together make up the extracellular fluid.

(3) The fluid within the cell walls forms the greatest proportion of the body fluid, amounting to 30 litres. This makes up the intracellular fluid.

Different factors help in maintaining the level of fluid in these three compartments. The plasma proteins, serum albumin, serum globulin, and fibrinogen are the chief factors that maintain the osmotic pressure within the capillaries and so keep the circulating fluid within the vessels. The salt content chiefly influences the tissue fluid and intracellular fluid.

Salts and Electrolytes

Within the body fluids are salts in solution. Salts are electrolytes, i.e. they are made up of *ions*. Ions are atoms that have lost or gained one or two electrons and as a result have become electrically charged. They are able to take part in chemical changes and the way in which they do so depends on the type of charge which they have.

There are two types of ion: those carrying negative charges, known as anions, and those carrying positive charges, known as cations. Cations unite chemically with anions to form molecules and herein lies the secret of electrolyte balance within the body.

The main salt of extracellular fluid is sodium chloride. This contains sodium (Na), which has a positive charge, and chloride (Cl), which has a negative charge. It is not only essential for health that these two elements are present and able to combine, but there must also be a balance between them. This fact is true of all other electrolytes. The balance is maintained by the action of both the respiratory system and the kidneys, which themselves are influenced by the nervous system and by hormones.

Hormones

The pituitary and adrenal glands both have an influence on the salt and water balance in the body. The antidiuretic hormone from the posterior lobe of the pituitary gland controls the final reabsorption of water in the renal tubules. If the hormone is lacking there is excessive diuresis. Aldosterone from the adrenal cortex increases the reabsorption of sodium by the renal tubules and reduces the sodium content of sweat.

Disturbance of the Fluid and Electrolyte Balance

Upset of the fluid and electrolyte balance may occur in many ways:

Water depletion
- when there is lack of intake
- when there is excessive loss from vomiting, diarrhoea, sweating or haemorrhage.

There is loss of fluid from the subcutaneous tissues and the skin becomes hot and dry and loses its elasticity. The circulating fluid becomes less, the capillary walls suffer from lack of oxygen and become more permeable, and further leakage from the vessels occurs, giving rise to the condition of shock.

Sodium depletion
- in excessive sweating
- in diarrhoea or where there is much faecal loss from a fistula or ileostomy
- in pathological conditions, such as Addison's disease or hypopituitarism, where the kidneys are unable to conserve sodium.

Chloride depletion
- persistent vomiting where heavy loss of chlorides from the hydrochloric acid will lead to the condition of alkalosis
- prolonged gastric aspiration.

Potassium depletion
This may arise whenever there is prolonged diarrhoea, vomiting, condition of shock, or lack of intake, and where there is excessive diuresis or continued use of diuretics such as chlorothiazide.

In prolonged loss of sodium and chloride, potassium migrates from the cells to replace extracellular salt. Potassium is slow to leave the cells but also is slow to permeate back into the cells when replacement is being carried out. Its lack leads to muscular weakness, cardiac arrhythmias, apathy and mental confusion. The kidneys still excrete potassium, making the condition worse.

Protein depletion
- where there is inadequate intake, malnutrition or starvation
- where there is excessive protein loss in renal disease or severe burns.

There is loss of osmotic pressure in the blood and great loss of fluid into the tissues.
- in severe haemorrhage where the only satisfactory replacement is by blood of the correct group.

It is seldom that any one of these depletions occurs alone. Fluid, sodium, and chloride are all lost together, but in severe diarrhoea more sodium is lost and in persistent vomiting it is the heavy loss of chlorides which upsets the acid–base balance.

Normally a diet containing an adequate protein and fluid content will also supply the necessary sodium, chloride and potassium.

Replacement of Fluid Loss

Oral fluids
Where there is a fluid lack, replacement is best by the oral route. It is unlikely there will be a lack of water only, and for excessive sweating a one-fifth strength normal saline may be taken by mouth. Most of the other conditions will not benefit from oral fluids and another route will have to be chosen.

Rectal fluids
These may be given for temporary relief of dehydration but their administration cannot be maintained over a period of days.

Subcutaneous infusion
Normal saline (a 0.9% solution of sodium chloride) may be given to replace salt and water loss.The use of hyaluronidase, the spreading factor, aids absorption. This is not now used when facilities for intravenous infusion are available.

Intravenous infusion
This is the commonest way of combating water and salt depletion and if due regard is paid to the electrolyte balance it can be maintained over long periods. It is most usual to give a 4% dextrose solution in one-fifth strength normal saline (0.18% solution). Hartmann's solution may also be used. This is an isotonic solution containing salts of sodium, potassium and calcium with lactic acid.

In any condition in which there is likely to be a depletion of water, salts or protein, or whenever parenteral fluids are given, there must be close observation of the patient with careful measurement and recording of all sources of fluid loss and fluid intake. Analysis of the blood chemistry will be carried out in all severe or prolonged cases.

Other Parenteral Fluids

Dextran infusion
Dextrans are polysaccharides produced by the action of bacteria on the disaccharide sucrose. They are plasma substitutes which increase the osmotic pressure in the circulation and have a combining power with water, so increasing the circulating volume of fluid. They are useful in treating hypovolaemic shock, moderate blood loss and severe burns.

Dextraven and *Intradex* have an average molecular weight of 110 000. Before infusion a sample of blood should be removed for blood grouping and cross-matching.

Macrodex has an average molecular weight of 70 000 and may be given in normal saline or dextrose solution.

Rheomacrodex has an average molecular weight of 40 000. This lower weight increases capillary blood flow and renal excretion, giving advantages if used during vascular or cardiac surgery. There is no interference with blood typing or cross-matching.

Intravenous nutrition

Carbohydrate. *Sorbitol* 30% solution is a sugar alcohol and supplies calories in a small volume of fluid (1 litre supplies 1200 calories). Sorbitol is metabolized into fructose and then utilized or stored in the liver as glycogen. It is not re-absorbed by the renal tubules and thus produces diuresis; but it is well utilized and the excretion rate is low. Sorbitol metabolism is not dependent on insulin.

Protein. *Aminosol-Vitrum* is an amino acid solution prepared from casein and dialysed to remove pyrogens and the large molecules that might cause allergy. It may be used alone as a 10% solution (50 g amino acids and 165 cal in 500 ml) or in combination with glucose or fructose and ethanol. Aminosol–fructose–ethanol solution provides 875 calories per litre.

Trophysan is a colourless solution of pure crystalline amino acids in a preparation containing vitamins and mineral salts. It may be given alone or with sorbitol to increase the calorie value.

Fat emulsions. These may be used in conjunction with protein solutions and provide a high calorie value in a small volume of fluid.

Intralipid is prepared from soya bean oil. A 20% solution provides 2000 calories per litre.

Lipiphysan is an isotonic solution of either 10 or 15% emulsion of cotton-seed oil with sorbitol and yields 1240 and 1780 calories per litre respectively.

BLOOD TRANSFUSION

Blood Groups

It is frequently necessary to replace blood when a patient has lost a large amount as the result of accidental haemorrhage or major surgery. Although this practice is common, it is not without its dangers. Thus it is of vital importance for the medical and nursing staff to make sure that blood of the correct group is given to each patient. Elaborate precautions are taken to ensure that errors do not occur, because the administration of blood which is not compatible with that of the recipient may well prove fatal.

All blood for transfusion is compared with that of the recipient in a procedure known as cross-matching. There are four major groups. A, B, AB and O. Fig. 13 shows their compatibility. Group O blood may be donated to a person of any group and for this reason a person with group O blood is known as a universal donor. Group AB can receive blood from any group and is therefore known as the universal recipient group.

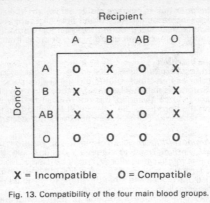

X = Incompatible O = Compatible

Fig. 13. Compatibility of the four main blood groups.

One other factor to be considered when cross-matching is the Rhesus factor, so named because it was discovered in the blood of rhesus monkeys in 1940. Some 85% of Caucasians possess this factor and are described as Rhesus-positive (Rh +ve). The 15% that do not possess it are termed Rhesus-negative (Rh −ve). A Rhesus-positive person may be transfused with positive or negative blood, but a Rhesus-negative person must receive blood which is also negative, or else he will produce antibodies to the factor.

If a Rhesus-negative women has a child by a Rhesus-positive man, there is a danger that some of the fetus's positive cells may cross the placental barrier and cause the mother to develop Rhesus antibodies. However, nowadays it is possible, immediately after the birth of the child, to give the mother serum which will destroy the antibodies and so eliminate the danger of a later child being harmed by exposure to them while he is still unborn.

Blood Transfusion Fluids

Fresh blood. This is particularly useful in cases of active sepsis or haemolytic disease because the cells will not have undergone change.

Stored blood. This is stored at 4°C and may be kept for up to 3 weeks. A slight reaction is likely if the blood has been kept for 3 weeks. It is particularly useful for all emergency cases of haemorrhage, and as a pre- or postoperative measure or during operation when special hazards are encountered.

Frozen blood. Liquid nitrogen held at a temperature of −79°C enables blood to be stored indefinitely. Several hours are needed to prepare it for use, by a process of washing and centrifugation.

Packed red cells. Part of the plasma is removed from whole blood. Using the closed sterile system (transfer unit attached to blood-pack unit) the packed red cells can be stored for 21 days, whereas bottled red cells must be used within 12 to 24 hours. It is used to increase the number of cells without overloading the circulation with fluids, as in some cases of anaemia.

Platelet-rich blood. This may be collected with silicone-treated equipment or in a disposable bag in which there is 50 ml of EDTA solution (a di-sodium salt of ethylene diamine tetra-acetic acid), an anticoagulant which is preferable to acid citrate dextrose solution in preserving the platelet content of blood. Platelets are required in controlling haemorrhage in haemolytic disease.

White cells. In certain diseases transfusions of white cells only are required. These can be prepared and infused in a similar manner to other fluids.

9
NORMAL VALUES

	SI units
Blood	
Bleeding time	60–360 s
Clotting time	240–600 s
Haemoglobin	12–18 g/dl
pH	7.35–7.45
PCO_2	5–6 kPa
PO_2	11–15 kPa
Platelets	$150–400 \times 10^9$/litre
Red cells	$4–6 \times 10^{12}$/litre
White cells	$4–11 \times 10^9$/litre
Plasma	
Calcium	2.10–2.60 mmol/l
Phosphate (as P)	0.8–1.5 mmol/l
Urate	0.40 mmol/l (male)
Urate	0.36 mmol/l (female)
Cholesterol	4.0–8.0 mmol/l
Magnesium	0.5–1.0 mmol/l
Glucose (fasting)	2.8–5.0 mmol/l
Sodium	135–146 mmol/l
Potassium	3.5–5.0 mmol/l
Chloride	95–105 mmol/l
Bicarbonate	21–30 mmol/l
Urea	3.3–7.5 mmol/l
Protein (total)	60–80 g/l
Albumin	30–50 g/l
Asp. transaminase	12 IU/l*
Phosphatase, tartrate labile	0–4.0 IU/l
Alan. transaminase	22 IU/l (male)
Alan. transaminase	17 IU/l (female)
Phosphatase, alkaline (adult)	25.92 IU/l
Bilirubin (total)	17 µmol/l
Bilirubin (direct)	NIL
Creatinine	44–106 µmol/l
Cortisol	180–720 µmol/l
Urine	
Creatinine	8800–17 600 µmol/24 hr
Urea	420–730 mmol/24 hr
Specific gravity	1002–1040
Cerebrospinal fluid	
Glucose	2.8–3.9 µmol/l
Protein	150–300 mg/l

*IU = International Unit

10
NUTRITION

The following section has been designed to provide useful information related to nutrition. Detailed dietary advice has been purposely omitted and readers are recommended to consult a dietician if this is required.

Definitions

Nutrition is the combination of processes by which the body receives and uses food for growth, development and maintenance.

Nutrients are substances that nourish the body. The six classes of nutrients are:

- fats
- carbohydrates
- proteins
- minerals
- vitamins
- water

Nutritional status is the condition of the body as a result of its receiving and using nutrients.

Dietetics is the science of applying the principles of nutrition to the feeding of individuals or groups.

Basal metabolic rate (BMR) is the energy requirement of the body when totally at rest at a comfortable ambient temperature 12–18 hours after food consumption. It is influenced by:

- age
- sex
- surface area
- body composition
- glandular activity
- nutritional status

Fever increases basal metabolism by about 10% for every 1°C rise in core temperature.

The **specific dynamic action** of food is the additional energy utilization arising from its ingestion and digestion.

There are two units which express the measurement of energy:

(1) The *Calorie* (Cal) or *kilocalorie* (kcal) is the amount of heat required to raise the temperature of 1 kilogram of water by 1° Celsius.

(2) The *joule* (J) represents the amount of energy which is released when 1 kilogram in weight falls through a height of 1 metre under the influence of gravity.

1 Calorie = 4.184 kilojoules (approx. 4.2 kJ)

Enteral nutrition is the administration of nutrients via the gastrointestinal tract. This includes the oral and nasogastric routes and administration via a gastrostomy or jejunostomy.
Parenteral nutrition is the administration of nutrients directly into the blood stream, via a central or peripheral vein.

Energy Value of Different Nutrients

1 g of carbohydrate yields 4 Calories = 17 kilojoules
1 g of protein yields 4 Calories = 17 kilojoules
1 g of fat yields 9 Calories = 38 kilojoules
1 g of alcohol yields 7 Calories = 29 kilojoules

Table 1 shows the energy and protein value of some common foods (from *The Composition of Foods* (4th edn.) by McCance & Widdowson, HMSO, 1979):

Table 1

Per 100 g	Energy		Protein
	(kcal)	(kJ)	(g)
Porridge	44	188	1.4
(60 g oatmeal/500 ml H$_2$O)			
Rice, white, boiled	123	522	2.2
Bread			
Wholemeal	216	918	8.8
Brown	223	948	8.9
Hovis	228	968	9.7
White	233	991	7.8
Cereals			
Allbran	273	1156	15.1
Cornflakes	368	1567	8.6
Muesli	368	1556	12.9
Rice Krispies	372	1584	5.9
Shredded Wheat	324	1378	10.6
Special K	388	1650	18.0
Sugar Puffs	348	1482	5.9
Puffed Wheat	325	1386	14.2
Weetabix	340	1444	11.4
Biscuits			
Cream Crackers	440	1857	9.5
Digestive Plain	471	1981	9.8
Digestive Chocolate	493	2071	6.8
Flour products			
Sponge cake with fat	464	1276	10.0
Sponge cake without fat	301	1280	4.2
Pastry shortcrust, cooked	527	2202	6.9
Desserts			
Custard (made with powder)	118	496	3.8
Ice cream dairy	167	704	3.7

Per 100 g	Energy		Protein
	(kcal)	(kJ)	(g)
Ice cream non-dairy	165	691	3.3
Jelly made with water	59	251	1.4
Jelly made with milk	86	363	2.8
Rice, canned	91	386	3.4
Dairy products			
Milk, fresh, whole	65	272	3.3
Milk, fresh, skimmed	33	142	3.4
Butter	740	3041	0.4
Cream, single	212	876	2.4
Cream, double	447	1841	1.5
Cheese: Cheddar type	406	1682	26.0
Danish blue type	355	1471	23.0
Edam	304	1262	24.4
Cottage cheese	96	402	13.6
Cream	439	1807	3.1
Yogurt Low Fat: Natural	52	216	5.0
Flavoured	81	342	5.0
Fruit	95	405	4.8
Eggs: Whole, raw	147	612	12.3
White, raw	36	153	9.0
Yolk, raw	339	1402	16.1
Boiled	147	612	12.3
Fried	232	961	14.1
Margarine, all kinds	730	3000	0.1
Meat			
Beef: Mince, stewed	229	955	23.1
Rumpsteak, grilled (lean only)	168	708	28.6
Lamb: Leg, roast (lean only)	191	800	29.4
Pork: Leg, roast (lean only)	185	777	30.7
Chicken, roast (meat only)	148	621	24.8
Liver, lamb, fried	179	748	20.1
Kidney, lamb, fried	155	651	24.6
Ham, canned	120	502	18.4
Sausages, pork, grilled	318	1320	13.3
Fish			
Cod, grilled	95	402	20.8
Haddock, steamed (fresh)	98	417	22.8
steamed (smoked)	66	279	15.1
Vegetables			
Beans, runner, boiled	19	83	1.9
broad, boiled	48	206	4.1
baked (canned in tomato sauce)	64	270	5.1
Brussel sprouts, boiled	18	75	2.8
Cabbage, Winter, boiled	15	66	1.7
Carrots, old, boiled	19	79	0.6
Cauliflower, boiled	9	40	1.6
Cucumber, raw	10	43	0.6
Lettuce, raw	12	51	1.0
Onions, raw	23	99	0.9
Peas, frozen, boiled	41	175	5.4
Potatoes, old, boiled	80	343	1.4
Potatoes, old, roast	157	662	2.8
Potatoes, old, chips	253	1065	3.8
Sweetcorn on the cob, boiled	123	520	4.1
Tomatoes, raw	14	60	0.9

Per 100 g	Energy		Protein
	(kcal)	(kJ)	(g)
Fruit			
Apples, eating (weighed with skin and core)	35	151	0.2
Bananas, raw (without skin)	79	337	1.1
Grapes, white, raw (skin and pips)	60	255	0.6
Grapefruit (flesh only)	22	95	0.6
Oranges (flesh only)	35	150	0.8
Pears (flesh only)	41	175	0.3
Sugar and related products			
Sugar, white	394	1680	Trace
Jam	261	1114	0.4
Marmalade	261	1114	0.1
Honey (in jars)	288	1229	0.4
Chocolate, milk	529	2214	8.4
plain	525	2194	4.7
Beverages			
Horlicks (powder)	396	1679	13.8
Ovaltine (powder)	378	1606	9.8
Tea, Indian, infusion	<1	2	0.1
Coffee, instant, powder	100	424	14.6
Marmite	179	759	41.4
Orange juice, canned, unsweetened	33	143	0.4
Ribena, undiluted	229	976	0.1
Lemonade (bottled)	21	90	Trace
Beer: Draught mild	25	104	0.2
Draught bitter	32	132	0.3
Lager (bottled)	29	120	0.2
Stout (bottled)	37	156	0.3
Cider, dry	36	152	Trace
sweet	42	176	Trace
White wine, dry	66	275	0.1
medium	75	311	0.1
sweet	94	394	0.2
Red wine	68	284	0.2
Spirits (70% proof)	222	919	Trace
Sherry, dry	116	481	0.2
medium	118	489	0.1
sweet	136	568	0.3

Table 2 shows the amounts of several different foods (in grams) containing 7 g of protein (useful in the administration of low protein diets):

Table 2

Animal sources		Vegetable sources	
Meat	30	Soya flour	15
Cheese	30	Bread (Hovis)	90
Poultry	30	Bread (white)	90
Bacon	30	Chocolate (milk)	90
Fish	45	Beans (baked)	120
Milk (dried, skimmed)	22	Beans (dry, boiled)	105
Milk (evaporated)	90	Peas (boiled)	150
Milk (fresh)	210	Lentils (boiled)	120

Table 3 shows amounts of food (in grams) containing 10 g carbohydrate (useful in the administration of diabetic diets):

Table 3

Cereals, etc.		Fruits	
Biscuits, plain	15	(weighed with stones and juice,	
Bread	20	but no peel)	
Breakfast cereal	15	Apple, raw	120
Oatmeal, dry	15	Apple, stewed	150
Rice, semolina, tapioca,		Apricots, fresh	180
cornflour, etc.	15	Apricots, dried, stewed	60
Milk, fresh	200 ml	Banana, raw	60
Milk, evaporated	90 ml	Cherries, raw	120
Bournvita, etc.	15	Cherries, stewed	120
Cocoa powder		Damsons, stewed	180
(unsweetened)	30	Gooseberries, raw, ripe	120
		Grapes	80
Vegetables		Greengages, raw	120
Beans, baked	60	Greengages, stewed	120
Beans, broad	150	Melon	210
Beans, haricot	60	Orange	120
Beetroot	120	Peaches, fresh	120
Parsnips	90	Pears, raw	120
Peas, fresh or frozen	120	Pears, stewed	150
Peas, dried	60	Plums, stewed	240
Potatoes	60	Prunes, stewed	60
Potato, chips	30	Raspberries, raw	180
		Strawberries, raw	180

Table 4 shows varieties of food containing little carbohydrate (useful in the administration of diabetic diets):

Table 4

Vegetables	Salads	Fruits
Artichokes, green	Cucumber	Blackcurrants
Asparagus	Lettuce	Gooseberries, stewed
Beans, french	Mustard and cress	Grapefruit
Beans, runner	Radishes	Loganberries
Broccoli	Watercress	Rhubarb
Brussels sprouts		
Cabbage	Beverages	Condiments
Cauliflower	Tea	Salt
Celery	Coffee	Pepper
Marrow	Soda water	Mustard
Mushrooms	Clear meat or chicken	Vinegar
Onions	soup	Saccharine
Spinach	Marmite	Vanilla
Tomatoes	Oxo, Bovril	Lemon juice
	Diabetic squash	Salad oil

Table 5 shows the role and sources of important vitamins and minerals in the diet.

Table 5

Vitamin	Functions	Deficiency	Chemical and physiological properties	Sources	Average daily requirements
Fat-soluble A (retinol)	For normal growth in children. To maintain a healthy condition of the skin and mucous membranes, particularly of the respiratory tract and conjunctiva. Aids night vision.	Roughened and dry skin. More liable to infection where mucous membranes in poor condition. Inability to see in dim light. Xerophthalmia leading to blindness.	Can be synthesized in the body from carotene present in coloured fruits and vegetables. May be stored in the liver.	Halibut- and cod-liver oil; liver; butter, margarine, cheese and egg yolk. Carrots, spinach, water-cress, dried apricots and tomatoes	750 µg (retinol equivalents)
D (calciferol)	Necessary for the absorption and metabolism of calcium and phosphorus in the body	Rickets. Osteomalacia. Defective deposition of enamel leading to dental caries.	Can be formed by the action of ultra-violet light on the ergosterol in the skin	Halibut- and cod-liver oil; fat fish; egg yolk. Butter, margarine, cheese and milk	2.5 µg cholecalciferol
E (tocopherol)	Related to reproduction in rats but no conclusive evidence that it plays any part in fertility in human beings	—	—	Wheat-germ; lettuce, green leaves and milk	—
K	Essential for the proper clotting of blood	Deficiency only temporary due to jaundice or sterilization of the gut by chemotherapy	Not absorbed from the gut if bile missing. Can be synthesized in the bowel	Green plants, cabbage and green peas	—

Vitamin	Functions	Deficiency	Chemical and physiological properties	Sources	Average daily requirements*
Water-soluble B1 (thiamine)	To obtain a steady and continuous release of energy from carbohydrate	Check in growth of children. Neuritis. Beri-beri.	Easily destroyed by high temperatures and baking soda	Brewers' yeast, bacon, liver. Wholemeal and national bread.	1.2 mg
B2 (riboflavine)		Checks growth. Cracks and soreness at corner of the mouth and of the tongue. Opacity of the cornea	Little lost during normal cooking	Vegetables Yeast, dairy produce, eggs and liver	1.7 mg
Nicotinic acid or niacin	Concerned with protein metabolism	Skin becomes rough and red. Diarrhoea and digestive upsets. Mental symptoms. Pellagra		Yeast, meat extracts, meat, offal. Wholemeal bread	18 mg
B6 (pyridoxine)		Unlikely	May be usefully given during radiotherapy treatment	Present in most foods	—
Folic acid	Aids in formation of red blood corpuscles	Some cases of macrocytic anaemia	—	Liver and green vegetables	—
B12 (cyanocobalamin, cytamen)	Necessary for development of red blood corpuscles	Pernicious anaemia	Cannot be absorbed unless the intrinsic factor is present in the stomach	Liver and other sources, as above. Prepared from streptomycin cultures	—

Biotin, choline, inositol, pantothenic acid and *para*-aminobenzoic acid are also members of the vitamin B complex

Vitamin	Functions	Deficiency	Chemical and physiological properties	Sources	Average daily requirements*
C (ascorbic acid)	Necessary for the proper formation of collagen in connective tissue and for formation of intercellular cement. Also for the formation of bones and teeth	Checks growth in children. Delays wound healing. Soreness of the mouth and gums. Capillary bleeding. Scurvy	Lost by long storage of fruit and vegetables; by cooking in the presence of air; by plant enzymes released by grating and chopping	Rose-hip syrup, blackcurrants, oranges and lemons. Green leaf vegetables and potatoes. High content in new potatoes, decreasing with age	30 mg

*For a moderately active man (excludes infants, pregnancy, lactation). Based on Report No. 120 of the Department of Health and Social Security, 1969 (HMSO).

Mineral	Functions	Deficiency	Chemical and physiological characteristics	Major sources	Recommended adult allowance
Calcium	Essential part of bone matrix and teeth. Major role in blood clotting, cell-permeability and enzyme systems	Rickets, including skeletal deformities, soft, fragile bones and retarded growth. Osteomalacia in adults. Dental caries. Tetany.	Uptake and utilization adversely affected by phytate, oxalate. Vitamin D essential for efficient utilization. Absorption enhanced by lactose and ascorbic acid	Milk and milk products. Canned fish eaten with bones. Fortified flour	500 mg

Mineral	Functions	Deficiency	Chemical and physiological characteristics	Major sources	Recommended daily adult allowance
Iron	Essential component of haemoglobin	Hypochromic anaemia. Moderate deficiency causes lethargy; in severe cases, palpitations and oedema	Poorly absorbed. Uptake further reduced by certain food components (e.g. phytate, oxalate); absorption enhanced by acid (ascorbic acid, gastric acidity)	Liver; red meat. Egg yolk. Dried apricots; raisins	10–12 mg
Magnesium	Essential component of several enzyme systems (in particular carbohydrate metabolism) and neuromuscular transmission	Irritability, muscle weakness, arrhythmias, depression	Normal component of sweat, therefore major losses in extremely hot climates and intense exercise	Milk; legumes; nuts; wholegrain cereals	300–350 mg Deficiency unlikely
Iodine	Constituent of thyroxine, which has profound overall effect on metabolism	Goitre. In areas of extreme deficiency cretinism can occur endemically	Radioactive form widely used as a diagnostic measure of thyroid activity	Sea foods; iodized salt	100–140 μg

(From *Nutrition and Dietetics in Health and Disease* by Joan M. Huskisson: Baillière Tindall, 1981)

Table 6 gives the recommended daily amounts of food energy and some nutrients for population groups in the UK.

Table 6 (cont. on facing page)

Age range[a] years	Occupational category	Energy (MJ)	Energy (kcal)	Protein[b] (g)	Thiamin (mg)	Riboflavin (mg)
Boys						
under 1					0.3	0.4
1		5.0	1200	30	0.5	0.6
2		5.75	1400	35	0.6	0.7
3–4		6.5	1560	39	0.6	0.8
5–6		7.25	1740	43	0.7	0.9
7–8		8.25	1980	49	0.8	1.0
9–11		9.5	2280	57	0.9	1.2
12–14		11.0	2640	66	1.1	1.4
15–17		12.0	2880	72	1.2	1.7
Girls						
under 1					0.3	0.4
1		4.5	1100	27	0.4	0.6
2		5.5	1300	32	0.5	0.7
3–4		6.25	1500	37	0.6	0.8
5–6		7.0	1680	42	0.7	0.9
7–8		8.0	1900	47	0.8	1.0
9–11		8.5	2050	51	0.8	1.2
12–14		9.0	2150	53	0.9	1.4
15–17		9.0	2150	53	0.9	1.7
Men						
18–34	Sedentary	10.5	2510	63	1.0	1.6
	Moderately active	12.0	2900	72	1.2	1.6
	Very active	14.0	3350	84	1.3	1.6
35–64	Sedentary	10.0	2400	60	1.0	1.6
	Moderately active	11.5	2750	69	1.1	1.6
	Very active	14.0	3350	84	1.3	1.6
65–74	Assuming a	10.0	2400	60	1.0	1.6
75+	sedentary life	9.0	2150	54	0.9	1.6
Women						
18–54	Most occupations	9.0	2150	54	0.9	1.3
	Very active	10.5	2500	62	1.0	1.3
55–74	Assuming a	8.0	1900	47	0.8	1.3
75+	sedentary life	7.0	1680	42	0.7	1.3
Pregnancy		10.0	2400	60	1.0	1.6
Lactation		11.5	2750	69	1.1	1.8

[a]Since the recommendations are average amounts, the figures for each age range represent the amounts recommended at the middle of the range. Within each age range, younger children will need less, and older children more, than the amount recommended.
[b]Recommended amounts have been calculated as 10% of the recommendations for energy.
[c]1 nicotinic acid equivalent = 1 mg available nicotinic acid or 60 mg tryptophan.
(HMSO: DHSS Report No. 120, 1969)

Table 6 (cont. from facing page)

Nicotinic acid equivalents (mg)c	Ascorbic acid (mg)	Vitamin A retinol equivalents (µg)d	Vitamin De cholecalciferol (mg)	Calcium (mg)	Iron (mg)
5	20	450	7.5	600	6
7	20	300	10	600	7
8	20	300	10	600	7
9	20	300	10	600	8
10	20	300	e	600	10
11	20	400	e	600	10
14	25	575	e	700	12
16	25	725	e	700	12
19	30	750	e	600	12
5	20	450	7.5	600	6
7	20	300	10	600	7
8	20	300	10	600	7
9	20	300	10	600	8
10	20	300	e	600	10
11	20	400	e	600	10
14	25	575	e	700	12g
16	25	725	e	700	12g
19	30	750	e	600	12g
18	30	750	e	500	10
18	30	750	e	500	10
18	30	750	e	500	10
18	30	750	e	500	10
18	30	750	e	500	10
18	30	750	e	500	10
18	30	750	e	500	10
18	30	750	e	500	10
15	30	750	e	500	12g
15	30	750	e	500	12g
15	30	750	e	500	10
15	30	750	e	500	10
18	60	750	10	1200f	13
21	60	1200	10	1200	15

d1 retinol equivalent = 1 µg or 6 µg β-carotene or 12 µg other biologically active carotenoids.

eNo dietary sources may be necessary for children and adults who are sufficiently exposed to sunlight, but during the winter children and adolescents should receive 10 µg (400 IU) daily by supplementation. Adults with inadequate exposure to sunlight, for example those who are housebound, may also need a supplement of 10 µg daily.

fFor the third trimester only.

gThis intake may not be sufficient for 10% of girls and women with large menstrual losses.

Doubts have been expressed about the validity of the recommended daily amounts for folate. The Committee on Medical Aspects of Food Policy has decided that there is too little information at present upon which to base a practical recommendation for folate until further research has been done.

Table 7 is a list of useful nutritional supplements and their manufacturers:

Table 7

Complete feeds and meal replacements	Addresses*
Build-up (Carnation)	Carnation Foods Co. Ltd, Danesfield House, Medmensham, Marlow, Bucks SL7 2ES.
Complan (Farley Health Products)	Farley Health Products Ltd, Torr Lane, Plymouth, Devon PL3 5UA.
Clinifeed range (Roussel)	Roussel Laboratories Ltd, Roussel House, Wembley Park, Middx HA9 0NF.
Ensure and Ensure plus (Abbott)	Abbott Laboratories Ltd, Queenborough, Kent ME11 5EL.
Express Supplement (Express Nutrition)	Express Nutrition, 430 Victoria Road, South Ruislip, Middx HA4 0HF
Isocal (Mead Johnson)	Mead Johnson, Division of Bristol Myers Co. Ltd, Station Road, Langley, Slough SL3 6EB.
Nutrauxil (KabiVitrum)	KabiVitrum Ltd, KabiVitrum House, Riverside Way, Uxbridge, Middx UB8 2YF.
Survade (Scientific Hosp. Supplies)	Scientific Hospital Supplies Ltd, 38 Queensland Street, Liverpool L7 3JG.
Fortison range (C & G)	Cow & Gate Clinical Products Div.,
Fortisip range (C & G)	Cow & Gate House,
Fortimel (C & G)	Trowbridge, Wilts. BA14 8YX.
Carbohydrate sources	
Maxijul (Scientific Hosp. Supplies)	see above
Caloreen (Roussel)	see above
Hycal (Beecham)	Beecham House, Great West Road, Brentford, Middx TW8 9BD.
Nutrical (Scientific Hosp. Supplies)	see above
Fortical (Cow & Gate)	see above
Protein sources	
Maxipro (Scientific Hosp. Supplies)	see above
Casilan (Farley Health Products)	see above
Fat sources	
Calogen (Scientific Hospital Supplies)	see above
Liquigen (Scientific Hosp. Supplies)	see above
MCT Oil (Mead Johnson)	see above
'Elemental' products	
Flexical (Mead Johnson)	see above
Nutranel (Roussel)	see above
Survimed (Scientific Hosp. Supplies)	see above
Vivonex (Norwich-Eaton)	Norwich-Eaton Pharmaceuticals Ltd, Regent House, The Broadway, Woking, Surrey GU21 5AP.

*Correct at time of going to press.

Table 8 sets out desirable weights for adults (medium frame):

Table 8

	Height (in bare feet)		Weight (without clothes)	
	ft. in.	cm	lb	kg
Men	5 5	165	122–135	55–61
	5 6	168	126–139	57–63
	5 7	170	130–144	59–65
	5 8	173	134–148	61–67
	5 9	175	138–152	63–69
	5 10	178	142–157	65–71
	5 11	180	146–162	66–74
	6 0	183	150–167	68–76
	6 1	185	154–172	70–78
	6 2	188	159–177	72–80
	6 3	191	164–182	75–83
Women	5 0	152	102–114	46–52
	5 1	155	105–117	48–53
	5 2	157	108–121	49–55
	5 3	160	111–125	50–57
	5 4	163	115–130	52–59
	5 5	165	119–134	54–61
	5 6	168	123–138	56–63
	5 7	170	127–142	58–65
	5 8	173	131–146	60–66
	5 9	175	135–150	61–68
	5 10	178	139–154	63–70

(From *Manual of Nutrition* (8th edn.) HMSO, 1982)

Table 9 supplies a list of commonly used methods of nutritional assessment and normal values:

Table 9

Dietary history	—
Appearance and fit of clothing	—
Body weight/height	see Table 8
Creatinine/height index	see Table 10
Triceps skinfold thickness (TSF)	see Table 11
Arm muscle circumference	see Table 12a & b
(= Arm circumference $-\pi \times$ (TSF))	
Grip strength	—
Serum albumin	39 g/dl
Serum transferrin	200 mg/dl
(= TIBC $\times$ 0.8) $-$ 43),	
where TIBC = total iron binding capacity	
Haemoglobin: Male	14 g/dl
Female	10 g/dl
Percentage body fat: Male	12%
Female	26%

(Calculated as follows:
Y = body density
X = log of Σ of skinfolds at four sites
Male $Y = 1.1610 - 0.0632^X$
Female $Y = 1.581 - 0.0720^X$

Percentage body fat $= \left(\dfrac{4.95}{Y} - 4.5\right) \times 100$

Table 10 gives the ideal urinary creatinine values for adults:

Table 10

| Male* | | Female† | |
Height (cm)	Ideal creatinine (mg)	Height (cm)	Ideal creatinine (mg)
157.5	1288	147.3	830
160.0	1325	149.9	851
162.6	1359	152.4	875
165.1	1386	154.9	900
167.6	1426	157.5	925
170.2	1467	160.0	949
172.7	1513	162.6	977
175.3	1555	165.1	1006
177.8	1596	167.6	1004
180.3	1642	170.2	1076
182.9	1691	172.7	1109
185.4	1739	175.3	1141
188.0	1785	177.8	1174
190.5	1831	180.3	1206
193.0	1891	182.9	1240

*Creatinine coefficient (males) = 23 mg/kg of ideal body weight
†Creatinine coefficient (females) = 18 mg/kg of ideal body weight
(From Kaminski M.V. and Winborn A.L. (1978) *Nutritional Assessment Guide*, Midwest Nutrition Education and Research Foundation Inc.)

Table 11 gives results of the triceps skinfold (in mm) for adults:

Table 11

Sex	Standard	90% standard	90%–60% standard	60% standard
Male	12.5	11.3	11.3–7.5	7.5
Female	16.5	14.9	14.9–9.9	9.9

(From Jelliffe D.B. (1966) *The Assessment of the Nutritional Status of the Community*. WHO Monograph No. 53, Geneva.)

Table 12 gives figures (in cm) for the mid-arm circumference (a) and mid-arm muscle circumference (b) for adults:

Table 12
(a)

Sex	Standard	90% standard	90%–60% standard	60% standard
Male	29.3	26.3	26.3–17.6	17.6
Female	28.5	25.7	25.7–17.1	17.1

(b)

Sex	Standard	90% standard	90%–60% standard	60% standard
Male	25.3	22.8	22.8–15.2	15.2
Female	23.2	20.9	20.9–13.9	13.9

(From Jelliffe, D.B. (1966) *The Assessment of the Nutritional Status of the Community*. WHO Monograph No. 53, Geneva.)

Useful Addresses

British Diabetic Association
10 Queen Anne Street
London W1M 0BD

British Dietetic Association
Daimler House
Paradise Street
Birmingham B1 2BJ

Coeliac Society
P.O. Box 181
London NW2

British Nutrition Foundation
15 Belgrave Square
London SW1

Useful References

Davidson Sir S., Passmore R., Brock J.F. and Trusswell A.S. (1979)
Human Nutrition and Dietetics. Churchill Livingstone.
Green M.L. and Harry J. (1981)
Nutrition in Contemporary Nursing Practice. Wiley Medical.
Paul A.A. and Southgate D.A.T. (1978)
McCance and Widdowson The Composition of Food. HMSO.
Huskisson J.M. (1981)
Nutrition and Dietetics in Health and Disease. Baillière Tindall.
Dickerson J.W.T. and Lee H.A. (1978)
Nutrition in the Clinical Management of Disease. Edward
Arnold.
Moghissi K. and Boore J. (1983)
Parenteral and Enteral Nutrition for Nurses. Wm. Heinemann.

Cultural Differences in Diet

Food habits vary according to race, religion and culture. It is
important to try and accommodate these individual preferences
when a patient is in hospital. The following points may be useful
guidelines although an effort should be made to discover personal preferences where possible.

Jews

Orthodox Jews eat a 'kosher' diet (kosher = clean or pure). This
refers to the method of food preparation including animal slaugh-
ter. The following are normally avoided:
(1) flesh from animals with cloven feet (e.g. pigs, deer);
(2) shellfish (e.g. crabs, oysters) and fish without fins and scales
(e.g. eels);
(3) the consumption of milk and meat products at the same meal;
(4) strict orthodox Jews may avoid ordinary cheese, which is
prepared from rennet obtained from the stomach of animals.

Roman Catholics

Meat may be avoided on Fridays, although this is no longer subject to papal decree.

Seventh Day Adventists

Members of this group are usually ovolactovegetarians. Intake of iron and calcium is potentially unsatisfactory unless the diet is well balanced.

Moslems

Pork is usually avoided. Traditionally eaten foods include rice and mutton (which is the preferred meat). The evening meal is often light and consists of white cheese, olives and bread. Some Moslems use their hands to eat in preference to cutlery. Scrupulous washing is normally performed before meals.

Hindus

The cow is usually regarded as a sacred animal. Some Hindus may eat fish, eggs and milk while others restrict themselves to milk as their only source of animal protein.

Vegans

A vegan eats no animal foods, or any product of an animal. Therefore, whereas vegetarians will eat dairy produce, vegans will not. A very carefully balanced and varied diet is required in order to avoid nutrient deficiency, especially in children.

11
URINE TESTING

Marked changes occur in the composition of urine when it is allowed to stand, and therefore only fresh specimens of urine should be tested.

Urine testing has now been made much easier by the development of multiple reagent strips by Ames. They are simple to use providing the instructions are followed carefully, and give clear indication of urinary abnormalities, which may then require more definitive tests in the laboratory.

It is essential that the nurse be aware of the possible causes of the most common urinary abnormalities so that the nursing care of the patient can be planned accordingly.

Urinary abnormality	Possible cause
Protein	Acute nephritis, nephrotic syndrome, damage due to toxins. Acute febrile conditions, congestive cardiac failure.
Glucose	Diabetes mellitus. Low renal threshold for glucose.
Acetone and diacetic acid	Incomplete fat metabolism usually associated with abnormality of carbohydrate metabolism. In patients with diabetes mellitus it may be indicative of the onset of diabetic coma.
Blood	Neoplasms, crush injury to genitourinary system, calculi, TB of kidney. Schistosoma infection.
Bile	Obstructive jaundice (gall stones). Liver disease (i.e. hepatitis).
Pus	Infection of the genitourinary system.

12
MEASUREMENT OF DRUGS

Arithmetical problems encountered by nurses using the metric system will be fairly simple, though the nurse will need to have a reasonable knowledge of the system. The following are examples which illustrate how calculations can be carried out.

Percentages, Fractions and Decimals

1 per cent equals 1 part in 100 or $\frac{1}{100}$

5 per cent equals 5 parts in 100 or $\frac{5}{100} = \frac{1}{20}$

Parts that are less than 1 can be written as fractions or decimals

1 divided by 2 = ½ or 0.5
1 divided by 4 = ¼ or 0.25
e.g. 1 g = 1000 mg
½ g or 0.5 g = 500 mg
¼ g or 0.25 g = 250 mg

Calculating Dosages

There sometimes occurs the need to calculate dosages of drugs because the prescribed strength is not available. There is a formula to meet this problem:

Divide the amount required by the amount available and multiply this by the amount in the stock solution:

$$\frac{\text{Amount required}}{\text{Amount available}} \times \text{Amount in stock solution}$$

This can be converted in the following manner: A dose of 100 mg of cortisone is required. The available solution is of 250 mg in 10 ml. Thus

$$\frac{100}{250} \times 10 = \frac{\cancel{100}^{2}}{\cancel{250}_{5}^{}} \times \cancel{10}^{2} = 4 \text{ ml}$$

Or, as another example, 5000 units of heparin are required when the available solution is 25 000 units in 5 ml. Thus

$$\frac{5000}{25\,000} \times 5 = \frac{5000}{\cancel{25\,000}} \times \cancel{5}^1 = 1 \text{ ml}$$

It is possible to calculate this by mental arithmetic as 5000 divides into 25 000 five times, and one-fifth of 5 equals 1. However, the nurse should always write the problem down if she is in any doubt at all and if necessary have the result checked by a colleague.

Should it be necessary to divide one fraction by another, it can be done in a similar fashion by using the same formula. It should simply be remembered that the second of the two fractions must be inverted, as follows. To prepare chlorhexidine 1 in 2500 from a stock solution of 1 in 500 in 1 litre.

Strength required = 1 in 2500
Strength available = 1 in 500
Amount of solution = 1 litre

Thus

$$\frac{1}{2500} \div \frac{1}{500} = \frac{1}{\cancel{2500}} \times \frac{\cancel{500}}{1} = \frac{5}{25} = \frac{1}{5}$$

Therefore one-fifth of a litre is required. Since 1 litre = 1000 ml, one-fifth of a litre = 1000 ÷ 5 = 200 ml of solution required.

To divide decimals the decimal point may be moved, provided that it is moved the same number of places in each figure. Thus, to measure a dose of digoxin 0.125 mg from a stock solution of 0.5 mg in 2 ml, the formula is written in the following manner:

Strength required = 0.125 mg
Strength available = 0.5 mg
Amount of solution = 2 ml

$$\frac{0.125}{0.5} \times 2 = \frac{\cancel{125}}{\cancel{500}} \times \cancel{2}^1 = \tfrac{1}{2} \text{ ml or } 0.5 \text{ ml}$$

Abbreviations Used in Prescriptions

Abbreviations of Latin terms are being replaced by English versions, which is considered safer. However, the nurse may still meet these Latin abbreviations:

Abbreviation	Latin	English
a.c.	ante cibum	before food
ad lib.	ad libitum	to the desired amount
b.d. *or* b.i.d.	bis in die	twice a day
c.	cum	with
o.m.	omni mane	every morning
o.n.	omni nocte	every night
p.c.	post cibum	after food
p.r.n.	pro re nata	whenever necessary
q.d.	quaque die	every day
q.d.s.	quater die sumendum	four times daily
q.i.d.	quater in die	four times a day
q.q.h.	quater quaque hora	every four hours
R	recipe	take
s.o.s.	si opus sit	if necessary
stat.	statim	at once
t.d.s.	ter die sumendum	three times a day
t.i.d.	ter in die	three times a day

13
DRUGS AND THEIR CONTROL

The two acts which control the use of poisons in medicine are: (1) The Misuse of Drugs Act 1971, which, with the Misuse of Drugs Regulations 1973, came into force on 1 July 1973. The Act combines and extends the Dangerous Drugs Acts 1965 and 1967 and the Drugs (Prevention of Misuse) Act 1964, which have been repealed; and (2) The Pharmacy and Poisons Act 1933 and the Poisons Rules (2). Additions are made to the drugs affected by these acts from time to time.

The Misuse of Drugs Act

This Act aims at checking the unlawful use of the drugs liable to produce dependence or cause harm if misused. Drugs affected by this Act are referred to as *Controlled Drugs* and are divided into 4 Schedules. Schedules 2 and 3 include those drugs which were previously controlled under the Dangerous Drugs Act and some additional ones. They include:

Cocaine	Amphetamine
Diamorphine (heroin)	Dexamphetamine
Levorphanol	Dihydrocodeine injection
Methadone	Mephentermine
Morphine	Methylphenidate
Opium	Methaqualone
Pethidine	Phenmetrazine

Medical practitioners and registered dentists may prescribe preparations containing these poisons. For exceptions see *The Misuse of Drugs (Notification of and Supply to Addicts) Regulations 1973.*

A prescription must bear:

- patient's name and address
- date
- signature of prescriber (*not only initials*)
- total quantity to be supplied, in words or figures

Every general practitioner is required to keep a record of all purchases of these drugs, and of the amounts issued to individual patients.

In hospitals the use of these drugs is under strict control, although minor variations in details may occur in individual institutions.*

(1) A special cupboard is used for storing such drugs, and this should be marked 'CD'.
(2) The cupboard is kept locked, and the key carried on the person of the State Registered Nurse in charge.
(3) Renewal of supplies can only be obtained by an order signed by a medical officer; and the drugs can only be given under the written instructions of such.
(4) Each dose of these drugs administered must be entered into a special Register provided for the purpose, with the date, patient's name and time of giving. The persons giving and checking the drug must sign this entry.

In most hospitals it is a rule that each dose given must be checked by two persons, one of whom should be a State Registered Nurse. This person should see the bottle from which the drug is taken, and check the dose with the written prescription.

All bottles containing controlled drugs should be marked conspicuously with a special label.

The hospital pharmacist usually checks at intervals the contents of the CD cupboard and compares its contents with the records of the Register.

In addition the nurse in charge of the ward should check controlled drugs and their records at least every seven days and report discrepancies to her superiors.

The Pharmacy and Poisons Act

Many substances are covered by this act and these are divided into 'Schedules', of which 1 and 4 are concerned with medicine.

In hospitals such drugs are kept under lock and key and they should be distinctively labelled and stored in bottles of special shape.

Schedule 1 lists all the preparations to which special restrictions apply under the Poisons Rules. These drugs may be sold only to persons known to the chemist, on a medical prescription or on a police order. The poisons book must be signed. The commoner ones, including their alkaloids or salts, which are used in hospitals are the following

Apomorphine	Digitalis
Arsenic	Emetine
Atropine	Ergot
Belladonna	Hyoscine
Carbachol	Methylpentynol (Oblivon)
	Strychnine

*See Department of Health and Social Security report of joint sub-committee on the Control of Dangerous Drugs and Poisons in Hospital.

Schedule 4 lists those substances to be sold by retailers only upon a prescription given by a duly qualified medical practitioner. These drugs are also included in Schedule 1. The group of drugs can be divided into Schedule 4A and 4B, the prescriptions for which must fulfil different requirements, Schedule 4A having rules similar to the Misuse of Drugs Act. This applies chiefly to pharmacists and doctors, but for nurses the same rules apply to all poisons.

Examples of Schedule 4A drugs:

Most barbiturate drugs   Cyclophosphamide
Gallamine injections   Mercaptopurine
Mustine injections

Examples of Schedule 4B drugs:

Chlorpromazine   Sulphonamide drugs
Milder sedatives   Thiazide diuretics
Tranquillizers   Thyroid preparations

The Therapeutic Substances Act 1956

This Act controls the manufacture, supply and sale of certain drugs and preparations. The provisions of the Act are similar to those controlling the Poisons Schedules. The preparations controlled are:

Antibiotics   Heparin
Blood   Insulin
Corticosteroids and corticotrophin   Surgical ligatures
Curare   Vaccines and sera

The Misuse of Drugs (Notification of and Supply to Addicts) Regulations 1973

Medical practitioners may not prescribe, administer or supply cocaine or diamorphine, or their salts, to addicted persons, except for the purpose of treating organic disease or injury, unless they have obtained a special licence and work in a specially licensed NHS hospital or similar institution. Addicts will have to undergo treatment in such a hospital or clinic. For further information apply to the Department of Health and Social Security, Alexander Fleming House, London SE1 6BY.

Intravenous Drugs

It is becoming increasingly common in many hospitals for nurses to prepare intravenous drugs and add them to infusions. No nurse should attempt this practice until she (a) has been properly trained in the procedure, (b) holds a recognized nursing qualification, (c) has the permission of her employing authority.

The nurse preparing the drugs must have them fully checked by a colleague before adding them to the infusion. Once they have been added a label stating time, date and drug added must be affixed to the container, and should bear the signatures of both nurses.

DRUG/AMOUNT ADDED	DATE	TIME	SIG.	CHECKED

DISCARD THIS BOTTLE IF UNUSED
12 HRS. AFTER ADDING DRUGS

14
THE NURSE AND THE LAW

The aim of this short appendix is to bring to the awareness of the nurse some legal aspects of nursing. Every student and nurse will do well to think seriously about the following points and to exert the utmost care both in carrying out all nursing procedures and in dealing with patients and their relatives since neglect may cause great distress to her patients and their families and damage the good name of the hospital. Carelessness or negligence may lead to an action in court and heavy damages could be awarded against the nurse or the hospital authority. Any nurse whether qualified or in training having a particular legal problem and who is a member of a professional organization, the Royal College of Nursing or any other trade union, should without delay consult its legal department whether she is working in a hospital or in the community. Fully paid membership entitles her to free advice and representation at any inquiry or inquest, and an indemnity insurance will protect her should costs or damages be awarded against her.

Consent for Operation

A patient coming into hospital still retains his rights as a citizen and his entry only denotes his willingness to undergo an investigation or a course of treatment. Any investigation or treatment of a serious nature, or an operation in which an anaesthetic is used, requires the written consent of the patient. A patient may give his own consent if he has attained the age of 16 years and is of sound mind.

No one should be asked to sign an operation consent form before he has full understanding of the procedures involved. The proposed operation is described on the consent form in general terms only, leaving the exact extent of the surgery to the discretion of the surgeon, but a patient has the right to refuse surgery going beyond the extent to which he has agreed to submit. If he does so, or wishes further explanation, the nurse should refer the question to the surgeon. It is the responsibility of the doctor to obtain written consent and not the nurse.

For patients under 16 years of age in England and Wales and for minors in Scotland (12 years for a girl and 14 years for a boy) the consent of the parent or guardian is normally obtained. In the event of any difficulty, the ward sister should inform the surgeon and the senior administrative officer. This also applies in those cases where the patient is unfit to give consent and no relative is available.

Correct Identity

The nurse or the midwife has the grave responsibility to make sure that all babies born in hospital are correctly labelled at birth and to ensure that at no time are they placed in the wrong cot or handed to the wrong mother.

All patients in general hospitals wear identity bands, in order that mistakes may be avoided. It is very important that the correct band is given to each patient and these are normally checked as part of the admission procedure. With young children or unconscious patients even greater care must be taken to ensure correct identity.

Every patient before being given premedication for an operation should be labelled in the manner approved by the hospital. The label should state the patient's name and hospital number. Moreover, a written request stating the same details should be brought to the ward by the theatre porters to ensure that the correct patient is taken to the right theatre. In the theatre it is the anaesthetist's and the surgeon's responsibility to see that they have received the proper patient and that the correct operation is carried out. It is not the nurses' duty to indicate the exact area of operation, which digit or whether the left or right side is to be operated on. But the ward sister or her deputy may be responsible for making sure that, before the patient is sent to the theatre, the medical staff have indicated clearly the site of operation, and for reporting to the surgeon if this has not been done.

In the Theatre

During operations the 'scrubbed' nurse must check the number of all instruments, needles, swabs and packs on her trolleys and, as the operation proceeds, check that each item used is returned to her. She will then have to carry out a final check before the body cavity is closed. If any doubt arises she must inform the surgeon, who should delay his final closure until a recount has taken place. At the conclusion the theatre nurse in charge and the surgeon sign the operation register stating that a correct final count was obtained.

Drugs

The legal requirements for the nurse in regard to the storage and administration of drugs are set out in Appendix 13.

Accidents or Injury

Should a patient sustain injury while in hospital he may bring an action against the hospital authority or against the person to whom he attributes the injury—this may be a member of the medical, nursing or ancillary staff. The hospital has a certain degree of responsibility for the actions of its staff, but a member of the staff who has been negligent or incompetent and has so caused loss or injury to a patient may be found guilty of culpable negligence and damages will then be awarded against her personally. In the case of a student nurse it may have to be shown that she has received proper instruction in the procedure undertaken, e.g. where a burn has been received from an unprotected hot-water bottle, if she is to be held responsible.

Accidents can arise to visitors or employees of the hospital through negligence in such matters as cleaning equipment placed on stairways, polish or grease left on the floor, faulty electrical equipment or torn furnishings. Hospital staff should constantly be alert to the risks entailed and bring them to the notice of the person concerned or the proper authority. In the case of a pure accident where no negligence or incompetence is involved there is no liability at law.

An action may be brought against the hospital several years after the accident has occurred. It is therefore necessary that at the time of the incident an accurate and full record should be made on the special form provided. This form should contain a complete factual statement of how the accident occurred, of the kind of steps taken, e.g. whether or not X-rays were made, and should list the names of witnesses and of the medical officer called to carry out an examination. The risk of accidents to staff, patients and visitors will be minimized if notice is taken of the Health and Safety at Work Act 1974. This lays down that Health and Safety Officers should be appointed and be responsible for ensuring that safe working conditions exist within the area in which they work. These Officers are responsible for ensuring that the 1974 Act is enforced.

Self-discharge of Patient

When the patient demands to discharge himself the nurse on duty should try to dissuade him and should inform the medical officer concerned with his care. If the patient is adamant, each hospital will follow its own procedure. It is probable that a senior administrative officer will see the patient and ask him to sign a written statement to the effect that he is discharging himself against medical advice. Should he refuse to sign, a note to this effect will have to be made and signed by two witnesses, one of whom is usually the administrative officer concerned and the other the nurse in charge at the time. The patient must be allowed to leave, except in the case of a mentally disordered patient who is subject to a restriction order or where it is felt he may be a danger to himself or others, when he may be detained for three days to enable an order to be obtained.

Mentally Disordered Patients

The proper care and treatment of these patients which includes those with *mental illness, mental impairment, severe mental impairment* and *psychopathic disorder*, and the safeguarding of their property and affairs is laid down in the *Mental Health Act 1983*, and the rules made thereunder. Most of these patients are now admitted without legal formality (*informal admission*) provided that they are not unwilling to enter hospital. They may leave when they wish unless detained for three days.

A person may be liable to detention in hospital or guardianship under the Act only if he is suffering from one of the *named* forms of disorder and if, for his own health or safety or for the protection of others, he needs restraint or control.

Unless subject to a Court Order, mentally impaired or psychopathic patients can first be made subject to detention or guardianship only before the age of 21 years. This ceases at 25 years unless a report has been furnished by the responsible medical officer that they would be likely to act in a manner dangerous to themselves or others. Except in criminal cases and subject to the aforesaid, detention in hospital or guardianship is for two consecutive periods of 1 year and then for 2-yearly periods. Renewal of authority in each instance is on report by the responsible medical officer that continuance of the detention or guardianship is necessary for the patient's own health or safety or for the protection of others.

Professional Confidence

Guarding the confidences of the patient is an ethical duty of the medical and nursing professions and nurses must take care never to discuss personal information received by nature of their position, except with senior members of the staff when the knowledge may help in the patient's treatment. Even then it will in many cases be wise to ask the patient's permission to pass on the relevant information. No confidential information should be divulged to relatives or friends, nor should details of the patient's condition be passed on to his employer as this may cause loss to the patient for which the nurse may be legally liable. This does not mean that near relatives should not be informed of the patient's progress: but discretion must be exercised.

Patient's Property

The Department of Health and Social Security requires all hospitals under its care to inform patients that the hospital cannot accept responsibility for valuables or money unless these have been handed over for safe keeping. Where it is known that a patient has an excess of money he should be invited to hand it over against a signed receipt so that it may be placed in the hospital safe. The valuables and money of an unconscious patient admitted as an emergency should be listed, checked by two nurses and put in safe keeping.

While a patient is in hospital, the nurse has no right to go through his locker or personal property without his consent. Searching his possessions may be justified if it is suspected that the patient intends to injure himself or others and has the means to do so. Yet, even in such a case, the nurse will be wise to have a witness.

When a patient dies in hospital his possessions must be recorded in the property book, but money and valuables should be listed and packed separately. The property will then be checked and the book signed by two persons, usually a nurse and the sister or her deputy. Strictly speaking, the property should be handed over to the executors of the deceased, but unless property of considerable value is involved it is usual to hand it over, against a receipt, to the next of kin. This may be the responsibility of an administrative officer and in this case the nurse should on no account give property or valuables to relatives or friends of the deceased. Care must be taken in the descriptive terms used; for example, yellow metal is a safer term to use than gold and white metal than silver or platinum since the relatives may refuse to accept an article made of base metal that has been incorrectly described.

Making of Wills and Signing of Legal Documents

Most hospitals have a rule against or discourage nurses from signing legal documents or witnessing signatures during their professional duties. This is to protect the nurse should the document be challenged later on the ground of the unfitness of the patient. However, the nurse has the duty to pass on immediately any request of this nature on the part of the patient so that the services of a solicitor may be obtained or those of a hospital administrative officer, who will assist the patient in every way, even in drawing up a simple will if so required.

Suspicion of Theft

The nurse is cautioned not to make accusations of theft against any hospital employee except to a senior trained colleague since without sufficient evidence she may easily lay herself open to an action for libel or slander. The nurse is also cautioned against the all too ready habit of borrowing as this could result in a charge of and conviction for theft. This refers to hospital property as well as borrowing from a private person. Conviction in turn leads to disciplinary action by the General Nursing Council, which means that her name may be removed from the Nurses Register.

Further Reading

Further information on the legal responsibilities of the nurse may be obtained from the following books and booklets, which are highly recommended to ward sisters and nursing administrators.

Speller S.R. (1976) *Law Notes for Nurses*, 6th ed. London: Rcn.
Whincup M.H. (1978) *Legal Aspects of Medical and Nursing Service*. 2nd ed. Ravenswood Publications.

Safeguards Against Failure to Remove Swabs and Instruments from Patients (1978) London: Medical Defence Council and Royal College of Nursing.

Safeguards Against Wrong Operations (1978) London: Medical Defence Council and Royal College of Nursing.

Watchdog: For the Record (1978) London: Royal College of Nursing.

Health and Safety at Work Act, etc. 1974. London: HMSO.

15

THE REORGANIZED HEALTH SERVICE

No profession has undergone more radical change in reorganization in recent years than that experienced by nursing.

It began in 1966 with the publication and hasty implementation of the Salmon report which led to much disquiet amongst the profession. This was followed by further reorganization in 1974 which maintained some of the changes introduced by Salmon whilst introducing further innovations, following which nursing was managed on a three-tier system at District, Area and Regional level.

The report of the Royal Commission on the National Health Service published in 1979 criticised the structure of the National Health Service, saying that there were too many tiers, too many administrators in all disciplines, a failure to make speedy decisions and too much money being wasted. They recommended the removal of one of the tiers. Consequently the government published a consultative document ('Patients First') followed by details of how the National Health Service was to be reorganized.

The major recommendation was that the Area tier of the system should be disbanded with as much decentralization of the health service as possible, with a devolution of power to District Authorities. The function of the Regional Authorities would remain as it was, serving the 14 regions of the country, each with its own administrative officers. The 90 Area Health Authorities were replaced by 193 new District Health Authorities.

'Patients First' laid down the ideal criteria for the new districts: 'An ideal District Health Authority would be responsible for a locality which is "national" in terms of social geography and health care, large enough to justify the range of specialities normally found in a District General Hospital, but not so large as to make members of the authority remote from the services for which they are responsible and from the staff who provide them. It would be co-terminous with the boundaries of social services, housing and education authorities.'

The management teams of the new District Health Authorities are similar to those of the abolished areas, namely District Nursing Officer, District Medical Officer, District Administrator, Finance Officer, hospital consultant and GP representative, teams of co-equals who would manage by consensus and advise the District Health Authority on policy and determine how DHA decisions should be implemented. District Health Authorities comprise 16 members and must include 1 nurse/HV/midwife, 1 Consultant, 1 GP, 1 nominee of the University, 1 Trade Union representative, 4 local authority representatives, the remaining seats being filled at the discretion of the Regional Health Authority. The Chairman of the DHA is appointed by the Secretary of State.

Below District level management of the nursing service is on a unit basis, with management by a Director of Nursing Services and a unit administrator. These structures are seen as being co-terminous. The size of the units is smaller than previous sectors and nursing divisions and would likely be the community services of the district as a single hospital of reasonable size, or the maternity or mental illness services of a district, or it may comprise a group of small hospitals. The function of each unit is to make as many decisions as possible delegated to them by the DHA. The Director of Nursing Services in charge of a unit is directly responsible to the District Nursing Officer, and controls the unit nursing budget with advice from the treasurer and in consultation with a senior medical representative.

Grades of senior staff and their salaries below District Nursing Officer are open for negotiation, are at the discretion of the district management team and will vary from district to district; they may be senior managerial posts or senior clinical posts, but the demise of the titles 'Senior Nursing Officer' and 'Nursing Officer' is inevitable. Similarly the roles of the ward sister and staff nurse may undergo modification as the new system of management increases in confidence.

The aim of the most recent reorganization was to ensure better management, a more cost-effective service, and an improvement in the standards of care offered to the patient.

16

STATUTORY BODIES AND
NURSING EDUCATION

On 30 June 1983 the existing statutory and training bodies were disbanded and their responsibilities taken over on 1 July 1983 by the United Kingdom Central Council (UKCC) and four national bodies representing England, Wales, Scotland and Northern Ireland. This change came about as a result of the Nurses, Midwives and Health Visitors Act 1979, which laid upon the new bodies the responsibilities of making provision for the education, training regulation and discipline of nurses, midwives and health visitors, and also for the maintenance of a single professional register. The new authorities were further charged with improving the standards of training and professional conduct of nurses.

The 1979 Act gives much greater powers to the new bodies, offering much more scope for all aspects of the development of the profession.

The Professional Register

The register, rolls and records of the disbanded statutory and training bodies have been merged to form the basis of the new single professional register. The recognized qualifications of any nurse, midwife or health visitor will be incorporated into the new register, which will become fully operational in 1984, and will also include recognized post-basic qualifications.

There are eleven parts to the new register:

Part 1
for Registered General Nurses (i.e. previous SRN/RGN)
Part 2
for Enrolled Nurses (General) (i.e. previous SEN)
Part 3
for Registered Mental Nurses (i.e. previous RMN)
Part 4
for Enrolled Nurses (Mental) (i.e. previous SEN(M))
Part 5
for Registered Nurses for the Mentally Handicapped (i.e. previous RNMS/RNMD)
Part 6
for Enrolled Nurses (Mental Handicap) (i.e. previous SEN(MS))
Part 7
for Registered Sick Children's Nurses (i.e. previous RSCN)

Part 8
for Registered Fever Nurses (opened only to admit those possessing this registration and then immediately closed)
Part 9
for Enrolled Nurses (i.e. previous EN in Scotland and Northern Ireland)
Part 10
for Registered Midwives (i.e. previous SCM)
Part 11
for Registered Health Visitors (NB: registration and consequent regulation is new for Health Visitors)

It should be understood that whilst the UKCC is responsible for maintaining the register, it is the responsibility of the National Boards to award the qualification. Therefore, from 1 July 1983, when sending out examination results the National Boards have been including with the results application forms for UKCC registration to the successful candidates.

The National Boards have not yet determined the terminology they intend to associate with qualifications, and until this happens the terminology set out in this section, e.g. RGN (for Registered General Nurse), will apply. Those who are already 'registered' prior to 1 July 1983 will be allowed to use their previous designation, e.g. SRN.

Nurse Training

Under the rules for training the content is made shorter, allowing National Boards to formulate guidelines for training for their own countries. These changes reflect a move of emphasis putting greater importance on the outcome of education rather than the process of education—this will result in greater academic freedom for the National Boards and offers exciting opportunities to experiment with some aspects of nurse education.

Entrance Requirements

In order to enter nurse training, applicants must be at least 17½ years of age (except in Scotland where applicants may enter at 17 years of age). Some Boards may not allow candidates to enter until 18 years of age.

Educational requirements vary quite widely between Schools of Nursing and these variations will be allowed to continue until 1986 when the minimum entrance requirement will be either 5 GCE 'O' level passes, or their equivalent, or successful completion of the Council's test. Under present educational systems applicants may enter either student or pupil nurse training, the differences being as follows:

Student Nurse Training (equates with 1st level nurse in EEC terms)
Basic student nurse training takes 166 weeks leading to

entrance to the appropriate part of the register. However, there are at present a variety of combinations of training, e.g. RGN/RSCN, RGN/RMN, and the training period for these will obviously be longer. Some courses associated with Universities are available which lead on successful completion to entry to the register and the award of a degree.

Pupil Nurse Training

Pupil Nurse Training at present lasts 110 weeks and leads to qualification as an Enrolled Nurse and entrance to the appropriate part of the register.

Further Training

Upon registration or enrolment nurses may seek to undertake further training for another part of the register. Such courses are shortened to take account of previous nursing qualifications.

Nurse training is currently available in general nursing, and nursing the mentally ill, the mentally handicapped or sick children.

In order to comply with EEC regulations nurse training must meet a required standard and therefore the criteria affecting nurse training may, in the future, undergo modification to meet the requirements of EEC legislation. The desired aim is that all member countries will eventually provide comparable training programmes to allow free passage of nurses within member states of the community.

Rules to allow this reciprocal recognition of nursing qualifications have already been laid down by the UKCC.

Continuing Clinical Education

Prior to the emergence of the new bodies the Joint Board of Clinical Nursing Studies was responsible for the co-ordination and supervision of numerous post-basic nursing courses in a wide range of specialities.

The courses are still available with the award of a recognized certificate on completion; however, the work of the JBCNS has now been assumed by the English and Welsh National Boards.

The curricula and criteria for these courses are very closely scrutinized to ensure that standards are maintained, and the developments within the speciality are continually being incorporated into the courses. Therefore, there is a constant review of the contents of these courses.

There are within the UKCC facilities for registering certificates of continuing clinical education.

District Nurse Training

Qualified nurses who wish to work in the community must apply for District Nurse Training, which since 1981 has been mandatory for those practising in the community. The course lasts approximately one year and is undertaken in a College of Further Education, with field work in the community supervised by a practical work teacher.

Nurses are seconded for these courses by health authorities who are responsible for paying salaries and college fees.

Health Visitor Training

Under the new Act, Health Visitors are required to register in order to be able to practise, so statutory rules for their training are required. Health Visitor training is available throughout the United Kingdom, and the substance of the training is at present based on that previously laid down by the now defunct Council for the Education and Training of Health Visitors' Regulations.

Midwifery Training

Following training for the register nurses may wish to proceed to midwifery training. Registered nurses may undertake an 18-month course leading to the qualification of Registered Midwife. Those who are not registered nurses may undergo a three-year period of training for a similar qualification. Following directions from the European Courts of Justice and a subsequent Act of Parliament, men are now eligible for midwifery training in the United Kingdom.

Clinical Teacher Training

Nurses who wish to teach in the clinical setting can undertake a teaching course during which they learn the skills associated with teaching in the clinical area and the classroom. These courses are available on a full or part-time basis.

The Diploma in Nursing

The Diploma in Nursing is moderated by the Department of Extra-Mural Studies of the University of London who award the Diploma to successful candidates. This is a three-year part-time integrated modular course which involves social sciences in a nursing-orientated discipline.

At present, it is essential to obtain the Diploma in Nursing before applying for most courses leading to registration as a nurse teacher.

Nurse Tutor Training

Those wishing to become registered nurse tutors must undertake specialized training. They may undertake either the University of London's Sister Tutor's Diploma course, or a course at a recognized College of Further Education, following successful completion of which the candidate can apply to the UKCC for recognition as a tutor.

Nursing Degrees

Many nurses choose to study for a degree after completion of their basic training, and, as previously mentioned, some obtain a degree in conjunction with their basic nurse training.

A number of Universities are now offering relevant degrees to qualified nurses on a part-time basis, and the Open University offers a number of courses which can be taken at the pace desired by the student.

17

PROFESSIONAL ORGANIZATIONS

Royal College of Nursing of the
United Kingdom

Known as the Rcn, this is the professional organization in the United Kingdom for nurses holding a statutory qualification or in training for such a qualification. The Rcn is also a certificated independent trade union. While the Rcn's UK headquarters are in London it has national headquarters in Scotland, Northern Ireland and Wales from which its National Boards operate; it also has various area offices in England. The Rcn is governed by a council elected by and from amongst its members.

The membership structure of the Rcn is based on some 200 local centres. The Rcn incorporates four associations, namely Associations of Nursing Education, Nursing Management, Nursing Practice and Nursing Students. It also incorporates the following six societies: Occupational Health Nursing, Oncology Nursing, Geriatric Nursing, Primary Health Care Nursing, Psychiatric Nursing and Research. Specialist Forums relating to more specific spheres of professional practice exist within the associations and societies.

The *Rcn Institute of Advanced Nursing Education* in London, Birmingham and Belfast offers a range of courses for qualified nurses, some of which prepare for an Rcn Certificate or for a University Diploma while many are short topic-centred or refresher courses. The Rcn Institute in London and Birmingham is recognized by the Department of Education and Science as an establishment of further eduction.

The *Professional Nursing Department* undertakes the work of the Rcn concerned with the advancement of nursing, the promotion of high standards of care and the formulation and presentation of the professional viewpoint on all matters relevant to professional practice in particular and to health service provision in general. The Rcn Centres, Associations, Societies and forums are staffed by expert nurse officers working within this department.

The *International Department* deals with the work arising from the Rcn's membership of the International Council of Nurses, the Commonwealth Nurses Federation and the European Nursing Group. The department is also much involved in activities within the EEC arising from the Rcn's role in representing the nurses of the UK on the Standing Committee of the EEC.

Programmes are arranged for nurses from overseas visiting the UK on study tours on either an individual or a group basis; arrangements are also made for Rcn members wishing to study or work abroad.

The *Labour Relations and Legal Department* provides a comprehensive service to members in relation to matters arising in their employment situation. It is concerned with salaries and conditions of service and with the work of the Rcn as a nationally recognized negotiating body. It administers the Rcn Steward Scheme which provides members with a workplace representative; it also administers the Rcn Safety Representative Scheme and provides, or commissions, the necessary training programmes for both these schemes. The Rcn provides professional indemnity insurance for all its members.

The *Press and Public Relations Department* is concerned with communications to the membership, the profession and the general public. It maintains close links with the media. It is also responsible for the production of the Rcn's official newspaper— *The Nursing Standard.* Since early 1979 this publication has been issued weekly and is free of charge to every nurse who applies for it. The department is also responsible for various other publications including a series of research reports.

The Rcn also offers a *Welfare Advisory Service* to all nurses experiencing personal problems.

Royal College of Midwives

The Royal College of Midwives is an educational and professional organization and trade union exclusively for midwives. The aim is to promote and advance the art and science of midwifery and to raise the efficiency of midwives. The College is the recognized negotiating body for midwives, having representation on the Nursing and Midwifery Staffs Negotiating Council. Under the Midwives Act, the College is approved by the National Boards of England and Wales to provide courses in preparation for the Midwife Teachers Diploma, the Advanced Diploma in Midwifery, and the majority of midwifery statutory refresher courses. Among other benefits of membership are professional indemnity insurance scheme and a personal accident insurance scheme.

International Council of Nurses (ICN)

Founded in 1899, the International Council of Nurses (ICN) is the oldest international professional organization in the health care field. ICN accepts into membership one association of nurses per country. There are 95 national nurses' organizations in membership. In addition ICN works with approximately 50 other national associations or groups of nurses with a view to their future membership.

The governing body of the ICN is the Council of National Representatives (CNR), composed on the principle of one country one vote. The CNR meets every two years to determine policy matters affecting the nursing profession. Every fourth year this meeting is held in conjunction with an ICN quadrennial Congress, open to nurses throughout the world.

ICN has one standing committee, the Professional Services Committee, which considers trends and problems in relation to nursing education, practice, service and the social and economic welfare of nurses. In addition there are frequent *ad hoc* committees.

The ICN Board of Directors consists of the President, three Vice-Presidents and 11 other members (seven are representatives and four members-at-large), elected by the CNR at the time of the ICN Congress. The area representatives on the Board are elected from the seven different ICN areas: Africa, the Eastern Mediterranean, Europe, North America, South and Central America, Southeast Asia, and the Western Pacific.

ICN's objectives are:

1. To promote the development of strong national nurses' associations.
2. To assist national nurses' associations to improve the standards of nursing and the competence of nurses.
3. To assist national nurses' associations to improve the status of nurses within their countries.
4. To serve as the authoritative voice for nurses and nursing internationally.

The activities of the ICN reflect the wide range of interests and needs of its international membership, focusing on such areas as nursing education, economic and general welfare of nurses, nursing practice and service, nursing legislation, nursing research, and co-operation with other health professions.

ICN is in official relationship with the World Health Organization (WHO), is included on the special list of non-governmental organizations maintained by the International Labour Organization (ILO), for consultative purposes is in relationship with the United Nations Educational, Scientific and Cultural Organization (UNESCO) and with the United Nations International Children's Emergency Fund (UNICEF), is on the Consultative Register of the Economics and Social Council (ECOSOC), and is in relationship with the International Committee of the Red Cross, the League of Red Cross Societies, the World Medical Association, the International Hospital Federation and the Union of International Associations.

Florence Nightingale International Foundation (FNIF)

This educational trust in memory of Florence Nightingale was founded in 1934 by the International Council of Nurses and now forms the Educational Division, aimed at improving nursing service by the furthering of nursing education. It has established a centre of information on educational opportunities in nursing in all countries. The Foundation arranges study programmes, research projects and advises individual nurses on nursing education.

PROFESSIONAL ORGANIZATIONS

King Edward's Hospital Fund for London

This fund was founded by King Edward VII for the support, benefit or extension of the hospitals of London. It makes grants to hospitals and convalescent homes serving the London area. It maintains the Hospital Centre for the dissemination of knowledge and improvements in design of hospital equipment. It has an extensive information and advisory service. The premises include a large reference library, a lecture hall, discussion rooms and a display area for hospital equipment.

The King Edward's Hospital Fund provides staff colleges for residential courses in preparation for senior positions in hospital. It also provides the Emergency Bed Service which in the London metropolitan regions aids doctors seeking a hospital bed for an acute case.

Nuffield Foundation

The objects of the Nuffield Foundation are the advancement of health and the prevention and relief of sickness, particularly by medical research and teaching; the advancement of social well-being, particularly by scientific research; the care and comfort of the aged poor; and the advancement of education.

A subsidiary organization is the Nuffield Provincial Hospitals Trust, the aim of which is to improve the organization and the efficiency of hospital, medical and health services in the provinces. It finances the Nuffield Centre for Hospital and Health Service Studies of the University of Leeds. The centre provides residential courses in hospital administration and supports research.

Whitley Councils for the Health Services
(Great Britain)

The Whitley Councils are the national organizations set up to negotiate salaries and conditions of service for persons engaged in the National Health Service. They consist of a General Council that deals with matters common to all personnel, such as travelling and subsistence allowance, and of nine functional councils which deal with remuneration and conditions of service applying to a particular group. These comprise:

Administrative and Clerical Staffs Council
Ambulance Men's Council
Ancillary Staffs Council
Dental Whitley Council (Local Authorities)
Medical and (Hospital) Dental Council
Nurses and Midwives Council
Optical Council
Pharmaceutical Council
Professional and Technical Staffs Council A and Council B

Council has a management side and a staff side. In the case of the Nurses and Midwives Council the members of the management side are appointed by the Ministry of Health, regional boards and employing authorities. The staff side represents the employees and the members are appointed by the participating organizations such as the Royal College of Nursing, Royal College of Midwives and national Unions of which nurses and midwives are members (e.g. COHSE, NUPE, NALGO).

18
NURSING RESEARCH

Nursing is regarded as both an art and a science. Put into simple terms, the art is the nursing action of doing what we do for our patients, the science is our nursing knowledge, or knowing why we do what we do; if nursing is to be regarded as a profession the two are indivisible.

A great deal of nursing action in the past was carried out because that was what nurses were taught to do—there was little scientific evidence other than the eventual survival of the patient to show that what was done was effective care. Therefore, nursing research developed in order to prove or disprove the validity of established nursing actions.

Initially there was a great mystique attached to nursing research, largely unwarranted, and due to an inability to conceptualize researchers as nurses, and to regard them as interlopers telling others how to do their jobs. This dichotomy appears to have been resolved and the value of this branch of science in improving the standards of our delivery of health care is becoming more apparent.

The increasing awareness of the importance of nursing research is reflected by the inclusion of 'research appreciation' in the curricula of the statutory nurse training bodies. This was essential if nurses were to be able to utilize the wealth of knowledge in the ever-increasing amount of published nursing research and apply it within the sphere of their daily professional activities.

For nursing research to be relevant and useful certain criteria have to be met: the researcher must be competent, and the research methods and design must be validated before a full research study is embarked upon. (This is of course true of any research programme.) Therefore it is apparent that research is a speciality within nursing, as is coronary care, and special training and aptitudes are necessary to perform the role.

The ultimate object of nursing research is to increase our knowledge in all areas of nursing—care, education and management—so that the profession might grow in stature and lay down a base of knowledge for future generations of nurses. In order to benefit from this, nurses must become research minded and ask 'why' as well as 'how', learn the not-so-difficult language of nursing research in order to implement research findings, and keep themselves informed of developments in nursing.

Further Reading

J.M. and Hockey L. (1979) *Research for Nursing—a Guide for Enquiring Nurse.* H.M. & M.

Research Reports (various)—Rcn Publications.

Calnan J. (1976) *One Way to do Research.* Heinemann.

19

THE NURSING PROCESS

The nursing process is probably the most controversial thing to happen to nursing in recent years, and there have been many problems associated with its introduction. Perhaps the greatest of these is a reluctance to change.

For many years delivery of nursing care centred around ward routine and was task allocated, e.g. one nurse took and recorded all temperatures, blood pressures and pulses and these were recorded both individually and centrally. This method of working de-personalized care, which in fact was dictated by the nurse in charge.

The nursing process seeks to individualize the delivery of care, so that the patient receives care to meet his particular needs, and so that effective nursing interventions can be made to prevent or minimize problems. In order for this to happen certain logical stages must be followed. These involve: i) the taking of a nursing *history* leading to ii) an *assessment* of the patient's individual needs and his actual and potential nursing problems, iii) the *planning* of individual care to meet these needs and to prevent or solve problems, iv) the *implementation* of that care, and v) an *evaluation* to ascertain if the needs have been met and the problems prevented or solved.

Nursing history

This is generally a record of social history, past relevant medical history and previous hospitalization, health problems such as allergies and the patient's normal activities of daily living.

Nursing assessment

This relates to the physical status of the patient as the nurse and the patient perceive it and includes: general appearance, mobility, hearing, vision, nutritional status, condition of the skin, the oral cavity, speech or language difficulty and mobility. Such an assessment may be a collaborative one made with total involvement of the patient.

Taking the nursing history and making the assessment will necessarily involve full patient and/or relative involvement. The use of closed-ended questions should be avoided, and this should be a relaxed and unhurried time when patients and relatives are encouraged to talk.

Planning care

Following the compilation of the nursing history and assessment the nurse will need to analyse the information in order (a) to

potential and actual problems, and (b) to plan the care
...ary to prevent or solve problems and to meet the patient's
... nursing needs. Again patients and, where relevant, rela-
th... should be involved in the planning of this care.

Implementation

Having planned or prescribed the care of the patient the nurse in
collaboration with her colleagues should ensure that the care is
carried out effectively and record accurately on the progress notes
that this has been done. Again, whenever possible patients
should be encouraged to participate in their own care. This often
gives them a sense of being in control in an often strange
environment.

Evaluation

The foregoing are a complete waste of time unless an effective
and regular evaluation of the care delivered is carried out. This
enables the nurse to assess the effectiveness of her nursing
interventions and to change a plan of care which is not achieving
the effect she desires. Evaluation is also a time when all members
of the nursing team can come together to discuss the care of their
patients and exchange ideas on suitable nursing strategies to
meet particular patient needs or problems.

Further Reading

There are many excellent books available which cover all aspects
of the nursing process and the nurse is encouraged to consult
these for greater in-depth information and a wide variety of ideas
on how individualized patient care can be effectively achieved.

Hunt J.M. and Marks-Maran D.J. (1980) *Nursing Care Plans*. H.M.
& M.
McFarlane of Llandaff and Castledine G. (1982) *A Guide to the
Practice of Nursing using the Nursing Process*. C.V. Mosby.
Kratz C.R. (1979) *The Nursing Process*. Baillière Tindall.
Roper N., Logan W.W. and Tierney A.J. (1981) *Learning to Use the
Process of Nursing*. Churchill Livingstone.
Roper N., Logan, W.W. and Tierney A.J. (1983) *Using a Model for
Nursing*. Churchill Livingstone.

In addition the library of the Royal College of Nursing provides a
reference list of articles published on this subject.

20

USEFUL ADDRESSES

Association of Nurse Administrators, 13 Grosvenor Place, London SW1X 7EN
Tel. 01-235 5258

Association of Nursing Students, Royal College of Nursing, 1a Henrietta Place, Cavendish Square, London W1M 0AB
Tel. 01-629 6441

British Association of Social Workers, 16 Kent Street, Birmingham B5 6RD
Tel. 021-622 3911

British Red Cross, 9 Grosvenor Crescent, London SW1X YEJ
Tel. 01-235 5454

Chartered Society of Physiotherapy, 14 Bedford Row, London WC1R 4ED
Tel. 01-242 1941/7

Chest and Heart Association, Tavistock House North, Tavistock Square, London WC1H 9JE
Tel. 01-387 3012

Department of Employment, St. Martin's Place, London WC2N 4JH
Tel. 01-930 7833

Department of Health and Social Security, Alexander Fleming House, Elephant and Castle, London SE1 6BY
Tel. 01-407 5522

Emergency Bed Service, Fielden House, 28 London Bridge Street, London SE1 9SG
Tel. 01-407 7181

English National Board for Nursing Midwifery and Health Visiting, Victory House, 170 Tottenham Court Road, London W1P 0HA
01-388 3131

Federated Superannuation Scheme for Nurses and Hospital Officers (Contributory), Rosehill, Park Road, Banstead, Surrey
Tel. 07373 57272

Haemophilia Association, PO Box 9, 16 Trinity Street, London SE1 1DE
Tel. 01-407 1010

Health Services Superannuation Division, Department of Health and Social Security, North Fylde Central Offices, Hesketh House, 200–220 Broadway, Fleetwood, Lancs FY7 8LG
Tel. 039-17 77123

Hospital Savings Association, 30 Lancaster Gate, London W2 3LT
Tel. 01-723 7601

International Council of Nurses, 37 Rue Vermont, 1202 Geneva, Geneva 20
Tel. Geneva 336400

...dward's Hospital Fund for London, 14A Palace Court,
...on W2 4HT
Tel. 01-727 0581

K...'s Fund Centre, 126 Albert Street, London NW1 7NF
Tel. 01-267 6111

King's Fund College, 2 Palace Court, London W2 4HS
Tel. 01-229 9361

National Association for the Welfare of Children in Hospital,
Argyle House, 29 Euston Road, London NW1
Tel. 01-833 2041

National Staff Committee for Nurses and Midwives, 168 Black-
friars Road, London SE1 8EU
Tel. 01-703 6380

Nation's Fund for Nurses, 1 Henrietta Place, Cavendish Square,
London W1M 0AB
Tel. 01-580 3965

Northern Ireland National Board for Nursing, Midwifery and
Health Visiting, 123/137 York Street, Belfast BT15 1JB
Tel. 0232-246333/247861

Nuffield Foundation, Regent's Park, London NW1 4RS
Tel. 01-722 8871/9

Nurses and Midwives Council of the Royal College of Nursing
(United Kingdom), 1 Henrietta Place, London W1M 0AB
Tel. 01-636 3866

Nursing and Hospital Careers Information Centre, 121/123
Edgware Road, London W2 2HX
Tel. 01-402 5296

Princess Mary's Royal Air Force Nursing Service, Ministry of
Defence, First Avenue House, High Holborn, London WC1V 6HE
Tel. 01-430 5639

Queen Alexandra's Royal Army Nursing Corps, Ministry of
Defence, First Avenue House, High Holborn, London WC1V 6HD
Tel. 01-430 5555

Queen Alexandra's Royal Naval Nursing Service, Ministry of
Defence, First Avenue House, High Holborn, London WC1V 6HD
Tel. 01-430 5555

Rcn Student Section, Henrietta Place, London W1M 0AB
Tel. 01-580 2646

Royal Association for Disability and Rehabilitation (RADAR), 25
Mortimer Street, London W1N 8AB
Tel. 01-637 5400

Royal British Nurses Association, 94 Upper Tollington Park,
London N4 4NB
Tel. 01-272 6821

Royal College of Midwives, 15 Mansfield Street, London W1M 0BE
Tel. 01-580 6523/5

Royal College of Nursing of the United Kingdom, 1 Henrietta
Place, Cavendish Square, London W1M 0AB
Tel. 01-580 2646

Royal College of Nursing of the United Kingdom (Scottish Board),
44 Heriot Row, Edinburgh EH3 6EY
Tel. 031-225 7231

USEFUL ADDRESSES

Royal College of Nursing of the United Kingdom (Northern Ireland Board), 17 Windsor Avenue, Belfast BT9 6EE
Tel. 0232 668236/7

Royal College of Nursing of the United Kingdom (Welsh Board), Tŷ Maeth, King George V Drive East, Cardiff CF4 4XZ
Tel. 0222 751374/5

Royal National Institute for the Blind, 224 Great Portland Street, London W1N 6AA
Tel. 01-388 1266

Royal National Institute of the Deaf, 105 Gower Street, London WC1
Tel. 01-437 8030

Royal National Pension Fund for Nurses, Burdett House, 15 Buckingham Street, Strand, London WC2N 6ED
Tel. 01-839 6785

Scottish Board for Nursing, Midwifery and Health Visiting, Trinity Park House, South Trinity Road, Edinburgh EH5 3SF
Tel. 031-552-6255

Sexual and Personal Relationships of the Disabled (SPOD), DIORAMA, 14 Peto Place, London NW1 4DT
Tel. 01-486 9823

Society of Chiropodists, 8 Wimpole Street, London W1M 8BX
Tel. 01-580 3227

United Kingdom Central Council for Nursing, Midwifery and Health Visiting, 23 Portland Place, London W1A 1BA
Tel. 01-380 0717

United Nursing Services Club, 40 South Street, London W1
Tel. Secretary 01-470 1564
Members 01-629 0896

Welsh National Board for Nursing, Midwifery and Health Visiting, 13th Floor, Pearl Assurance House, Greyfriars Road, Cardiff CF1 3AG
Tel. 0222-395 535

Whitley Council for Nurses and Midwives, Staff Side Secretary, 1 Henrietta Place, Cavendish Square, London W1M 0AB
Tel. 01-636 3866

Women's Royal Voluntary Service Headquarters, 17 Old Park Lane, London W1Y 4AJ
Tel. 01-499 6040

21
DEGREES, DIPLOMAS, ORGANIZATIONS, ETC.

ABPN	Association of British Paediatric Nurses
ADMS	Assistant Director of Medical Services
ADNS	Assistant Director of Nursing Services
AIMSW	Associate of the Institute of Medical Social Workers
ARRC	Associate, Royal Red Cross
ASTMS	Association of Scientific Technical and Managerial Staffs
BA	Bachelor of Arts
BAO	Bachelor of the Art of Obstetrics
BC,BCh,BChir	Bachelor of Surgery
BChD,BDS	Bachelor of Dental Surgery
BDA	British Dental Association
BM	Bachelor of Medicine
BMA	British Medical Association
BP	British Pharmacopoeia
BRCS	British Red Cross Society
BS	Bachelor of Surgery
BSc	Bachelor of Science
ChB	Bachelor of Surgery
CCD	Central Council for the Disabled
CCHE	Central Council for Health Education
CM,ChM	Master of Surgery
CMB	Central Midwives' Board
CNN	Certificated Nursery Nurse
CoHSE	Confederation of Health Service Employees
CPH	Certificate of Public Health
CSP	Chartered Society of Physiotherapists
CU	Casualties Union
DA	Diploma of Anaesthetics
DCh	Doctor of Surgery
DCH	Diploma of Child Health
DCP	Diploma in Clinical Pathology
DDA	Dangerous Drugs Act
DDMS	Deputy Director of Medical Services
DDS	Doctor of Dental Surgery
DHyg	Doctor of Hygiene
DIH	Diploma in Industrial Health
DipN	Diploma in Nursing
DipNEd	Diploma in Nursing Education
DM	Doctor of Medicine (Oxford University)
DNA	District Nursing Association

DEGREES, DIPLOMAS, ETC.

DNS	Director of Nursing Services
DO	Diploma in Ophthalmology
DObstRCOG	Diplomate of the Royal College of Obstetrics and Gynaecologists
DPH	Diploma in Public Health
DPhil	Doctor of Philosophy
DPM	Diploma in Psychological Medicine
DR	Diploma in Radiology
DSc	Doctor of Science
DTM&H	Diploma in Tropical Medicine and Hygiene
EN(G)	Enrolled Nurse (General)
EN(M)	Enrolled Nurse (Mental)
EN(MH)	Enrolled Nurse (Mental Handicap)
FACP	Fellow of the American College of Physicians
FACS	Fellow of the American College of Surgeons
FCSP	Fellow of the Chartered Society of Physiotherapists
FDS	Fellow in Dental Surgery
FETC	Further Education Teaching Certificate
FFARCS	Fellow of the Faculty of Anaesthetists, Royal College of Surgeons
FNIF	Florence Nightingale International Foundation
FPS	Fellow of the Pharmaceutical Society
FRACP	Fellow of the Royal Australasian College of Physicians
FRACS	Fellow of the Royal Australasian College of Surgeons
FRCGP	Fellow of the Royal College of General Practitioners
FRcn	Fellow of the Royal College of Nursing
FRCOG	Fellow of the Royal College of Obstetricians and Gynaecologists
FRCP	Fellow of the Royal College of Physicians
FRCPE	Fellow of the Royal College of Physicians, Edinburgh
FRCPI	Fellow of the Royal College of Physicians of Ireland
FRCPath	Fellow of the Royal College of Pathologists
FRCPsych	Fellow of the Royal College of Psychologists
FRCS	Fellow of the Royal College of Surgeons
FRCSE	Fellow of the Royal College of Surgeons, Edinburgh
FRCSI	Fellow of the Royal College of Surgeons of Ireland
FRFPS	Fellow of the Royal Faculty of Physicians and Surgeons
FRIPHH	Fellow of the Royal Institute of Public Health and Hygiene
FRS	Fellow of the Royal Society
FRSE	Fellow of the Royal Society of Edinburgh
FRSH	Fellow of the Royal Society of Health
FRSM	Fellow of the Royal Society of Medicine

	Fellow of the Society of Radiographers (Radiography)
	Fellow of the Society of Radiographers (Radiotherapy)
GMC	General Medical Council
HSA	Hospital Savings Association
HV	Health Visitor
ICN	International Council of Nurses
ICW	International Council of Women
IHF	International Hospitals Federation
LDS	Licentiate in Dental Surgery
LMRCP	Licentiate in Midwifery of the Royal College of Physicians
LMSSA	Licentiate in Medicine and Surgery of the Society of Apothecaries, London
LRCP	Licentiate of the Royal College of Physicians
LRCPE	Licentiate of the Royal College of Physicians of Edinburgh
LRFPS	Licentiate of the Royal Faculty of Physicians and Surgeons
LSA	Licentiate of the Society of Apothecaries
MA	Master of Arts
MAO	Master of the Art of Obstetrics
MAOT	Member of the Association of Occupational Therapists
MB	Bachelor of Medicine (other than from Oxford)
MC,MCh,MChir	Master of Surgery
MCSP	Member of the Chartered Society of Physiotherapists
MChOrth	Master of Orthopaedic Surgery
MChS	Member of the Society of Chiropodists
MD	Doctor of Medicine (other than from Oxford)
MIND	National Association for Mental Health
MRCOG	Member of the Royal College of Obstetricians and Gynaecologists
MRCP	Member of the Royal College of Physicians
MRCPath	Member of the Royal College of Pathologists
MRCPsych	Member of the Royal College of Psychiatrists
MRCS	Member of the Royal College of Surgeons
MRSH	Member of the Royal Society for the Promotion of Health
MS	Master of Surgery
MSA	Member of the Society of Apothecaries
MSRG	Member of the Society of Remedial Gymnasts
MSR(R)	Member of the Society of Radiographers (Radiography)
MSR(T)	Member of the Society of Radiographers (Radiotherapy)
MSc	Master of Science
MTD	Midwife Teachers' Diploma
NALGO	National Association of Local Government Officers

NAMCW	National Association for Maternal and Child Welfare
NAMH	National Association for Mental Health
NAWCH	National Association for the Welfare of Children in Hospital
NHS	National Health Service
NHSR	National Hospital Service Reserve
NNEB	National Nursery Examination Board
NUPE	National Union of Public Employees
ONC	Orthopaedic Nursing Certificate
PMRAFNS	Princess Mary's Royal Air Force Nursing Service
PhD	Doctor of Philosophy
QARANC	Queen Alexandra's Royal Army Nursing Corps
QARNNS	Queen Alexandra's Royal Naval Nursing Service
QHP	Queen's Honorary Physician
QHNS	Queen's Honorary Nursing Sister
QHS	Queen's Honorary Surgeon
QIDN	Queen's Institute of District Nursing
RADC	Royal Army Dental Corps
RAMC	Royal Army Medical Corps
RCM	Royal College of Midwives
Rcn	Royal College of Nursing and National Council of Nurses of the United Kingdom
RCNT	Registered Clinical Nurse Teacher
RFN	Registered Fever Nurse
RGN	Registered General Nurse
RHA	Regional Health Authority
RHV	Registered Health Visitor
RM	Registered Midwife
RMO	Resident Medical Officer
RMN	Registered Mental Nurse
RN	Registered Nurse (USA and other overseas countries)
RNMD	Registered Nurse for Mental Defectives
RNMH	Registered Nurse for the Mentally Handicapped
RNMS	Registered Nurse for the Mentally Subnormal
RNT	Registered Nurse Tutor
RRC	Royal Red Cross
RSCN	Registered Sick Children's Nurse
StAAA	St Andrew's Ambulance Association
StJAA	St John Ambulance Association
StJAB	St John Ambulance Brigade
SCM	State Certified Midwife
SEN	State Enrolled Nurse
SPoD	Sexual and Personal Relationships of the Disabled
SRN	State Registered Nurse

SSStJ	Serving Sister of the Order of St John of Jerusalem
VAD	Voluntary Aid Detachment
WHO	World Health Organization
WPHOA	Women Public Health Officers' Association
WRVS	Women's Royal Voluntary Service